ADMINISTRATION OF HEALTH AND PHYSICAL EDUCATION PROGRAMS, INCLUDING ATHLETICS

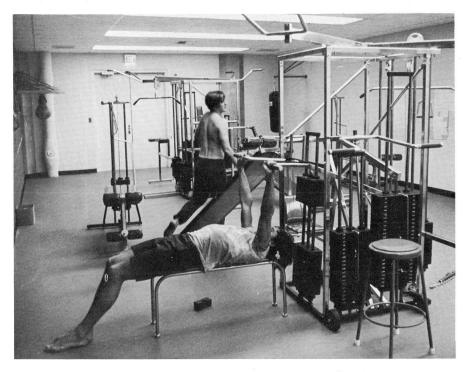

Weight Training Room, Trinity College, Hartford, Conn.

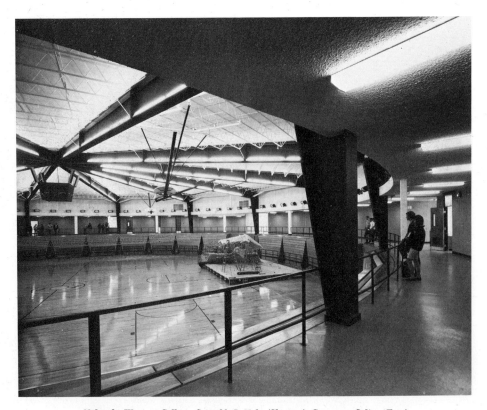

Nebraska Western College, Scottsbluff, Neb. (Shaver & Company, Salina, Kan.)

ADMINISTRATION OF

Health and physical education programs

INCLUDING ATHLETICS

CHARLES A. BUCHER, A.B., M.A., Ed.D.

Professor of Education, New York University,
New York, N. Y.

FIFTH EDITION

With 362 illustrations

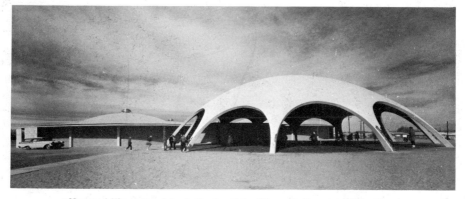

Sherwood Elementary School, Greeley, Colo. (Shaver & Company, Salina, Kan.)

THE C. V. MOSBY COMPANY

Saint Louis   1971

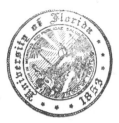

To my wife JACKIE

and

my children DIANA, RICHARD, NANCY, *and* JERRY

Preface

The role of administration is becoming increasingly significant in determining the success of health and physical education programs. The manner in which these specialized programs are organized, structured, and supervised determines the results and objectives achieved.

Administration is rapidly becoming a science with a subject matter of its own. If health and physical education specialists are to have outstanding programs in their fields, they must be familiar with administrative theory regarding the structure of organizations, the role of the leader, and the ingredients of outstanding programs. They must also be knowledgeable regarding such administrative functions as community relations, facility management, fiscal accounting, curriculum development, and pupil, teacher, and program evaluation. This fifth edition examines the administration of health, physical education, and athletic programs as a science and brings significant subject matter in administration to the attention of the reader.

This text has been completely revised. All chapters have been brought up to date, with the latest developments and trends in health and physical education included in each subject discussed. For example, new information on administrative theory, personnel administration, adapted physical education, crowd control, health education, facility management, supplies and equipment, audiovisual aids, and pupil, teacher, and program evaluation has been added. Two new chapters — Chapter 1, The

Changing Nature of Administration, and Chapter 6, Student Leadership in Physical Education — have been added. Finally, the book has been completely reorganized so that the material is presented in a more meaningful and logical sequence.

The fifth edition is divided into five parts: Part One, The Changing Nature of Administration; Part Two, Administration of Physical Education Programs; Part Three, Health Programs for Students; Part Four, Administrative Functions; and Part Five, Administration of Recreation, Club, and Outdoor Education and Camping Programs. Appendices have also been developed that include such valuable information as sources of equipment and supplies; procedures for care, repair, and storage of equipment; school laws and regulations relating to health and physical education programs; and athletic field and court diagrams.

I would like to thank all the individuals, schools, colleges, and other organizations who contributed photographs, charts, and other materials for this revision.

Dr. Jean Tallman, Chairman, Physical Education Department, Davis and Elkins College, Elkins, West Virginia, is responsible for preparing the excellent Instructor's Manual that the publisher gives to each instructor who adopts this text. The author wishes to thank Dr. Tallman for preparing a manual that will help each instructor to offer a more meaningful course to his or her students.

Charles A. Bucher

Contents

one

THE CHANGING NATURE OF ADMINISTRATION

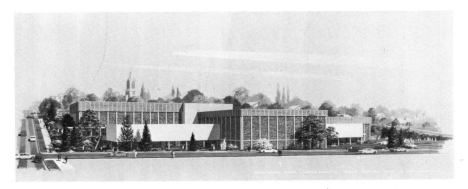

Physical Education Bldg., Seattle University, Seattle, Wash.

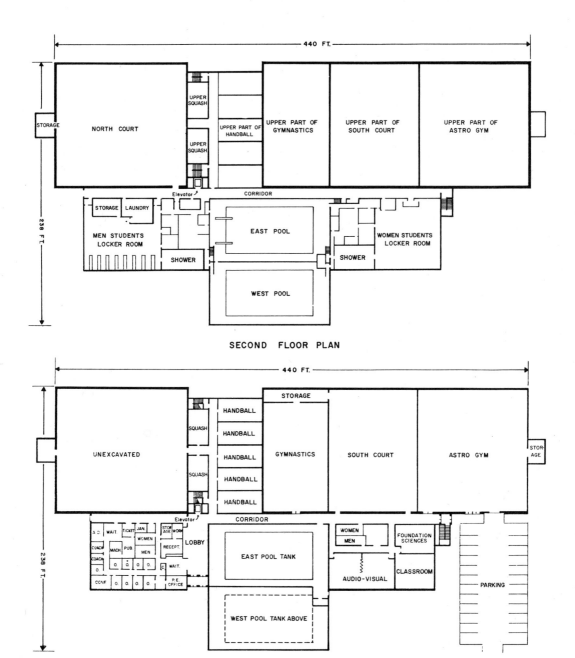

SECOND FLOOR PLAN

FIRST FLOOR PLAN

Physical Education Bldg., Seattle University, Seattle, Wash.

By analyzing several definitions of administration a reader may be better able to understand what a text in administration is designed to cover. Some of the definitions proposed by experts in this field represent analyses of the administrative process based on research; others have been formulated as a result of experience as an administrator or observation of administrators at work.

Based upon Hemphill, Griffiths, and Frederickson's[*] research, Jenson and Clark[†] propose the following as a definition of administration: "The administrative process is the way an organization, through working with people, makes decisions and initiates action to achieve its purposes and goals." Halpin,[‡] after analyzing administration in education, industry, and government, states that administration refers to a human activity involving a minimum of four components: (1) the *functions or tasks* to be performed, (2) the *formal organization* within which administration must operate, (3) the *work group* or groups with which administration must be concerned,

and (4) the *leader* or leaders within the organization. Administration has also been defined as a means of bringing about effective cooperative activity to achieve the purposes of an enterprise.

After considerable research and the formulation of a philosophy of administration that is stated later in this chapter, I propose the following definition: *Administration is concerned with the functions and responsibilities essential to the achievement of established goals through associated effort. It is also concerned with that group of individuals who are responsible for directing, guiding, coordinating, and inspiring the associated efforts of individual members, so that the purposes for which an organization has been established may be accomplished in the most effective and efficient manner possible.*

THE SCOPE OF ADMINISTRATION

It has been estimated that there are more than 5 million individuals in the United States today performing administrative work as their main function. This number is large, but as the technology and the specialized functions of this country advance, there will be an increasing number of individuals needed to perform the myriad administrative duties characteristic of the thousands of organizations in society. There are at least as many administrative positions in physical education and health as there are schools and colleges. This, of course, runs into several thousands of positions. In addition, there are many large educational institutions with several persons who assist in the administrative process

---

[*]Hemphill, J., Griffiths, D., and Frederickson, N.: Administrative performance and personality, New York, 1962, Bureau of Publications, Teachers' College, Columbia University. (This study is sometimes referred to as the "Development of Criteria of Success in School Administration" project.)

[†]Jenson, T. J., and Clark, D. L.: Educational administration, New York, 1964, The Center for Applied Research in Education, Inc. (The Library of Education).

[‡]Halpin, A. W.: A paradigm for research on administrative behavior. In Campbell, R. F., and Gregg, R. T., editors: Administrative behavior in education, New York, 1957, Harper & Row, Publishers, p. 161.

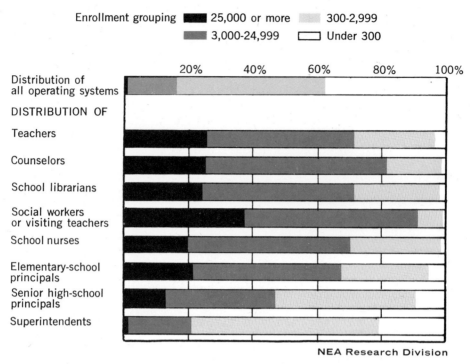

Distribution of personnel by school enrollment, 1968-69. (From Research Division, National Education Association, NEA Research Bulletin **47**:82, 1969.)

concerned with health and physical education programs. Also, there are many agencies such as the YMCAs and Boys' Club, who also have administrative positions. Administration offers many career opportunities for both women and men.

It is essential that individuals who perform administrative work know the many aspects of this particular field. If they are not aware of certain basic facts and are not acquainted with acceptable administrative procedures, many errors may be made. This could result in loss of efficiency, production, and staff morale and in poor human relations, to mention only a few of the possible outcomes. Administration is rapidly becoming a science with a body of specialized knowledge that should be known by all who would administer in a wise and effective manner. Plato in his book, *Laws,* summed it up in a few words that still hold true today: ". . . that God governs all

things, and that chance and opportunity cooperate with Him in the government of human affairs. There is, however, a third and less extreme view, that art should be there also; for I should say that in a storm there must surely be a great advantage in having the aid of the pilot's art. You would agree?"

A PHILOSOPHY OF ADMINISTRATION

People represent the most important consideration in the world. The real worth of a field of endeavor, organization, or idea is found in what it does for human beings. The most important and worthwhile thing that can be said about a particular vocation, organization, or movement is that it contributes to human betterment.

People have goals that represent a variety of human objectives. They include the need for security for oneself and one's family, the desire to be employed in a worth-

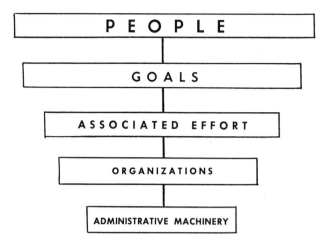

Graphic representation of a philosophy of administration.

while and gainful occupation, the wish to worship one's God, the enjoyment of recreation, and the need to obtain an education.

People do not miraculously work together. They do not, as a natural phenomenon, band together and strive to accomplish common objectives. Since many groups of people have common goals, however, they do work together and through associated effort help each other to achieve goals that would be impossible for them to accomplish alone. No one person can establish a school for his children's education, for example, but through the cooperative effort and support of many people a school is made possible. Thus individuals have similar goals that they will work together to attain.

People form organizations to help them fulfill their desires and wishes; they join together and establish a church, a business enterprise, a health association, a governmental agency, a country club, a hospital, or some other type of organization that will help them achieve the goals that they desire. Thus there are thousands of different types of organizations that have been created by human beings who have banded together to achieve objectives that they consider worthwhile.

Organizations, in order to function most

effectively, must have some type of machinery to help them run efficiently, to organize and execute their affairs, and to keep them running smoothly, so that the goals for which they have been created will be achieved. This machinery is administration. It is the framework of organizations. It is the part that helps organizations implement the purposes for which they have been established.

Administration, therefore, exists to help people achieve the goals they desire in order to live happy, productive, healthful, and meaningful lives. It is not an end in itself; rather, it is a means to an end—the welfare of the people for whom the organization exists. Administration exists for people, not people for administration. Administration can justify itself only as it serves the people who make up the organization, helping them to achieve the goals they have as human beings.

It can be seen, then, that in an organization, where the associated efforts of many individuals are necessary, there is no spontaneous and automatic working together of the individuals involved. There are no miraculous thought and planning that result in the achievement of goals and purposes. It is not a natural trait of human beings to cooperate and work side by side in a happy and purposeful manner. This is accomplished through direction, and administration gives this direction.

To a considerable degree, the actions of human beings in society are determined through their association with formal organizations. Formal organizations have leaders and purposes. They depend upon the cooperative efforts of individuals to achieve the objectives that have been set. Many times organizations have failed when their leaders have been of low caliber, when there has been a lack of cooperative effort among 'members, or when the objectives have not been in conformance with what is essential and good for society.

Administration determines in great measure whether an organization is going to progress, operate efficiently, achieve its objectives, and have a group of individuals within its framework who are happy, cooperative, and productive. Administration has to do with directing, guiding, and integrating the efforts of human beings so that specific aims may be accomplished. It refers particularly to a group of individuals, many times called executives, who have as their major responsibility this direction, guidance, integration, and achievement.

Administration is especially concerned with achievement—proof that the organization is producing those things for which it has been established. To be able to achieve these results in a satisfactory manner presupposes an understanding of human relationships and the ability to foresee the future and plan for any eventuality. It demands the capacity to coordinate many different and conflicting types of human personalities. Good administration should ensure that the associated efforts of individuals are productive. To accomplish this, administrators should possess those attributes that are conducive to bringing out the most creative and best efforts on the part of the members of the organization.

Administration also requires close supervision of the facilities, materials, supplies, and equipment essential to the life of the organization. It implies a logical formulation of policies and the effective operation of the organization.

THE IMPORTANCE OF ADMINISTRATION

A study of administration is important for all teachers of health and physical education. A few of the more significant reasons why teachers should understand administration are discussed in the following paragraphs.

1. *The way in which schools and colleges are administered determines the course of human lives.* The lives of both students and teachers are affected by administration. It affects the type of education offered, the climate in which the education takes place, and the goals that are sought. It vitally affects the happiness and achievement of every teacher.

2. *Administration provides an understanding and appreciation of the underlying principles of the science of this field.* Methods, techniques, devices, and procedures used by the administration can be evaluated more accurately and objectively by faculty and staff if they possess administrative understanding. Also, sound administration will be better appreciated and unsound practices more easily recognized. Human resources will have less chance of being exploited, and efficient management and organization will be furthered through such understanding.

3. *A study of administration will assist in deciding whether a person wishes to select this area on a career basis.* Personal qualifications may be better evaluated and possibilities of success better predicted with increased understanding and appreciation of the administrative process.

4. *Most physical education and health educators perform some types of administrative work and therefore an understanding of administration will contribute to better performance in this area.* Adminis-

tration is not restricted to one group of in-dividuals. Most teachers and staff members have reports to complete, equipment to or-der, evaluations to make, and other duties to perform that are administrative in na-ture. An understanding of the science of administration will assist in carrying out these assignments.

5. *Administration is fundamental to as-sociated effort.* Goals are reached, ideas are implemented, and an esprit de corps is developed with planning and cooperative action. A knowledge of administration fa-cilitates the achievement of such aims.

6. *An understanding of administration helps to assure continuity.* A fundamental purpose of administration is to carry on that which has proved successful rather than to destroy the old and attempt a new and untried path. An appreciation of this concept by all members of an organization will help to ensure the preservation of the

best traditional practices that exist in the organization.

7. *A knowledge of administration helps to further good human relations.* An under-standing of sound administrative principles will better assure the cooperation of the various members who make up the organ-ization in order that the greatest efficiency and productivity will be assured.

Outstanding individuals in various walks of life have recognized the importance of administration. *Charles A. Beard,* a famous historian, referred to administration as the key science of the present day. *Henri Fayol,* French engineer and industrialist, stressed the great need for studying admin-istration scientifically, since it is one of the most important elements in all vocations and professions. *Paul Pigors,* American so-ciologist, felt that the main contribution of administration was to preserve the status quo in society. *Brooks Adams,* American

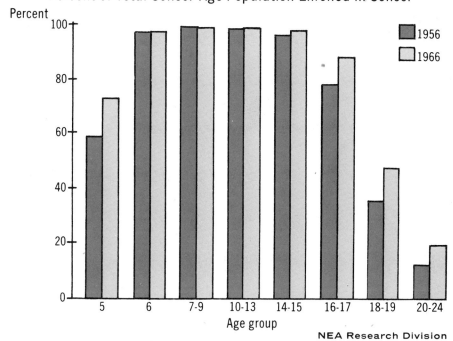

Percent of Total School-Age Population Enrolled in School

NEA Research Division

A higher percentage of young people are in school.

lawyer and historian, took an almost opposite view from Pigors' when he advocated administration as being most important because it can help in social change. *James Burnham,* American political philosopher, went further and pointed to the fact that the chief administrators in present-day society had assumed so much power that the social revolution was already in evidence. *Charles E. Merriam,* American political scientist, contended that administration was another outcome of human technology that made it possible for man to better adapt to his complex environment.

The evidence is ample that administration is rapidly becoming a science and that the study of this science is essential to everyone. A study of administration can result in a better-ordered society through more efficiently run organizations. Every individual belongs to formal organizations. Through a democratic approach to administration the individual can aid in carrying on what has proved to be good in the past and steer a course that will ensure progress in the future.

THE DEVELOPMENT OF A THEORY OF ADMINISTRATION

It is increasingly being recognized that administration is not something that is hit or miss, trial and error, or a matter of expediency. Instead, there is evidence to show that a theory of administration is emerging. It is recognized that from a study of this administrative theory one will gain the ability to act wisely in specific situations, and since theory is practical, it provides an accurate picture of how human beings work. Administrative theory will also help in the identification of problems that need to be solved if an effective working organization is to exist.

Textbooks and the professional literature on administration indicate a search for a substance of administration and for a framework of theory that would make the substance a meaningful whole. The traditional emphasis has been upon the form rather than upon the substance. Organizations such as the National Conference of Professors of Educational Administration, the Cooperative Program in Educational Administration, and the University Council for Educational Administration are helping to give impetus to this new movement and thereby helping to make administration much more of a science than has existed in the past. Although there are some educators who oppose such a trend, it seems assured that administration is in the process of becoming more scientific and thereby characterized by more objectivity, reliability, and a systematic structure of substance. Such theory is explaining what administration is and providing guides to administrative action.

The traditional and modern views of administration

The traditional view of administration revolved around the idea that administration existed in order to carry out the policies that had been developed by the duly constituted policy-forming group, such as a board of education. Modern administration not only carries out policy but also plays an important role in the development of policy, utilizing the knowledge and expertise that come from training and experience.

A study of the history of administration shows that policy-forming groups, such as boards of education, were once held accountable for how the schools were administered, whereas the modern approach delegates administrative responsibilities to the trained school administrator. The old concept of leadership in administration was a sort of passive type of leadership that remained in the background while the policy-forming group provided the strength and skill that were needed to run the schools. Under the modern view of administration, however, strong administrative leadership is a requirement so that technical and ex-

Table 1-1. Instructional organization and practices, 154 middle schools in systems enrolling over 12,000 pupils, 1968-69*

Instructional organization and practices	Number and percent of schools by grade level†							
	Grade 5 (20 schools)		Grade 6 (146 schools)		Grade 7 (154 schools)		Grade 8 (148 schools)	
	Num-ber	Per-cent	Num-ber	Per-cent	Num-ber	Per-cent	Num-ber	Per-cent
Organization								
Self-contained classrooms	10	50.0%	31	21.2%	3	1.9%	3	2.0%
Partial departmentalization	7	35.0	74	50.7	55	35.7	36	24.4
Total departmentalization	3	15.0	35	24.0	91	59.1	105	70.9
No reply	—	—	6	4.1	5	3.3	4	2.7
Practices								
Subject area teams	4	20.0	45	30.8	51	33.1	52	35.1
Interdisciplinary teams	2	10.0	19	13.0	29	18.8	25	16.9
Small group instruction	7	35.0	55	37.7	63	40.9	66	44.6
Large group instruction	4	20.0	35	24.0	45	29.2	47	31.8
Flexible scheduling	5	25.0	39	26.7	44	28.6	43	29.1
Closed-circuit TV	1	5.0	22	15.1	25	15.6	25	16.9
Independent study	3	15.0	30	20.5	39	25.3	40	27.0
Individualized instruction	4	20.0	39	26.7	47	30.5	48	32.4
Tutorial programs	3	15.0	32	21.9	33	21.4	31	20.9

*From NEA Research Bulletin 47:51, 1969.
†Percentages are based on the total number of middle schools in the survey, which includes each of the grades. The number of schools with each grade is shown in the column headings.

pert judgments can be made to help the schools to achieve their objectives more effectively. The traditional view of administration claimed the best way to prepare to administer was to practice administering: experience was seen to be the best teacher. The modern view of administration, however, recognizes the value of experience but at the same time maintains that there exists a body of knowledge or theory that, when mastered, can help the administration play a more effective role in the organization with which it is associated.

According to Jenson and Clark,* new perspectives of educational administration are the result of six phenomena:

1. Administration is a science and the administrator is a professional person.
2. An intensive study of administration includes such phenomena as behaviors, social interactions, and human relationships.

3. Application of theory and model constructs are included in the study of administration.
4. Administration is differentiated into two dimensions: content and process.
5. New forces shape new perspectives in administration: new technologies, population trends, value systems, knowledge explosion, ideological conflicts, and so on.
6. Interest of scholars and researchers in the scientific study of the field of administration is increasing.

The preparation of administrators

The modern view of administration is that a professional preparation program for the person who desires to enter the field of administration should include such essentials as: taking foundation work in cognate fields, knowing himself as an individual and as a potential administrator, having competency in administrative skills to be performed, understanding the community, recognizing the importance of instruction, studying and practicing decision making,

*Jenson and Clark, op. cit., p. 37.

and realizing the importance of human relations. Finally, there should be on-the-job learning experience that is closely supervised by an experienced professor.

Several types of content, all of which are pertinent to physical education and health administrators, are suggested by Culbertson[*] as being needed in the preparation of administrators in order to fulfill the following responsibilities.

Making decisions. Content should include a study of concepts and theories that relate to individual, group, and organization decision making. The relationship of such items as basic research, computer technology, and value systems to decision making would also be considered.

Communication. A study of communication—one-way, two-way, and group, as well as organizational communications—should be included. Mass communications and opinion change should also be considered.

Coping with change. A study of the dynamics of change in relation to individuals, groups, and organizations should be made. A study should also be made of barriers to change, how change can be effected, the leadership needed, conflicts, and related topics. For example, Table 1-1 indicates a number of types of instructional organization and practices. The administration plays a key role in bringing about such changes and practices.

Building morale. Content should include how morale is achieved in a modern organization. Special attention should be given to motivation, interpersonal relations, values, organizational loyalty, perception, and so on.

Such content material and preparation, if offered, would produce well-educated administrations, according to the American Association of School Administrators.[*] The AASA, for example, feels that an administrator (in this case a superintendent of schools, but the points are equally applicable to administrators of physical education and health programs) as a result of his professional training should:

1. Have a deep devotion to the human values that are at the heart of America's purpose and upon which her destiny rests and an understanding of the galaxy of relationships and ethical beliefs upon which those values and ethical principles are based.
2. Be able to make wise and sound decisions toward the improvement of teaching and toward more efficient learning.
3. Know laboratory and classroom environments, tools for teaching, and the structural organization for deployment of staff and pupils.
4. Be well schooled in what science and research show about the expectations, drives, fears, interests, and personal diversities that exist in groups of teachers, children, and young people.
5. Understand the American public—what it is, what it wants, how it is organized, how it can make itself felt, and who leads it.
6. Be efficient in using public funds.
7. Have a combination of personal power, insight, and skill that enables him to get a team of associates to work closely and effectively with him. Some of the most energetic and intellectually astute superintendents (administrators) find themselves carrying more and more burdens because they unknowingly tie in knots the energies and abilities of the men and women closest to them.
8. Have wisdom and good judgment, as well as skill, in oral and written communication.
9. Possess creative, imaginative, and realistic competence in sensing society's evolutionary and emerging aspirations and needs.
10. Have the vision, courage, and patience needed to plan wisely for the future.
11. Be professionally competent in many areas of evaluation.
12. Comprehend the educational needs of adults, children, and youth.

[*]Culbertson, J.: The preparation of administrators. In Behavioral science and educational administration, the Sixty-Third Yearbook of the National Society for the Study of Education, Chicago, 1964, University of Chicago Press.

[*]The education of a school superintendent, Washington, D. C., 1963, American Association of School Administrators, pp. 11-12.

13. Have an education that feeds upon education, that generates an unquenchable thirst for more understanding, and that keeps him far out in front of the doggedly pursuing menace of obsolescence.

The anatomy of administrative leadership

Being the head of a department, division, or school of physical education and health and being the leader of these organizations are two different things. The head can be a person who takes care of the clerical details and occupies the main office in a department or division, but he may not necessarily be the leader of the organization. The administrative leader of an organization is one who helps and influences others in a certain direction as problems are solved and goals achieved. In a school, college, or agency situation the persons influenced are teachers, pupils, clerks, parents, custodians, and any person involved with the organization.

The question as to what makes a leader is a provocative one. Much research has been done in recent years as to what constitutes the administrative leader. Years ago it was felt that combinations of personality characteristics or traits were the ingredients that determined who was a leader. However, research such as that of Gouldner,* indicates that: "At this time there is no reliable evidence concerning the existence of universal leadership traits."

Other studies have provided further information in regard to leadership. Stogdill† states as a result of his research that "the qualities, characteristics, and skills required in a leader are determined to a large extent by the demands of the situation in which he is to function as a leader." In other words, a health or physical education administrative leader in one situation may

not necessarily be a leader in another situation. Different styles of leadership are needed to meet the needs of different settings and situations. Administration therefore is a social process.

Certain traits and attributes that influence leader behavior have been identified. For example, Pierce and Merrill,* in examining research on leadership, found that such qualities as popularity, originality, adaptability, judgment, ambition, persistence, emotional stability, social and economic status, and communicative skills were very important for a person to possess if he hoped to lead. The traits that were found to be most significant were popularity, originality, and judgment.

Goldman† examined the research on leadership and suggests that certain factors are significant. When these factors are related to physical education and health administrative leaders, the following guidelines are worth considering:

1. The administrators of physical education and health programs who possess such traits as ambition, ability to relate well to others, emotional stability, communicative skill, and judgment have greater potential for success in leadership than persons who do not possess these traits.
2. The administrators of physical education and health programs who desire to be leaders of their organization must have a clear understanding of the goals of the organization. The direction in which they desire to lead the organization must be within the broad framework of the goals and objectives of the school district and consonant with the needs of the community they serve.
3. The administrators of physical education and health programs who desire to be leaders of

*Gouldner, A. W., editor: Studies in leadership, New York, 1950, Harper & Row, Publishers, p. 34.
†Stogdill, R. M.: Personal factors associated with leadership: a survey of the literature, Journal of Psychology **25**:63, 1948.

*Pierce, T. M., and Merrill, E. C., Jr.: The individual and administrative behavior. In Campbell, R. F., and Gregg, R. T., editors: Administrative behavior in education, New York, 1957, Harper & Row, Publishers, p. 331.
†Goldman, S.: The school principal, New York, 1966, The Center for Applied Research in Education, Inc. (The Library of Education), pp. 88-89.

their organizations must understand each of the persons who work with them, including their personal and professional needs.

4. The administrators of physical education and health programs who desire to be leaders of their organizations need to establish a climate within which the organization goals, personal needs of each staff member, and their own personality traits can operate harmoniously.

Administrative tasks

Administration is a process involving pertinent tasks that must be performed if an organization is to progress and achieve its goals. These tasks represent the mission of the organization as delineated into subtasks. For example, the task of the school is to educate, and in order to accomplish this mission certain subtasks are essential. Campbell and his associates[*] analyzed administrative tasks and came to the conclusion that there were seven operational task areas. These are: (1) school-community relationships, (2) curriculum development, (3) pupil personnel, (4) staff personnel, (5) physical facilities, (6) finance and business management, and (7) organization and structure. In Part Four of this text the following administrative tasks and functions in regard to school health and physical education programs are discussed in detail: the physical education plant, budget making and financial accounting, purchase and care of supplies and equipment, legal liability and insurance management, curriculum planning, professional, school and community relations, office management, measurement of pupil achievement, and teacher and program evaluation. The task of organization and structure is covered in Chapter 3.

Administrative skills

Some administrators are successful and some fail because of the administrative skills they lack. Jenson and Clark,[*] as a result of their research, have identified three types of administrative skills that are essential: conceptual, technical, and human relations. These skills are necessary for the successful administration of physical education and health programs.

Conceptual skills include the abilities to see the organization as a whole, to originate ideas, to sense problems, and to work out solutions to these problems that will benefit the organization and establish the right priorities and organizational direction. It reduces the risk factor to a minimum.

Technical skills are the administrative skills that relate to the various tasks that must be performed. For example, such tasks as budgeting, curriculum planning, communication, preparing reports, group dynamics, policy development, and public relations, to name only a few, require certain specialized skills if they are to be performed efficiently and accurately.

The third type of skills, *human relations skills,* refers to the administration's ability to have good working relationships among the staff, to get along with people, and to provide a working climate where individuals will not only produce but also grow on the job.

Stages of the administrative process involving decision making

Decision making in the administrative process requires that certain steps be followed. The ordinary problem-solving approach that has been traditionally used includes the recognition of the problem, identifying the alternatives, gathering and organizing facts, weighing alternatives, and finally arriving at a decision. Jenson and Clark,[†] however, feel that the administration should not stop at the point of arriving at a decision but, instead, feel that it is es-

---

[*]Campbell, R. F., and others: Introduction to educational administration, ed. 2, Boston, 1962, Allyn and Bacon, Inc.

[*]Jenson and Clark, op. cit., pp. 56-57.
[†]Jenson and Clark, op. cit., pp. 53-55.

sential to go on to the stages that involve implementation and assessment. The sequential stages of this process, they feel, are well stated by Burr and his associates*:

1. *Deliberating*   The problem is discussed, facts on the problem are gathered, and the problem is carefully analyzed.

2. *Decision making*   As a result of the deliberation a decision is made. Alternatives are carefully weighed and a choice is made based on the facts.

3. *Programming*   After the decision is made the program is developed so that it is ready for implementation. Questions are asked and actions taken in regard to the resources that are available, the planning that needs to be done, the budget, equipment, and material requirements that exist, and the needs in regard to staff and so on. In other words, information is researched that will provide a successful program and the right direction, in light of the decision that was made.

4. *Stimulating*   After the programming has been developed, it is set into operation. This requires the involvement of people, arousing interest, obtaining commitments, and initiating action. Motivation needs to be encouraged and attitudes developed in this process.

5. *Coordinating*   To effectively implement a program requires the coordination of staff efforts, material resources, proper communication, and other essentials that will assure that the program will be successfully launched.

6. *Appraising*   The last stage in the continuum is evaluating and appraising all stages of the process and the results obtained. It attempts to analyze where the process was successful or where it failed and the reasons for the success or failure. The information gath-

ered will be used in future endeavors.

Rules of administrative organization

Bartholomew* suggests certain rules of organization that he gathered from a study of the field of public and business administration. These have implications for organizing and administering physical education and health programs.

1. *Administrative work may be most efficiently organized by function.* This rule of organization refers to the "doctrine of unity" that holds that all officers engaged in a particular type of work should function under a single authority.

2. *Unified direction should be embodied in the organization.* This refers to the "unity of command," which in essence means that no staff member should be subject to the orders of more than one superior.

3. *Organization may be according to purpose.* Staff, auxiliary, and line activities may be separated.

4. *Organization should be done on a hierarchical basis.* A vertical type of structure that begins at the bottom with production personnel and then goes upward through section heads, division heads, to the organization head should exist. Such units are differentiated on the basis of level of authority and responsibility.

5. *Organization and social purpose cannot be disassociated.* The organization (structure) is a means and not an end in itself.

6. *There is no single correct form of organization.* Such things as size, geography, personnel, and funds available will determine at any given time what is the best organization for a particular situation.

7. *Span of control should be definitely considered in organizational structure.* This

---

*Burr, J. B., and others: Elementary school administration, Boston, 1963, Allyn and Bacon, Inc., pp. 398-402.

*Bartholomew, P. C.: Public administration, Paterson, N. J., 1959, Littlefield, Adams & Co., pp 4-8.

rule of organization refers to the number of subordinates who can be adequately supervised by one individual. In other words, the number of communication contacts that can be effectively carried on by any administrative office and subordinates will determine the span of control.

ADMINISTRATION AND POLICY FORMATION

Policy serves as a guideline for successful administration. In the areas of health education and physical education, specifically, policy would represent a series of statements that guide the director or administrator and his staff when making decisions so that their program shows organization with a directed purpose.

Policy, whether it represents the philosophy of the total school or college program or merely the department of health and physical education, has the purpose of guiding those persons associated with the program. Wherever there is a successful organization there will be a sophisticated administration supported by well-designed policies. These policies outline the manner in which the organization will operate and are accepted principles of administration set to guide courses of action. Examples of policies are as follows:

> The Department of Health and Physical Education will periodically test its students to determine their physical fitness levels.

> The Department of Health and Physical Education will hold monthly departmental meetings.

Policy should not be confused with rules and regulations that are more specific in nature and designed to implement or carry out policy. For example, the policy above, in reference to physical fitness testing, could also have regulations regarding the test to be used, when the test will be conducted, and what will be done with the results.

The need for written policies

Policy, as previously outlined, is a series of statements used to guide the administration and the staff in achieving a successful program. Some schools and colleges operate with a minimum of policy guiding their program. Consequently, this can create a series of small crises when the instructional staff has a number of problems for which they have no predetermined course of action. Policy is the best answer for administrative success since it eliminates chaos and confusion.

Each department in the school or college program needs to develop policies unique to its own area of specialization. School and college health and physical education programs are no exception, and administrators as well as staff in these areas should have the knowledge and ability to formulate policy that best fits their programs.

It should be recognized, however, that too many written policies may be just as ineffective as having no written policies at all. Consequently, there is an urgent need to continuously review and appraise existing policies and practices.

How policy is developed

Policy formation in the public school or college is guided by certain national philosophic concepts. Many of the goals that a school or college hopes to achieve, for example, are dictated by forces greater than the separate schools or colleges. These guided principles were developed many years ago and embodied in the Constitution and the Declaration of Independence and affect and control the major goals of educational institutions. Therefore, regardless of what policies an administrator would like to issue, he has certain boundaries within which he must operate. He is also subordinate to state edicts, whether it be written law or by statements issued through the office of the State Commissioner of Education.

Policy development in public schools and

colleges is basically determined by federal and state constitutions, state educational officials, and the local college board of trustees or school board of education. For example, the federal courts have recently interpreted policy on prayers in the public schools relative to the national constitution. The state constitution has policies governing such procedures as when students may enter or leave school. State education officials set policy on such items as minimum salary schedules and centralization or decentralization of school districts. However, all courses of action that have not been predetermined by the state or federal government concerning the local school are left to the local school board of education, the superintendent, the principal, and the school instructional staff.

When developing policy within the Department of Health and Physical Education, there are many steps to be taken that will culminate in an intelligent, purposeful departmental policy. Whenever policy is under consideration, it is of primary importance that those persons who might be affected by the policy should share in the determination of its nature. Group formulation of policies utilizes the intelligence of more persons and thereby should result in better policy. Also, to be most effective, policy making should be continuous, involving widespread participation of administrators, teachers, and other persons where desired. Old policies often fail to serve as guides in a changing organization, department, school, college, and world.

Why is it important for teachers to share in the policy-making process? Teamwork in the teacher-administrator relationship is a must for an efficient organization and, as such, in the sharing by all the staff in the school or college policy-making procedure. Some of the values of teacher participation in policy making are that as teachers share they will care more about effectively executing the policy they helped to develop. It will bring out many different points of view, which will result in better pretesting of policy and thus eventually make for a sounder policy. It will improve teacher-administrator relationships. It will give the teacher a better feeling of belonging and thereby give the school or college a more enthusiastic supporter.

Although teachers should be involved in policy development, it should be remembered that there is a basic difference between staff participation in decision making and the duties and responsibilities concerned with policy execution.

How to write policy

The actual formation of policy involves a logical organization and administration of philosophic concepts to a meaningful conclusion. This may be the most important task the administrator will have to consider when organizing his or her program; that is, how to construct policy.

Objective policy formation may be determined by values and mandates of our culture, human relations, knowledge of teaching and learning, staff suggestions by such means as a suggestion box, staff meetings, advisory council, and curriculum or other committees.

Regardless of who is selected to help write policy, the basic technique is the same. Those persons who are responsible must research the area for which the policy is to be written. This may be done by such means as reviewing previous policies, surveying the personnel of the department for suggestions, finding out what other outstanding school or college systems are doing, or studying recommendations of professional committees and commissions. After the research has been done and the subject thoroughly studied, the formulation of the policy takes place using wording that is clear, concise, and unambiguous. When a possible policy statement is ready, it can be reviewed by the staff and changes made where necessary. If there is a difference of opinion that cannot be resolved, it may be necessary for the head of the department to make a decision. Furthermore, the upper echelons of administrative authority are consulted and, of course, they should review and approve the final draft of policy.

Where policy needs to be established

Policy needs to be written in the broad areas of administration. The following paragraphs cite a few examples.

Personnel. In a well-designed educational institution, those persons who are associated with the proper functioning of the program must be selected and guided by intelligent policy. There should be policy statements in regard to personnel management. Such policies might include how personnel are appointed to the system. Also, for those individuals whom the organization expects to employ as teachers, there should be written policy available for them to study relative to such matters as what they will encounter in the system in respect to tenure provisions, promotion, transfer, leaves of absence, and sabbatical leaves.

Curriculum. When an educational institution has an intelligent and well-directed staff, it still needs a well-designed curriculum to be a meaningful program. Curriculum organization and development are an important function of any department. Therefore, it is recommended that a set of policies related to curriculum development be designed and written for use as practical guidelines.

Student evaluation. Once a significant curriculum has been adopted, an evaluation process must follow. This involves evaluating student progress toward the stated objectives of the program. Again, there must be policy to serve as a guideline for such evaluation. In addition to such matters as grading, there should be a well-developed policy on promotion, graduation, and successful completion of assigned work.

There are many other areas where policies need to be developed. In the health area, for example, there should be policy on such matters as exclusion from school for health reasons, on matters affecting the psychologic as well as the physical environment, and on how the health science instruction program should be conducted. In physical education there is need for policy in regard to such things as athletics and extra pay for coaching. In addition, a problem such as excuses needs to be governed by written policy.

The department of health and physical education should have a series of policy statements governing its organization and administration. With intelligent and coordinated development a successful and more meaningful program can be offered. One further point should be mentioned. The administration should recognize that in addition to the development of policy there must also be proper dissemination of the information about approved policy. All statements should be in writing and recognized as official acts. In some cases it might be helpful to prepare a handbook on policies concerned with departmental activities.

DEMOCRATIC ADMINISTRATION

The administration should recognize certain steps in the democratic process of a staff and organization working together in order to accomplish group goals. Some of the steps that should be considered are as follows:

1. Goals should be developed through the group process. The goals that are set should be attainable, challenging, and adapted to the capacities of the members.

2. Good morale should be developed among the entire staff. This is essential to constructive group action. A permissive climate must be established in group deliberations. All must feel a sense of belonging and recognize their important contribution in the undertaking. A feeling of "oneness" should pervade the entire group.

3. Group planning must be done in a clearly defined manner. A stated procedure

should be followed. It should be a cooperative undertaking, based upon known needs and flexible enough to allow for unforeseen developments. The fulfillment of plans should bring satisfaction and a feeling of success to all who participated in their formulation and accomplishment. All should share in recognition for a completed job.

4. In staff meetings and other group discussions the administration must encourage the utilization of democratic principles. Each member's contribution must be encouraged and respected. Differences of opinion must be on a "principle" basis rather than on a "personal" basis. The organization's objectives and purposes must be continually kept in mind. All members must be encouraged to facilitate the group process by accepting responsibility, alleviating conflict, making contributions, respecting the opinions of others, abiding by the will of the majority, and promoting good group morale.

5. There must be periodic evaluation of progress. The group should evaluate itself from time to time as to its accomplishments in terms of the organization's goals and the effectiveness of the group process. Each individual must evaluate his own role as a member of the organization in respect to contributions made to the group process and the accomplishments of the group.

Many problems arise when the democratic process is used. Application of the democratic process to the functioning of an organization does not solve all problems. Instead, many situations and difficulties arise because of elements that are inherent in the application of democratic principles. It is important to recognize these problems and cope with them as they arise. Despite such dilemmas, the advantages of the democratic process far outweigh the disadvantages.

The problem of divided opinion

In a democratic organization, it is assumed that the wishes of the majority prevail. There is a question that often arises in this connection: Is the majority always right? Very often an important issue will be determined by one vote. Students of history remember that during post-Civil War days one vote kept Andrew Johnson from being removed from office. Every individual can recall similar situations within organizations where like results have occurred. Is this a weakness of democracy? Should important problems, plans, and issues be decided by such a small difference of opinion?

It seems that the reasoning behind such a dilemma is clear. All who believe in democracy recognize the importance of having as much unanimity of thinking as possible. However, they also recognize that it is much better to have a majority make a decision than to have it made by one person who is an autocrat.

The problem of subjective personal opinion as opposed to scientific fact

In many democratic discussions it appears to some individuals that scientific evidence should dictate policies and that personal opinions must not become involved. On complicated issues situations develop where certain individuals are acquainted with scientific data that in themselves define the issue. Therefore, the conclusion is reached that discussion, voting, or other devices are useless since the course of action is very clear as indicated by known fact.

The answer to such a problem seems to be that there will be acceptance if individuals know and recognize the facts. Generally, acceptance fails to materialize when evidence is not conclusive or when it has not been properly publicized. The democratic process can contribute immeasurably to such enlightenment. Through discussion, facts can be presented and understanding reached. Individuals with reasonable intelligence will accept scientific fact as against personal opinion, if the presentation is clear and the evidence is convincing. William Gerard Hamilton during the late eighteenth century made a statement which has a bearing on this point: "Two things are always to be observed; whether what is said is true in itself, or being so, is applicable. In general, things are partly true, and partly not; in part applicable, and in part not. You are careful therefore to distinguish; and to show how far this is true and applies, and how far not." The democratic process is the most effective method yet devised to show what is true and applies.

The problem of standards

A question that is often raised in connection with the utilization of the democratic process is: What does it do to standards of performance? There is a belief in some quarters that by allowing majority opinion and decisions to prevail, standards of performance are lowered to a "middle level." The individuals who have a low set of standards tend to pull down those with high standards. In effect, this results in a compromise on middle ground. The standards take on mediocrity rather than remain at a high level.

The answer to this problem is difficult. A democracy rests upon the worth of the individual. It has faith in the individual, the goals that he will set, and the standards he wants to follow. The challenge presents itself to those whose standards are high to bring the rest up to their level, rather than to allow themselves to be relegated to a lower one. Such a process may take time. Results are not always immediate in a democracy. Nevertheless, the principles upon which it is based are sound. By utilizing such principles as freedom of discussion and assemblage, it is possible to educate and to elevate standards.

The problem of time

Democratic discussions with their need for deliberation and agreement take time.

Such delay often creates problems, sometimes with serious consequences. There is often too much delay between the need for action, decision, and execution. Democracy is based upon the necessity for individuals to see the need for a course of action and then, after seeing this need, deliberate on it, and finally see that the decision that they have made is put into effect.

It is true that this dilemma often works to the disadvantage of many individuals. However, it does not necessarily have to be this way. It has been seen how rapidly the federal government will act in case of emergency. For example, it did not take long for Congress to declare war after the attack on Pearl Harbor or to vote the necessary supplies and help once our country was at war. The delay occurs when there is misunderstanding, when a situation is not meaningful, and when the course of action is confusing. Perhaps it is wise in many cases to have this lag of time. Hasty action also results in many mistakes.

The element of time is usually important in cases of emergency. Democratic organizations make provisions for action under such conditions. Members of an organization can vest such powers in qualified individuals when necessary. John Locke in his *Treatise on Civil Government* pointed out that sometimes it is inevitable that decisions be made quickly by the executive in charge. It would seem logical that the wise administrator and organization would provide for such emergency action.

The problem of discussion with uninterested and noninformed individuals

Another problem that frequently arises in democratic deliberations is that some individuals who participate in group discussions are many times not interested or competent to discuss intelligently and constructively the subject at hand. Such a situation may be very helpful as an educational device. As individuals become better informed on various topics they contribute more. Many minds are better than one or two. Any group should welcome as much help as possible in solving problems.

The problem of authority

Criticism has often been directed against the democratic process from the standpoint that it results in confusion and poor direction. The authority for certain acts is not clearly established. Furthermore, it is conducive to a conflict of ideas, which results in indecisiveness.

It seems important to recognize the part that democratic principles play in such a problem. A democratic organization vests in its members the right to help determine policies, purpose, and methods. They want a "say" in these important factors that vitally affect their lives. At the same time, however, they vest authority for execution of policy and purpose in administrators who are responsible to the group for their actions. Any democratically run organization has to recognize clearly the definite lines that exist between policy formation and execution. If an individual has been placed in an administrative position, the wherewithal to perform his duties effectively must also be granted. In a sense, all individuals have authority in their respective positions. Authority goes with the job and not with the individual. This is true from the top to the bottom of the organization. There is no "final authority" except as it exists in the entire membership. All organizations that are to be efficient and effective must clearly recognize these principles upon which the functioning of an organization rests.

The future of democracy

The problems that have been listed should not be used to deter the application of democratic principles to any organization. If one takes any other method of government, it would readily be found that problems of much greater magnitude and seriousness exist. Furthermore, the administrator as a leader can do much toward solving and alleviating the difficulties that are associated with democratic dilemmas. Outstanding leadership is essential to any democratic organization. High-quality leadership will stress the importance of group participation, freedom of action, good human relations, and the importance of each individual member. This is important and far outweighs any advantages associated with systems that are not democratic.

ADMINISTRATION AND THE CHALLENGE OF MODERN EDUCATION

Education is America's largest industry. This country has nearly 60 million people in classrooms from coast to coast. There are approximately 2 million teachers in the elementary and secondary schools of the nation. More than $50 billion are spent each year on educational programs. The United States government is investing billions of dollars to ensure a quality education for each of its citizens. Educational construction costs more than $5 billion a year. Expenditures on classroom equipment, such as books, audiovisual devices, and desks, amount to $1 billion a year. Certain leading corporations in the United States have linked themselves to the educational business in such areas as copying machines, microfilms, texts and reading material, programmed instruction, electronics, language laboratories, and learning systems. More than 60% of the antipoverty program in the Economic Opportunity Act is estimated as being allocated directly to education. Job Corps centers rely heavily on educators for help and guidance.

The growth of education during the last few years has been phenomenal. For example, expenditures in 1950 were about $9.3 billion, or 3.5% of our gross national product (the sum of all goods and services). A rise to 6.1% of the gross national product has been projected by the middle 1970's. Ten years ago school and college enrollments were under 40 million. The United States Office of Education foresees enrollments of 62 million by the middle 1970's. Textbook sales have risen from about $200 million to $600 million annually in the past decade, or an annual growth of about 12%. Two-year college enrollments have jumped from less than 300,000 students in 1954 to nearly 1 million today. The following statistics are outlined by the United States Office of Education in a publication that projects the education of the present into the education of the future (1974-1975):

A 71 percent increase in students getting bachelor's degrees, up from 525,000 to 899,000.

Almost twice as many persons getting master's degrees, from 111,000 to 210,000.

Twice as many persons getting doctoral degrees from 15,300 to 31,900.

An 89 percent increase in total spending by colleges and universities, from $11.9 billion to $22.5 billion.

A 74 percent increase in students seeking degrees at colleges and universities, up from 5 million in the fall of 1964 to 8.7 million in the fall of 1974.

A 13.5 percent increase in enrollment at public and private elementary and secondary schools, from 48.1 million in 1964 to 54.6 million in 1974.

A 25.9 percent increase in public and private high school graduates, from 2.7 million to 3.4 million.

An increase of 507,000 public and private elemen-

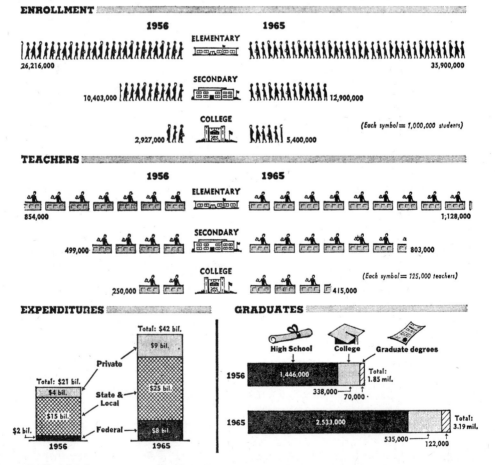

The nation's school system — a decade of growth. (© 1965 by The New York Times Company. Reprinted by permission.)

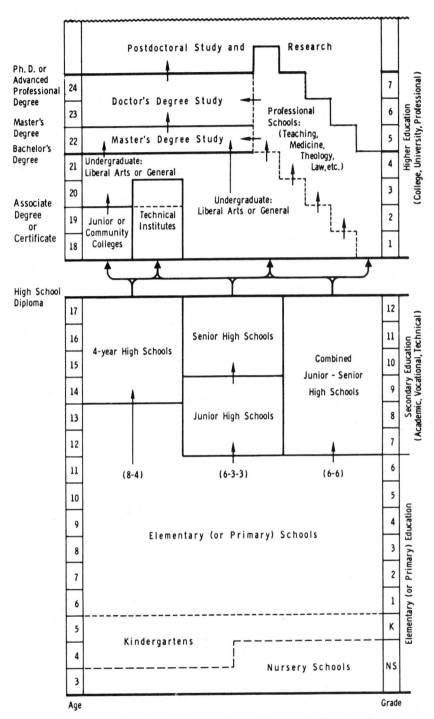

The structure of education in the United States. (From Digest of educational statistics, Washington, D. C., 1965 edition, U. S. Department of Health, Education and Welfare, Office of Education.)

tary and secondary school teachers, from 1.9 million to 2.4 million.

A 47 percent increase in expenditures for elementary and secondary schools, from $26.1 billion to $38.4 billion in the 1974-1975 school year.

The projections indicate that in 1974, the number of high school students will have more than doubled, and the number of degree-seeking college students will have more than tripled the 1954 totals. A decade from now, an estimated 16.4 million students will be in high school.*

The growth in education during recent years and the future expansion predicted place a heavy responsibility upon those persons who provide leadership in this area to offer a program that will preserve the democratic foundations upon which this nation was built, to help develop the potentials of each young person, and to devise educational programs that keep abreast of the times. This Herculean task falls not only upon those individuals who are la-

beled administrators but also upon all educators, whatever role they play in the schools. As such, a study of the facts that comprise the components of educational administration is essential to all, teachers and administrators alike.

THE CHANGING NATURE OF EDUCATION

In addition to the phenomenal growth in enrollments and the cost of running our schools, there have been many significant changes in the manner in which schools and colleges educate our young people. The schools and colleges of America are undergoing a major overhaul. A sampling of some new innovations follows*:

1. The ungraded system in elementary schools that eliminates grade lines in respect to subject matter and student progress

---

*Projections of educational statistics of 1974-75, Washington, D. C., 1965 edition, U. S. Department of Health, Education and Welfare.

*For further discussion of new innovations, see Chapter 3.

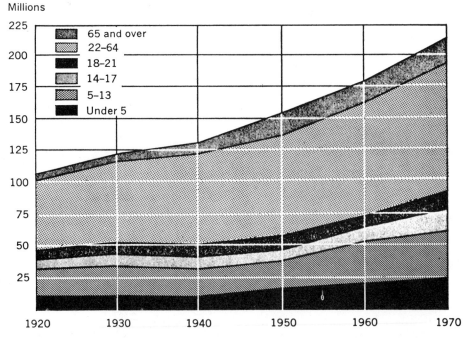

Fifty years of population growth – 1920 to 1970 – has many implications for education. (From NEA Research Bulletin 39:91, 1961.)

2. "Shared time" projects in which both public and parochial school students participate
3. Cooperative buying of school supplies and equipment by several school districts
4. Area schools for rural students desiring modern industrial training
5. Foreign languages offered in the elementary grades
6. Project Head Start—a federally aided program to help slum youngsters enter school better prepared for their new experience
7. Children taught to read with the assistance of a computerized typewriter
8. The new alphabet (Pitman or Initial Teaching Alphabet) with forty-four symbols that represent various sounds being used to provide children with their first experience in reading
9. The new mathematics
10. The new physics
11. The new grammar
12. Team teaching—employing two, three, or more teachers
13. Educational television
14. Teaching machines—giving a student knowledge bit by bit and at his own pace
15. Extension of the school day from 9 A.M. to 5 P.M.
16. Extension of the school year
17. Flexible scheduling with class time ranging from 20 minutes to 1½ or 2 hours
18. Independent study to enable students to carry out advanced work
19. Facilities built underground to cut expense costs
20. The use of educational parks to bring elementary and secondary schools together on campuses
21. Special programs for the gifted students
22. Aid for slum children

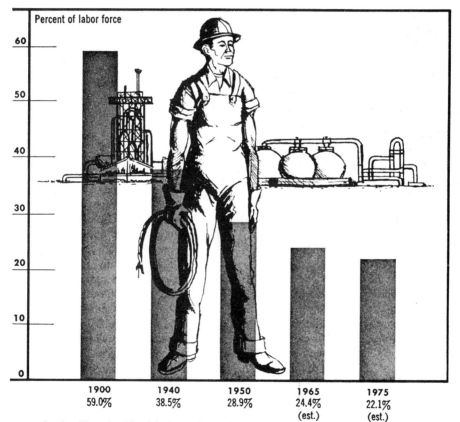

Based on "Occupational Trends in the United States," 1900 to 1950, Working Paper No. 5 of the U. S. Department of Commerce, Bureau of the Census; and unpublished data of the U. S. Department of Labor, Bureau of Labor Statistics.

The falling demand for unskilled labor. (From NEA Research Bulletin 38:12, 1960.)

Education is on the move. New ways of doing things, new facilities, new programs, and the emphasis upon research have become bywords in school systems across the country. Education is not static but instead is a dynamic, constantly changing entity. Educators need to be aware of the changes taking place in the schools and to adapt their own efforts and special fields accordingly. Administration should help in the evaluation of these new innovations, checking the advantages against the disadvantages and weighing their implications for each teacher's field of specialization.

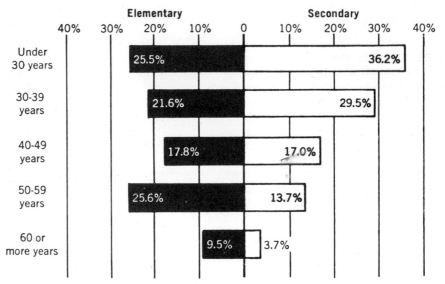

Age distribution of teachers by school level, February, 1965. (From NEA Research Bulletin **43:**68, 1965.)

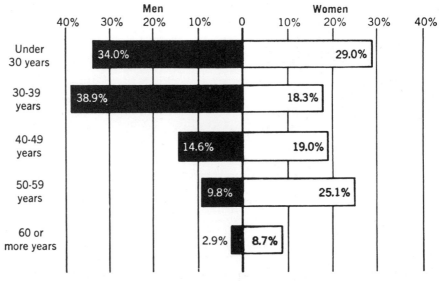

Age distribution of teachers by sex, February, 1965. (From NEA Research Bulletin **43:**68, 1965.)

Education exists in and out of the schools

There is an educational revolution going on in education outside the schools. Business organizations have their education departments. Communications media such as television and radio are in the business of education. Youth groups such as the Campfire Girls and Boy Scouts provide educational experiences, and a multitude of other agencies are also involved. It is therefore important to be realistic about education in America and to be concerned with it in its broadest sense—in and out of the schools. This means teachers, administrators, and educators, in general, must prepare themselves to give leadership to out-of-school programs as well as those with which they are directly involved in the schools.

Equality of education for everyone

The civil rights movement, Project Head Start, the Job Corps, and other national developments indicate that this country is striving to provide each person, regardless of race, color, creed, or economic means, with a quality education. The implications of such a worthy goal mean federal funds, broadened programs, and educational consumers with different needs and interests.

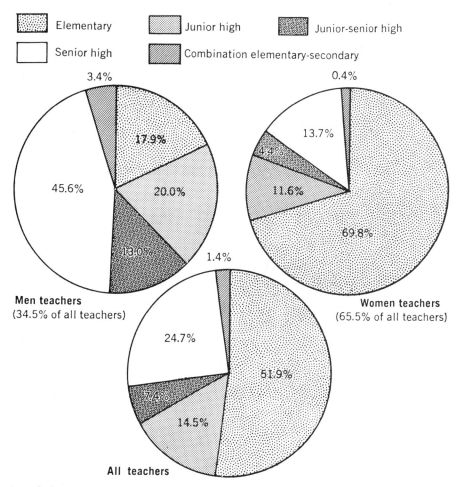

Distribution of classroom teachers by teaching assignment, February, 1965. (From NEA Research Bulletin **43:**68, 1965.)

The curriculum reform movement

Knowledge and truth change with history and with the application of the scientific method to social and educational problems. Young people today need to be acquainted with truths that are truths today. The new mathematics and new physics are only a few of the changes in the curriculum reform movement that are taking place in our schools in an attempt to get at the truth. The trivia must be abolished, the overlap and duplication eliminated, and a new look provided where deficiencies and weaknesses exist. There is a need to debate ways of doing this, a need to test results, a need to experiment, a need for new programs, and a need for alternatives.

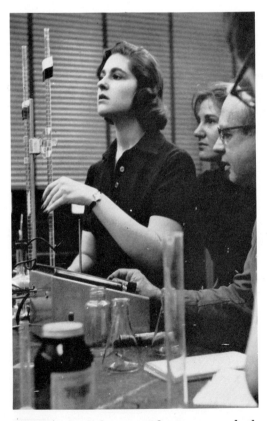

Education and the arts and sciences are both in the business of education. (Yeshiva University, New York, N. Y.)

The scientific study of teaching and learning

There is a realization that the teaching and learning processes can be improved. New techniques can be utilized, new assignments given, and new projects developed. In the preparation of teachers, all parts of a university must work together. Schools of education and the arts and the sciences are both in the business of education whether they like it or not. Learning can be done more efficiently, and the answers will be learned only as constant experimentation takes place and research and testing are done.

The trend toward more public control

The increase of state and federal outlays for education means that control is also shifting from local to federal sources. Federal and state grants mean that the conditions under which such monies are expended for educational purposes must meet the approval of the upper echelons of governmental authority.

Closer working relationship among the home, school, and community

The community is voicing increased concern about the education of its children. Parent-teacher organizations, advisory councils, and other lay groups want to have a say about how their educational systems are run. Educators can no longer live a cloistered existence and be oblivious to the public voice. Avenues of communication must be established and educational problems aired if they are to be solved effectively.

The belief that all problems can be solved through education

The fact that many Americans are killed each year on the nation's highways has resulted in Americans turning to schools for a solution to this problem. The fact that tests have shown that American children are not physically fit has resulted in the public asking the schools to help remedy the problem. Education is increasingly being looked upon as a panacea for many of the problems with which our society is vexed. Consequently, there are pressures for time in the school schedule, personnel to do the job, and budget allocations to support the suggested reforms.

The internationalization of education

The exchange programs involving faculty and students, the increased speed of transportation, the junior-year abroad, the great amount of travel by Americans to other countries, and the creation of international centers and other evidences of cross-cultural intermingling have resulted in educational concern for people and problems outside the continental United States. Americans no longer live by themselves. What they do and how they think affects not only Americans but also other people around the globe. Education is not limited to the United States but involves the entire globe.

THE CHALLENGE OF THE FUTURE AND THE ADMINISTRATION OF HEALTH AND PHYSICAL EDUCATION PROGRAMS

The changes taking place in education and the goals being sought have vital implications for school health and physical education programs.

1. *Health educators and physical educators must be aware of new developments in general education.* There are so many changes taking place in education today that unless a person continually makes a determined effort to keep abreast of these changes, he is likely to find that he is out of pace with the times. Each health educator and physical educator should read current literature that concerns itself with new trends and practices in education. There are many excellent publications that cover the latest thinking in education. Keeping abreast of new innovations does

not simply mean possessing a superficial knowledge of each development, but, instead, it means being informed as to the nature and scope of the innovation, where and why it is being used, its advantages and disadvantages, and its implications for health and physical education programs.

In addition to being knowledgeable about what is happening in education, some of the new trends may have special implications for school health and physical education programs. For example, in regard to the nongraded elementary school, one might ask the following questions: Should a student be permitted to proceed at his own rate of speed in areas that have a unique relationship to his physical growth and development in the same way that he would proceed in a course in mathematics where the learning involves primarily the mental mechanisms? What is the ideal type of schedule for physical education and health education? Should all class periods be the same length or be of varying lengths? If so, what are they? In what way can programmed instruction be used most effectively in health education and physical education? The answers to such questions will require much thought and investigation, but the end results are very important to the most effective administration of these special fields.

2. *Health educators and physical educators should be continually studying their present programs and practices to determine if they are keeping up with the times.* Just as programs are changing in mathematics, English, and science, so also should programs of school health education and physical education be studied for possible needed changes. Changing for the sake of change itself should not be the case, but sometimes traditional ways of doing things become outmoded and consequently new innovations are needed to keep up with the times. For example, such ideas as the following have been suggested and may possibly warrant further study:

a. Physical education classes meeting in the classroom as well as in the gymnasium
b. Health science classes being taught only by teachers trained and interested in this area
c. A textbook in classes of physical education
d. A conceptualized approach to the teaching of health
e. A program of educational athletics
f. A national curriculum in physical education
g. A movement education emphasis in physical education
h. Perceptual motor skills as a means of improving reading in the early grades
i. New approaches to the teaching of critical health areas such as alcohol, tobacco, narcotics, and sex education
j. Team teaching

3. *Health educators and physical educators should recognize that new challenges to education have administrative implications for their programs.* The tremendous growth and emphasis upon education have special implications for the field of administration. Such factors as policies developed, budgets approved, personnel appointed, facilities and equipment purchased, curricula planned, and special subject matter and activity programs encouraged will determine the direction of school health and physical education programs in the future. The challenge of the increased role for education in American life, with increased funds, personnel, and facilities to accomplish the objectives that have been established, will be met only as sound administrative practices are followed. The challenge means that all health educators and physical educators should understand what does and does not constitute sound administrative practice.

4. *Health educators and physical educators should place more emphasis on research.* There is an urgent need for more emphasis upon research in the fields of health education and physical education. Research is needed to advance the frontiers of knowledge in regard to these special fields, their contributions to mankind, their role in academic achievement, the function they have in personality develop-

ment, and the tangible impacts they have on the health, productivity, and leadership of Americans. These are only a few areas that need to be investigated. In addition to more research being conducted, there needs to be greater emphasis on the training of research workers in professional preparation programs. Also, there should be more outlets for publicizing the research findings. At present, the *Research Quarterly* of the American Association of Health, Physical Education and Recreation (about sixty studies a year), *The Journal of School Health,* and *The School Health Review* are the main outlets, although certain psychologic and physiologic publications do provide other means of communication. However, there should be more outlets with greater implementation of findings at the grass roots level.

5. *Health educators and physical educators must become more scholarly.* Excellence in educational undertakings means that the educators involved—the persons who are doing the teaching and administering—must themselves be scholarly individuals. There is so much cross fertilization in educational endeavors that each teacher and administrator can contribute to the education of our young people in many areas other than his own specialty. This can only be possible as each educator becomes a scholarly individual in his own right. Furthermore, it is important for health education and physical education to be able to stand on an equal footing with academic subjects and not be found wanting when more scholarly discussions are held.

Questions and exercises

1. Define the term *administration* in your own words. Give illustrations to point out the various facets of your definition.
2. Prepare an organization chart for some department, school, or agency with which you are familiar. Discuss significant aspects of the administrative setup of this organization.
3. Prepare a rating sheet that could be utilized

by students to determine the extent of their qualifications for the field of administration.

4. Write an essay discussing the role of the administrator in achieving cooperation from members of an organization.
5. What are some basic principles that should be observed in respect to channels of communication?
6. Why is a study of administration important to you as a physical educator or health educator?
7. Compare the traditional and the modern views of education. What do we mean by a theory of administration, and how does theory help in the practice of administration?
8. What type of preparation should potential administrators receive according to the administrative theorists?
9. What are the qualities that make for administrative leadership? Will the administrative leader be a success in whatever job he assumes?
10. In respect to policy formation discuss the following: (a) what is policy? (b) why is policy needed? (c) how should policy be developed and written? Prepare a sample policy in physical education.
11. Describe a democratic administrator. Compare his characteristics with those of an autocratic administrator.
12. Why is education playing an increasing role in American life?
13. Project health education or physical education 20 years into the future and describe the type of program you would like to see.

Reading assignment in *Administrative Dimensions of Health and Physical Education Programs, Including Athletics:* Chapter 1, Selections 1 to 4.

Selected references

American Association for Health, Physical Education, and Recreation: Developing democratic human relations through health education, physical education and recreation, Washington, D. C., 1951, The Association.

Bender, J. F.: The technique of executive leadership, New York, 1950, McGraw-Hill Book Co.

Bucher, C. A.: Foundations of physical education, ed. 5, St. Louis, 1968, The C. V. Mosby Co.

Bucher, C. A., Koenig, C., and Barnhard, M.: Methods and materials for secondary school physical education, ed. 3, St. Louis, 1970, The C. V. Mosby Co.

Center for the Advanced Study of Educational Administration: Perspectives of educational administration and the behavioral sciences, Eugene, 1965, The University of Oregon.

Educational Personnel Administration Number, Education, December, 1954. (A compilation of fourteen articles on educational personnel administration.)

Goldman, S.: The school principal, New York, 1966, The Center for Applied Research in Education, Inc. (The Library of Education).

Griffiths, D. E.: The school superintendent, New York, 1966, The Center for Applied Research in Education, Inc. (The Library of Education).

Gulick, L., and Urwick, L., editors: Papers on the science of administration, New York, 1937, Institute of Public Administration.

Halpin, A. W., editor: Administrative theory in education, New York, 1958, The Macmillan Co.

Jenson, T. H., and Clark, D. L.: Educational administration, New York, 1964, The Center for Applied Research in Education, Inc. (The Library of Education).

Knezevich, S. J.: Administration of public education, New York, 1962, Harper & Row, Publishers, pp. 223-226.

Kozman, H. C., editor: Group process in physical education, New York, 1951, Harper & Row, Publishers.

Morphet, E. L., and others: Educational organization and administration, Englewood Cliffs, N. J., 1967, Prentice-Hall, Inc.

Simon, H. A.: Administrative behavior, New York, 1957, The Free Press.

Tead, O.: The art of leadership, New York, 1935, Whittlesey House.

Tead, O.: The art of administration, New York, 1951, McGraw-Hill Book Co.

Thompson, J. D., editor: Approaches to organizational design, Pittsburgh, 1966, University of Pittsburgh Press.

Urwick, L.: The elements of administration, New York, 1943, Harper & Row, Publishers.

Willower, D. J., and Culbertson J., editors: The professorship in educational administration, Columbus, Ohio, 1964, The University Council for Educational Administration.

CHAPTER 2 ADMINISTRATIVE RELATIONSHIPS AND OBJECTIVES

Each person associated with the schools and colleges of this country should view himself first as an educator and second as a health educator, physical educator, recreation supervisor, history teacher, or other type of specialist. Each person should see himself working to achieve goals that are common to general education and toward which the schools and colleges are directing their efforts. Each person should view his own special field with a perspective that gives balance to the total enterprise. Each person should strive to appreciate fully what all areas of specialization are attempting to accomplish and the contribution each makes toward helping our young people develop into mature, well-educated adults.

A field of endeavor is characterized by the objectives for which it exists. Objectives help the members of a group to know where they are going, what they are striving for, and what they hope to accomplish. Physical educators and health educators have clearly stated objectives toward which they are working. The student preparing for a career in these fields or administrators and leaders working in these fields should understand the objectives and be guided by them. Objectives, therefore, represent the aims, purposes, and outcomes that are derived from participating in physical education and health education programs.

HEALTH EDUCATION AND PHYSICAL EDUCATION DEFINED

The term *health* as defined by the World Health Organization refers to the total health of the person, including mental, emotional, physical, and social health, and not merely the absence of disease and infirmity. The school health program is designed to achieve this objective through a plan of health instruction, health services, and healthful school living. A definition of school health education as included in the report of the Joint Committee on Health Education Terminology,* is: "The process of providing or utilizing experiences for favorably influencing understandings, attitudes, and practices related to safe living."

The term *physical education* as used in this text is defined as follows: *Physical education, an integral part of the total education process, is a program aimed at the development of physically, mentally, emotionally, and socially fit citizens through the medium of physical activities that have been selected with a view to realizing these outcomes.*

GENERAL EDUCATION

Since school and college health and physical education should first be viewed within the concept of general education, it is appropriate to first define what is meant by general education and second to delineate the role of health and physical education within general education.

The purposes for which education exists have been set forth by many individuals and many organizations. One group of pur-

---

*Report of the Joint Committee on Health Education Terminology, Journal of Health, Physical Education, and Recreation 33:27, 1962.

poses reflects the socioeconomic goals for education as presented in ten characteristics that are desired for the individual American. These characteristics were stated in 1937 by a committee that included a philosopher, a lawyer, a sociologist, a superintendent of schools, and two secretaries of state education associations.

1. Hereditary strength
2. Physical security
3. Participation in an evolving culture
   a. Skills, techniques, and knowledges
   b. Values, standards, and outlooks
4. An active, flexible personality
5. Suitable occupation
6. Economic security
7. Mental security
8. Equality of opportunity
9. Freedom
10. Fair play

Also included in the report of this committee, which included John Dewey and Willard E. Givens, were statements that "education must be universal in its extent and application, universal in its materials and methods, and universal in its aims and spirit." When analyzing and studying this list, one cannot but realize the great implications each of the items has for the fields of school health and physical education.

In 1938 the Educational Policies Commission also set forth certain purposes of education that they felt included a summarization and enlargement of statements that had been published previously by various committees and individuals representing the National Education Association. These purposes were (1) the objectives of self-realization, which are concerned with developing the individual to his fullest capacity in respect to health, recreation, and philosophy of life, (2) the objectives of human relationship, which refer to relationships among people on the family, group, and society levels, (3) the objectives of economic efficiency, which are concerned with the individual as a producer and a consumer, and (4) the objectives of civic responsibility, which stress the individual's relationship to his local, state, national, and international forms of government.

Today, general education is looked upon as preparing the individual for a meaningful, self-directed existence. For a student to be prepared to accomplish this goal means that he must have an understanding of (1) his cultural heritage and the ability to evaluate it, (2) the world of nature and the ability to adapt to it, (3) the contemporary social scene and the values and skills necessary for effective participation, (4) the role of communication and skill in communicating, (5) the nature of self and others and growth in capacity for continuing self-development and for relating to others, and (6) the role of esthetic forms in human living and the capacity for self-expression through them. Thus the role of general education is a multifaceted undertaking requiring many different experiences and specialties.

HEALTH AND PHYSICAL EDUCATION PROGRAMS CONTRIBUTE TO GENERAL EDUCATION

Health education and physical education are integral parts of general education. Science indicates that these fields of endeavor contribute in many ways.

1. *The mind and body are inseparable.* Physical, mental, social, and emotional development are closely interwoven into the fabric of the human being. A person can think himself into being sick just as sickness can affect his thinking; *psychosomatic* has become an important word in our vocabulary. Intellectual, physical, and emotional developments are closely associated. Endocrinology has shown that mentality changes as body chemistry changes. Biology has linked the cell to the learning experience. Psychology points to the fact

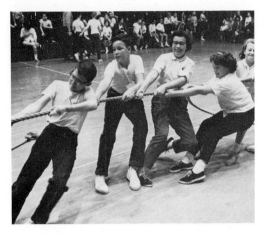

Davenport, Iowa, Public Schools.

that the child's earliest learnings are tactual and kinesthetic.

2. *Motor skills contribute to learning.* Intelligence is not the only answer to achievement in school. Motor learning is involved in readiness skills that are basic to perception, symbolic manipulation, and concept formation. If motor learning during the early years of childhood is deficient, more complex and advanced learning will be impeded. Psychologists Radler and Kephart * point out that motor activity of some type forms the foundation for all behavior, including the higher thought processes. They further stress that human behavior will function no better than the motor skills that are a part of the individual's makeup.

3. *Health and physical education contribute to academic achievement by developing physical fitness.* Research indicates that students who are achieving academically are also physically above average. It appears that physical fitness, at least up to a certain minimum level, is essential for good health and necessary for academic achievement.

4. *Health education and physical education contribute to academic achievement*

*Radler, D. H., and Kephart, N. C.: Success through play, New York, 1960, Harper & Row, Publishers.

through their contribution to social development. Research shows a relationship between scholastic success and the degree to which a student is accepted by his peer group. Similarly, the boy or girl who learns and applies sound principles of personality development or who is well grounded in motor skills, for example, usually possesses social status among his or her peers.

5. *Health education and physical education contribute to the emotional development of educationally subnormal students.* The value of health and physical education programs for educationally subnormal students may be greater than for average boys and girls. Dr. James N. Oliver, lecturer in education at the University of Birmingham, England, has done much research on educationally subnormal boys and has found that systematic and progressive physical conditioning yields marked mental and physical improvement. He believes much of the improvement results from a boy's feelings of achievement that has the side effect of influencing his academic work for the better.

6. *Health education and physical education are integral parts of general education since they possess a subject matter essential to human beings.* Just as it is important to teach English so that people can communicate articulately, history so that they will appreciate their cultural heritage, and fine arts so that they can appreciate and enjoy Picasso and Beethoven, so it is also important to educate people regarding their physical selves so that they may function most efficiently as human beings. A very intelligent group of young people in our schools and colleges today are not going to be physically active, develop skill, stop their sexual promiscuity, drinking, smoking, and use of narcotics unless given some good reasons. They are going to have to understand and know that the time spent in the pursuit of these goals has its rewards. Thus facts and subject matter become a necessity.

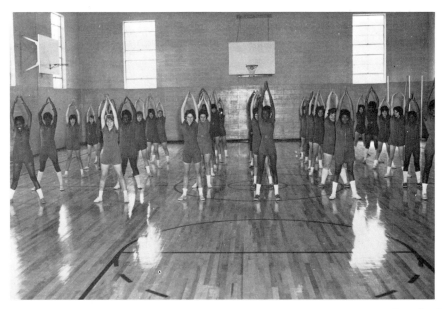

Physical education is a part of general education. (Emma Woerner Junior High School, Louisville, Ky.)

RELATIONSHIP OF HEALTH EDUCATION AND PHYSICAL EDUCATION

Health education and physical education as professional fields of endeavor are closely allied, especially in respect to their administrative aspects. In many schools and colleges, both come under one administrative head. They are concerned with the accomplishment of similar objectives. In many small communities both health education and physical education, although not always desirable, are taught by the same person. Professional preparation institutions usually incorporate both areas in the same schools or departments. In the American Association for Health, Physical Education, and Recreation, they are linked together professionally. Individuals working in these specialized areas share facilities, personnel, funds, and other items essential to their programs. General school administrators feel they are closely related.

These are only a few of the reasons why a close administrative relationship should and must exist between these specialized fields. Although professional persons realize the place of each and the need for specialists in each area, at the same time they also recognize the importance of maintaining a close and effective working relationship. The administrator is a key person in seeing that such a relationship is maintained. In some quarters there has been disunity and strained relations between these areas because the administrator did not assume his role of appeaser and unifier.

In recent years educational thinking has been more and more cognizant of the place of health education and physical education in school and college programs. Each is closely related to the other, but at the same time each is distinct. Each area has its own specialized subject matter content, its specialists, and media through which it is striving to better the living standards of human beings. In the larger professional preparation institutions each has its own separate training program. There is continual agitation for separate certification of its leaders in the various states. Some sections of the country have recognized this

need and have established state certification standards for employment of these
specialized workers.

Although many educators and others feel
that physical education has traditionally
reflected the thinking and work of both
areas, this is an erroneous belief. There is
a definite need for the specialist in each of
the areas of health and physical education.
Each can render a service to humanity.
Each can make a contribution that is distinct and separate from the other's. Each
has its own destiny.

A close relationship among teachers in
these areas, however, is evidenced by the
fact that, to a great degree, they work on
committees together and have professional
books and magazines that cover the literature of both fields. Both are concerned
with the total health of the individual. Both
recognize the importance of activity in developing and maintaining good personal
health. Both are concerned with the physical as well as the social, mental, emotional,
and spiritual aspects. Both recognize the
importance of developing good human relations as a basis for effective living in a
democracy. Both are interested in promoting the total health of the public at large
as a means to enriched living, accomplishment of worthy goals, and increased happiness.

OBJECTIVES OF HEALTH AND PHYSICAL EDUCATION PROGRAMS

The ultimate objectives of school and
college health and physical education programs are similar. The essential difference
lies in the fact that each area attempts to
achieve its goals by utilizing different skills,
media, and approaches. The objectives of
each of the two areas are discussed in the
pages to follow.

Objectives of health education programs

The long-term, overall objective of a
health program is to maintain and improve
the health of human beings. This refers to
all aspects of health, including physical,
mental, emotional, and social. It applies to
all individuals, regardless of race, color,
economic status, creed, or national origin.
Schools and colleges have the responsibility to see that all students achieve and
maintain optimum health, not only from a
legal point of view but also from the standpoint that the educational experience will
be much more meaningful if optimum
health exists. A person learns easier and
better when in a state of good health.

A synthesis of some of the objectives of
the school and college health programs that
have been listed by leaders in the field include the following:

1. To teach scientific health knowledge so that
   the individual can make intelligent health
   decisions
2. To develop desirable health attitudes in
   order that the individual will have an interest in applying health knowledge to his
   own daily regimen of living
3. To convey to the consumer that health is a
   three-dimensional entity, embodying social,
   mental, and physical aspects
4. To contribute to the physical, social, and
   emotional development of each boy and
   girl
5. To further good personality development
   among students
6. To encourage the student to be a wise
   consumer and producer with respect to
   health goods and services
7. To encourage the correction of remediable
   defects among those persons where they
   exist
8. To help students and teachers to live
   healthfully at school and college
9. To reduce the incidence of communicable
   disease in the school, college, and community
10. To appreciate the many health services
    available in the school, college, and com-
    munity
11. To further home-school cooperation in
    health matters

The commonly mentioned objectives
concerned with the development of health
knowledge, desirable health attitudes, and
desirable health practices deserve further
discussion.

Development of health knowledge. In order to accomplish the health knowledge objective, health education must present and interpret scientific health data for purposes of personal guidance. Such information will help individuals to recognize health problems and to solve them by utilizing information that is valid and helpful. It also will serve as a basis for the formulation of desirable health attitudes. In the complex society that exists today there are so many choices confronting an individual in regard to factors that affect his health that a reliable store of knowledge is essential.

Individuals should know how their bodies function, causes and methods of preventing disease, factors that contribute to and maintain health, and the role of the community in the health program. Such knowledge will aid the individual to live correctly, help protect his body against harm and infection, and impress upon him the responsibility for his own health and the health of others.

Knowledge of health will vary with different ages. For younger children there should be an attempt to provide experiences that will show the importance of living healthfully. Such settings as the cafeteria, lavatory, and medical examination room offer these opportunities. As the individual grows older, the scientific knowledge for following certain health practices and ways of living can be presented. Some of the areas of health knowledge that should be understood by students and adults include nutrition, the need for rest,

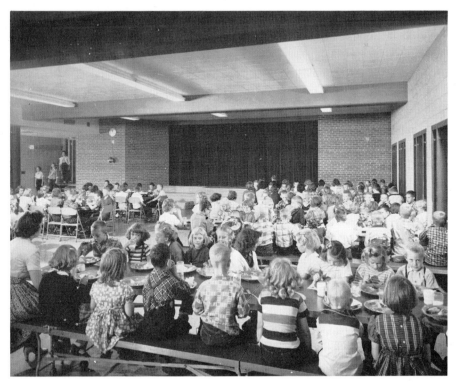

Burnett and Logan, Chicago.

One objective of health education is the cultivation of those habits of living which will promote present and future health. (Washington Irving Elementary School, Waverly, Iowa.)

sleep, and exercise, protection of the body against changing temperature conditions, contagious disease control, drugs, environmental pollution, family living, human sexuality, the dangers of self-medication, and community resources for health.* If such topics are brought to the attention of persons everywhere and if the proper health attitudes and practices are developed, better health will result.

There should also be an adequate knowledge of what constitutes healthful living and adequate health services.

Both the physical and nonphysical environment should be considered in healthful living. School and college buildings, homes, and other places where people congregate should be clean, sanitary, well lighted, and ventilated, provide ample space, and be adjusted to the various health needs of individuals. In addition, the importance of the nonphysical environment should be recognized. This environment reflects how teachers and pupils get along with each other, incentives, organization and administrative structure and procedures, and other items that greatly affect mental and emotional health.

Knowledge of what constitutes adequate health services should also be understood. Such health services as health appraisal, health counseling, communicable disease control, education of the handicapped, and emergency care of injuries should be appreciated by all. Only as this knowledge is imparted will the various services be utilized in a manner most conducive to the health of students.

Development of desirable health attitudes. The term *health attitudes* refers to the health interests of the individual or the motives that impel him to act in a certain way. All the health knowledge that can be accumulated will have little worth unless the individual is interested and motivated to the point that he wants to apply this

knowledge to everyday living. Attitudes, motives, drives, or impulses, if properly established, will result in the individual's seeking out scientific knowledge and utilizing it as a guide to living. This interest, drive, or motivation must be dynamic to the point where it results in behavior changes.

School and college health programs must be directed at developing those attitudes that will result in optimum health. Students should have an interest in, and be motivated toward, possessing a state of buoyant health, being well rested and well fed, having wholesome thoughts free from anger, jealousy, hate, and worry, and feeling strong and possessing physical power to perform life's routine tasks. They should have the right attitudes toward health knowledge, healthful school living, and health services. If such interests as these exist within the individual, proper health practices will be followed. Health should not be an end in itself except in cases of severe illness. Health is a means to an end, a medium that aids in achieving noble purposes and contributes to enriched living.

Another factor that motivates individuals to good health is the desire to avoid the pain and disturbances that accompany ill health. They do not like toothaches, headaches, or indigestion because of the pain or distraction involved. However, developing health attitudes in a negative manner, through fear of pain or other disagreeable conditions, is a questionable approach.

A strong argument for developing proper attitudes or interests should center around the goals one is trying to achieve in life and the manner in which optimum health is an aid in achieving such goals. This is the strongest incentive or interest that can be developed in the individual. If one wishes to become a great artist, an outstanding businessman, or a famed dancer, it is greatly beneficial if he or she has good health. This is important so that the study,

---

*See also Chapter 12.

training, hard work, trials, and obstacles that one encounters can be met successfully. Optimum health will aid in the accomplishment of such goals. As Jennings, the biologist, has pointed out, the body can attend to only one thing at a time. If its attention is focused on a toothache, a headache, or an ulcer, it cannot be focused satisfactorily on some essential work that has to be done. Centering health attitudes or interests on life goals is a dynamic thing because these represent an aid to accomplishment, achievement, and enjoyable living.

Development of desirable health practices. Desirable health practices represent the application of those habits that are best, according to the most qualified thinking in the field, to one's routine of living. The health practices that an individual adopts will determine in great measure the health of that person. If practices or habits harmful to optimum health are engaged in, such as failure to obtain proper rest or exercise, overeating, overdrinking, oversmoking, and the use of harmful drugs and failure to observe certain precautions against contracting diseases, then poor health is likely to follow.

Knowledge does not necessarily ensure good health practices. An individual may have at his command all the statistics as to the results of speeding at 70 miles per hour and of using seat belts, but unless this information is applied it is useless. The health of an individual can be affected only by applying that which is known. At the same time, knowledge will not usually be applied unless an incentive, interest, or attitude exists that impels its application. It can be seen, therefore, that in order to have a good school health program, it is important to recognize the close relationship that exists among health knowledge, health attitudes, and health practices. One contributes to the other.

Another health objective that is sometimes listed is that of skill development.

This refers to the development of such skills as those involved in first aid and safety. A mastery of such skills enhances good health.

Recent significant health studies. A significant study in the field of health education was the School Health Education Study,* which was initiated in September, 1961, under a grant from the Samuel Bronfman Foundation of New York City. This study included a synthesis of research in selected areas of health instruction, a national study of health instruction in the public schools, and the development of a concept approach to the teaching of health that identified the key concepts in the teaching of health, statements of concepts for organizing the curriculum, and substantive elements that delineated the subject matter content. All of these concepts are directed at certain behavioral outcomes that are deemed desirable for the student. The School Health Education Study is discussed at greater length in Chapter 12.

Another significant step forward at the state level has developed in New York State. As a result of the increased awareness of health problems, including the widespread use of drugs and narcotics, tobacco, and alcohol, Governor Nelson Rockefeller signed the Speno-Brydges Bill in May, 1967. This law required the teaching of health in all grades throughout the state of New York. A new health curriculum was developed and the program introduced in 1970. As a result of this legislation and the increased interest in health on the part of the citizens of this state, schoolchildren are receiving instruction in the critical

---

*The following reports were published by the School Health Education Study, 1201 16th St. N.W., Washington, D. C.: Synthesis of research in selected areas of health instruction, July, 1963; School Health Education Study: A summary report, June, 1964; School Health Education Study: A call for action, February, 1965; and School Health Education Study: A conceptual approach, February, 1965.

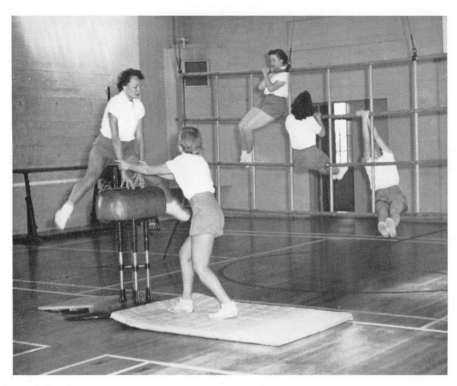

The physical development objective. (Department of Physical Education, University of California at Berkeley.)

health areas of tobacco, drugs, alcohol, and family living and also in such areas as nutrition, mental and emotional health, disease prevention and control, and accident prevention.

What is developing in New York State is increasingly being felt throughout the nation. More and more state departments of education and health, larger and larger groups of citizens, and more governmental officials are beginning to recognize that education is vital to the nation's health and well-being.

Objectives of the school and college physical education programs*

A study of the individual reveals four general directions or phases in which

*Bucher, C. A.: Foundations of physical education, ed. 5, St. Louis, 1968, The C. V. Mosby Co.

growth and development take place—physical development, motor development, mental development, and human relations development. Physical education plays an important part in contributing to each of these phases of human growth and development.

The physical development objective. The physical development objective deals with the program of activities that builds physical power in an individual through the development of the various organic systems of the body. It results in the ability to sustain adaptive effort, the ability to recover, and the ability to resist fatigue. The value of this objective is based on the fact that an individual will be more active, have better performance, and be healthier if the organic systems of the body are adequately developed and functioning properly.

Muscular activity plays a major role in the development of the organic systems of the body. The term *organic* refers to the digestive, circulatory, excretory, heat regulatory, respiratory, and other systems of the human body. These systems are stimulated and trained through such activities as hanging, climbing, running, throwing, leaping, carrying, and jumping. Health is also related to muscular activity; therefore, activities that bring into play all of the fundamental "big muscle" groups in the body should be engaged in regularly. Furthermore, the activity should be of a vigorous nature so that the various organic systems are sufficiently stimulated.

Through vigorous muscular activity several beneficial results take place. The trained heart provides better nourishment to the entire body. The trained heart beats slower than the untrained heart. It pumps more blood per stroke, with the result that more food is delivered to the cells and there is better removal of waste products. During exercise the trained heart's speed increases less and has a longer rest period between beats. After exercise it returns to normal much more rapidly. The end result of this state is that the trained individual is able to perform work for a longer period of time, with less expenditure of energy and much more efficiency, than the untrained individual. This trained condition is necessary for a vigorous and abundant life. From the time an individual rises in the morning until he goes to bed at night, he is continually in need of vitality, strength, endurance, and stamina to perform routine tasks, be prepared for emergencies, and lead a vigorous life. Therefore, physical education aids in the development of the trained individual so that he will be better able to perform his routine tasks and live a healthy, interesting, and happy existence.

The motor development objective. The motor development objective is concerned with performing physical movement with as little expenditure of energy as possible and in a proficient, graceful, and esthetic

manner. This has implications for one's work, play, and anything else that requires physical movement. The name *motor* is derived from relationship to a nerve or nerve fiber that connects the central nervous system, or a ganglion, with a muscle. Movement results, as a consequence of the impulse it transmits. The impulse it delivers is known as the motor impulse.

Effective motor movement is dependent upon a harmonious working together of the muscular and nervous systems. It results in greater distance between fatigue and peak performance; it is found in activities involving running, hanging, jumping, dodging, leaping, kicking, bending, twisting, carrying, and throwing; and it will enable one to perform his daily work much more efficiently and without reaching the point of being "worn out" so quickly.

In physical education activities, the function of efficient body movement, or neuromuscular skill as it is often called, is to provide the individual with the ability to perform with a degree of proficiency. This will result in greater enjoyment of participation. Most individuals enjoy doing those particular activities in which they have acquired a degree of mastery or skill. For example, if a child has mastered the ability to throw a ball consistently to a designated spot and has developed batting and fielding power, he will like to play baseball or softball. If he can swim 25 or 50 yards without tiring and can perform several dives, he will enjoy being in the water. If an adult can consistently serve tennis "aces," he will like tennis; if he can drive a ball 250 yards straight down the fairway, he will like golf; and if he can throw ringers, he will like horseshoes. A person enjoys doing those things in which he or she excels. Few individuals enjoy participating in activites in which they have little skill. Therefore, it is the objective of physical education to develop in each individual as many physical skills as possible so that interests will be wide and varied. This will

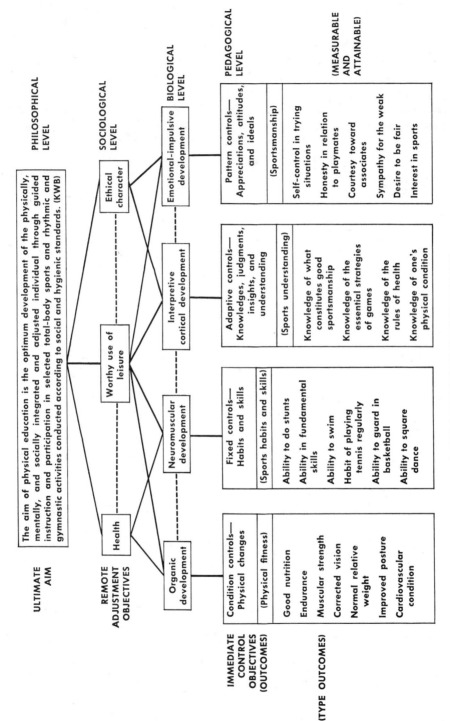

THE PURPOSES OF PHYSICAL EDUCATION

Objectives of physical education. (From Bookwalter, K. W.: Physical education in the secondary schools, Washington, D. C., 1964, The Center for Applied Research in Education, Inc.)

not only result in more enjoyment for the participant, but at the same time will allow for better adjustment to group situations.

Physical skills are not developed in one lesson. It takes years to acquire coordinations, and the most important period for development is during the formative years of a child's growth. The building of coordinations starts in childhood, when an individual attempts to synchronize his muscular and nervous systems for such movements as creeping, walking, running, and jumping. A study of kinesiology shows that many muscles of the body are used in even the most simple of coordinated movements. Therefore, in order to obtain efficient motor movement or skill in many activities, it is necessary to start training early in life and to continue into adulthood. Furthermore, a child does not object to the continual trial-and-error process of achieving success in the performance of physical acts. He does not object to being observed as an awkward, uncoordinated beginner during the learning period. Most adults, however, are self-conscious when going through the period of learning a physical skill. They do not like to perform if they cannot perform in a creditable manner. The skills they do not acquire in their youth are many times never acquired. Therefore, the physical education profession should try to see that this skill learning takes place at a time when a person is young and willing and is laying the foundation for adult years.

The motor development objective also has important implications for the health and recreational phases of the program. The skills that children acquire will determine to a great extent how their leisure time will be spent. One enjoys participat-

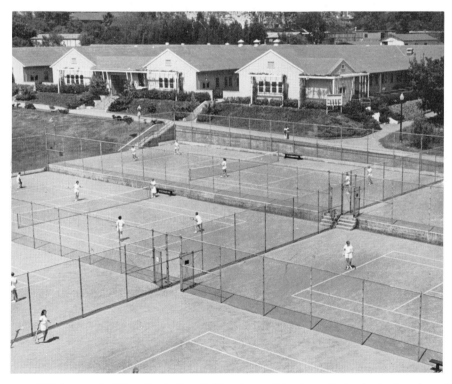

Developing skill in worthwhile physical activities is an objective of physical education. (Department of Physical Education, University of California at Berkeley.)

ing in those activities in which one excels. Therefore, if a child excels in swimming, a great deal of his leisure time is going to be spent at a pool, lake, or beach. If he excels in tennis, he will be found on the courts on Saturdays, Sundays, and after dinner at night. There is believed to be a correlation between juvenile delinquency and lack of constructive leisure-time activity. If we want children to spend their leisure moments in a physically wholesome way, we should see that skills are gained in physical education activities.

The mental development objective. The mental development objective deals with the accumulation of a body of knowledge and the ability to think and interpret this knowledge.

Physical activities must be learned; hence, there is a need for thinking on the part of the intellectual mechanism, with a resulting acquisition of knowledge. The coordinations involved in various movements must be mastered and adapted to the environment in which the individual lives, whether it be in walking, running, or wielding a tennis racquet. In all these movements the child must think and coordinate his muscular and nervous systems. Furthermore, this type of knowledge is acquired through trial and error. Then, as a result of experience, there is a changed meaning in the situation. Coordinations are learned, with the result that an act once difficult and awkward to perform becomes easy to execute.

The individual should not only learn coordinations but should also acquire a knowledge of rules, techniques, and strategies involved in physical activities. Basketball can be used as an example. In this sport a person should know the rules, the strategy in offense and defense, the various types of passes, the difference between screening and blocking, and finally the values that are derived from playing in this sport. Techniques that are learned through experience result in knowledge that is also

acquired. For example, a ball travels faster and more accurately if one steps with a pass, and time is saved when the pass is made from the same position in which it is received. Furthermore, a knowledge of followership, leadership, courage, self-reliance, assistance to others, safety, and adaptation to group patterns is very important.

Knowledge concerning health should play an important part in the program. All individuals should know about their bodies, the importance of sanitation, factors in disease prevention, the importance of exercise, the need for a well-balanced diet, values of good health attitudes and habits, and the community and school agencies that provide health services. This knowledge will contribute greatly to physical prowess as well as to general health. Through the accumulation of a knowledge of these facts, activities will take on a new meaning and health practices will be associated with definite purposes. This will help each individual to live a healthier and more purposeful life.

A store of knowledge will give each individual the proper background for interpreting new situations that confront him from day to day. Unless there is knowledge to draw from, he will become helpless when called upon to make important decisions. As a result of participation in physical education activities, an individual will be better able to make discriminatory judgments, by which knowledge of values is mentally derived. This means that he has greater power for arriving at a wise decision and that he can better discern right from wrong and the logical from the illogical. Through his experience in various games and sports, he has developed a sense of values, an alertness, the ability to diagnose a tense situation, the ability to make a decision quickly under highly emotionalized conditions, and the ability to interpret human actions.

In physical education activities one also gains insight into human nature. The various forms of activity in physical education are social experiences that enable a participant to learn about human nature. For all children and youth this is one of the main sources of such knowledge. Here they discover the individual's responsibility to the group, the need for followership and leadership, the need to experience success, and the feeling of "belonging." Here they learn how human beings react to satisfactions and annoyances. Such knowledge contributes to social efficiency and good human relations.

The human relations objective. The human relations objective is concerned with helping an individual make personal adjustments, group adjustments, and adjustments as a member of society. Activities in the physical education program offer one of the best opportunities for making these adjustments, if there is proper leadership.

Social action is a result of certain hereditary and derivative tendencies. There are interests, hungers, desires, ideals, attitudes, and emotional drives that are responsible for everything we do. A child wants to play because of his drive for physical activity. A man will steal food because of the hunger drive. America is opposed to totalitarian governments because of its desire for personal freedom. The responses to all these desires, drives, hungers, and the like may be either social or antisocial in nature. The value of physical education reveals itself when we realize that play activities are one of the oldest and most fundamental drives in human nature. Therefore, by providing the child with a satisfying experience in activities in which he has a natural desire to engage, the opportunity is presented to develop desirable social traits. The key is qualified leadership.

All human beings should experience success. This factor can be realized through play. Through successful experience in play activities, a child develops self-confidence and finds happiness in his achievements. Physical education can provide for this successful experience by offering a variety of activities and developing the necessary skills for success in these activities.

If children are happy, they will usually make the necessary adjustments. An individual who is happy is much more likely to make the right adjustment than the individual who is morbid, sullen, and unhappy. Happiness reflects friendliness, cheerfulness, and a spirit of cooperation, all of which help a person to be content and to conform to the necessary standards that have been established. Therefore, physical education should instill happiness by guiding children into these activities where this quality will be realized.

In a democratic society all individuals should develop a sense of group consciousness and cooperative living. This should be one of the most important objectives of the physical education program. Whether or not a child will grow up to be a good citizen and contribute to the welfare of society will depend to a great extent upon the training he receives during his youth. Therefore, in various play activities, the following factors should be stressed: aid for the less-skilled and weaker players, respect for the rights of others, subordination of one's desires to the will of the group, and realization that cooperative living is essential to the success of society. In other words, the golden rule should be practiced. The individual should be made to feel that he belongs to the group and that he has the responsibility of directing his actions in its behalf. The rules of sportsmanship should be developed and practiced in all activities that are offered in the program. Courtesy, sympathy, truthfulness, fairness, honesty, respect for authority, and abiding by the rules will help a great deal in the promotion of social efficiency. The necessity for good leadership and followership should also be stressed as important to the interests of society.

The needs and desires that form the basis for people's actions can be controlled

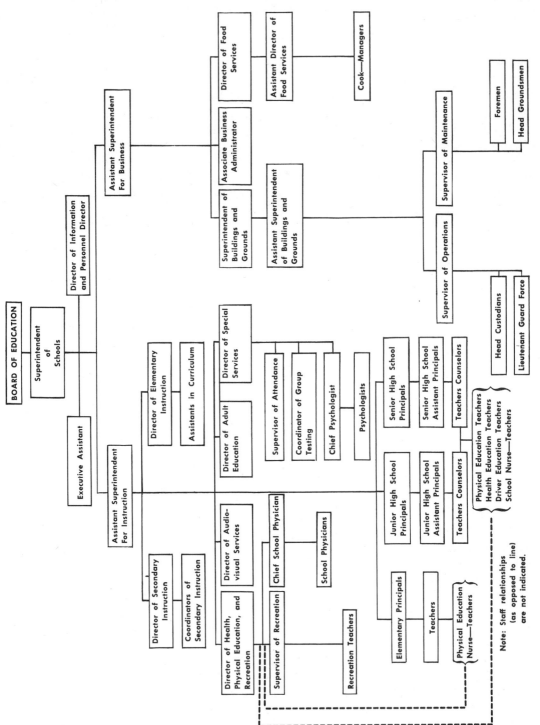

An organization chart for a public school system.

through proper training. This training can result in effective citizenship, which is the basis of sound, democratic living. Effective citizenship is not something that can be developed by artificial stimuli. It is something that is achieved only through activities in which individuals engage in their normal day-to-day routine. Since play activities have such a great attraction for youth, and since it is possible to develop desirable social traits under proper guidance, physical education should realize its responsibility. It should do its part in contributing to good citizenship, the basis of our democratic society. In this chaotic world with its cold wars, hot wars, hydrogen bombs, racial strife, student unrest, imperialistic aims, human ambitions, and class struggles, human relations are more and more important to personal, group, and world peace. Only through a better understanding of one's fellowman will it be possible to build a peaceful and democratic world.

THE ROLE OF ADMINISTRATION IN ACHIEVING OBJECTIVES

Good administration is an essential in the fields of school and college health education and physical education if the goals that have been set for these professions are to be realized. Harmony must be encouraged among the various members of the staff, adequate facilities provided, the program planned and continually reevaluated, a public relations plan established, leadership provided, and many other essentials and details attended to with dispatch if the objectives are to be achieved.

The administrator is a key person; he sets the pace and provides the leadership. If this individual does not assume the responsibilities that go with such a position, there will be apathy and indifference all along the line and consequently the aims for which the professions exist will not be realized. Administrators must continually keep in mind the goals toward which they are working. With these in mind they

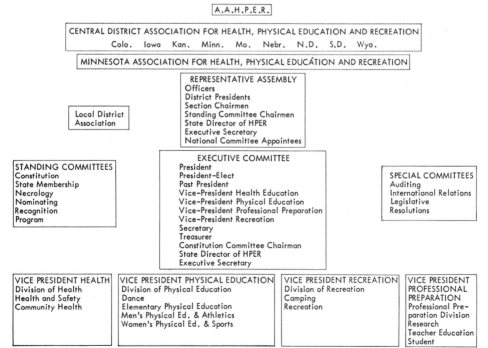

Structure of a state association. (From Minnesota Association for Health, Physical Education, and Recreation News Letter 2:3, 1965.)

should gear their staff relationships, programs, and other factors in a way that will
be most efficient and productive from the
standpoint of realizing such goals.

Administrators frequently have the areas
of both health and physical education
within their administrative division. This
affords the opportunity to promote the kind
of cooperation that is needed to achieve
the aims of each. One cannot be promoted
at the expense of the other. One cannot be
recognized as being more important than
the other. If such is the practice progress
will be obstructed. Administrators must
recognize the important place that each
area has in the total picture. All administrative policies must preserve this balance.

If the administrators have only one of
these specialized areas within their division, this should not limit their relationship
with the other. Both areas are closely allied
and it is very important that they work
closely together. Administrators will determine in large measure whether or not this
becomes a reality.

PROFESSIONAL ORGANIZATIONS

The administrator should be familiar
with the role of professional organizations
in his work. He should realize that these
associations help in the achievement of objectives, promote professional ethics, scholarship, leadership, and high educational
standards.

Some of the organizations with which
the health educator and physical educator
should be familiar are listed below.*

National Education Association
American Association for Health, Physi-
cal Education, and Recreation
National Recreation and Park Association
American Academy of Physical Educa-
tion

American School Health Association
National College Physical Education As-
sociation
National Association of Physical Educa-
tion for College Women
National Junior College Athletic Associa-
tion
American Physical Therapy Association
Society of State Directors of Health,
Physical Education, and Recreation
American Youth Hostels, Inc.
Young Women's Christian Association
Physical Education Society of the Young
Men's Christian Associations of North
America
Boys' Clubs of America
National Collegiate Athletic Association
National Association of Intercollegiate
Athletics
Canadian Physical Education Association
Delta Psi Kappa
Phi Delta Pi
Phi Epsilon Kappa
American College of Sports Medicine

Questions and exercises

1. Survey ten schools or colleges in your area
   to determine the administrative relationship
   of health and physical education.
2. Why is it important for health and physical
   educators to work closely together?
3. Prepare a research paper on the reasons why
   health and physical education were incorporated in the national association.
4. Why are both health education and physical
   education specialists needed in the schools?
5. Define health and physical education.
6. List and discuss the objectives of both
   school and college health and physical
   education.
7. Interview or correspond with five health educators and five physical educators on the main
   problems confronting their professions.
8. To what extent are the objectives of school
   and college health and physical education
   being achieved today?
9. Define the term *school health program*. Discuss the various aspects of the program.
10. Why are health attitudes so important?
11. What are the goals of physical education in
    addition to developing an individual phys-
    ically?

---

*For a detailed discussion of these organizations,
refer to Chapter 22 in Bucher, C. A.: Foundations of physical education, ed. 5, St. Louis, 1968,
The C. V. Mosby Co.

12. What are some of the benefits to an individual that come from physical activity?
13. How can physical education contribute to the development of good citizenship?
14. Why must there be cooperation to achieve the objectives in health and physical education? What part does the administrator play?

Reading assignment in *Administrative Dimensions of Health and Physical Education Programs, Including Athletics:* Chapter 2, Selections 5 to 10.

Selected references

American Association for Health, Physical Education, and Recreation: Health concepts—guides for health instruction, Washington, D. C., 1966, The Association.

American Association for Health, Physical Education, and Recreation: Knowledge and understanding in physical education, Washington, D. C., 1969, The Association.

American Association for Health, Physical Education, and Recreation: Physical education for college men and women, Washington, D. C., 1965, The Association.

Bauer, W. W.: Teach health, not disease, Journal of Health and Physical Education **12:**296, 1941.

Bookwalter, K. W.: Physical education in the secondary schools, New York, 1964, The Center for Applied Research in Education, Inc. (The Library of Education).

Bucher, C. A.: Foundations of physical education, ed. 5, St. Louis, 1968, The C. V. Mosby Co.

Bucher, C. A.: Physical education for life, St. Louis, 1969, McGraw-Hill Book Co. (A textbook for high school courses in physical education.)

Bucher, C. A., and Dupee, R. K., Jr.: Athletics in schools and colleges, New York, 1965, The Center for Applied Research in Education, Inc. (The Library of Education).

Bucher, C. A., Koenig, C., and Barnhard, M.: Methods of materials for secondary school physical education, ed. 3, St. Louis, 1970, The C. V. Mosby Co.

Bucher, C. A., Olsen, E. A., and Willgoose, C. E.: The foundations of health, New York, 1967, Appleton-Century-Crofts.

Bucher, C. A., and Reade, E. M.: Physical education and health in the elementary school, ed. 2, New York, 1971, The Macmillan Co.

Joint Committee of National Education Association and American Medical Association: The physical educator asks about health, Washington, D. C., 1951, American Association for Health, Physical Education, and Recreation.

Joint Committee on Health Problems in Education of National Education Association and American Medical Association: School health services, Washington, D. C., 1964, National Education Association.

Byrd, O. E.: School health administration, Philadelphia, 1964, W. B. Saunders Co.

Grout, R. E.: Health teaching in schools, ed. 4, Philadelphia, 1963, W. B. Saunders Co.

Hillson, M.: Change and innovation in elementary school organization, New York, 1965, Holt, Rinehart & Winston, Inc.

Irwin, L. W., and Mayshark, C.: Health education in secondary schools, St. Louis, 1968, The C. V. Mosby Co.

Joint Committee on Health Problems in Education of National Education Association and American Medical Association: Healthful school living, Washington, D. C., 1969, National Education Association.

Joint Committee on Health Problems in Education of National Education Association and American Medical Association: Health education, Washington, D. C., 1961, National Education Association.

National Committee on School Health Policies of the National Conference for Cooperation in Health Education: Suggested school health policies, ed. 3, Washington, D. C., 1966, National Education Association.

Neff, F. C.: Philosophy and American education, New York, 1966, The Center for Applied Research in Education, Inc. (The Library of Education).

Oberteuffer, D., and Beyrer, M. K.: School health education, ed. 4, New York, 1966, Harper & Row, Publishers.

Smolensky, J., and Bonvechio, L. R.: Principles of school health, Boston, 1966, D. C. Heath & Co.

Van Dalen, D. B.: Health and safety education, New York, 1963, The Center for Applied Research in Education, Inc. (The Library of Education).

Willgoose, C. E.: Health education in the elementary school, ed. 2, Philadelphia, 1964, W. B. Saunders Co.

CHAPTER 3 THE ADMINISTRATIVE SETTING

The administrator, teacher, and leader of physical education and of health education must be cognizant of the roles played by those who administer our educational institutions and the administrative structure of the school, college, and community. Many changes are taking place in the area of educational administration. Since health and physical education programs constitute integral parts of this administrative setting, it is important to understand the changes taking place.

Educational administrators increasingly must have special qualifications and preparation for their duties. School and college administrators need to be well-educated persons who are knowledgeable about the major aspects of managing an educational system or institution. They need to be "idea" men—thinkers with a vision of the future. They should possess a multitude of qualities that enable them to wear the hat of a teacher, architect, speaker, human relations expert, philosopher, and business executive. The administrator should train for his position through an intensive study of the science and theory of administration, and he should also have practical experience as an intern on the job.

ADMINISTRATIVE CHANGES IN SCHOOL ORGANIZATION
School districts

The school administration carries out its duties in a larger school district than was formerly the case, as a result of reorganization, centralization, and consolidation. The number of districts employing only a few teachers is declining rapidly. Enlargement of school districts has been necessary because of (1) the teacher shortage, (2) small district financial problems, and (3) inadequate curricula.

The school district is the basic administrative unit for the operation of local elementary and secondary schools and is a quasimunicipal corporation established by the state. This basic educational unit ranges through the United States from a one-teacher rural system to a large metropolitan system serving thousands of pupils. A system may be an independent governmental unit or part of a state government, county, or other local administrative unit. The governing body of the system is the school board. The chief administrative officer is the superintendent of schools. The number of basic administrative units reported in 1931 and 1932 was 127,531. Today, there are approximately 30,000 administrative units.

State and federal control

Traditionally, local communities have exercised almost complete control over local education, and the state has not interfered with local operations of school programs. Today, however, local communities have transferred some of their influence over education to state and federal governmental units. The control has advanced proportionately as the amount of state and federal financial aid to schools has increased. If school systems do not have quality educational programs as outlined by the state, fail to follow state and federal laws in such matters as civil rights, or fail to meet certain stipulations as attached to the use of

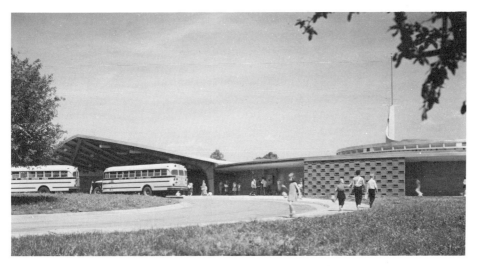

Shaver & Company, Salina, Kan.

The administrative setting for health and physical education programs. (Valley Winds Elementary School, St. Louis, Mo.)

governmental funds, such financial help can be withheld. This threat of withholding monies is proving to be a strong means of bringing local school districts into line with what is desired by state and federal authorities.

Patterns of school organization

The pattern of school organization at the elementary and secondary levels is in a period of transition. Some of the present patterns of school organization are as follows:

1. The traditional high school or 8-4 system— Under this type of organization the 4-year high school is preceded by the 8-year elementary school.
2. The combined junior and senior high school or 6-6 or 7-5 plan—Under this type of organization the junior and senior high schools are combined under one principal.
3. The emphasis upon junior high school or 6-3-3 system—Under this plan the junior high schools are grouped separately under one principal. Although the junior high school usually includes grades seven through nine, there are exceptions to this type of organization.
4. The 4-year high school or 6-2-4 system— Under this plan the 4-year high school is

similar to the traditional high school in organization, and the junior high school consists of two grades.
5. The middle school or 4-4-4 plan—This type of organization is a new development that retains the old high school idea but usually groups the early elementary grades together and the fifth to eighth (or other) grades in one unit.

There are many arguments that can be set forth for each plan of school organization or such other plans as the 6-3-3-2 or the 8-4-2, which includes 2 years of community college. The physical, psychologic, and sociologic aspects of the school setting and of child growth and development, the need for effective communication between schools, the range of subjects, the facilities provided, and the preparation of teachers are all pertinent to the type of administrative organization selected.

SCHOOL AND COLLEGE STRUCTURE

In this section the roles of the board of trustees, board of education, president of a college, superintendent of schools, principal and other administrative personnel, and lay groups will be discussed, as well as

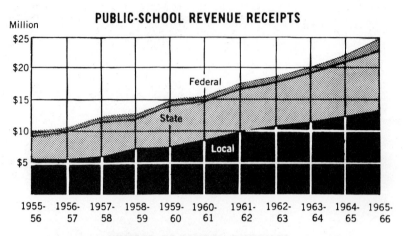

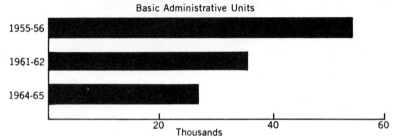

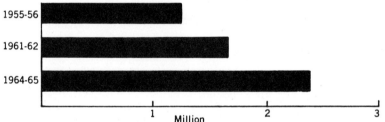

Changes taking place in public school systems in the United States. (From NEA Research Bulletin 44:23, 1966.)

the place of physical education and health education within the educational framework. Much of this information applies directly to the school structure where most health education and physical education personnel are employed.

The college and university structure is analogous in some ways to the structure of the school system. For example, many of the administrative functions of a board of trustees of a college are similar in scope to those of a board of education, and the pres-

ident of a college has duties similar in some respects to a superintendent of schools. The director of physical education or the director of health education needs to perform many of the same duties in a college as the director does in a school system. A brief discussion of the college and university structure is included here to show the aspects of the structure that are especially unique to higher education.

A college or university is characterized by a governing board, usually known as a

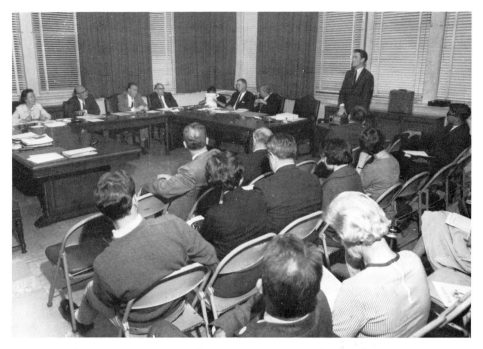

School board meeting. (Mamaroneck, N. Y.)

board of trustees, which is granted extensive powers of control by legislative enactment or by its charter. The governing board of a college usually delegates many of its powers to the administration and faculty of the institution. The administrative officers, usually headed by a president, are commonly organized into such principal areas of administration as academic, student personnel services, business, and public relations. The members of the faculty are usually organized into colleges, schools, divisions, and departments of instruction and research. In large institutions one frequently finds a university senate that is the voice of the faculty and that serves as a liaison between faculty and administration. Health and physical education can have school, division, or department status. The duties of a dean, director, or chairman correspond in many ways to those of a director of health education and/or physical education in a school system.

Board of education, school committee, or board of directors*

The board of education is the legal administrative authority created by the state legislature for each school district. The responsibility of the board is to act on behalf of the residents of the district it represents. It has the duty of appraising and planning the educational program on a local basis. It selects executive personnel and performs duties essential to the successful operation of the schools within the district. The board develops policies that are legal and in the interest of the people it serves. It devises financial means within the legal framework to support the cost of the educational plan. It keeps its constituents informed of the effectiveness and needs of the total program.

Some of the more specific powers of boards of education include purchasing

*The term *board of education* is used in this discussion although *school committee* and *board of directors* are used in some sections of the country.

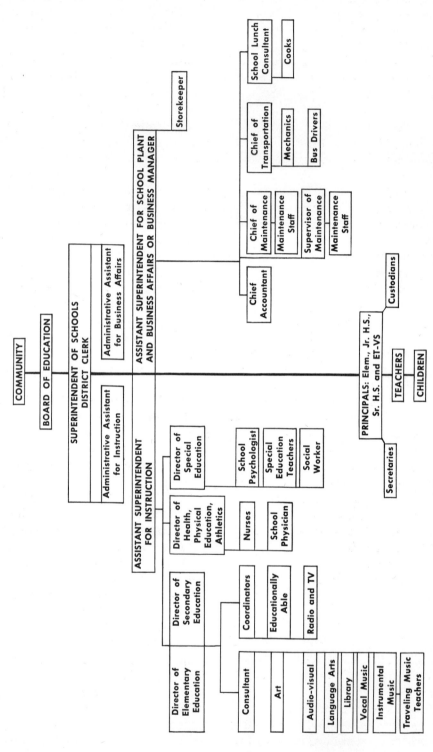

The operational organization chart clarifies channels of communication for the employees of the school district. The superintendent administers school district policies through the assistant superintendents, and they in turn utilize intermediate staff members in the process.

property, planning school buildings, determining the educational program, securing personnel, levying taxes for school purposes, approving courses of study, determining the school calendar, and providing for the school census. The powers of boards of education are fixed by state statutory enactment.

The qualifications for board members are very few. There are usually general requirements that specify citizenship, age, residence, and sometimes ownership of property. In many communities women as well as men are playing very prominent roles. According to surveys that have been conducted, boards of education usually include individuals who are past middle age, have been successful in their community, and are conservative in nature. There has been an improvement in recent years in the organization and composition of boards of education. The addition of women and individuals who are nonpartisan in their outlook, the organization of smaller and less cumbersome boards, and provisions for longer terms of office are resulting in a more stable educational policy.

Boards of education vary in size. There is the usual three-member board in the common-school district that represents the independent one- or two-room school setup. Township boards of education range from five to nine members, county boards from three to fifteen, and city boards from three to sixteen. The trend is toward small boards of education.

Board of education members are appointed in some cases, and in others they are elected.

The National School Boards Association has indicated the following characteristics of school boards in forty-two cities throughout the nation having more than 300,000 population.

Most school boards have seven, five, or nine members, in that order. Three cities have boards with fifteen members. The composition of school board members (3%

women and 13% Negroes) is broken down as follows: businessmen, 103; lawyers, 66; housewives, 51; physicians, 22; ministers, 11; and college professors, 8.

Most of the 137,000 members of the nation's 25,000 school boards are elected. Among the large cities, only Philadelphia, Pittsburgh, and Washington, D.C., choose boards through a committee of court judges. In Boston, Detroit, Los Angeles, and St. Louis, school boards are elected.

There is a growing feeling among professional and lay leaders alike for the need of reform in respect to school board operations. Reforms have been advocated by such an important group as the New York Committee on Educational Leadership and are receiving support in some of the more progressive sections of the country. These reforms include (1) the transfer of all administrative functions that encumber school board operations to the superintendent of schools, (2) better procedures for screening school board members so that the "office seeks the man rather than the man seeks the office," (3) elimination of the annual public vote on the school budget where required and substituting budget hearings in its place, and (4) improved procedures for selecting superintendents of schools.

General administrative personnel

The administrative personnel that will be discussed include the superintendent of schools, assistant superintendent, clerk of the board, principal, supervisor, director, and lay groups.

Superintendent of schools. Within a large school system where many schools are involved there is a superintendent who has overall charge of the school program. Associate or assistant superintendents are in charge of technical detail, management, or various phases of the program, such as secondary education. There is also a superintendent's position associated with smaller schools. These officers are known as district superintendents. They are responsible for many schools extending over a wide geographic area.

The superintendent's job is to carry out the educational policies of the state and the board of education. He acts as the leader in educational matters in the community. He also provides the board of education with the professional advice it needs as a lay organization. From an executive standpoint, he appraises the entire educational program over which he has control, working closely with the board of education to eliminate weaknesses and to establish a strong system of education. Any large organization needs leadership; so too does the educational system of any community.

The qualifications for the position of superintendent vary in different communities. In some villages and cities the individual must be a resident and in others this is not necessary. The educational requirement varies a great deal. Some communities require a doctorate and others require a minimum of professional training. There is a trend, however, in the direction of increased training. Most superintendents of schools have their bachelor and master's degrees and an increasing number have taken work beyond the master's. Many have their doctorates. Both teaching and administrative experience are frequently listed as requirements.

Assistant superintendent for business services or school business administrator. The business administrator serves as director of business affairs and of buildings and grounds. In a college or university there is also one administrative officer who carries out similar duties. The business administrator usually has direct supervision of the business office staff, the building service and maintenance staff, and general supervision of the custodial staff. He has responsibility for supervising the operation and maintenance of all buildings and grounds. He may perform the duties of the superintendent as directed in the superintendent's absence. (Chapter 4 is devoted to a de-

tailed discussion of the school business administrator.)

Assistant superintendent or director of instructional services. The director of instruction has under his direct supervision the divisions of elementary education, secondary education, adult education, health and physical education, music education, vocational and practical arts, summer school education, and inservice training of teachers. He gives major consideration to the development of curriculum materials, to organization, and to the supervision of instruction and teaching. He may perform the duties of the superintendent of schools as directed in the superintendent's absence. In a college or university the administrative officer in charge of the academic program could be a vice-president, dean, provost, or other officer.

Assistant superintendent or director of personnel services. The director of personnel supervises both professional and nonprofessional employees. He recruits and interviews candidates for positions. He is usually responsible for all pupil personnel services, guidance and psychologic services, handicapped children and special services, as well as attendance and adjustment, including pupil accounting. He may supervise and coordinate the medical services, including medical, dental, and nurse-teacher services. He may coordinate and direct the publications and information services and carry on testing and research activities. He may perform the duties of the superintendent as directed in the superintendent's absence. In a college or university many of these responsibilities are carried out by a dean of men or a dean of women.

Clerk of the board. The clerk of the board of education is usually under the direction of the superintendent of schools. He has custody of the seal of the board, notifies members of the board of regular and special meetings, and has charge of files and records of the board. He sees that all files and records are properly maintained, presents a periodic financial statement, and supervises accounting for tuition pupils. He preaudits and certifies all bills, examines and certifies all payrolls, and keeps an active insurance register. He usually conducts the annual school election and keeps the bond and coupon register of the board and public library, together with necessary reports of bonds and interest due.

Principal. The position of principal is very similar to that of the superintendent. It differs mainly in respect to the extent or scope of responsibility. Whereas the superintendent is usually in charge of all the schools within a particular community, the principal is in charge of one particular school. The duties of the principal include responsibility for executing educational policy as outlined by the superintendent, appraising the educational offering, making periodic reports on various aspects of the program, directing the instructional program, promoting good relationships between the community and the school, and supervising the maintenance of the physical plant.

In many school situations, principals teach in addition to their administrative responsibilities. Some conduct extracurricular activities such as leading the band or coaching a varsity athletic team. Some principals have responsibilities on only one school level, but where various levels are combined in one structural unit, this responsibility may extend from the high school level down through the junior high school and even to the elementary school.

The qualifications for the position of principal vary. There is in evidence a trend toward increased training for such positions. Some communities feel that the principal should have more training than the teachers.

Boards of education must select school administrators from the individuals available. The prestige, money, security, and other factors that the position offers play an important part in determining the quality of individual that can be secured.

Supervisor. This position usually implies a responsibility associated with the improvement of instruction. In some cases the assignment might be much broader in scope and in corporate responsibility for the entire elementary or secondary instructional program. In most cases, however, it usually applies to specific subject matter areas.

Director. The role of the director involves responsibility for functions of specific subject matter area or a particular educational level. The responsibilities have administrative as well as supervisory implications.

Director of health, physical education, and recreation. A common position to be found in educational systems is that of director of health, physical education, and recreation. One state, for example, grants a special certificate for a director of health, physical education, and recreation after a stated program of studies has been accomplished, a stated amount of experience has been had, and other requirements met. Other communities and states have directors of health and physical education. Some have directors of physical education, directors of health, and directors of recreation where the fields of specialization are completely separated.

In a college or university there may be a director who heads up the entire physical education program and a director in charge of the health program, or the two fields may be combined into the same administrative unit, whether it be a college, school, division, or department.

A director's position exists to provide leadership, program, facilities, and other essentials in these special areas. Specific areas of responsibility for a director of health, physical education, and recreation in general include the following:

General duties
1. Implement standards established by the state Department of Education and the

local board of education. (In a college it would be the university administration.)

2. Interview possible candidates for positions in the special areas and make recommendations for these positions.

3. Work closely with the assistant superintendent in charge of business affairs, assistant superintendent in charge of instruction, and subject matter and classroom teachers.

4. Coordinate areas of health, physical education, and recreation.

5. Supervise all inside and outside facilities, equipment, and supplies concerned with special areas—this responsibility includes maintenance, safety, and replacement operations.

6. Maintain liaison with community groups—this responsibility includes such duties as holding educational meetings with doctors and dentists to interpret and improve the school health program, scheduling school facilities for community groups, and serving on various community committees for youth needs.

7. Prepare periodic reports regarding areas of activity.

8. Coordinate school civil defense activities in some school systems.

9. Serve on the school health council.

Health

1. Health services—in some cases includes the supervision of school nurse teachers and dental hygiene teachers and coordination of the work of school physicians. Other responsibilities include preparation of guides and policies for the program of health services, organization of health projects, and obtaining proper equipment and supplies.

2. Health science instruction—includes supervision of health education programs throughout the school system, preparation of curriculum guides and research studies, and upgrading the program in general.

3. Healthful school living—includes general supervision of school plant, psychologic aspects of school program, and formation of recommendations for improvement.

Physical education

1. Supervise total physical education program (class, adapted, intramurals, extramurals, and varsity interscholastic or intercollegiate athletics).

2. Administer schedules, practice and game facilities, insurance, and equipment.

3. Maintain liaison with county, district, and state professional groups.

4. Upgrade program in general.

Recreation

1. Supervise various aspects of the recreation program that, in addition to school program, may include summer and vacation playgrounds, teen centers, and so on.

2. Obtain, where necessary, facilities, equipment, personnel, and supplies.

3. Plan and administer program.

Lay groups

The general public is participating more and more in the work of schools and colleges. Parent-teacher associations, citizens' councils, alumni groups, and study groups are a few of the organizations that express the lay opinion of the community in regard to educational matters. This interest on the part of the public should be encouraged and helped in every way possible. There are more than 10 million members of parent-teacher associations alone throughout the country. The public school program should reflect what the public wants and thinks is best for their children. This can be accomplished only through active "lay" participation. Administrators and other school personnel should make sure that the citizens of the community are adequately informed in respect to educational matters so that the best type of program may be developed.

HEALTH WITHIN THE SCHOOL AND COLLEGE STRUCTURE*

The superintendent and principal or president and dean have the main responsibility for school and college health programs. The attitude they have toward health and the degree to which they recognize the importance of achieving professional objectives will determine the success of the school health program.

Administrators must recognize certain important principles in regard to health so that it may have an important place in the total school and college program. The following are basic concepts: Health should

---

*See also Chapters 12, 13, and 14.

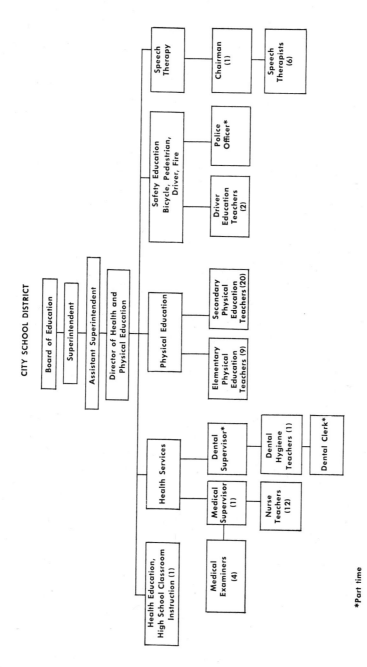

CITY SCHOOL DISTRICT

*Part time

The director of health and physical education in the school structure. (From Bucher, C. A., Koenig, C. R., and Barnhard, M.: Methods and materials for secondary school physical education, ed. 3, St. Louis, 1970, The C. V. Mosby Co.)

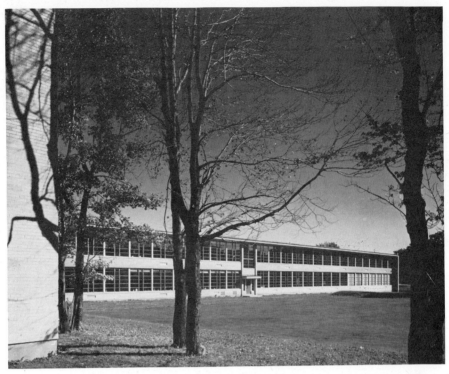

Superintendents and principals have important responsibilities for promoting health within the school. (Chandler Street Junior High School, Worcester, Mass.)

be an important and integral part of the overall educational program. All teachers and other personnel should understand and appreciate the importance of promoting health and the contributions they can make through their own work toward realizing such a goal. There should be individuals on the staff who have had special training in this field so that they may take the leadership in developing and promoting an adequate program. There should be coordination of the various instructional aspects of the educational program to ensure adequate coverage of health information and to avoid unnecessary overlapping. There should be provision for concentrated health teaching. Adequate facilities, time, money, and personnel should be provided to carry on this special work properly. A close working arrangement with the community should be recognized as an essential to a well-developed program. There should

be a statement of policies in regard to health that is clear and understood by all.

Terminology for the school and college health program. The following definitions were drawn up by the Committee on Terminology that represented the American Association for Health, Physical Education, and Recreation, the Society of Public Health Educators, and the American Public Health Association. It is presented here for the reader's information.[*]

Dental examination—The appraisal, performed by a dentist, of the condition of the oral structures to determine the dental health status of the individual.

Dental inspection—The limited appraisal, performed by anyone with or without special dental preparation, of the oral structures to determine the presence or absence of obvious defects.

[*]Report of the Joint Committee on Health Education Terminology, Journal of Health, Physical Education, and Recreation 33:27, 1962.

Health appraisal—The evaluation of the health status of the individual through the utilization of varied organized and systematic procedures such as medical and dental examinations, laboratory test, health history, teacher observation, etc.

Health observation—The estimation of an individual's well-being by noting the nature of his appearance and behavior.

Medical examination—The determination, by a physician, of an individual's health status.

Screening test—A medically and educationally acceptable procedure for identifying individuals who need to be referred for further study or diagnostic examination.

Cumulative school health record—A form used to note pertinent consecutive information about a student's health.

School health program—The composite of procedures used in school health services, healthful school living, and health science instruction to promote health among students and school personnel.

Healthful school living—The utilization of a safe and wholesome environment, consideration of individual health, organizing the school day, and planning classroom procedures to favorably influence emotional, social, and physical health.*

Health school environment—The physical, social, and emotional factors of the school setting which affect the health, comfort, and performance of an individual or a group.*

Health science instruction—The organized teaching procedures directed toward developing understandings, attitudes, and practices relating to health and factors affecting health.

School health services—The procedures used by physicians, dentists, nurses, teachers, etc. designed to appraise, protect, and promote optimum health of students and school personnel. (Activities frequently included in school health services are those used to (1) appraise the health status of students and school personnel; (2) counsel students, teachers, parents, and others for the purpose of helping school-age children get treatment or for arranging education programs in keeping with their abilities; (3) help prevent or control the spread of disease; (4) provide emergency care for injury or sudden sickness.)

School health education—The process of providing or utilizing experiences for favorably influencing understandings, attitudes, and practices relating to individual, family, and community health.

Safety education—The process of providing or utilizing experiences for favorably influencing understandings, attitudes, and practices relating to safe living.

Health counseling—A method of interpreting to students or their parents the findings of health appraisals and encouraging and assisting them to take such action as needed to realize their fullest potential.

School health coordination—A process designed to bring about a harmonious working relationship among the various personnel and groups in the school and community that have interest, concern, and responsibility for development and conduct of the school health program.

Essential aspects of the school and college health program. Health within the educational structure will be discussed under three headings: health science instruction, health services, and healthful school and college living.

*Health science instruction.** In the area of health science instruction, scientific knowledge is imparted and experiences are provided so that students may better understand the importance of developing good attitudes and health practices. Information concerning such subjects as nutrition, communicable disease, rest, exercise, sanitation, drugs, alcohol, tobacco, environmental pollution, human sexuality, first aid, and safety is presented.

On the elementary level the responsibility for such health education rests primarily on the shoulders of the classroom teacher, although in some school systems trained specialists are provided as resource persons. On the secondary and college levels, it is recommended that individuals who have had special training in health education be responsible for concentrated health instruction. This is not always the case. Sometimes, in the absence of a trained specialist, the teacher of physical education, home economics, or science or some other teacher is given the responsibility. This procedure, however, is not always desirable

---

*See also Chapter 14.

*See also Chapter 12.

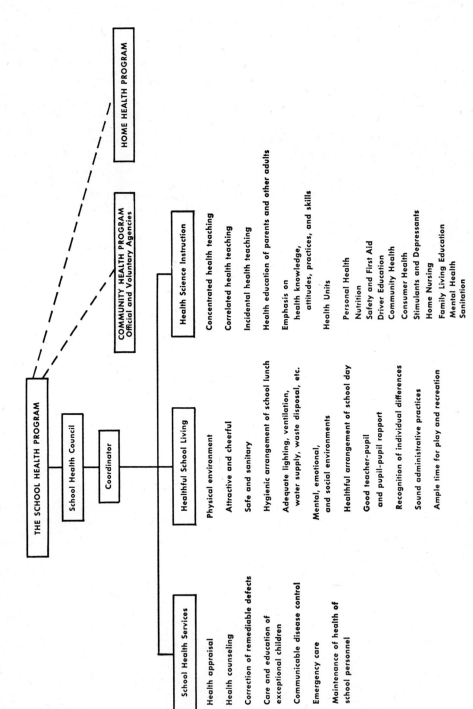

Suggested health education for the schools of the United States. (From Bucher, C. A.: Foundations of physical education, ed. 5. St. Louis, 1968, The C. V. Mosby Co.)

because of the lack of necessary qualifications by persons other than a specialist.

A concentrated course in health education should be required of all students for at least 1 and preferably 2 years at the secondary level. Some states are now requiring health in every grade. At the college level there should be at least a one-semester health course for all students. Health educators should teach such courses, and these subjects should be given the same credit and time allotments as other important ones in the curriculum. Again, this recommendation is not followed in many schools and colleges because of the lack of trained personnel, the fact that other subjects are given a priority listing, and the lack of an appreciation on the part of school and college administrators of the importance of health education. Some schools incorporate health education in the physical education class. When this is the case, it quite often becomes a "rainy day" proposition. Some feel that it is adequately cared for in other subjects, such as science and home economics. Correlating health instruction in various subject matter areas is to be encouraged. However, this in itself is not sufficient.

The emphasis in health education at the primary grade level should be on how to live healthfully, at the intermediate grade level on *why* certain types of health practices are important, and at the secondary level on personal and community health. It should be reiterated that although there is a place for concentrated teaching at the secondary and college levels, at the same time it is important for all subject matter areas to also recognize their possibilities and responsibilities for teaching health.

The possibilities for health education should also be recognized in the various experiences the child has in school. When the school physician gives the medical examination, the dental hygienist examines the child's teeth, an emergency concerned with health exists in the community, or the curiosity of the child is aroused, "teachable moments" for imparting health information are presented. This type of health education often leaves a greater impression upon young minds than the more formal classroom type.

*Health services.** The health services phase of school and college health programs includes health appraisal, health counseling, correction of defects, provision for the exceptional child, prevention and control of communicable disease, and emergency care of injuries.

In this phase of the health program it is important to recognize concern for mental, emotional, social, and physical health. In providing health services that include all these phases of health, several persons in addition to the health educator play prominent parts.

The classroom teacher has an important responsibility in health services. He or she is probably closer to the child than any other person on the staff and therefore can detect deviations from the normal. The teacher also is in a position to give good advice, provide first aid when necessary, administer certain screening tests, and oversee the general welfare of the child.

The nurse plays a prominent role in the administration of the health program. Through counseling, acting as a resource person for other staff members, developing close relationships with parents, helping physicians, and other responsibilities peculiar to her profession, the nurse is a key person.

The physician has the potential for playing a very important part in school and college programs. Through medical examinations, health guidance, protection of students from communicable diseases, development of health policies, and consultations with parents, it is possible for the physician to exercise a great force for good in the health of the students and parents

---

*See also Chapter 13.

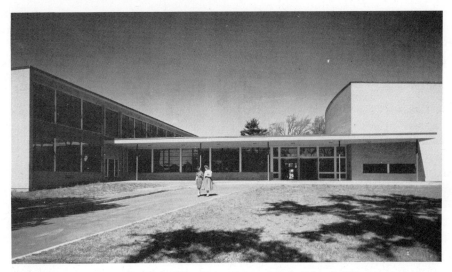

Healthful school living. (Chandler Street Junior High School, Worcester, Mass.)

with whom he comes in contact. It has been the observation of many educators, however, that the physician often does not realize the educational implications of his role in the health program. As a result, he does not take advantage of "teachable moments" that occur whenever a student is being given a medical examination or when conferences are held with parents.

Dentists and dental hygienists play an important role wherever their services are provided. These specialists appraise the dental needs of students. Here again there is an unlimited opportunity to educate the student and the parent on the importance of proper oral hygiene.

Psychologists, psychiatrists, social workers, guidance counselors, speech correctionists, and others are increasingly being brought into school and college health services programs. All have an important part to play and contribution to make to the total health of young people who attend schools and colleges in this country.

Healthful school and college living.* Healthful living is also an important part of the total health program. In addition to a healthful physical environment, a wholesome emotional environment must also be provided. Both are important to the health of the student.

The physical environment should provide an attractive, safe, and wholesome place for students to congregate. This implies that such important considerations as lighting, ventilation, heating, location, sanitary facilities, play space, equipment, and other essentials are adequately provided for in the buildings and areas that are used for educational purposes. It also means there is proper maintenance by the custodial staff and includes any other factors that influence the physical arrangements of the school or college plant.

The emotional environment is just as important to the student's health as the physical one. To ensure a wholesome emotional environment, proper rapport must exist between the teacher and pupils and among the pupils themselves; educational practices pertinent to such matters as grades, promotions, assignments, schedules, play periods, attendance, class conduct, and discipline must be sound; and the teachers themselves must be well adjusted.

---

*See also Chapter 14.

Other phases of health administration.
There are two other aspects of the health
program that need special attention—the
health council and the health coordinator.

The health council. Every school and
every school system should have health
councils or committees to help ensure a desirable and adequate health program. This
means that there should be a health council for each school and one central health
council for all the schools in a particular
school system. The number of members
comprising such councils may vary from
three or four persons in a small school to
fifteen or sixteen in a larger school. Potential members of such councils are the school
principal, health coordinator, nurse, psychologist, guidance person, custodian, dental hygienist, physician, dentist, physical
education teacher, science teacher, home
economics teacher, classroom teacher,
teacher of handicapped persons, nutritionist, students, parents, public health officer,
mayor, clergymen, and any other individual who is particularly related to the
health of the school or community and has
something to contribute.

Health councils are responsible for coordinating the entire health program of the
school. This would include determining
subject matter to be taught, resources to be
utilized, and experiences to be provided;
securing a healthful environment in which
to live; arranging inservice training for
teaching personnel; encouraging closer
school-parent relationships in respect to
such important health procedures as medical examinations; promoting sanitary conditions; providing for the safety of children;
and distributing health literature.

Representatives from various community
and school groups that are interested in
health can accomplish much when sitting
around a conference table discussing their
problems. A spirit of cooperation and "oneness" will aid in developing procedures and
taking action that will promote better
health for all.

Health coordinator. Health affects many
subject matter areas, the school plant,
educational practices, and practically every
aspect of school life. It is important therefore to have coordination. This means that
responsibility must be fixed in one person.
By having someone responsible it is possible to integrate health into the total education program and the total community
health program.

As a result of the need for coordination of the various phases of health, many
schools have appointed health coordinators. In some places this individual is
known by another title such as health consultant or health educator. This person, in
most cases, is appointed by the administration and has particular qualifications for
the job.

The responsibilities of the health coordinator include such duties as integrating and
correlating the various phases of health education in the subject matter areas, chan-
neling health information to staff members,
keeping records, preparing reports periodically on pertinent health matters, providing
leadership for health councils, seeing that
established health policies are carried out,
appraising and evaluating the total health
program, arranging special health examinations when needed, counseling students on
health problems, aiding the physician in
the performance of his duties, helping in
the maintenance of a healthful environment, organizing safety and other programs
that promote health, and helping in furthering school-home relationships.

PHYSICAL EDUCATION WITHIN THE SCHOOL AND COLLEGE STRUCTURE

Physical education is increasingly occupying a more important role in the school
and college offering. During its early history, physical education was regarded by
general school administrators as a fad, an
appendage to the educational program, or
a necessary evil to be tolerated. In recent

years, however, it has been viewed by an increasing number of educators as an integral part of the total educational offering with many potentialities for contributing to enriched living.

Terminology in physical education. Components of the physical education program are characterized by many and varied terms. Since there has been no committee established to work out descriptive terms for the various phases of the program, as in the case of the health program, there is lack of uniformity within the profession. I would like to suggest that the four components of the physical education program, into which it logically divides itself, be called (1) the required class or basic instruction program, (2) the adapted pro-

gram, (3) the intramural and extramural athletics program, and (4) the varsity interschool or intercollegiate athletics program.

The *required class* or *basic instruction program* is the provision of physical education for all students and is characterized by instruction in such matters as the rules, strategies, and skills of the various activities that comprise the program.

The *adapted program* refers to that phase of physical education that meets the needs of the individual who, because of some physical inadequacy, functional defect capable of being improved through exercise, or other deficiency, is temporarily or permanently unable to take part in the regular physical education program.

SCHOOL AND COLLEGE PHYSICAL EDUCATION PROGRAM			
Chairman of Department			
The Basic Instructional Class Program	**Adapted Program**	**Intramural and Extramural Athletics Program**	**Varsity Interscholastic or Intercollegiate Athletics Program**
Instructional in nature	For special students including those with:	Competitive leagues and tournaments, play and sports days, etc.	For skilled students
Required of all students	Faulty body mechanics	Voluntary in nature	Voluntary in nature
Daily period	Nutritional disturbances (over- and underweight)	For all students	Conducted during out-of-school hours
Credit given	Heart and lung disturbances	Conducted during out-of-class hours	Organized and administered with needs of participant in mind
Variety of activities	Postoperative and convalescent cases	Laboratory period for required class program	Rec.: For high school and college students only
Team games	Hernias, weak and flat feet, menstrual disorders, etc.	Wide variety of activities based on needs and interests of students	Wide variety of activities based on needs and interests of students
Dual and individual games	Nervous instability	Rec.: Intramural athletics— fourth grade through college	
Rhythms and dances	Poor physical fitness	Rec.: Extramural athletics— seventh grade through college	
Games of low organization	Crippling conditions (infantile paralysis, etc.)		
Gymnastics	Provision for physical, mental, emotional, and social welfare of student		
Aquatics	Provision for program during regular class and special classes		
	Restricted and remedial physical activity		
	Utilization of special conditioning exercises, aquatics, and recreational sports		
	Harmonious working relationships with medical and nursing personnel		

The *intramural and extramural athletics program* is voluntary physical education for all students within one or a few schools or colleges. It is characterized by such events as competitive leagues and tournaments and play and sports days and acts as a laboratory period for the required class program. In the intramural program activities are conducted for students of only one school or college, while in the extramural program students from more than one school or college participate.

The *varsity interschool or intercollegiate athletics program* is designed for the skilled individuals in one school or college who compete with skilled individuals from another school or college in selected physical education activities.

Organization. The various departments of physical education throughout the country have many different plans of organization. A few years ago it was quite common to see such titles as Department of Physical Culture or Hygiene. The term *physical training* was also used as a descriptive term for the work performed in this special area.

Today, one also sees a variety of titles associated with physical education work. In some schools and colleges it is the "physical education department," in others the "health and physical education department," and in others it is the "health, physical education, and recreation division." Camping and safety may also be included.

The titles that are given also show to some degree the particular work that is performed within these phases of the total program. In some schools and colleges physical education is organized into a separate unit with the various physical activities, intramural, extramural, and interschool or intercollegiate athletics—comprising this division. In other schools and colleges, health and physical education are combined in one administrative unit. In some cases, although the word *health* is used, there is little evidence of the particular specialized type of health work as it is known

today. This is also true where the word *recreation* is used in the title. In the discussion to follow, the term *physical education* will be used.

There is usually a person designated as head or chairman of the physical education department. The title of director of physical education is also used. In smaller schools, it is quite common to have only one man and one woman on the physical education staff, each acting as the head of his or her separate division.

The duties of the head of a physical education department include coordinating the activities within his particular administrative unit, requisitioning supplies and equipment, preparing schedules, making budgets, holding departmental meetings, teaching classes, coaching, hiring and dismissing personnel, developing community relations, supervising the intramural, extramural, and interscholastic programs, evaluating and appraising the required class program, representing the department at meetings, reporting to the principal, and having overall general responsibility for the activities carried on.

The required class or basic instruction program.[*] The required class or basic instruction program refers to the instructional program. In some states this phase of the program is required by state law, and in others it is governed by a local regulation. In a few schools and colleges participation is not required but voluntary. Classes are scheduled in much the same way as other subjects. Students, however, are too often assigned on the basis of administrative convenience rather than homogeneously. Physical education people have advocated assigning students to classes in a way that would result in their realizing the greatest physical, social, and other benefits pertinent to this field of work. However, too few schools and colleges have followed these recommenda-

---

[*]See also Chapter 7.

tions. The emphasis in the class program is instructional and various games and activities are offered at different levels in the school program. On the elementary level, rhythmic activities and simple games are stressed, whereas on the secondary level there is a change to more highly organized games and sports.

A survey of the country will show many inferior programs of physical education if they are compared to the standards that have been set for the profession. In many communities the required class program, although serving the entire student body, is hampered by lack of time, facilities, and leadership. Stress on varsity sports and lack of administrative support have also been influential factors. The leadership that is found in many physical education programs is not resourceful, dynamic, and capable of promoting a sound program.

Where excellent required class or basic instruction programs of physical education exist, they have been developed on the basis of the physical, social, mental, and emotional needs of the students. A broad and varied program of activities, both outdoor and indoor, progressively arranged and adapted to the capacities and abilities of each student, is offered.

The adapted program.* One of the weakest phases of modern physical education programs is the lack of an effective adapted program at all educational levels. Since pupils should be required to take physical education each day they are in school, regardless of their physical condition or how they feel, the program must be adapted to their needs. The boy or girl should not be made to fit the physical education program. Instead, the physical education program should fit the individual. The child with a rheumatic fever history, the boy who has just returned from having an operation to remove his appendix, the girl who suffers menstrual difficul-

ties, mentally retarded and culturally disadvantaged students, and pupils with other health problems can all receive benefits from the physical education program, provided it is geared to their individual differences. To ensure the cooperation of parents, administrators, and others and to work out the best possible program, there should be a close working relationship between the nursing, medical, and other health professions. This procedure will also help to ensure that the prescription recommended properly fits the student's needs. Another consideration that cannot be overlooked is having qualified teachers assigned to the adapted program. The effectiveness of such a program will depend to a great extent upon the type of leadership that is provided.

The intramural and extramural athletics program.* The goal of the intramural and extramural program is to provide competition in games, sports, and other physical activities for the rank and file of the student body. This program is in addition to the required class or basic instruction program. Whereas the required class or basic instruction program is designed to be largely instructional in nature so that basic fundamentals for playing various activities can be learned, the intramural and extramural program is designed to provide an opportunity for students to utilize these learned skills in actual competitive situations.

There is a place in the intramural and extramural program for all students, regardless of degree of skill, strength, age, or field of specialization. It offers an opportunity for friendly competition between groups from the same school or college. Sometimes "sports" and "play" days are also included. These special events involve students from one or many schools who are invited to participate. Teams are composed of students from the same school

---

*See also Chapter 8.

*See also Chapter 9.

and college and from many different schools and colleges.

As many as 90% or 95% of the students participate in the intramural and extramural programs where there is an active interest. Since these programs are conducted on a voluntary basis, this indicates the amount of enthusiasm and interest that can be generated through a well-organized program. High attendance in such a program usually reflects a broad offering of activities, with leagues or some other unit of competition, organized in a manner that appeals to the interest and needs of the students.

In small schools and colleges, intramural and extramural programs are usually conducted by one or two persons who are also in charge of the required class or basic instruction program. This places an additional load on such individuals and consequently some fail to develop the type of program that could be offered if more personnel were available. In larger schools and colleges it is quite common to have a director of intramural athletics. This places the responsibility on one person and usually results in a better-organized and more effective program.

Close coordination should exist between the required class and intramural and extramural programs. Furthermore, department members, student managers, and interested faculty members should be encouraged to help in the conduct of the program. For the best administration of intramural and extramural programs, most schools also give careful consideration to units of competition; a program of fall, winter, and spring activities; eligibility requirements; provisions for medical examination; preliminary training periods; scheduling; variation in types of tournaments; coaching; and awards.

The varsity interschool and intercollegiate athletics program.* The varsity in-

---

*See also Chapter 10.

ter-school program in athletics is designed for the individuals most highly skilled in sports. It is one of the most interesting and receives more publicity than the other two phases of physical education in the school setup. The reason for this is not that it is more important or renders a greater contribution; instead, it is largely the result of its popular appeal. The fact that sports writers and others discuss it in glowing terms and that it involves competition that pits one school or college against another school or college also increases its public appeal. A spirit of rivalry develops. This seems to be characteristic of the American culture.

The varsity interschool and intercollegiate athletics program has probably had more difficulties attached to it than any of the other phases of the program. The desire to win and to increase gate receipts has resulted in evil practices. Large stadia and sports palaces have been constructed that require large financial outlays for their upkeep.

For many years there has been much controversy over whether or not girls should engage in interscholastic and intercollegiate sports. Some advocate such activities for the girls because they feel they should also be offered the advantages that accrue to boys. On the other hand, others feel that physiologic and social implications indicate that girls should not participate in such activities. As a result of this controversy, some schools and colleges do not have interscholastic and intercollegiate competition for girls and in their place have stressed "sports" and "play" days.

In some schools and colleges the interschool phase of the program comes under a director of athletics. It is his responsibility to arrange the schedules, make the necessary arrangements for athletic events, such as securing officials, and care for the numerous details essential to a well-organized program. For many schools and colleges smaller in size, the individual or individuals who administer the required class and intramural and extramural programs also administer the interschool phase of the total physical education program. Since all are closely related, utilize the same personnel in most cases, share the same facilities, and are interested in achieving the same objectives, it is important that they all come under the jurisdiction of the same department. Such an organization makes it possible for all to accomplish their purposes under the leadership of an individual who recognizes the value and place of each in a well-rounded program.

In connection with financing athletic programs, many schools have what is called a general organization, which is in charge of the finances not only for the athletic program but also for other school activities, such as dramatics and music. This has been used with success in some schools and takes the financial responsibility out of the physical education department and places it in an impartial organization.

Other items of particular importance that should be arranged for in the administration of athletics are provision for medical supervision and an accident plan. Both should be carefully considered by any school desiring to have a sound athletics program.

The organization of physical education in colleges and universities

Physical education is organized as one administrative unit for men and women in a majority of colleges and universities in the United States. The administrative unit

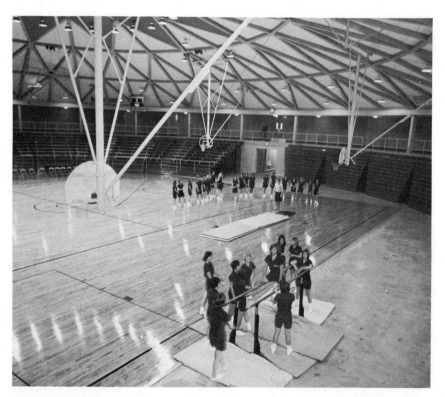

Shaver & Company, Salina, Kan.
A phase of the physical education program. (McPherson High School, McPherson, Kan.)

State College Board of Trustees

President of the College

Vice President

or

Dean of the College

Associate Dean or Head ———— Executive Committee: All Department Chairmen

School of Physical Education, Health, and Recreation

Chairman, Department of Physical Education, Men	Chairman, Department of Physical Education, Women	Chairman, Department of Health Education	Chairman, Department of Recreation	Chairman, Department of Intercollegiate Athletics, Men (Director of Athletics)
Advisory Committee	Advisory Committee	Advisory Committee	Advisory Committee	Advisory Committee
Basic Instruction for Men	Basic Instruction for Women	Undergraduate Professional Curriculum	Undergraduate Professional Curriculum	Administration of Intercollegiate Athletics
Undergraduate Professional Curriculum	Undergraduate Professional Curriculum	Service Courses in First Aid	Service Courses, General Elementary Teachers	Coordination of Athletic Coaching Courses
Graduate Professional Curriculum	Graduate Professional Curriculum	State Field Service	Campus Recreation	Coordination of Intercollegiate Athletic Schedules
Intramural Sports	Intramural Sports	Coordination With Community Health Services	State Field Service	Coordination of Teaching Services of Coaches
Supervision of Sports Facilities	Extramural Sports	Health Education Institutes and Workshops	Administration of Outdoor Education Center	Coordination of Maintenance and Use of Athletic Facilities
Supervision of Aquatics	Dance Productions	Public and Private School Consultations	Recreation Institutes and Workshops	Coordination of Conference Affiliation, National Collegiate Athletic Association, American Amateur Athletic Union, etc.
Faculty-Staff and Community Instructional Services	Faculty-Staff and Community Instructional Services		Coordination with Community Recreation Services	
Research Laboratory	Research Laboratory		Public, Private, and Commercial Recreation Consultations	

Organization chart for a school of physical education, health, and recreation. (Developed by Don Adee.)

may be either a college, school, division, or department; the administrator in charge of the physical education program may be called a dean, director, supervisor, or chairman. In many institutions of higher learning this administrator is responsible directly to the president or to a dean, but in a few instances, he is responsible to the director of athletics. (In a majority of colleges, athletics are included as part of the same administrative setup with the rest of the physical education program.) In many cases the duties of the athletic director and the administrator of the physical education program are assigned to the same person. Many colleges and universities have intra-

Table 3-1. Total and first-time opening fall degree-credit enrollment in junior colleges, by sex: United States, 1954 to 1974 (adapted)*†

	Total fall enrollment			First-time fall enrollment		
Fall	Total	Men	Women	Total	Men	Women
(1)	(2)	(3)	(4)	(5)	(6)	(7)
1954	282,433	171,752	110,681	129,349	76,517	52,832
1955	308,411	196,671	111,740	139,969	86,176	53,793
1956	347,345	225,635	121,710	162,810	101,610	61,200
1957	369,162	237,679	131,483	167,640	104,037	63,603
1958	385,609	248,040	137,569	174,949	107,744	67,205
1959	409,715	259,754	149,961	181,679	111,257	70,422
1960	451,333	282,155	169,178	213,976	128,570	85,406
1961	517,925	320,156	197,769	243,777	145,665	98,112
1962	589,529	365,624	223,905	260,440	156,163	104,277
1963	624,789	386,660	238,129	271,673	163,062	108,611
1964	710,868	439,509	271,359	322,241	193,407	128,834
1965	791,000	492,000	299,000	384,000	230,000	154,000
1966	866,000	535,000	331,000	383,000	229,000	154,000
1967	944,000	587,000	357,000	388,000	232,000	156,000
1968	1,016,000	631,000	385,000	400,000	239,000	161,000
1969	1,048,000	651,000	397,000	419,000	251,000	168,000
1970	1,086,000	675,000	411,000	448,000	269,000	179,000
			Projected			
1971	1,150,000	714,000	436,000	474,000	284,000	190,000
1972	1,220,000	756,000	464,000	498,000	299,000	199,000
1973	1,291,000	799,000	492,000	519,000	312,000	207,000
1974	1,350,000	832,000	518,000	542,000	325,000	217,000

*Sources and method: Enrollment data from U. S. Department of Health, Education and Welfare, Office of Education circulars: Opening (fall) enrollment in higher education (1954 through 1970). Population data used are consistent with Series B projection in U. S. Department of Commerce, Bureau of the Census, Current population reports: projections of the population of the United States by age and sex to 1985, Series P-25, No. 179.

The projections of total and first-time opening fall degree-credit enrollment in junior colleges are based on the assumptions: (1) Attendance rates of men and of women aged 18 to 21 years in junior colleges will follow the 1954-1970 trends; (2) entrance rates of 18-year-old men and of 18-year-old women into junior colleges will follow the 1954-1970 trends.

Note: Data include 50 states and District of Columbia for all years. Because of rounding, detail may not add to totals.

†From U. S. Department of Health, Education and Welfare, Office of Education: Projections of educational statistics to 1947-75, Washington, D. C., 1965 edition, The Department, p. 12.

mural athletic directors, since in most of these institutions intramural athletics are a part of the physical education program.

Professional programs in physical education are a part of the physical education program at both the undergraduate and the graduate levels. Physical education and health *education* are frequently combined into the same administrative unit, but health *services,* as a general rule, are not organized as part of the physical education unit. Physical education is commonly responsible for the administration of recreation programs for both students and faculty.

THE TWO-YEAR COLLEGE

The junior college, or community college as it is sometimes called, deserves special mention because this type of institution is expanding at such a rapid rate and will continue to do so as the number of college-bound students rise. This means that more and more high school boys and girls upon graduation will find their educational opportunities in this kind of college.

Though there are exceptions, most junior colleges (and by this term the community college is included) have the following three functions:

1. To give 2 years of preprofessional training or general education. A student may graduate with a degree of associate in the arts or sciences after these 2 years or transfer to a 4-year institution for a bachelor's degree. This transfer program is sometimes called the university parallel curricula. Most 4-year colleges and universities will accept transfer students from accredited junior colleges if the academic achievement of the student is high and if the subjects studied mesh with the curricula of the higher institution.
2. To provide a complete program in a semiprofessional field such as secretarial work, home economics, medical laboratory techniques, drafting, and business education.
3. To provide classes for adults who want more education to help them in their jobs or who simply want to study subjects they never had a chance to study before.

The type of curricula offered by junior colleges is usually controlled by the needs and interests of the students they serve. Some junior college curricula are planned almost entirely for students who want a general education and who plan to transfer to a 4-year institution. Other junior colleges enroll the majority of students in semiprofessional courses.

A junior college in an agricultural area may feature agricultural courses, while another junior college in an industrial community may specialize in courses that prepare young people for jobs in nearby factories.

In respect to physical education and health education in the 2-year college, surveys conducted indicate that the pattern of 2 hours weekly for ½ unit credit is the most frequent procedure for physical education. Objectives in most cases stress the students' competence in maintaining good health and balanced personal adjustment. Some colleges are seriously attempting to meet these objectives, but others have not yet developed their programs sufficiently to accomplish this task. Athletics appear to be an especially strong point of physical education at the junior college level because of the great student and public interest. Some colleges provide broad programs of team competition in many sports, whereas others are very limited.

Most 2-year colleges have a health service program for their students, but instruction in personal and community hygiene or health is less usual than instruction in physical education. Where a health course is offered it is usually a one-semester course for 2 credits.

Interviews with deans of instruction, faculty, and students of 2-year colleges indicate that they prefer to have one department chairman in charge of both the health and physical education programs. The department chairman usually is responsible to the dean of students or dean of instruction.

Four-fifths are men

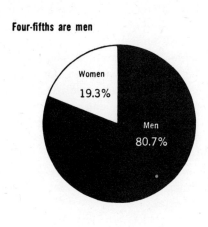

More than half have doctor's degrees

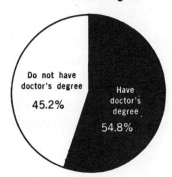

3 in 10 are assistant professors

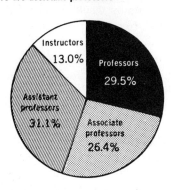

3 in 10 teach humanities

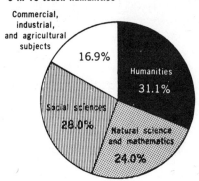

More than half teach in publicly controlled institutions

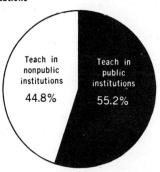

Distribution of faculty members by region

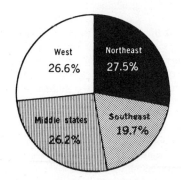

Faculty members in degree-granting institutions. (From NEA Research Bulletin 44:8, 1966.)

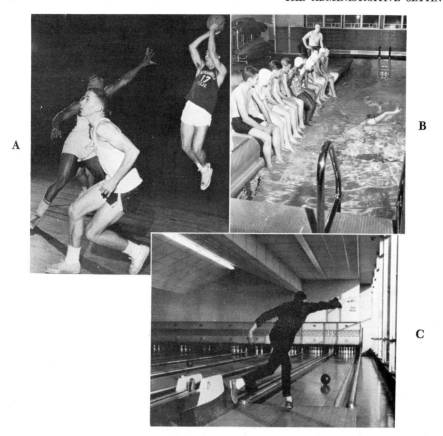

The physical education program in the 2-year college at Flint Community College, Flint, Mich. **A,** Defense is not stressed by all teams in the intramural league. **B,** All swimming classes are coeducational. Classes for beginning swimmers through water safety instructor course are offered in Durham Pool. **C,** Commercial alleys for their bowling classes.

COMMUNITY ORGANIZATION FOR HEALTH

It is important to understand not only the structure of the school and college but also that of the larger community of which it is a part. If programs of health and physical education are to render the most valuable service at the community level, their leaders must clearly understand its structural organization. This important level of government touches human lives to a great degree.

Public health organization at the local level

Health department. There are few, if any, local departments with more impor-
tant functions than the health department. In spite of this, the amount of money set aside and the emphasis placed on this phase of government are usually less than that spent on many other areas, such as for police or fire protection.

The department of health also works more closely with other branches of local government than most other departments. For example, it is closely related to bureaus having control of water supply and purification, garbage collection and disposal, sewerage system and street cleaning, and police department enforcement of the sanitary code. It also works with officers in charge of education, especially in regard to medical and dental inspection of school children. Such essential relationships make it imperative to have a local health department that is efficient and functions properly.

In some cities governed by a commission, health is combined with police and fire administration to form a department of public safety. However, in most cities, especially the larger ones, there is a separate department of health. At the head of the health department in these larger cities there is usually a board of health or a commission, headed by a health commissioner. In a few cities the health activities are guided by a single commissioner, who is appointed by the mayor or city council.

In many cases small or medium-sized cities and villages do not employ full-time health officers, and the public health activities are cared for by a physician who devotes only part time to this work. Under such conditions, a health department in the full sense of the phrase does not exist and the public health activities are bound to be limited.

On some occasions, two or three small communities have felt the need for full-time health personnel and consequently have pooled their efforts and resources and have combined to develop a joint health administration with a full-time health officer. This has resulted in advantages to all communities concerned. It is hoped that this policy will be used to a greater extent by small villages, towns, and cities located within a short enough radius to make such a system practical.

The recognized, successful health departments in larger cities have boards of health presided over by a commissioner of health. These boards enact the sanitary code of the city, issue emergency health orders, and have been given broad powers in all health matters. In some emergency situations such a group has been given the power to imprison persons, destroy property, forbid traffic, and perform similar duties to prevent the spread of disease.

The health department in larger communities is usually divided into certain specialized divisions, each having control over various health aspects of the community. Some of these divisions are as follows:

The *bureau of administration,* which coordinates all the various activities performed and serves as a central communication point with other city functions.

The *division of records,* which collects, preserves, and publishes vital statistics, issues burial permits, registers physicians, assists in enforcing child labor and school attendance laws, and performs statistical work for the department.

The *sanitary division* or *bureau,* which has jurisdiction over sanitary conditions and looks into such matters as reported nuisances and the sanitation of slaughterhouses and stables.

The *bureau of preventable diseases,* which is concerned with preventing and controlling communicable disease, holding tuberculosis and other clinics, disinfecting premises and goods, and supervising a staff of field nurses.

The *division of child hygiene,* which is concerned with child and infant care, eye and dental clinics, supervision of day nurseries, and placement and care of dependent children.

The *food and drug bureau,* which has control over the food and drug supply in the city and inspects premises where foods are stored, handled, sold, or prepared. It also is especially concerned with the persons who prepare or serve food in public eating places.

The *bureau of laboratories,* which carries on research work, maintains supply stations for diphtheria antitoxin and vaccine, and makes scientific studies of various diseases and combats them whenever possible.

The *bureau of hospitals,* which supervises the various hospitals which in large cities are maintained by the department for the care of individuals who have communicable diseases.

Last, but not least, there is the *bureau of public health education.* This bureau is gradually being added to more and more departments of health because it is becoming increasingly evident that individuals are not going to develop good health practices without an educational program. This bureau sends out various types of information concerning health matters, promotes cooperation between department officials and the public, publishes health literature for professional and lay persons, gives health lectures, and organizes exhibitions and other media for publicizing the importance of certain health practices.

The health department, as can be seen from the preceding description, provides many essential and important functions for a community. Unfortunately, many of the activities listed are not carried on by all cities. An analysis of the functions performed indicates a change of emphasis from that of merely eliminating nuisances and fighting epidemics to one of prevention and providing information and services essential for good health.

Health councils. One of the best ways to ensure that all the health resources in a community are being utilized effectively for the benefit of most people is to have a community health council.

A community contains many groups and individuals who are interested in health. With so many interested in such an endeavor, there is need for coordination and a clearinghouse for the solution of health problems. A council or committee that is composed of representatives of various community groups can serve a very useful purpose. Much progress can be made if representatives from such groups as voluntary and professional health agencies, schools, industry, merchants, and others interested in health meet to discuss health problems. Group discussion can take place,

problems can be aired, plans can be made, and work can be done that would never be possible without some type of cooperative effort. The health council is a comparatively new organization but has been found to be most helpful in promoting health in the community. As an agency through which many groups may cooperate to promote health, it has great possibilities for mobilizing public support for necessary health measures.

Voluntary health agencies. Some voluntary health agencies usually exist in communities of any size. These are organizations concerned with health that receive their support from public drives for funds, gifts, membership fees, and donations. Some examples of these are the American Cancer Society, National Tuberculosis Association, National Committee for Mental Hygiene, and the American Red Cross. Voluntary agencies in the field of health take the leadership for solving particular health problems that affect great numbers of American people. Through voluntary contributions and work, these agencies attempt to meet the problems.

Many voluntary health agencies exist now and new ones are being formed periodically. The greatest need at the present time is to coordinate the work that all the various agencies for health—whether they be official, voluntary, or private—are doing. There is considerable confusion in the public's mind because of the numerous agencies that are asking for financial help and support. If the work were better coordinated and organized, the public would have a clearer picture of what is needed and consequently would lend greater support.

Relationship between public health and school health programs

The health of the school child is a major consideration of our educational systems. In 1918 it was placed first on the list of "Cardinal Principles for Education." In 1938 it was reemphasized by the Educational Policies Commission. Conferences have been held, legislation passed, personnel appointed, and programs planned for the express purpose of promoting the health of the youth in our schools. This great emphasis focused on the health of the child and the happiness and fitness of future citizens of the United States means that every effort must be made to accomplish this objective in the most efficient and best way possible. Therefore, all the personnel and resources that are available in the community must be mobilized for this purpose. This is not a one-agency job. Instead, it requires the help and assistance of all organizations affecting the health of the child. Voluntary and official agencies, hospitals, boards of education, and other interested individuals and organizations must pool their resources, facilities, equipment, and knowledge in order that the health of the child may receive utmost consideration.

On the other hand, the solution of community health problems outside the school needs the concerted effort of every agency. Public health programs are to a great degree based upon an enlightened public that understands the health problems of the community and gives its support to the solving of these problems. The school can play a major part in helping to educate the citizens of the community so that health progress may be realized. The school health program should fit into the total community health program in a well-coordinated manner so as to render utmost service to all concerned.

In discussing interrelationships between school and public health programs, it is important to consider the controversy between community health groups and the schools as to who is responsible for administering the various phases of the school health program.

There are primarily three points of view as to where the responsibility lies. One group feels that the board of education should be responsible, another that public

health officials should assume the responsibility, and a third group thinks that school health is a joint responsibility of both the board of education and public health officials. It is advisable to consider briefly some of the arguments in favor of each point of view.

Those individuals who advocate board of education control for the school health program set forth many pertinent arguments in their behalf. These arguments can be summed up in the following statements. Board of education supporters point to the fact that the Tenth Amendment to the Constitution of the United States places the authority for education in the hands of the states. The states delegate this authority to the local communities, which in turn vest the authority in the board of education. The board of education, in the absence of legislation to the contrary, is responsible for all education, and health education, therefore, falls logically under their jurisdiction. They point to the fact that teachers, as a result of their training in such areas as psychology and methodology, are much better prepared to instruct children in health matters than are public health officials. They are better prepared to make health services meaningful educational experiences for all pupils. As another argument, they maintain that if public health officials were responsible for the school health program, the teachers would have two bosses, thus making for inefficient administration.

Those individuals who advocate that the school health program should be controlled by public health officials also list many pertinent arguments in their favor. Public health supporters say that health is logically a province of the medical profession and should therefore be under supervision of medical personnel, such as those found in most public health departments. They point to the fact that the school is part of the total community, and therefore such an important matter as health is a responsibility of community health officials. Furthermore, the pupil is in school only 5 days of each week and 180 or so days per year. The rest of the time he is in the larger community outside the school environment. They argue that public health nurses, as a result of their training and experience, are the best qualified to develop and administer a health services program, especially in respect to home-school-community relationships. They maintain that according to law the control of communicable diseases is a prerogative of public health officials and that they can do the job much more efficiently than can the board of education.

Finally, there is a group of persons who maintains that the school health program should be controlled jointly by both the board of education and public health officials. These point out that there will be better utilization of personnel, facilities, and community resources and that, consequently, greater health progress can be made if there is joint control with both working together for the good of all.

There does not seem to be a simple solution to this controversy as to where the responsibility for school health lies. Probably the answer to this problem will vary according to the community. The solution would seem to depend upon how each community can best meet the health needs of the people who inhabit its particular geographic limits. The type of administrative setup that most fully meets the health needs and makes for greatest progress should be the one that is adopted. Vested interests should not be considered, and the health interests of the consumer should be the primary concern. *Health is everybody's business*, and everyone should strive for the best health program possible in his community, state, nation, and world.

COMMUNITY ORGANIZATION FOR PHYSICAL EDUCATION

Physical education within the larger community outside of the school is usually in-

corporated in the programs sponsored by recreation people or by voluntary and private agencies such as the Boys' Club, YMCA, churches, and camps. Since these organizations and programs are considered in detail in the last two chapters of this book, they will not be discussed here.

Questions and exercises

1. Draw a structural organization chart for your school or college showing the various administrative divisions. Discuss the responsibilities of each of the divisions. Give special attention to the health and physical education divisions.
2. In regard to the board of education of the community in which you live, list the composition of the board, powers of the board, and qualifications of board members.
3. Discuss the role of the superintendent of schools, principal, and college administrators in a selected community.
4. Define each of the following: (a) health program, (b) health services, (c) health appraisal, (d) health counseling, (e) health education, (f) healthful school living, (g) health coordination, (h) health council, and (i) health educator.
5. What part does a health coordinator play in the school health program?
6. Describe in detail the three main divisions of the total school physical education program.
7. Discuss the relationship of local government to school health. What administrative provisions have been made for these important considerations?
8. Discuss in detail the organization and administration of a program of physical education in a junior college of your choice.

Reading assignment in *Administrative Dimensions of Health and Physical Education Programs, Including Athletics:* Chapter 3, Selections 12 to 15.

Selected references

Blackwell, T. E.: College and university administration, New York, 1966, The Center for Applied Research in Education, Inc. (The Library of Education).

Bookwalter, K. W.: Physical education in the secondary schools, Washington, D. C., 1964, The Center for Applied Research in Education, Inc. (The Library of Education).

Brickman, W. W.: Educational systems in the United States, New York, 1964, The Center for Applied Research in Education, Inc. (The Library of Education).

Brimm, R. P.: The junior high school. New York, 1963, The Center for Applied Research in Education, Inc. (The Library of Education).

Bucher, C. A.: Foundations of physical education, ed. 5, St. Louis, 1968, The C. V. Mosby Co.

Bucher, C. A.: Physical education for life, St. Louis, 1969, McGraw-Hill Book Co.

Bucher, C. A., and Dupee, R. K., Jr.: Athletics in schools and colleges, Washington, D. C., 1965, The Center for Applied Research in Education, Inc. (The Library of Education).

Bucher, C. A., Koenig, C., and Barnhard, M.: Methods and materials for secondary school physical education, ed. 3, St. Louis, 1970, The C. V. Mosby Co.

Bucher, C. A., Olsen, E., and Willgoose, C. The foundations of health, New York, 1967, Appleton-Century-Crofts.

Bucher, C. A., and Reade, E. M.: Physical education and health in the elementary school, ed. 2, New York, 1971, The Macmillan Co.

Byrd, O. E.: School health administration, Philadelphia, 1964, W. B. Saunders Co.

Educational Policies Commission: School athletics —problems and policies, Washington, D. C., 1954, National Education Association.

Eichhorn, D. H.: The middle school, New York, 1966, The Center for Applied Research in Education, Inc. (The Library of Education).

Ferguson, D. G.: Pupil personnel services, New York, 1963, The Center for Applied Research in Education, Inc. (The Library of Education).

Gauerke, W. E.: School law, New York, 1965, The Center for Applied Research in Education, Inc. (The Library of Education).

Goldhammer, K.: The school board, New York, 1964, The Center for Applied Research in Education, Inc. (The Library of Education).

Hillson, M.: Change and innovation in elementary school organization, New York, 1965, Holt, Rinehart & Winston, Inc.

Jenson, T. H., and Clark, D. L.: Educational administration, New York, 1964, The Center for Applied Research in Education, Inc. (The Library of Education).

Joint Committee on Health Problems in Education of National Education Association and American Medical Association: School health services, Washington, D. C., 1964, National Education Association.

Joint Committee on Health Problems in Education of National Education Association and American Medical Association: Healthful school living, Washington, D. C., 1969, National Education Association.

Joint Committee on Health Problems in Education of National Education Association and American Medical Association: Health education, Washington, D. C., 1961, National Education Association.

Linder, I. H., and Gunn, H. M.: Secondary school administration: problems and practices, Columbus, Ohio, 1963, Charles E. Merrill Books, Inc.

Morphet, E. L., Johns, R. L., and Reller, T. L.: Educational administration, Englewood Cliffs, N. J., 1967, Prentice-Hall, Inc.

Reynolds, J. W.: The junior college, New York, 1965, The Center for Applied Research in Education, Inc. (The Library of Education).

Willgoose, C. E.: Health education in the elementary school, ed. 2, Philadelphia, 1964, W. B. Saunders Co.

Wynn, R. D.: Organization of public schools, New York, 1964, The Center for Applied Research in Education, Inc. (The Library of Education).

CHAPTER 4

THE BUSINESS ADMINISTRATOR*

In recent years the position of school or college business administrator has grown extensively. The exact position, with its inherent responsibilities, is still in a stage of development. The business administrator is a person trained and experienced in the field of education with a background of business—or a person trained in business with a knowledge of educational techniques. The business administrator is part of the administrative team. He is a specialist making a contribution to the united efforts of the group in supporting the procedures of improving the educational opportunity of the pupils and the staff. School business administration has long been accepted to mean "that phase of school administration having responsibility for the efficient and economic management of the business affairs of the schools."†

The American Association of School Administrators and the Association of School Business Officials of the United States and Canada have now jointly agreed that school business administrators may be defined as follows:

The school business administrator shall be that employee member of the school staff who has been designated by the Board of Education and/or the Superintendent to have general responsibility for the administration of the business affairs of a school district. In any type of administrative organization, he shall be responsible for carrying out the general administration of the district and such other duties as may be assigned to him. Unless otherwise provided by local law or customs (as in dual control areas), he shall report to the Board of Education through the Superintendent of Schools.*

The school or college business administrator is an important member of the administrative team who has a significant contribution to make in the decision-making process as well as in executing business functions. He is well versed in education matters as well as in business management, and teaching experience is highly desirable. He is in a position to participate under the superintendent's or president's leadership and in making educational decisions as well as doing an efficient job of serving the district or college by providing educational activities for the staff and pupils.

Since health educators and physical educators must work closely with school business administrators, special consideration is given to this key school or college administrator and the role he plays in the administration of school and college programs in general and in school and college health and physical education programs in particular.

THE COLLEGE BUSINESS MANAGER

The college business manager, or the vice president of business affairs as he is sometimes called, is responsible for budget

*Thanks are due Mr. H. J. Stevens, Assistant Superintendent of Business Affairs, Nanuet, New York Public Schools, for his help in writing this chapter.

†Linn, H. H.: School business administration, New York, 1956, The Ronald Press Co., p. 21.

*Association of School Business Officials: The school business administrator (Bulletin 21), Evanston, Ill., 1960, The Association.

preparation and fiscal accounting, investment of endowment and other monies,
planning and construction of buildings,
data processing, management of research
and other contracts, business aspects of
student loans, and intercollegiate activities.

Most key business officers have earned a
master's or a doctor's degree, usually in
business administration. However, some
are certified public accountants and some
have taken courses in management institutes. Most college business managers are
recruited outside the academic world.

For the purposes of this chapter, the
term *business administrator* is used, and
the duties of such an educational officer
are discussed in terms of schools and the
school district. However, the functions that
are outlined for the business administrator,
the problems discussed, and the working
relationship with health and physical ed-

ucation personnel are similar to or have
implications for college as well as for school
health educators and physical educators.

RESPONSIBILITIES OF THE BUSINESS ADMINISTRATOR

The business administrator's responsibilities are varied. He is as familiar with employee health insurance problems as he is
with the butterfat content in milk. In the
smaller school district, the business responsibilities are incorporated into the duties of
the chief school administrator. As districts
enlarge, there is a need to hire a person to
oversee all the nonteaching areas of the
district so that the chief school administrator is free to devote more time to the
educational program of the district. No
two districts are alike in the handling of
business responsibilities.

Following are some of the administra-

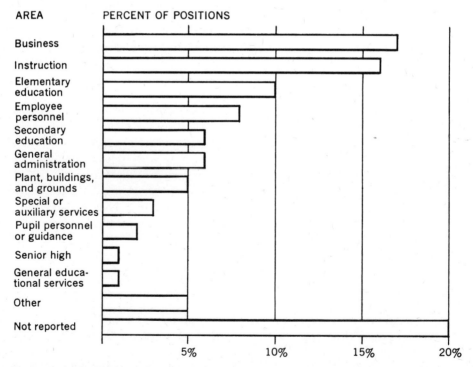

Major areas of assignment of 935 associate and assistant superintendencies. (From NEA Research
Bulletin **40:**26, 1962.)

tor's duties as listed by Frederick W. Hill,* past president of the Association of School Business Officials:

1. Budget and financial planning—This is an area in which the business official has to be sensitive to the needs of the staff in order to carry out a program. He also has to have a sixth sense to understand how much the community can expend on the program. This can be related to the accompanying isosceles triangle. There has to

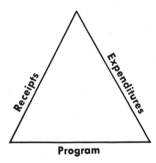

be a direct relationship among all the components that make up the three sides of the triangle.

2. Purchasing and supply management —The business official must utilize the best purchasing techniques to obtain maximum value for every dollar spent. After purchases are made and goods received, he is responsible for warehousing, storage, and inventory control. An article offered at the cheapest price is not always the most economical to purchase.

3. Plans—The business official works with administrators, teachers, architects, attorneys, and citizens of the community in developing plans for expansion of building facilities.

4. Personnel—The business official's duties vary in relation to the size of the district. In a small district he may be in charge of the nonteaching personnel, and in a large district he may be in charge of all personnel. In this capacity he has to

*Hill, F. W.: The rightful role of the school business official, School Business Affairs **29**:63, 1963.

maintain records, pay schedules, retirement reports, and other personnel records.

5. Staff improvement—The business official is always interested in upgrading the people under his jurisdiction by providing workshops and inservice courses concerning latest developments in the field.

6. Community relations—Without community support the school would not operate. Some administrators tend to forget this when they become too far removed from the community. There is always a need to interpret the business area to the public.

7. Transportation—It has often been said that boards of education find themselves spending too much time on the three B's—buses, buildings, and bonds. When this occurs, it is time to look into the hiring of a business official.

8. Food services—The business official is

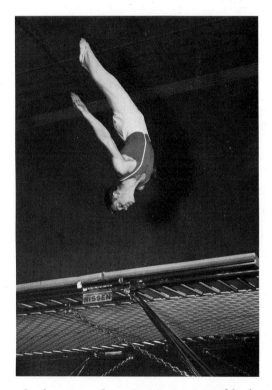

The business administrator is responsible for purchasing supplies and equipment. (Courtesy Nissen Corporation, Cedar Rapids, Iowa.)

responsible for the efficient management of the lunchroom.

9. Accounting and reporting—The business official establishes and supervises the financial records and accounting procedures.

10. Debt service—The business official is involved with various capital developments and financial planning through short-term and long-term programs. Part of the financial rating of a school or a college district is judged on the way its debt service is handled.

11. Insurance—The business official must be familiar with a large schedule of insurance provisions ranging from fire and liability to health insurance. He has to maintain records for proof in case of loss.

12. Legal matters—The business official has to be familiar with education law and he has to know when to consult with attorneys.

13. System analysis—The business official must constantly question existing systems to see if they can be changed so that the job can be done more efficiently. New methods are being introduced utilizing data processing that will be a challenge as well as an aid to the business official.

FUNCTIONS OF BUSINESS MANAGEMENT IN THE EDUCATIONAL PROGRAM

The business administrator is in a position to serve the educational program. His function is strictly limited by the size of the educational triangle—program, receipts, expenditures. The greater the perimeter of the triangle, the larger will be his sphere of operations. This applies to all departments in the system. Likewise, in times of inflation, the expenditures and receipts may increase, the program side will also increase, but the actual program could remain the same. Hence, it is obvious that the business administrator must project expenditures and receipts ahead if a constant program is going to be maintained.

The business office represents a means

to an end, and it can be evaluated in terms of how well it contributes to the realization of the objectives of education.

OBJECTIVES OF BUSINESS MANAGEMENT

In serving schools and colleges, the business administrator constantly has a goal to help them obtain the greatest educational service possible from each tax or aid dollar spent. He should take a democratic approach on decisions affecting others. A decision will then be reached that will be for the best, with the assurance that the educational benefits are worth the cost.

The business administrator is part of the team of administrators—along with presidents, principals, superintendents, and board members—who may be expected to look into the years ahead and have some ideas in regard to the future plans of the school or college.

RELATIONSHIP WITH HEALTH AND PHYSICAL EDUCATION DEPARTMENTS

The business administrator has a very close working relationship with physical educators and health educators.

Director of health and physical education

In a large school district the business administrator works directly with the director of the department on budgetary and financial matters. It is important that all matters concerning physical education programs in the various buildings of the school district be approved by the building principal before they go to the central office. This is especially true in the secondary school because the physical education program is one part of the total curriculum. After the programs have been approved by the principal, they should be presented by the principal to the central office. If any program is to be modified, the principal is notified accordingly. Purchasing of materials is done on a bid basis, and when substitutes are offered for specified items, the business administrator should consult with the director of the department. The director then acts as a consultant in determining the quality of the items being purchased. One of the most serious mistakes that can be made when working with the business administrator is to "pad" the budget request for supplies and materials. The old expression "murder will out" comes to the fore at this point. The physical education person may decide that he needs twenty-four basketballs for next year, but he decides to list thirty-six on his budget request—hoping for the twenty-four—and if he receives thirty-six, he will have that many extra in the storage closet. Likewise, the business administrator should not make blind deletions in the requisitions without a consultation. There has to be a feeling of rapport between the two areas—so when the physical educator requests twenty-four basketballs, he will know he will receive twenty-four, unless a mutual budget change has been made.

A teacher in the physical education department should analyze the community and school philosophy to determine how much emphasis is to be placed on the program. This will have a direct bearing on the expenditures. In some school districts the academic program is a runner-up to the athletic program. A new teacher to a school system soon finds out how liberal or conservative the district is when he commences to submit purchase requisitions. An early meeting with the business administrator would be very helpful in determining the financial philosophy of the school district toward the health and physical education program. Such a meeting would also spare some embarrassment in the future.

The health educator

The health educator plays a significant role in the school and college curriculum today. Educational growth is most effective when the students are progressing health-fully as well as intellectually. It has been found that one of the reasons for the lack of educational attainment has been the physical inability to cope with the school or college program. Many items come to the business office that can be passed on to the health educator such as teaching aids for the health program.

The myth of the school nurse-teacher functioning as a school nurse—minus the teaching—is now being overcome. In today's modern school the nurse-teacher is looked upon as a resource person to be brought into the classroom as a specialist to augment teaching units.

The business administrator and the school nurse-teacher must work together at all times. New schools are now being equipped with furnishings in color that have replaced the characteristic standard white equipment. The waiting rooms for health suites are now equipped with comfortable lounge furniture. The medications, equipment, and other supplies are not purchased at the local drug stores but on a bid basis through national supply houses.

The business administrator, as a member of the administrative team, has to be sensitive to change in growing school districts. Perhaps it was acceptable for the school nurse-teacher to combine her duties and become the attendance officer when the school district was small, but can her salary be justified if she has to use several hours a day on the telephone verifying absences or making home visits of truants? A non-teaching clerical person could be utilized for these duties at a considerable saving in salary, and this would also relieve the school nurse-teacher to perform other duties that would be more effective in the curriculum.

The dental hygienist

The dental hygienist is a relatively new addition to the health education team. Until recent years most school districts have utilized the services of the local dentists to make an annual dental inspection. In some districts the dentists were paid for this service. In other districts the dentists did it on a volunteer basis. In the latter school districts it is more difficult to initiate the idea of hiring an individual to make dental inspections. It must be emphasized that a dental hygienist is more than just a tooth inspector. A dental hygienist should be utilized in the classroom as a consultant, similar to the school nurse-teacher. At the time the dental hygienist's schedule is prepared, consideration should be made for classroom visitations to discuss dental hygiene with the students. It is the responsibility of the school business administrator to provide a means for the dental hygienist to obtain materials and equipment to carry out her function in the school district.

OTHER AUXILIARY SERVICES

The business administrator renders many additional services that have a direct bearing on health and physical education programs.

Team transportation

The business administrator is usually responsible for the transportation program. A good business administrator, with an educational background, will be cognizant of the importance of exercise of not only the mind but also of the body. He will, therefore, make a provision in his transportation program for buses to carry athletic teams to sport contests so that they will arrive safely on time at their destinations. The director of athletics must be informed as to the type of facilities that will be available to him so that he can plan accordingly. This involves a direct relationship between the director of athletics and the transportation supervisor. All requests for special athletic trips should be in writing and acknowledged by the secondary school principal or college administrator where he is involved. This is necessary since the principal or college administrator will be aware of any conflicts with other parts of

his program. The business administrator finds it very difficult to schedule special athletic trips on a moment's notice, although it is understandable when games are canceled for reason of weather or other unforeseen events. The director of athletics should submit a monthly calendar of athletic events, listing the date, time and place of departure, event, destination, number of participants, time of pickup, and remarks (see accompanying sample).

Month of April

April 8

Depart: 3:00 P.M.
From: Senior High School
Team: Junior Varsity Baseball
To: Jones High School
Students: 35
Pickup: 5:30 P.M.
Remarks:

April 9

Depart: 3:00 P.M.
From: Junior High School
Team: Varsity Tennis
To: Albany High School
Students: 5
Pickup: 5:00 P.M.
Remarks: Station wagon requested;
Coach Lewis will drive.

April 10

Depart: 3:00 P.M.
From: Senior High School
Team: Varsity Baseball and
Varsity Tennis
To: Baseball to Jones High School
Tennis to Albany High School
Students: 40
Pickup: Baseball—5:00 P.M.
Tennis—5:30 P.M.
Remarks: One bus for both teams—
drop off baseball first.

The events scheduled on April 8 are very routine and the transportation supervisor can request a bus accordingly. The events on April 9 are a little more complex and the director of athletics can state a preference for a station wagon. It is much more economical for a school district or college to furnish a station wagon to transport five students rather than a sixty-passenger bus. The events on April 10 are more complex, and the remarks indicate that one bus can be utilized for both teams. It is necessary to list the number of participants so that the proper size bus, or buses, can be assigned. This calendar should be submitted in triplicate (carbons) to the business administrator. After the transportation department has scheduled the trips, the business administrator initials all three copies and returns two copies to the athletic director. The director keeps one copy and the other copy is sent to the principal or college administrator. The procedure for submitting transportation requests could vary in different schools. The administrator might receive the schedule for approval before the business office.

Facilities, equipment, and supplies

The business administrator has a responsibility to provide adequate indoor and outdoor facilities and sufficient equipment and supplies for the health and physical education department, and the latter has the responsibility to keep these items in the best condition possible.

There are three phases related to facilities, equipment, and supplies.

The first phase is to secure needed items in order to provide a program. The size of the health suite and gymnasium, the field acreage, and the quantity and quality of the equipment are all related to money. The health educator and physical educator can present to the business administrator alternate programs with price tags for the business administrator to transfer into tax rates for the board of education or board of trustees. This is usually done prior to a building program.

The second phase is in regard to a main-

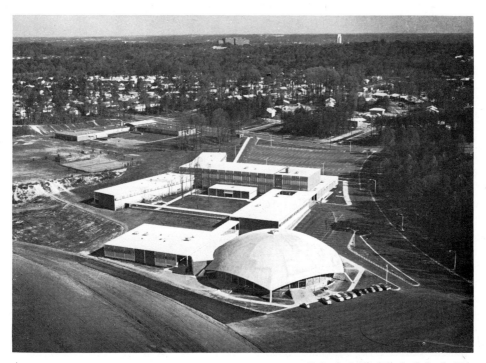

Bethesda Public Schools, Bethesda, Md.

tenance program. The director of health and physical education is usually the custodian of all the equipment and supplies. He has an obligation to the district to see that health supplies, uniforms, bats, balls, and other equipment are not unnecessarily damaged. He should delegate responsibility to the various teachers and coaches to supervise all participants at all times. Locker room damage can be extensive after a game if the players are not under continual supervision. Damaged uniforms can be repaired if the physical education personnel are aware of deteriorating conditions. Usually it is much more economical to repair them rather than to replace them.

The use of the grounds requires cooperation between the physical educator and the superintendent of buildings and grounds. There must be a direct line of communication between these two positions. The former is primarily interested in a first-rate physical education program, and the latter is primarily interested in first-rate facilities. Neither one can be first rate without cooperation between the two individuals involved and a mutual understanding of each other's problems.

The third phase of the utilization of facilities, equipment, and supplies relates to replacement of existing units. Equipment does wear out, and the life of the equipment does depend somewhat on the second phase. The business administrator, in his capacity as the director of the budget, prefers to replace items over a period of years—not all at once. It is a budget hardship to replace all football uniforms, for example, in 1 year, whereas the budget can absorb the cost if a few uniforms are replaced annually.*

At times there are some large replacement expenses that cannot be avoided, for example, replacing bleachers. The business administrator is in a position to include this in the budget as a capital expense or perhaps add it to a bond issue. But such a large budget item does merit special consideration from the business administrator. Too many special considerations added to the budget from the department will soon give people the impression that the program receives greater emphasis than the other phases of the instructional program. One of the ways to obtain economical and efficient use of the facilities, equipment, and supplies is for the business administrator and health and physical educators to reside as taxpayers in the community where they are employed.

Insurance*

The business administrator has to maintain a constant vigil on developments in the health and physical education insurance programs. Athletics represent one of the most important areas of coverage. Some schools and colleges do not provide an athletic insurance program. If a student is injured in an athletic event, the family would then be responsible for all medical expenditures. There would be be no provision for the school or college to reimburse the family for its expense. Of course, the school or college is always open to a lawsuit by the parents in an effort to reclaim expenses. This is expensive for the school or college, for if the claim is settled in favor of the parents, the school's or college's insurance premiums for the next few years are increased. If the lawsuit is settled in favor of the school or college, the insurance company has already placed a sum of money in reserve until the final decision is reached. This is also costly because the premium is increased during the time the money is in reserve. An intangible effect is the damage to the school's or college's public relations.

An alternative is to provide an opportunity for the students to purchase athletic insurance or, better yet, for the school or

---

*See also Chapter 17.

*Insurance is also discussed in Chapter 18.

college to purchase a policy for students participating in sports. Of course, the latter is the best method because all students are covered, regardless of their wealth, and the students' liability policy is not subject to suit. Most parents are only interested in recovering monies actually spent, and they are satisfied accordingly. Usually a blanket policy purchased by the school or college can be obtained at a lesser unit cost than a policy purchased by individuals. The athletic insurance program can be administered by a local or regional broker, relieving the school or college of going into the insurance business.

It is the responsibility of the director of physical education to supply accurate lists of participating students to the business office prior to the starting time of the sports. It is imperative for the various coaches to become aware of the insurance coverage so that when accidents do happen, they can inform the athletes as to the proper procedure to follow in filing reports and claims. Usually the business office will supply policies for every participant in a covered athletic team. The coach should not only be knowledgeable, but he should also show concern for accident victims. This is not only a form of good public relations, but it may also make the difference in the parents minds concerning a lawsuit. The coaches then must be instructed in the proper attitude to take when such mishaps occur.

Medical examinations

The business administrator has a responsibility to the department to ascertain that there are enough physicians appointed by the board of education or that the health services are adequate to serve the needs of the school district or college. Every student participating in physical education should have a medical examination before he enters into activities. In athletics there should be a medical examination before each sport season. This means that if a student is participating in football, basketball, and baseball, he would have three medical examinations.

A student was injured in a sectional wrestling meet and later died from the injury. Even though the school's liability carrier was not involved in the case, the adjuster was collecting material. His first request was the boy's medical examination that permitted him to participate in wrestling.

Coaches must be made aware of the significance of allowing a student to participate in a sport without a proper medical examination.

It is obvious that there is a direct relationship between the school or college business administrator and health and physical educators. They are dependent on the business administrator not only for supplies but also for guidelines in carrying out their program within the policies of the board of education or board of trustees. The purchase and care of supplies and equipment are discussed in detail in Chapter 17, but all the procedures usually originate in the office of the school business administrator. The staff of the health and physical education department can work with the business administrator in order to reach their objectives. It is important to realize that the business administrator and health and physical education personnel do have the same objective—to educate each child to the maximum of his ability. With that premise in mind, all the insignificant petty grievances, political overtones, and selfish desires will disappear into oblivion.

All personnel should respect the organizational structure and philosophy of the school or college. Subordinates that bypass their department heads, for instance, do not make good leaders. The first criterion of a good leader is that he must be a good follower. It is one thing to read the various school philosophies, but it is still another to be able to carry out the philosophy. Before joining the staff of a particular school or college, a teacher should become familiar with its philosophy and be prepared to live by it.

PROBLEMS IN WORKING WITH BUSINESS ADMINISTRATORS

Some of the pitfalls and problems encountered by business administrators in working with health and physical educators, as seen through the eyes of business administrators, are as follows:

1. Overestimation of budget requests with the idea of expecting a reduction in the request
2. Not being able to justify budget requests as they relate to the total educational program
3. Deadlines not met in submitting requests for transportation, supplies, and so on
4. Lack of awareness of the school district or college philosophy in regard to the place of the athletic program in the curriculum; hence, budget complications
5. Lack of cooperative planning in regard to the transportation equipment that is available and the scheduling of special athletic events away from school or college necessitating the use of buses
6. Late notification to the business administrator's office when a special athletic event is cancelled that requires the cancellation of a prearranged bus
7. Negligence in filing accident reports on students injured in sports or classes, no matter how insignificant an accident may seem at the time
8. Incomplete records on students participating in sports—especially in regard to the requirement that all students receive a physical examination *before* trying out for the sport
9. Lack of concern for accident victims
10. Lack of knowledge as to an injured student's rights and privileges under the student accident policy
11. Failure to realize that the educational goals represented in the philosophy of the school or college take priority over selfish, petty, and political interests
12. Lack of respect for the "chain of command" —a health and physical education teacher should not bypass the director of the department when communicating with the business office
13. Lack of interest in the facilities at his disposal, causing breakdowns and extra added expense

GUIDELINES FOR HEALTH AND PHYSICAL EDUCATORS

Some of the guidelines for health and physical educators to follow as viewed by business administrators are as follows:

1. All matters concerning health and physical education programs in the buildings of the district should be approved by the building principal before going to the school business administrator.

2. The school business administrator should also keep the central administration informed of any budget changes for the athletic programs since the curriculum will also be affected.

3. Supplies that are to be purchased should be accompanied by a complete specification, including model, catalogue size, and so on. Bids must be accepted on equivalents, but sometimes bids are received on substitutes. Health and physical educators should make themselves available to the business administrator to evaluate bids submitted.

4. Requisitions should be submitted after a careful study of the needs of the health and physical education department.

5. A teacher in the health and physical education department should be aware of the community's sentiment toward health and physical education programs and let that be one guideline for the curriculum.

6. The director of the health and physical education program should meet with the business administrator to determine the financial philosophy of the school or college toward the educational program.

7. The director of the health and physical education programs should keep the business administrator informed on new materials and ideas in his field.

8. All requests for special trips should be in writing on forms provided by the business office.

9. A monthly calendar should be submitted by the director of health and physical education, listing all athletic events and all pertinent transportation details.

10. The director of health and physical education should cooperate with the insurance program by submitting lists of students participating in sports, reporting accidents, and following through with physical examinations.

11. All personnel should be instructed in regard to administrative policies for dealing with accidents.

Questions and exercises

1. Interview a business administrator to obtain the following information: (a) the relations he has with health educators and/or physical educators, (b) how the business aspects of health education and/or physical education programs can be most effectively carried out, and (c) what a new teacher of health education and/or physical education should know about business administrators.
2. Why is a person who is a specialist in business management needed in school or college systems today?
3. Read one book or one article in a school or college administration magazine of your choice that concerns itself with the role of the business administrator in schools or colleges. Give a report to the class.
4. How is business management of health education and/or physical education carried on at the college level?

Reading assignment in *Administrative Dimensions of Health and Physical Education Programs, Including Athletics:* Chapter 3, Selection 11.

Selected references

Casey, L. M.: School business administration, New York, 1964, The Center for Applied Research in Education, Inc. (The Library of Education).

Hill, F. W.: The school business administrator, Evanston, Ill., 1960, American Association of Business Officials of the United States and Canada.

Hill, F. W.: The rightful role of the school business official, School Business Affairs 29:63, 1963.

Hill, F. W., and Colmey, J. W.: School business administration in the smaller community, Minneapolis, Minn., 1964, T. S. Denison & Co., Inc.

Knezevich, S. J., and Fowlkes, J. G.: Business management of local school systems, New York, 1960, Harper & Row, Publishers.

Linn, H. H.: School business administration, New York, 1956, The Ronald Press Co.

Naughton, J. J.: Profile of the chief school business administrator, Connecticut Teacher 34:16, April, 1967.

Roe, W. H.: School business management, New York, 1961, McGraw-Hill Book Co.

Stevens, H. J.: Are you issuing blank checks? School Management 9:80, 1965.

Personnel administration requires the recognition of, and adherence to, sound principles. Some important principles essential to effective personnel administration are discussed in the following paragraphs.

PRINCIPLES OF PERSONNEL ADMINISTRATION

Cooperation

To achieve cooperation implies that the specialties and unique abilities of individuals must be noted and utilized in situations where their services will be rendered under optimum conditions. The permanency of cooperation will depend upon the degree to which the purposes of the organization are achieved and individual motives are satisfied. The function of administration is to see that these essentials are accomplished.

The individual as a member of an organization

Administration should seek to imbue the organization with the theme that every individual has a stake in the enterprise. The undertakings can be successful only as all persons contribute to the maximum of their potentials, and with success will then come increased satisfaction to each individual. Above all, it must be recognized that submergence of self is necessary for the achievement of the organization's goals.

The fallacy of final authority

The authority that does exist belongs to the job and not to the person. The admin-

istrator should never feel powerful and all-important. Authority does not reside in one human being but in the best thinking, judgment, and imagination that the organization can command. Every individual has the authority that goes with his position and only that much. In turn, this authority is conditioned by other members whose work is closely allied to his achieving the objectives for which the organization exists. Authority comes from those who perform the more technical aspects of the organization's work as well as from those who, because of their positions, are responsible for the ultimate decisions. Department heads, foremen, and staff consultants issue reports interpreting the facts. Their judgments, conclusions, and recommendations contribute to the formulation of the final decisions that are the responsibility of the administrator. If these interpretations, judgments, conclusions, and recommendations are not accepted, the organization may fail. Its best thinking has been ignored. Furthermore, individuals cannot be induced to contribute their efforts in an organization that has little respect for their thinking. Authority is not resident in one person. Instead, it permeates the entire organization from top to bottom.

Staff morale

There are certain conditions that are known to contribute to staff morale. Some of the more important of these will be discussed. The administration should continually strive to create such conditions in their organizations. The degree of good staff morale that exists will be in direct proportion to the degree to which such conditions are satisfied.

Leadership. The quality of the leader will determine staff morale to a great degree. From the top down, there should be careful selection of all individuals who act in leadership capacities. Other things being equal, individuals will contribute better service, produce more, have an overall better morale, and have more respect for individuals who are leaders in the true sense of the word.

Physical and social environment. A healthful physical and social environment is essential to good staff morale. The health of the worker must be provided for. There must be good lighting to protect the eyes, good air to protect the lungs, and adequate safety precautions to protect the body. There must be provisions for mental health that include proper supervision, provision for advancement, provision for any emergency that may arise, and provision for intellectual improvement. Anything that is conducive to physical, mental, and emotional health is important to the morale of the individual and in turn to his efficiency as a member of the organization.

The social environment is also an important consideration. The individuals with whom one works and the activities in which one engages can strengthen or dampen the spirit. An individual is the product of his interactions with others. Therefore, in order to improve oneself it is very important to associate with those who can contribute to this improvement. Since the working day represents, to a great degree, the majority of an individual's social relationships, it is important that these relationships be wholesome and conducive to individual improvement.

Advancement. Human beings like to feel that they are "getting ahead in the world." This is an important consideration in developing and continuing a high de-gree of staff morale. This consideration necessitates informing each member of an organization as to what is essential for progress. Opportunities should be provided for self-improvement in learning new skills, gaining new knowledge, and having new experiences. In addition, encouragement should be given those who are anxious to improve and are willing to devote extra time and effort for such a purpose.

Recognition of meritorious service. Another requirement, similar to advancement, which is requisite for staff morale, is recognition for outstanding contributions to the organization. As has been previously pointed out, all human beings need to be recognized. Those who make outstanding contributions to the organization should be so honored. This is very important to further greater achievements.

Individual differences. An important principle of personnel management is the recognition of individual differences and different types of work. Individuals differ in many ways—abilities, skills, training, and physical, mental, and social qualities. There are also various types of work that require different skills, abilities, and training.

These differences in individuals and types of work must be recognized by the administrator. One of his or her main duties in respect to personnel should be to make sure that the right person is in the right niche. An individual who is a "round peg in a square hole" does not contribute to his own or the organization's welfare. To be placed in a position that should be held by a person with lesser qualifications or vice versa is unjust and devastating in its results.

It is important for the administrator to recognize in some formal way individual differences that exist in the organization. A system of status must exist for purposes of communication and orderly procedure. Such systems of status must be readily understood, authoritative, and authentic. These systems of status not only make for better communication but also provide the basis for personnel improvement and advancement within the organization. Furthermore, they help to develop a sense of responsibility in the individual. The status that is granted any one person should be in line with capacities and importance of the function he performs. Many disruptive features can develop in status systems if there is not recognition of individual abilities, if the system is allowed to become an end rather than a means to an end, and if proper incentives are not provided at each level.

QUALIFICATIONS OF THE ADMINISTRATOR

Although the qualities of a good administrator need to be considered in relation to the qualities of the persons in the or-

ganization he is attempting to lead, nevertheless it is helpful to recognize certain leadership characteristics that appear to be necessary if an administrator is to be successful on the job. The identification of these qualities is essential to help determine whether or not one should go into this important field if the occasion arises. This identification will also help in evaluating the type of administration one is experiencing in his own organization, whether he be an administrator or hold another position.

The qualifications of an administrator are many. Some (administrative mind, integrity, ability to instill good human relations, ability to make decisions, health and fitness for the job, willingness to accept responsibility, understanding of work, command of administrative technique, and intellectual capacity) are discussed in the following sections. There has been no at-

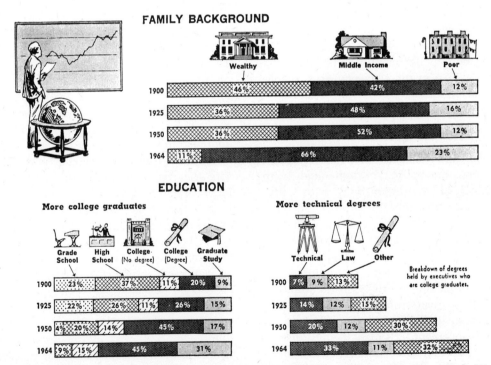

Nation's executives: changes in background and education. (© 1965 by The New York Times Company. Reprinted by permission.)

tempt to list these in order of importance, although in the discussion of each, one may be able to discern the most essential and important qualifications.

Administrative mind

A research project that involved a self-analysis of nearly 1,000 executives, all of whom were presidents of industrial organizations, pointed up the following important considerations for the person who wants to be a good administrator. Using time effectively, ability to get other people to do things, building a team, setting the direction, finding expert advice, making crisis decisions, negotiating, and effective self-improvement were considered important. Personal improvement, especially

directed along lines involving public speaking, planning work, memory skills, conference leadership, writing, producing better ideas, and reading, were also considered necessary.

Some individuals have qualities that, perhaps, have been developed through training and experience and that peculiarly adapts them to administrative work. These individuals are able to analyze situations objectively, have the ability to clarify generalizations, and possess the quality of administering in a constructive manner rather than in an exploitative way. Such persons are sensitive to human relations and the important part they play in the successful functioning of any organization. These individuals think in imagina-

Table 5-1. Mean maximum scheduled salaries,* teacher and administrative personnel, 1952-63 to 1968-69 (reporting systems with enrollments of 25,000 or more)†

Position	School year							Percent increase, 1968-69 over 1962-63
	1962-63	1963-64	1964-65	1965-66	1966-67	1967-68	1968-69	
Classroom teachers	$ 7,819	$ 8,213	$ 8,611	$ 9,025	$ 9,788	$10,530	$11,254	43.9%
Supervisory personnel assigned to individual buildings								
Supervising principals								
Elementary	10,597	11,345	11,732	12,499	13,295	14,378	15,428	45.6
Junior high	11,297	11,981	12,301	13,115	14,058	15,120	16,289	44.2
Senior high	12,064	12,682	13,236	14,062	14,973	16,188	17,408	44.3
Assistant principals								
Elementary	9,882	10,129	10,649	11,316	12,027	12,825	13,596	37.5
Junior high	10,186	10,419	10,820	11,460	12,120	13,207	14,128	38.7
Senior high	10,298	10,770	11,298	11,889	12,656	13,776	14,766	43.4
Counselors	9,094	9,183	9,421	10,314	10,960	11,844	12,525	37.7
Central-office admnistrators								
Supervisors	11,040	12,286	11,756	12,469	13,572	14,492	15,716	42.4
Consultants and/or coordinators	. .	. .	. .	. .	13,938	15,094	16,140	. .
Directors	13,043	13,520	14,184	14,853	16,011	17,061	18,252	39.9
Assistant superintendents	15,990	16,669	17,675	18,415	19,246	20,466	21,746	36.0

*Highest salaries scheduled, exclusive of long-service increments or special supplements.
†From NEA Research Bulletin, May, 1969, p. 42.

tive terms. They are able to see into the future and plan a course of action with an open mind. They recognize problems in order of importance, are able to analyze a situation, develop various plans of action, and reach logical conclusions. They have the ability to organize.

Integrity

One of the most important qualifications of any administrator is integrity. Whether or not a leader can inspire the staff, have their cooperation, and achieve the purposes of the organization will depend to a great degree upon his or her integrity. Everyone likes to feel that an administrator is honest and sincere, keeps promises, can be trusted with confidential information, and is an individual in whom one has faith. Such confidence cannot emanate from administrators unless they have integrity. Failure to fulfill this one qualification will result in low morale and an inefficient organization.

Ability to instill good human relations

Ray O. Duncan, former president of the American Association for Health, Physical Education, and Recreation (AAHPER), suggested the following as considerations for administrators: be friendly and considerate, be alert to the opinions of others, be careful what you say and how you say it, be honest and fair, be wise enough to weigh and decide, be able to tolerate human failings and inefficiency, be able to acquire humility, and plan well for staff meetings.

The ability to get along with associates in work is an essential qualification for an administrator. Only through cooperative effort is it possible for an organization to achieve its goals. This cooperative effort is greatest when the individuals responsible for the coordination of human efforts have the welfare of the various members of the organization at heart. This means that an administrator must be able to con-

vert the abilities of many individuals into coordinated effort. This is done in many ways. Some of these methods include setting a good example, inspiring confidence, selecting proper incentives, possessing poise, making the right decisions in tense moments, having an impersonal attitude, cooperating and helping others when necessary, and developing and practicing ethical standards. The administrator must be adept at the art of persuasion, which takes into consideration such important items as the points of view, interests, and other factors characterizing those to be persuaded.

There is very little associated effort without leadership. The administrator must be a leader and possess the attributes and qualities that people expect if they are to follow and contribute their best to achieve the purposes for which the organization has been established.

Ability to make decisions

The administrator must be able to make decisions when the situation necessitates such action. This presumes an understanding of what constitutes the important and the unimportant in the particular situation that is in question, the ability to foresee future developments and the results of a decision, and a knowledge of what is reasonable and what is unreasonable. It also assumes knowledge as to what is in the best interests of the organization and what is not, and what has the best chance for success and what has the least chance.

Decision is essential in order to accomplish objectives at the most opportune time. The administrator should have the capacity and be willing to make a decision. Many times if a decision is not forthcoming lethargy, suspense, and poor morale are created. The administrator who procrastinates beyond a reasonable time, is afraid of making the wrong decision, thinks only of his or her own security, and is oblivious to the organization's needs

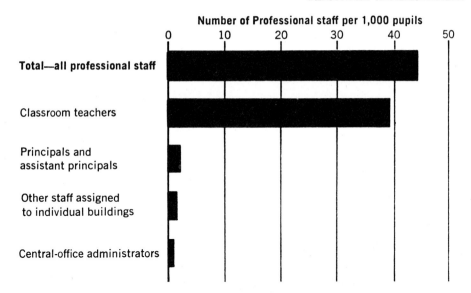

Professional employees per 1,000 pupils. (From NEA Research Bulletin **43**:77, 1965.)

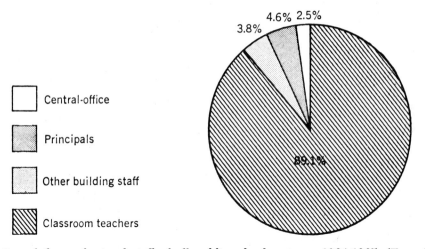

Distribution of the professional staff of all public school systems, 1964-1965. (From NEA Research Bulletin **43**:77, 1965.)

should never hold an administrative position.

Health and fitness for the job

Good health and physical fitness are essentials for the administrator. They often have a bearing on making the right decisions. Socrates once said that people in a state of bad health often made the wrong decisions in regard to affairs of state. Jennings, the famous biologist, pointed out

that the body can attend to only one thing at a time. Therefore, if attention is focused on a pain in the chest, a stomach ailment, or a nervous condition, it is difficult to focus it on the functions that an administrator must perform. Poor health may cause poor administration.

Vitality and endurance are essential to the administrator. They affect one's manner, personality, attractiveness, and disposition. Administrative duties often require long hours of tedious work under the most trying conditions. Failure to have the necessary strength and endurance under such conditions could mean the inability to perform tasks that are essential to the welfare of the organization. Members of an organization have confidence in those administrators who watch over their interests at all times. It is possible for an administrator to retain this confidence continuously only if he or she is in good health and physically fit to perform arduous duties.

When considering health and fitness for the job, it is important to recognize the many facets of health. The administrator should possess not only physical but also mental, emotional, and social health. Emotional stability, especially, is a must.

Willingness to accept responsibility

Every administrator must be willing to accept responsibility. There are duties to be performed that greatly influence the welfare of many individuals. Plans have to be fulfilled if the purposes of the organization are to be accomplished. Action is required to ensure production and render services. The person who accepts an administrative job is morally bound to assume the responsibility that is part and parcel of that position. A good administrator will experience a feeling of dissatisfaction whenever hc fails to meet responsibilities.

Understanding of work

The administrator will benefit from having a thorough understanding of the specialized work in which the organization is engaged. If it concerns a particular industry, it will be an advantage to know the production process from the ground up. If it is government, knowledge of related legislative, executive, and judicial aspects will help. If it is education, familiarity with that particular field will be an asset. If it is a specialized field within education or other area, it is necessary to have a knowledge of the particular specialty and also the part it plays in the total educational process. It is difficult to guide purposefully unless the individual knows his particular educational specialty and how it relates to other subject-matter areas. One often reads about the Congressman who was once a page in the Senate, the railroad executive who was a yard worker, the bank president who started as a bookkeeper, and the superintendent of schools who many years before started as a teacher. The technical knowledge and understanding of the total functioning of an organization are best gained through firsthand experience. An administrator will find that detailed knowledge of an organization's work is of great help in successfully guiding its operations.

Command of administrative technique

Administrative technique in many ways is similar to the first qualification listed —administrative mind. There is one essential difference. Administrative mind refers more to the "know how" and temperament of the individual, whereas *administrative technique* refers to the application of this knowledge and ability. An individual who possesses this quality can plan and budget his or her time and effort and also the time and work of others, in the most effective way possible. Time is not spent on details when more important work should be done. Tasks arc performed in a relaxed, efficient, calm, and logical manner. Work is accomplished in conformance with established standards. Duties are effectively executed, including those that involve strong pressure and great amounts of time. Resources for performing the job are utilized.

It has been said there are three conditions that burn out an administrator in a short length of time: performing his own duties in a tense, highly emotional manner, performing too many details, and being part of an organization that is not considerate of its administrators.

Intellectual capacity

Intellectual capacity in itself will not guarantee a good administrator. In fact, the so-called intellectual often makes a very poor administrator. Such traits as absent-mindedness and tardiness are often not compatible with acceptance of responsibility. The intellectual sometimes cannot make decisions because he visualizes so many sides of an issue. Furthermore, such an individual is often not interested in people but in books, figures, or other data instead. This makes a poor leader since lack of interest in human beings results in poor followership.

However, one should not gain from this discussion that intellectual capacity should be disregarded. To be a good administrator one must be intellectually competent. One should be able to think and reason logically, to apply knowledge effectively, to communicate efficiently, and to possess other factors that are closely allied to the intellectual process. There have been many so-called "brains" who failed miserably as administrators, whereas most good administrators can be classified as at least average in respect to their intellectual capacities.

Space has not permitted a discussion of all the qualifications of the administrator. Others, such as courage and initiative, are also important. There is in addition the ability to be an ambassador for the organization. Liaison work with higher echelon groups in the organization and also with outside groups is important. It is necessary at times to stand up and fight for one's own department or division. To a great degree this will determine whether it is respected and has equal status with other administrative divisions.

THE ADMINISTRATOR AS A LEADER

In the last 25 years research findings have indicated that some beliefs, such as certain qualities per se indicate who the leaders are, that leaders are born and not made, and that some of us will lead and others will follow, are not exactly true. Instead, in recent years research seems to indicate that personal characteristics must be related to the characteristics of the followers, because of the interaction of the two that takes place. The identification of qualities of certain individuals as leaders without relating these qualities to the persons they are going to try to lead has little meaning.

Stogdill* studied the relationship of personality factors to leadership and found that the leader of a group exceeds the average of the group in respect to such characteristics as intelligence, scholarship, acceptance of responsibility, participation, and socioeconomic status.

Berelson and Steiner† surveyed the scientific findings in the behaviorial sciences and formulated some propositions and hypotheses relating to leadership. In essence some of these are as follows:

1. The closer an individual conforms to the accepted norms of the group, the better liked he will be; the better liked he is, the closer he conforms; the less he conforms, the more disliked he will be.
2. The higher the rank of the member within the group, the more central he will be in the group's interaction and the more influential he will be.
3. In general, the "style" of the leader is determined more by the expectations of the membership and the requirements of the situation than by the personal traits of the leader himself.
4. The leadership of the group tends to be vested in the member who most closely conforms to the standards of the group of the matter in question or who has the most information and skill related to the activities of the group.
5. When groups have established norms, it is extremely difficult for a new leader, however capable, to shift the group's activities.

*Stogdill, R. M.: Personal factors associated with leadership, a survey of the literature, Journal of Psychology **25**:63, 1948.

†Berelson, B., and Steiner, G. A.: Human behavior: an inventory of scientific findings, New York, 1964, Harcourt, Brace & World, Inc., pp. 341-344.

6. The longer the life of the leadership, the less open and free the communication within the group and probably the less efficient the group in the solution of new problems.
7. The leader will be followed more faithfully the more he makes it possible for the members to achieve their private goals along with the group goals.
8. Active leadership is characteristic of groups that determine their own activities, passive leadership of groups whose activities are externally imposed.
9. In a small group, authoritarian leadership is less effective than democratic leadership in holding the group together and getting its work done.

Other studies that provide pertinent information on leadership include those of Myers,[*] Hemphill,[†] Homans,[‡] and Halpin.[§]

The physical educator or health educator who desires to exercise a leadership role in his or her organization should study the administrative theory reflected in the research studies available on this subject. This will help to better assure success as a leader in any particular situation.

MAJOR ADMINISTRATIVE DUTIES

Gulick and Urwick[‖] have utilized the word POSDCORB to outline the functions of an administrator. This is based on Henri Fayol's work, *Industrial and General Ad-*

---

[*]Myers, R. B.: The development and implications of a conception for leadership education, Unpublished doctoral dissertation, University of Florida, 1954.

[†]Hemphill, J. K.: Administration as problem solving. In Halpin, A. W., editor: Administrative theory in education, Chicago, 1958, Midwest Administration Center, University of Chicago.

[‡]Homans, G. C.: The human group, New York, 1950, Harcourt, Brace and World, Inc.

[§]Halpin, A. W.: A paradigm for the study of administrative research in education. In Campbell, N. R., and Gregg, R. T., editors: Administrative behavior in education, New York, 1957, Harper & Row, Publishers.

[‖]Gulick, L., and Urwick, L., editors: Papers on the science of administration, New York, 1937, Institute of Public Administration.

ministration. An organization of duties under these major headings is apropos to the section under discussion although the semantics of the subject in some cases is not appropriate to modern administration. POSDCORB refers to the functional elements of (1) planning, (2) organizing, (3) staffing, (4) directing, (5) coordinating, (6) reporting, and (7) budgeting.

Planning

Planning is the process of outlining the work that is to be performed, in a logical and purposeful manner, together with the methods that are to be utilized in the performance of this work. The total plan will result in the accomplishment of the purposes for which the organization is established. Of course this implies a clear conception of the aims of the organization.

In order to accomplish this planning, the administrator must have vision to look into the future and to prepare for what he sees. He must see the influences that will affect the organization and the requirements that will have to be met.

Organizing

Organizing refers to the development of the formal structure of the organization, whereby the various administrative coordinating centers and subdivisions of work are arranged in an integrated manner, with clearly defined lines of authority. The purpose behind this structure is the effective accomplishment of established objectives. Organizational charts aid in clarifying such organization.

This formal structure should be set up in a manner that avoids red tape and provides for the clear assignment of every necessary duty to some responsible individual. Whenever possible, standards should be established for acceptable performance for each duty assignment.

The coordinating centers of authority are developed and organized chiefly on the basis of the work to be done by the organization, services performed, individuals available in the light of incentives offered, and efficiency of operation. A single administrator cannot perform all the functions necessary, except in the smallest organizations. Hence, responsibility must be assigned to others in a logical manner. These individuals occupy positions along the line, each position being broken down in terms of its own area of specialization. The higher up the line one goes, the more general is the responsibility; the lower down the line one goes, the more specific is the responsibility.

Staffing

The administrative duty of staffing refers to the entire personnel function of selection, assignment, training, and providing and maintaining favorable working conditions for all members of the organization. The administrator must have a thorough knowledge of the staff. He or she must select with care and ensure that each subdivision in the organization has a competent leader and that each employee is assigned to the job where he can be of greatest service. Personnel should possess energy, initiative, and loyalty. The duties of each position must be clearly outlined. All members of the organization must be encouraged to utilize their own initiative. They should be rewarded fairly for their services. The mistakes and blunders of employees must be brought to their attention and dealt with accordingly. Vested interests of individual employees must not be allowed to endanger the general interests of all. The conditions of work should be made as pleasant and as nearly ideal as possible. Both physical and social factors should be provided for. Services rendered by the individual increase as the conditions under which he works improve.

Directing

Directing is a responsibility that falls to the administrator as the leader. He or she must direct the operations of the organization. This means distinct and precise decisions must be made and embodied in instructions that will ensure their completion. The administrator must direct the work in an impersonal manner, avoid becoming involved in too many details, and see that the organization's purpose is fulfilled according to established principles. Executives have a duty to see that the quantity and quality of performance of each employee are maintained.

The administrator is a leader. His or her success is determined by his ability to guide others successfully toward established goals. Individuals of weak responsibility and limited capability cannot perform this function successfully. The good administrator must be superior in determination, persistence, endurance, and courage. He must clearly understand his organization's purposes and keep them in mind as he guides and leads the way. Through direction, it is essential that faith be created in the cooperative enterprise, in success, in achievement of personal ambitions, in the integrity of the leadership provided, and in the superiority of associated efforts.

Coordinating

Coordinating means interrelating all the various phases of work within an organization. This means that the organization's structure must clearly provide for close relationships and competent leadership in the coordinating centers of activity. The administrator must meet regularly with chief assistants. Here arrangements can be made for unity of effort, reports can be submitted on progress, and obstacles to coordinated work can be eliminated. Good coordination also means that all factors must be considered in their proper perspective.

This duty requires the development of a faith that runs throughout the organization. Coordination can be effective only if there is faith in the enterprise and in the need for coordinated effort. Faith is the motivating factor that stimulates human beings to continue rendering service so that goals may be accomplished.

There should also be coordination with administrative units outside the organization where such responsibilities are necessary.

Reporting

Reporting is the administrative duty of supplying information to administrators or executives higher up on the line of authority or to other groups to which one is responsible. It also means that subordinates must be kept informed through regular reports, research, and continual observation. In this respect the administrator is a point of intercommunication. In addition to accepting the responsibility for reporting to higher authority, he must continually know what is going on in the area under his jurisdiction. Members of the organization must be informed on many topics of general interest, such as goals to be achieved, progress being made, strong and weak points, and new areas proposed for development. This information will come from various members of the organization.

Budgeting

As the word implies, budgeting refers to financial planning and accounting. It is the duty of the administrator to allocate to various subdivisions the general funds allotted to the organization. This must be done in a manner that is equitable and just. In carrying out this function, he must keep the organization's purposes in mind and apportion the available money to those areas or projects that will help most in achieving these purposes. It also means that controls must be established to ensure that certain limits will be observed, so-called budget padding will be kept to a minimum, and complete integrity in the handling of all the budgetary aspects of the organization will be maintained.

QUALIFICATIONS OF HEALTH AND PHYSICAL EDUCATORS

The most important consideration in administration is personnel. The members of an organization determine whether it will succeed or fail. Administration must take into account the qualifications of health and physical educators, factors that promote cooperation, principles of good human relations, the fallacy of final authority, the importance of decisiveness, the need for good staff morale, and other principles to be observed in personnel management.

Qualifications for health educators

The qualifications of health educators based on the recommendations from five national conferences on professional preparation as presented in adapted form are as follows*:

Health education

Knowledge of (1) what constitutes well-balanced and well-functioned health teaching and (2) implications of different age and developmental levels of human beings for teaching health and also for curricular organization of materials.

Skill in (1) detecting health interests and needs and motivating students to achieve and maintain an optimum level of personal health and (2) selecting and using acceptable methods, materials, and resources for health education as well as skill in health counseling.

School health services

Knowledge of the roles played by various professional health personnel in the referral and follow-up duties of teachers and the opportunities afforded in school health services for health education.

Skill in establishing school health policies for various health services, such as emergency care, observing children for deviations from good health, using screening techniques and health records, encouraging health corrections, and cooperating with home and community in child health problems.

---

*Preparing the health teacher, recommendations from five national conferences on professional preparation, Washington, D. C., 1961, American Association for Health, Physical Education, and Recreation, p. 26.

Healthful school living

Awareness of opportunities that exist in the school environment for the teaching of health, the relationship of facilities and other aspects of the physical environment to health, and the relationship of discipline, promotion, and other such practices to psychologic health.

Skill in the improvement of environmental conditions, the development of potentialities of the school lunch program as a medium of education, and the application of sound mental health principles to the school setting.

The personality of the health educator is of particular concern. The individual must be well adjusted and well integrated emotionally, mentally, and physically if he or she is to do a good job in developing these characteristics in others. Such a person must also be interested in human beings and possess skill and understanding in human relations so that health objectives may be realized.

It is very important that the health educator have a mastery of certain scientific knowledge and specialized skills and have proper attitudes. Such knowledge, skills, and attitudes will help the health educator identify the health needs and interests of individuals with whom he comes in contact, provide a health program that will meet these needs and interests, and promote the profession so that human lives may be enriched. This means that many experiences should be included in the training of persons entering this specialized field. These experiences can be divided into general education, professional education, and specialized education.

General education experiences should provide knowledge and skill in the communicative arts, understanding in sociologic principles, an appreciation of the history of various peoples with their social, racial, and cultural characteristics, and the fine and practical arts that afford a means of expression, a means of releasing the emotions, a medium for richer understanding of life, and a medium for promoting mental health. The behavioral sciences are espe-

cially important for the health educator. The science area is also very important to the health educator and should include anatomy and kinesiology, physiology, bacteriology, biology, zoology, chemistry, physics, and also such behavioral sciences as child and adolescent psychology, human growth and development, general psychology, mental hygiene, and sociology.

In professional education it is important for the health educator to have a mastery of the philosophies, techniques, principles, and evaluative procedures that are characteristic of the most advanced and best thinking in education.

The specialized health education area should include personal and community health, nutrition, family and child health, first aid and safety, sex education, drugs and narcotics, tobacco and alcohol, methods and materials, organization and administration of school health programs, public health, including the basic principles of environmental sanitation and ecology, communicable disease control, and health counseling. The qualifications for teachers of health to be certified in New Jersey are listed on p. 102.

Qualifications for physical educators

The following are some special qualifications of the physical educator.

The physical educator should be a graduate of an approved teacher training institution that prepares teachers for physical education. The college or university should be selected with care.

Since physical education is based upon the foundational sciences of anatomy, physiology, biology, kinesiology, sociology, and psychology, the leader in this field should be well versed in these areas.

The general education of physical educators is under continuous scrutiny and criticism. Speech, knowledge of world affairs, mastery of the arts, and other aspects of this area are important in the preparation of the physical educator. Since his

HEALTH EDUCATION

AUTHORIZATION. This certificate is required for teaching health education in the elementary and secondary schools.

REQUIREMENTS

I. A bachelor's degree based upon a four-year curriculum in an accredited college

II. Successful completion of *one* of the following:

    A. A college curriculum approved by the New Jersey State Department of Education as the basis for issuing this certificate

OR

    B. A program of college studies including:

general background

    1. A total of thirty semester-hour credits in *general background* courses distributed in at least three of the following fields: English, social studies, science, fine arts, mathematics, and foreign languages. Six semester-hour credits in English and six in social studies will be required.

    2. A minimum of eighteen semester-hour credits in *professional education* courses distributed over four or more of the following groups including at least one course in each starred area. A maximum of three semester-hour credits will be accepted in health education. These eighteen credits do not include student teaching.

       * Methods of teaching health education

professional education

       * Educational psychology. This group includes such courses as psychology of learning, human growth and development, adolescent psychology, educational measurements, and mental hygiene.

       * Health education. A maximum of three semester-hour credits will be accepted in this area. This group includes such courses as personal health problems, school health problems, nutrition, health administration, and biology.

       Curriculum. This group includes such courses as principles of curriculum construction, the high school curriculum, a study of the curriculum in the specific field, and extracurricular activities.

       Foundations of education. This group includes such courses as history of education, principles of education, philosophy of education, comparative education, and educational sociology.

       Guidance. This group includes such courses as principles of guidance, counseling, vocational guidance, educational guidance, research in guidance, and student personnel problems.

    3. A minimum of forty semester-hour credits in the *field of specialization* distributed among the following four areas, and covering both the elementary and secondary fields, with major emphasis on health education.

       Bacteriology, biology, and chemistry

       Psychology and sociology, including mental hygiene, adolescent psychology, sociology, and educational sociology

specialized field

       Health education, including anatomy, physiology, child growth and development, personal and community health, foods and nutrition, health aspects of home and family life, health counseling, safety and first aid, and organization, administration, and supervision of school health programs

       Methods of teaching, including a study of the public school health education curriculum

student teaching

    4. One hundred and fifty clock hours of *approved student teaching*. At least ninety clock hours must be devoted to responsible classroom teaching; sixty clock hours may be employed in observation and participation. This requirement is in addition to the eighteen credits in professional education.

PHYSICAL EDUCATION

AUTHORIZATION. This certificate is required for teaching physical education in elementary and secondary schools. (Health education shall be included in this authorization if the curriculum contains at least eighteen semester-hour credits in this field.)

REQUIREMENTS

I. A bachelor's degree based upon a four-year curriculum in an accredited college

II. Successful completion of *one* of the following:

A. A college curriculum approved by the New Jersey State Department of Education as the basis for issuing this certificate

OR

B. A program of college studies including:

general background
1. A minimum of thirty semester-hour credits in *general background* courses distributed in at least three of the following fields: English, social studies, science, fine arts, mathematics, and foreign languages. Six semester-hour credits in English and six in social studies are required.

professional education
2. A minimum of eighteeen semester-hour credits in *professional education* courses distributed over four or more of the following groups, including at least one course in each starred area. A maximum of three semester-hour credits will be accepted in health education. These eighteen credits do not include student teaching.

* Methods of teaching physical education in elementary and secondary schools

* Educational psychology. This group includes such courses as psychology of learning, human growth and development, adolescent psychology, educational measurements, and mental hygiene.

* Health education. A maximum of three semester-hour credits will be accepted in this area. This group includes such courses as personal health problems, school health problems, nutrition, health administration, and biology.

Curriculum. This group includes such courses as principles of curriculum construction, the high school curriculum, a study of the curriculum in the field of specialization, and extracurricular activities.

Foundations of education. This group includes such courses as history of education, principles of education, philosophy of education, comparative education, and educational sociology.

Guidance. This group includes such courses as principles of guidance, counseling, vocational guidance, educational guidance, research in guidance, and student personnel problems.

student teaching
3. One hundred and fifty clock hours of *approved student teaching*. At least ninety clock hours must be devoted to responsible classroom teaching; sixty clock hours may be employed in observation and participation. This requirement is in addition to the eighteen credits in professional education.

4. A minimum of forty semester-hour credits in the *field of specialization*, distributed among the following areas and covering both the elementary and secondary fields:

Anatomy, physiology, kinesiology

Coaching, development of personal skills, nature and function of play

History, principles, and organization and administration of physical education

specialized field
Materials and methods in physical education for the elementary grades and materials and methods in physical education for the high school

Health education including personal and community hygiene, first aid, and safety position requires frequent appearances in public, adequate knowledge and skill in the art of communication are essential.

Physical education work is strenuous and therefore demands that members of the profession be in a state of buoyant, robust health in order that they may carry out their duties with efficiency and regularity. It should also be remembered that physical educators are supposed to build healthy bodies. Therefore, they should be a good testimonial for their preachments.

Many moral and spiritual values are developed through participation in games and other physical education activities. It is essential, therefore, that the teacher of physical education have a proper background and possess such qualities that he or she will stress fair play, good sportsmanship, and a sound standard of values. The nature of his or her leadership should be such that the highest standards of moral and spiritual values are developed.

The physical educator should have a sincere interest in the teaching of physical education. Unless the individual has a firm belief in the value of his work and a desire to help extend the benefits of such an endeavor to others, he will not be an asset to the profession. A sincere interest in the teaching of physical education means that one enjoys teaching individuals, participating in the gamut of activities incorporated in such programs, helping others to realize the happiness and thrilling experiences of participation that he himself enjoys, and helping to develop citizenship traits conducive to democratic living. One must have a sincere love of the out-of-doors and of all the activities that make up the physical education program either indoors or out in the open. This means that anyone interested in physical education should enjoy sports and other activities. If there is not a liking for these activities, the individual is in the wrong profession.

The physical educator should possess an acceptable standard of motor ability. Physical skills are basic to the profession. To be able to teach various games and activities to others, it is necessary to have skill in many of them. The physical educator must enjoy working with people, with whom there is continuous association in an informal atmosphere when teaching physical education activities. The values of such a program will be greatly increased if the physical educator teaches in a manner conducive to happiness, cooperation, and a spirit of friendship. The qualifica-

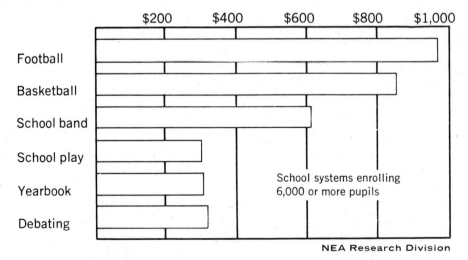

Average maximum annual salary supplements 1967-1968 for the physical educator qualified to coach selected pupil-participating activities. (From NEA Research Bulletin **46:**79, 1968.)

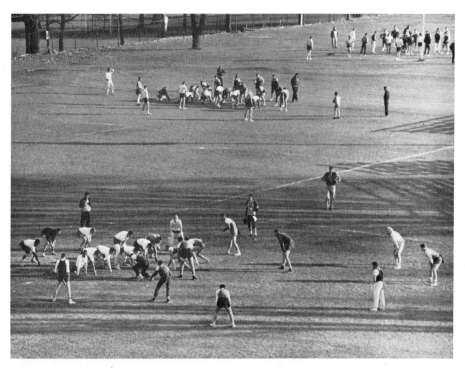

Freshman majors in health and physical education at Illinois State University working in flag football under the direction of experienced faculty members.

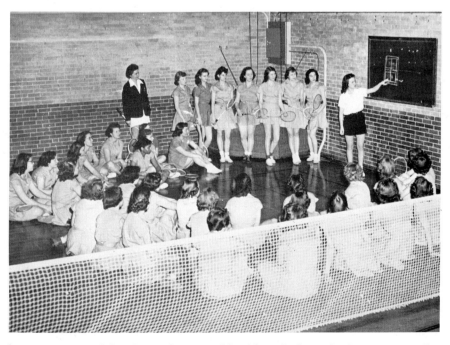

Leadership is an essential for the professions of health and physical education. An Illinois State University senior gives a demonstration lesson on badminton to a group of high school girls. Observing in the background is the supervising staff member.

HOW DO YOU MEASURE UP AS A MEMBER OF THE UNITED TEACHING PROFESSION?*

As a first step in determining your professional stature, place a check mark beside the questions you can answer *yes*.

As an individual, do you—

_____Join the united teaching profession — local, state, and national associations — and promote unified professional membership among your colleagues?

_____View your dues as an investment in your profession rather than just another expense?

_____Believe that being a member of the united teaching profession involves more than paying dues — that it includes participating actively, familiarizing yourself with the objectives of your associations, sharing in goal setting, and being a change agent?

_____Identify with your positional organizations (classroom teachers, principals, supervisors, or administrators)?

_____Identify with the associations representing your subject matter area?

_____Keep informed on educational issues through professional journals?

_____Abide by the Code of Ethics of the Education Profession?

_____Participate in political action by discussing issues, campaigning for candidates, and running for offices if you are so inclined?

_____Inform yourself about the economic benefits which may be offered by your local and state organizations?

_____Credit union__Life insurance__Health and accident insurance__Personal liability insurance__Income protection insurance__Tax-deferred annuity program__Installment financing__Home mortgage loans__Discount buying

As a member of your local association, do you—

_____Attend meetings?

_____Volunteer for assignments?

_____Accept committee appointments?

_____Participate in in-service education programs?

_____Lend your efforts in negotiations with the school board by contributing your ideas, serving on the negotiating team, or working on supportive committees?

_____Have a thorough knowledge of grievance procedures so that you can help in referring aggrieved colleagues to the proper persons?

_____Defend teacher rights?

_____Do your part to see to it that classroom teachers, as the largest segment of your association, have an impact commensurate with their number?

_____Work for minority-group involvement in your association program?

_____Reach out to the new teacher, acquaint him with your association's services, encourage him to participate in its activities, and accept him as a member of the team?

_____Support candidates for professional offices who have a record of service to the association; who are committed to the association's goals rather than to their own personal advancement; who speak for the membership?

_____Encourage your association to work with Student NEA chapters in nearby colleges?

_____Promote the Future Teachers of America by supporting FTA chapters and by serving as a sponsor?

_____Make sure your association is represented at meetings of your state education association as well as at those of the state classroom teachers association?

_____Make sure that your association uses its full quota of delegates to the Representative Assemblies of the NEA and of its Association of Classroom Teachers?

_____Serve as a delegate to state and national conventions if named?

*From Heflin, J.: How do you measure up? Today's Education, NEA Journal 5:64, 1969.

HOW DO YOU MEASURE UP AS A MEMBER OF THE UNITED TEACHING PROFESSION?—cont'd

As a member of the state association, do you—

_____Participate in state and regional meetings?

_____Accept committee assignments?

_____Prepare yourself for office?

_____Read your state association journal and newsletter?

_____Keep abreast of progress in your state association's legislative program?

_____Vote for candidates for public offices who are favorable to the state legislative program?

_____Join your state positional association?

_____Familiarize yourself with its program and services?

As a member of the National Education Association, do you—

_____Make your influence felt in the NEA Representative Assembly by studying NEA resolutions and reports and discussing them with delegates?

_____Attend regional and national conferences?

_____Identify with the Association of Classroom Teachers or your positional association and take advantage of its services?

_____Read TODAY'S EDUCATION and the *NEA Reporter*?

_____Support the NEA DuShane Emergency Fund?

_____Inform yourself and your colleagues about NEA services?

   __Life insurance__Accident insurance__Tax-deferred annuity program__NEA Mutual Fund__Auto leasing__Research__Publications and other materials__Field service__Salary and negotiation consultant services__Instructional activities__Legislative work __Travel program__Job referral service__Public relations__Promotion of high standards of teacher preparation, certification, and performance__Protection of professional, civil, and human rights

Next, write the names of the following in the blanks provided:

Your local association president_____

Your state education association president_____

The president of your state association of classroom teachers or of your positional association_____

Your NEA state director(s)_____

The NEA president_____

The president of NEA's Association of Classroom Teachers or of your positional association

_____

The NEA executive secretary_____

The NEA headquarters city_____

See how you measure up as a member of the united teaching profession.

tions for teachers of physical education to be certified in New Jersey are listed on p. 103.

QUALITIES THAT MAKE FOR SUCCESSFUL TEACHING

Several persons were interviewed as to the qualities and characteristics they thought existed in the best teachers to whom they were exposed. A list of those qualities that were mentioned most frequently are as follows:

1. Teacher knew his subject matter well.
2. Teacher took a personal interest in each student.
3. Teacher was well respected and respected his students.
4. Teacher stimulated his students to think.
5. Teacher was interesting and made his subject matter come to life.

6. Teacher was an original thinker and creative in his methods.
7. Teacher was a fine speaker, presented a neat experience, and was generally well groomed.
8. Teacher had a good sense of humor.
9. Teacher was fair and honest in his dealings with his students.
10. Teacher was understanding and kind.

PROBLEMS OF BEGINNING TEACHERS

Beginning teachers need considerable encouragement and help. The administration should be aware of this need and work to ensure that it is met. As a guide to some of the problems of beginning teachers, a survey of fifty teachers indicated the following:

1. Difficulties arising as a result of the lack of facilities
2. Large size of classes, making it difficult to teach effectively
3. Teaching assignments in addition to the primary responsibility of teaching health education or physical education
4. Discipline problems with students
5. Conflicting methodology between what the beginning teacher was taught in professional preparing institution and established patterns of experienced teachers
6. Clerical work—difficulty in keeping records up to date
7. Problems encountered in obtaining books and supplies
8. Problems encountered in obtaining cooperative attitude from other teachers
9. Lack of departmental meetings to discuss common problems
10. Failure to find time for personal recreation

WORKING EFFECTIVELY WITH GENERAL SCHOOL AND COLLEGE ADMINISTRATORS

School and college health and physical education programs are part of general education. Consequently, such items as the budgets allocated, facilities provided, and personnel appointed are subject to the thinking and decisions of general educators. Presidents of colleges, deans, superintendents of schools, principals, and administrators of instructional and business services, through their decisions and actions, affect these special programs in elementary and secondary schools and in colleges and universities of the nation. It is therefore important to get the thinking of these general administrators in respect to programs of school health, physical education, and recreation. The information that follows was taken from a review of general administration books and interviews with general administrators for the purpose of determining what constitutes effective working relationships between general school administrators and health and physical educators.

What constitutes effective working relations between general school administrators and health and physical educators?

Effective working relationships between general administrators and health and physical educators may be discussed under the headings of (1) responsibilities of gen-

Table 5-2. Major problems of teachers*

	Urban	Suburban	Rural
Large class size	40.4%	33.4%	30.6%
Classroom management and discipline	23.3	10.8	12.1
Inadequate assistance from specialized teachers	22.5	21.0	30.3
Inadequate salary	34.9	24.5	30.3
Inadequate fringe benefits	27.7	22.3	31.3
Ineffective grouping of students into classes	24.3	18.2	24.2
Lack of public support for schools	27.8	17.4	23.7
Ineffective testing and guidance program	21.1	14.2	20.8

*From NEA Research Bulletin 46:116, 1968.

eral administrators, (2) responsibilities of health and physical educators, (3) common points of conflict, and (4) checklist for effective working relationships.

Some responsibilities of general administrators. There are many responsibilities of general administrators that have an impact upon good working relationships. A few of the more important are listed in the following paragraphs:

1. *Administrators should possess a sound understanding of human nature so as to work effectively with people.* General administrators should not look upon the administrative process in an impersonal manner but, instead, should always keep in mind the human dimensions. As such, human problems should be given high priority.

2. *Administrators should understand their own administrative behavior.* They should see conflicts where they exist and not fabricate them where they do not exist. They should give an accurate account of group expectations although they may not be in agreement with them. They should recognize the differences and rationale between their own views and those of other people.

3. *Administrators should exercise wisely the authority vested in the administrative position.* The authority goes with the office and not with the person. Administrators should recognize that the administrative position exists to further the goals of the school system and the education of children and youth. It should never be used as a personal vendetta.

4. *Administrators should establish effective means of communication among members of the school system.* Opportunities should be readily available for a discussion of personal and/or professional problems, new ideas, and ways of improving the effective functioning of the organization.

5. *Administrators should provide maximum opportunity for personal self-fulfillment.* Each person has a basic psychologic need of being recognized, having self-respect, and possessing a feeling of belonging. Within organization requirements, general administrators should make this possible for each teacher on the job and every member of the school organization, regardless of subject area or job role.

6. *Administrators should provide leadership.* General administrators speak for their schools. They are the acknowledged leaders both in the internal and external functioning of the educational program. Such responsibility implies leadership qualities that will bring out the best individual effort on the part of each member of the staff and a total coordinated endeavor working toward common goals.

7. *Administrators should provide clearcut policies and procedures.* Policies and procedures are essential to efficient functioning of the school organization; therefore, they should be carefully developed, thoroughly discussed with members who are concerned, put in written form in clear concise language, and then followed.

8. *Administrators should plan meaningful faculty meetings.* Meetings of the staff should be carefully planned and efficiently conducted. Meetings should not, as a regular rule, be called on impulse and dominated by the general administrator. Plans and procedures agreed upon should be carried out.

9. *Administrators should make promotions on the basis of merit with an absence of politics and favoritism.* Promotions should be arrived at through a careful evaluation of each faculty member's qualifications and objective criteria.

10. *Administrators should protect and enhance the mental and physical health of the faculty and staff.* In carrying out this responsibility the general administrator should eliminate petty annoyances and worries that can weigh heavily upon staff members, attempt to increase the satisfactions that each person derives from the or-

ganization, promote friendly relationships, develop an esprit de corps, improve respect for and social status of staff members in the community, and establish a climate of understanding that promotes goodwill.

Some responsibilities of health and physical educators. All the responsibilities of health educators and physical educators cannot be discussed in the limited space available for this subject. A few of the more important responsibilities that affect good working relationships with general administrators are listed:

1. *Health and physical educators should lend thought and energy to supporting the total educational program.* Each staff member must see his or her responsibility to the total educational program. This means serving on committees, attending faculty meetings, contributing ideas, and giving support to worthy new developments regardless of the phase of the total program to which it belongs. Also, the staff member should view his or her own field of specialization in proper perspective with the total educational endeavor.

2. *Health and physical educators should take an interest in the administrative process.* Such interest can be tangibly shown by participating in policy making and decision making, doing some role playing as to the problems and pressures faced by the general administrator in his job, and contributing ideas that will help cut down on administrative red tape and thus streamline the educational process.

3. *Health and physical educators should carry out their individual responsibilities with dispatch and efficiency.* Each teacher or staff member has a job to do. If each job is performed effectively, the total school organization will function more efficiently. Only as each person assumes the responsibility for doing his or her own job in a responsible manner can the educational effort be accomplished effectively.

4. *Health and physical educators should get their reports in on time.* Purchase req-

uisitions, attendance, excuse, accident, and the multitude of other forms and reports that have to be completed and then collated in the general administrator's office must be done on time. Punctuality on the part of all staff members makes the general administrator's life much easier.

5. *Health and physical educators should be loyal to the administration.* Each staff member has the responsibility to be loyal to the administrators of his school organization. There can be differences of opinion and disagreement on the administrative process and the way it is conducted, but loyalty to the leaders is essential.

6. *Health and physical educators should observe proper administrative protocol.* Administrators do not appreciate a teacher going over their heads to a higher authority without their knowing about it. There are lines of authority that must be recognized and followed in every organization. Schools are no exception to the rule.

7. *Health and physical educators should be professional.* In relationships with colleagues, general administrators, or the public in general, a staff member should recognize that there is a professional way of behaving. Confidences are not betrayed, professional problems are ironed out with the people concerned, and personality conflicts are discussed with discretion.

Common points of conflict between general administrators and health and physical educators. Although there are many implications for conflict in the listing of responsibilities for general administrators and for health and physical educators, some additional areas where poor working relationships occur are listed as follows:

1. The failure on the part of general administrators to recognize health and physical educators as vital subjects of the academic and educational process
2. A failure on the part of general administrators to see health education and physical education as two distinct and separate fields
3. The existence of an authoritarian and un-

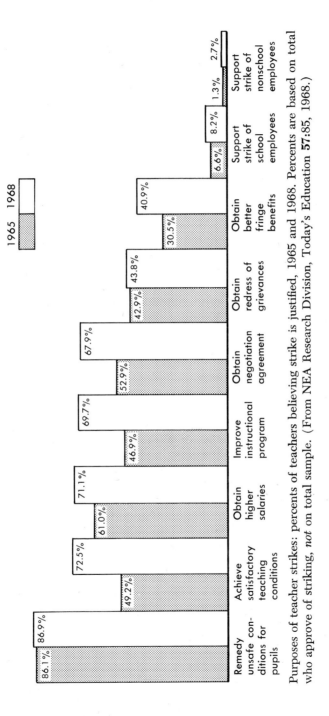

Purposes of teacher strikes: percents of teachers believing strike is justified, 1965 and 1968. Percents are based on total who approve of striking, *not* on total sample. (From NEA Research Division, Today's Education **57**:85, 1968.)

democratic administration with the general administrator ruling with an iron hand

4. The failure to outline clearly goals and responsibilities for the organization and for each member of the organization
5. The existence of some teachers' unions and organizations that obstruct rather than further the democratization of administration
6. The failure of general administrators to provide dynamic leadership
7. The failure of the administrator to provide clearly defined policies
8. The practice of administrators encroaching upon classes and schedules without good reason or adequate previous announcement
9. The assignment of unreasonable teaching loads and extra class assignments
10. The failure of teachers to read bulletins that contain important administrative announcements
11. The failure of teachers to conscientiously assume the duties and responsibilities associated with administrative routine, such as the checking of attendance
12. The failure of teachers to handle disciplinary cases properly
13. The existence of unsatisfactory plant, buildings, and working conditions
14. The lack of adequate teacher materials and equipment
15. Overemphasis upon athletics

What administrative groups worry about

The professional magazine, *Nation's Schools,** conducted an opinion poll to determine what schoolmen worry most

*Schoolmen worry most about teacher, money shortages, Nation's Schools 81:81, 1968.

about. A 4% sampling was done of 16,000 school administrators in 50 states that brought a 54% response. An 8% sampling was done of 8,000 school board members, which brought a 22% response. Presented here in adapted form are some of the main worries of school officials.

Superintendents of schools

Shortages of teachers
Inadequate funds
Militant teachers
Overcrowded conditions
Relations with school board
Transportation problems
Student problems of dress
Desegregation
New curricula
Community pressures
Use of drugs

School board members

Inadequate funds
Shortages of teachers
Militant teachers
Overcrowded conditions
Transportation problems
Relations with school administrators
Desegregation
Vandalism
Community pressures
New curricula
Student problems of dress
Use of drugs

CHECKLIST FOR EFFECTIVE WORKING RELATIONSHIPS BETWEEN GENERAL ADMINISTRATORS AND HEALTH AND PHYSICAL EDUCATORS

	Yes	No
1. Job descriptions of all school personnel are formulated, written, and disseminated to each individual involved.		
2. Policies are cooperatively formulated.	___	___
3. Teachers are encouraged to participate in the determination of policies. Administration utilizes committees of faculty to develop policies.	___	___
4. Policies cover priorities in the use of physical education facilities.	___	___
5. Policies have been developed and are in writing for the major areas of the educational enterprise as well as specifically for the fields of health education and physical education.	___	___

CHECKLIST FOR EFFECTIVE WORKING RELATIONSHIPS BETWEEN GENERAL ADMINISTRATORS AND HEALTH AND PHYSICAL EDUCATORS —cont'd

		Yes	No
6.	Departmental policies and procedures are up to date and complete.	___	___
7.	Board of education establishes and approves policies and programs.	___	___
8.	Health and physical educators know the policies for their school system and work within this framework.	___	___
9.	Open channels of communication are maintained between administrator and teacher.	___	___
10.	Inservice education is provided teachers.	___	___
11.	Teachers are encouraged to participate in the activities of professional organizations.	___	___
12.	Supervisors act in an advisory and not an administrative capacity.	___	___
13.	The teaching load of all teachers is equitable in that the following factors are considered: work hours per week, number of students per week, and number of after-school activities scheduled.	___	___
14.	Athletics are open to all students and conducted according to sound educational principles.	___	___
15.	Policies are in writing and disseminated and cover the organization and administration of varsity interscholastic athletics.	___	___
16.	Coaches are certified in physical education.	___	___
17.	The group process is effectively used in faculty and committee meetings.	___	___
18.	There is a strong belief in and a willingness to have a democratic administration.	___	___
19.	Faculty meetings are well organized.	___	___
20.	New staff members are oriented in respect to responsibilities, school policies, and other items essential to their effective functioning in the school system.	___	___
21.	Departmental budgets and other reports are submitted on time and in proper form.	___	___
22.	Staff members attend faculty meetings regularly.	___	___
23.	Staff members participate in curriculum studies.	___	___
24.	Classroom interruptions are kept to an absolute minimum.	___	___
25.	Proper administrative channels are followed.	___	___
26.	Relationships with colleagues are based on mutual integrity, understanding, and respect.	___	___
27.	The administration is interested in the human problems of the school organization.	___	___
28.	Maximum opportunity is provided for personal self-fulfillment consistent with organization requirements.	___	___
29.	Department heads are selected on the basis of qualifications rather than seniority.	___	___
30.	Staff members are enthusiastic about their work.	___	___
31.	All personnel are provided opportunities to contribute to the improved functioning of the school system.	___	___
32.	The school board's executive officer executes policy.	___	___
33.	Faculty and staff assignments are educationally sound.	___	___
34.	The administration works continually to improve the working conditions of school personnel.	___	___
35.	Out-of-class responsibilities are equitably distributed.	___	___
36.	The administration provides recreational and social outlets for the staff.	___	___
37.	The administration recognizes and records quality work.	___	___
38.	Health and physical educators seek to improve themselves professionally.	___	___

Continued.

CHECKLIST FOR EFFECTIVE WORKING RELATIONSHIPS BETWEEN
GENERAL ADMINISTRATORS AND HEALTH AND PHYSICAL EDUCATORS
—cont'd

	Yes	No
39. Health and physical educators view with proper perspective their special fields in the total educational enterprise.		
40. Health and physical educators organize and plan their programs so as to best meet the needs and interests of their students.		
41. Health and physical educators continually evaluate themselves and the professional job they are doing in the school system.		
42. Budgetary allocations are equitably made among departments.		
43. The administration is sensitive to the specific abilities and interests of teachers and staff.		
44. Health and physical educators take an active role in school planning.		
45. Health and physical education objectives are consistent with general education objectives.		
46. The administration recognizes and gives respect and prestige to each area of specialization in the school system.		
47. Health and physical educators are consulted when new facilities are planned in their areas of specialization.		
48. Funds are available for professional libraries, professional travel, and other essentials for a good inservice program.		
49. Health and physical educators carefully consider constructive criticism when given by the administration.		
50. The administration is skilled in the organization and administration of a school system.		

Questions and exercises

1. Draw up a list of competencies that you consider essential for all teachers.
2. Draw up a list of competencies that in your opinion are essential for teachers of health and/or physical education.
3. Define the term *administration* in your own words and give illustrations to point out the various facets of your definition.
4. Discuss the qualifications of a good administrator, giving concrete examples to support the importance of each qualification listed.
5. Prepare an organization chart for some department, school, or agency with which you are associated. Discuss significant aspects of the administrative setup of this organization.
6. Prepare a rating sheet that could be utilized by students to determine the extent of their qualifications for the field of administration.
7. From your own experience, prepare a list of principles that you feel are essential to good personnel relations.
8. Prepare two skits, one dramatizing some aspects of good personnel relations and the other pointing up some poor practices in regard to such relations.

9. What is meant by the term *fallacy of final authority?* Cite two illustrations to support the idea involved.
10. Interview five general administrators and summarize their feelings about health education and physical education.
11. Write an essay of approximately 500 words on the subject: "Ways in which health education and/or physical education can become more important in the eyes of general administrators."
12. Read one general administration book and summarize its comments on health education and/or physical education.
13. What do you feel are the responsibilities of health educators and/or physical educators in the total educational program?
14. If you were a general administrator, what kind of a health educator or physical educator would you hire for your school or college system? Outline the type of person you would want working for you.

Reading assignment in *Administrative Dimensions of Health and Physical Education Programs, Including Athletics:* Chapter 4, Selections 16 to 20.

Selected references

Bucher, C. A.: Foundations of physical education, ed. 5, St. Louis, 1968, The C. V. Mosby Co.

Byrd, O. E.: School health administration, Philadelphia, 1964, W. B. Saunders Co.

Douglass, H. R.: Modern administration of secondary schools, Boston, 1963, Ginn & Co.

Jenson, T. J., and Clark, D. L.: Educational administration, New York, 1964, The Center for Applied Research in Education, Inc. (The Library of Education).

Moore, H. E.: The administration of public school personnel, New York, 1966, The Center for Applied Research in Education, Inc. (The Library of Education).

NEA Report of the Project on Instruction: Schools for the sixties, New York, 1963, McGraw-Hill Book Co.

CHAPTER 6   STUDENT LEADERSHIP IN PHYSICAL EDUCATION

One of the major responsibilities of all educators is to develop the leadership essential to the democratic society in which we live. All phases of the educational process should be concerned with carrying out and fulfilling this function. A democratic form of government depends upon an enlightened populace capable of assuming responsibility for its own governance and self-direction.

Physical educators have the ability to develop leadership qualities in the students who participate in their programs. Many opportunities exist in curricular and extracurricular physical education programs to enable students to assume leadership responsibilities under the direction and guidance of experienced physical educators. Under qualified supervision students can develop such attributes as cooperation, self-control, and good human relations and become imbued with the desire to serve other people. In addition, students can become involved with such responsibilities as planning and evaluating the programs in which they participate. To achieve the best results, however, the climate in which they participate should be friendly and permissive, be a place where initiative and creativity are encouraged, and provide frequent opportunities to discuss problems with their classmates and teachers and to understand clearly the meaning of good leadership. Finally, certain principles must be recognized if successful student leadership is to be developed. These principles include a clear delineation of student and staff responsibilities and a leadership program where

individual development and self-direction are encouraged.

When a program of student leadership is established with such principles and conditions in mind, it will not only help each student to grow and develop but it will also be of value to the fields of physical education and health. Students frequently become more interested in these specialized fields and often decide to pursue a career in them as a result of seeing firsthand the opportunities they provide. Student leadership also renders a valuable service to the department by making it possible for more students to receive individualized instruction from their better skilled classmates; by providing better safety conditions under which activity participation can take place, since more spotters and other staff members are available; and by providing for the maximum utilization of class time as a result of a larger and more effective instructional staff. Many times student leadership also enables the teacher to spend more of his or her time in teaching rather than having to give attention to small clerical details such as attendance taking and equipment and supply management. Furthermore, it helps to enrich the program by providing expanded leadership for such extras as exhibitions, demonstrations, and intramural and interscholastic athletics.

ADVANTAGES AND DISADVANTAGES FOR THE STUDENT

I have spoken to many students who have engaged in student leadership responsibilities in their respective physical education programs. As seen through their eyes, there are many advantages and disadvantages to serving in a student leadership capacity. An analysis of their evaluations of such a responsibility indicates that many of the disadvantages, however, can be eliminated if the program is conducted in a sound educational manner.

Students who have taken on student leadership responsibilities find that they are recognized by classmates and faculty as leaders who have special skills and personal attributes that qualify them for such a role. They also mention some of the more tangible material rewards that go with such a responsibility, for example, special uniforms, lockers, award dinners, assembly programs, and other forms of recognition. Those students who are interested in physical education or health as a possible career point out that they are provided an opportunity to learn more about the field and to get experience as a leader in this area of specialization. Furthermore,

they point out that leadership qualities are developed with such experience, such as the ability to think, analyze problems, and make judgments concerning how a class should be conducted. The social experiences, such as associating with other leaders within their own school as well as student leaders in other schools, are also rewarding.

Student leaders feel that they gain a sense of duty and responsibility from their experience. They learn to abide by a code of ethics that has been established so that their responsibilities as a leader can be carried out as effectively as possible. They enjoy the responsibilities that are given to them and find that the additional duties help to develop their health and bodies.

Student leaders have also commented on the disadvantages that accrue from taking on such responsibilities. Some students indicate that they are asked to take on duties in order that the teacher may get an additional rest period. Others say they are requested to assume duties for which they are not qualified, for ex-

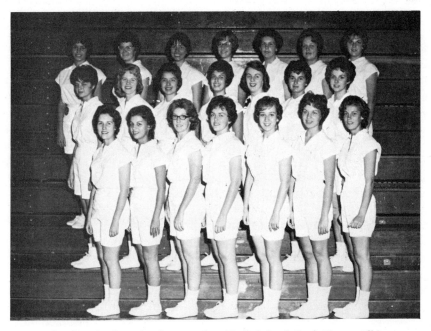

Student leaders. (Rich Township High School, Park Forest, Ill.)

ample, teaching certain skills in which they are not proficient. Some students have found that the leadership program is poorly organized and administered and as a result they are not motivated to develop leadership qualities. In addition, they point out that some of the jobs assigned are menial in nature and not related to the development of leadership traits. In addition to pointing out disadvantages that evolve from the teacher's actions, they also point the finger at certain students who are autocratic and undemocratic in the execution of their responsibilities, thus preventing the achievement of desirable educational goals.

An interesting observation of some student leaders is that at times they feel that only a few select students are given the opportunity to have leadership experiences and, as a result, many potential leaders are overlooked. Students feel that more persons should be provided with the opportunities to develop leadership traits through such an experience. A last observation of students is that the actual leaders who have gone through the training program are sometimes combined with the leaders-in-training in many of the experiences, social and curricular, that are provided. The students who make this observation indicate that they do not feel this procedure is the best one to follow since there is much duplication in the program provided.

QUALIFICATIONS OF THE STUDENT LEADER

The student leader obviously must have certain qualifications if he is to achieve the goals for which a leadership program is established. Since the student leader will have an impact on all the students with whom he works, it is important that such exposure yield sound educational results. Therefore, it is important to have established standards by which student leaders are selected. There are five quali-

fications that should be used as a guide in the selection of student leaders.

Personality

The personality of the student leader should be conducive to interaction with the other students and faculty in a harmonious and desirable manner. A student leader should be cheerful and friendly, possess a sense of humor, and be able to smile at himself. He should be enthusiastic about and enjoy his work, but at the same time he must command the respect of his classmates and be viewed as the leader who must guide and make decisions for the welfare of the entire class.

Intelligence and scholarship

Above-average intelligence and the application of this intelligence as demonstrated by getting passing grades in all subjects should be a requirement of the student leader. Intelligence and sound judgment are needed as a basis for making wise decisions, solving problems, and gaining the respect of one's classmates.

Interest in other people

Leadership cannot be exercised by a person unless he has a sincere interest in other people. The student leader should have an understanding of the needs of human beings and possess a desire to serve them. In addition, he should have a sympathetic attitude toward classmates with less skill who are awkward and uncoordinated in physical movement. Also, he should demonstrate qualities of good sportsmanship at all times.

Health and a love of physical activity

The student leader in physical education should exemplify the qualities that he is trying to develop in other students. Good health and sport skills and general motor ability are important considerations for the student leader in this field of specialization. In addition to providing a desirable image of the physical education leader, these qualities are prerequisites to the energy and productivity that are needed to carry out the responsibilities associated with the job of student leader.

Leadership qualities

In addition to the qualities that have been discussed as essential to a student's leadership role, other qualities are also necessary. These qualifications include the need to recognize the importance of the democratic process in teaching, the ability to efficiently organize classes and groups for activities, and other attributes such as dependability, desire, resourcefulness, initiative, industriousness, and patience.

METHODS OF SELECTING THE STUDENT LEADER

There are several methods utilized by physical educators to select student leaders. Some physical educators advocate the appointment of temporary leaders during the first few sessions of a class until the students become better known to their classmates and instructor. Some of the methods by which student leaders are selected are discussed in the following paragraphs.

Volunteers

Students are asked to volunteer to become a student leader. It may happen that the least qualified persons are the ones who volunteer. If this method is used, it should probably be used with the understanding that the student leader will serve for only a relatively short period of time. Also, there can be a rotation of student leaders with this method so that all volunteers may have such an experience.

Appointment by the teacher

The physical education instructor may appoint the student leader, utilizing his experience and judgment as a basis for his selection, based upon the qualities that are needed for such a position. One of the limitations of this procedure is that it is not democratic since it does not involve the students who are going to be exposed to the student leader. However, if the teacher has the objective of letting each student in the class have a student leadership experience, he can overcome this limitation.

Election by the class

Another method of selecting student leaders is to have the students in the physical education class vote and elect the person or persons they would like to have serve in this capacity. A limitation of this method is that the person selected is often the most popular student as a result of his participation in sports, student government, or some other school activity. Being the most popular student does not mean that he is qualified to be a leader. This is a democratic procedure, however, and if the guidelines for selection of a leader are established and if the proper climate prevails, it can be an effective method.

Selection based on test results

A battery of tests is sometimes used by physical educators as a means of selecting student leaders. Tests of physical fitness, motor ability, sports skills, and/or other instruments that indicate leadership and personality characteristics yield useful information. They provide tangible evidence that a person has some of the desirable qualifications that are needed by a student leader in a physical education class. In addition, if the physical educator desires to have the entire class participate in the student leadership program, the test results may also be of value to the teacher in helping each student to identify weaknesses that need to be overcome during the training period.

Selection by Leaders' Club

Physical educators sometimes organize Leaders' Clubs as a means of providing a continuing process for the selection of student leaders. The students who are members of the Leaders' Club, under the supervision of a faculty advisor, select new students to participate as leaders-in-training. Then, after a period of training, these students in turn become full-fledged student leaders. This method, with its advantages and disadvantages, is discussed at greater length in the paragraphs to follow.

TRAINING THE STUDENT LEADER

One method of selecting and training student leaders is through a Leaders' Club. These clubs commonly have their own constitution, governing body, faculty advisor, and training sessions.

The written constitution of a Leaders' Club usually states the purpose of the club, requirements for membership, qualifications and duties of officers, financial stipulations, procedures for giving awards and honors, and other rules governing the organization.

The governing body of the Leaders' Club may consist of a president, vice-president, treasurer, and secretary, all of whom are elected by the members of the club.

The faculty advisor is a teacher who works closely with the leaders to ensure that the objectives of the Leaders' Club are accomplished. The faculty advisor exercises close supervision over the affairs of the club and, in addition, provides inspiration and motivation to the leaders, encouraging creativity, and helping the students to achieve their goals.

The Leaders' Club usually has regular meetings on a weekly, biweekly, or monthly basis.

The Leaders' Club involvement in the selection and training of student leaders

In some schools, the students who are interested in becoming student leaders apply for membership in the Leaders' Club. Certain requirements are usually established

as a means of judging whether or not a student is eligible for membership in the Club. In one school these requirements are listed as follows:

1. Grade of 80% or above in physical education
2. Scholastic average of at least 70% in major subjects
3. Passing grades in all subjects
4. Satisfactory health record
5. Membership in school's general organization
6. Recommendation of the physical education teacher as to personality, character, and quality of work
7. All-around physical performance
8. Good rating on physical fitness tests

When a student's application to membership in a Leaders' Club is accepted, a period of training for one semester usually follows. During this period students learn the requirements and responsibilities of a student leader, practice demonstrating and leading as an assistant in physical education classes, and become familiar with the rules of games, the techniques of officiating, and other responsibilities that go with the role of student leader.

After the training period has ended, the qualifications of the trainees are again reviewed by the Leaders' Club. Such items as scholastic average, health and medical record, character, recommendations of physical education teachers, performance on skill tests, scores on written tests of rules, ability to officiate, and skill proficiency are examined. The next step may be the personal interview. The big hurdle is frequently a visit before the entire governing body of the Leaders' Club. Here the candidate's record is reviewed, pertinent questions are asked, and action is taken. The faculty advisor, however, usually makes the final judgment.

Some physical educators feel that the Leaders' Club involvement in the selection and training of student leaders is quite formal and not in the best interests of the goals of the leadership program. These critics especially question the personal interview at the end of the training period and action being taken by a student's peers in determining whether or not a student should become a member of the Leaders' Club. Furthermore, some physical educators object to clubs and societies in general as being contrary to the democratic ideals that should guide any leadership program.

Methods of guiding the student leader

There are several methods that have proved effective in guiding student leaders, either during their training period or while they are actually serving as full-fledged student leaders. These methods include movies, guest lecturers, leaders' physical education period, and meetings. *Movies* can be shown on such subjects as strategies involved in sports or how to play a game or sport. *Guest lecturers,* such as visiting physical education teachers, sports personalities, and educational specialists in such areas as motor learning and teaching techniques, can be utilized advantageously. A *leaders' physical education period,* where the student leaders themselves comprise the class and the faculty advisor covers various duties that the student leader must assume, can be helpful. *Meetings* in which the faculty advisor offers advice and instruction, problems are discussed, and other matters involving the student leader are covered are also an excellent medium of guiding student leaders.

HOW THE STUDENT LEADER MAY BE UTILIZED

Student leaders may be used in the physical education program in several capacities.

Class leaders

There are many opportunities in the basic physical education instructional class period where student leaders can be utilized to advantage. These include:

1. Acting as squad leader, where the student takes charge of a small number of students for an activity
2. Being a leader for warm-up exercises at the beginning of the class period
3. Demonstrating how activities—skills, games, strategies—are to be performed
4. Taking attendance
5. Supervising the locker room
6. Providing safety measures for class participation, such as acting as a spotter, checking equipment and play areas, and providing supervision
7. Assuming measurement and evaluation responsibilities, such as helping in the testing program, measuring performance in track and field, and timing with a stop watch

Officials, captains, and other positions

Student leaders can gain valuable experience by serving as officials within the class and intramural program, being captain of an all-star or other team, coaching an intramural or club team, and acting as scorers and timekeepers.

Committee members

Many committee assignments should be filled by student leaders so that they gain valuable experience. These include being a member of a *rules committee,* where rules are established and interpreted for games and sports; serving on an *equipment and grounds committee,* where standards are established for the storage, maintenance, and use of these facilities and equipment; and participating on a *committee for planning special days or events* in the physical education program, such as play, sports, or field days.

Supply and equipment manager

Supplies and special equipment are needed in the physical education program when the various activities are being taught. This includes such equipment as basketballs, archery, golf, and hockey equipment, and audiovisual aids. The equipment must be taken from the storage areas, transferred to the place

STUDENT LEADERSHIP SURVEY OF NINE NEW YORK STATE SCHOOLS

Questions

1. Do you use any kind of student leadership in your physical education classes?

2. If yes, do you use boys or girls or both?

3. What are their duties?
    Squad leaders, demonstrators, etc.

4. Do you use student leaders during athletic events at your school?

5. Do your student leaders in any way help formulate curriculum through suggestions to the teacher?

6. Do you use your athletic captains in a leadership role during practice or game situations? How?

7. Do you find the work of student leaders beneficial to the overall implementation of the program?

8. How do you select your leaders—teacher-appointed, class-elected, squad-elected classes, athletics?

9. How long do they serve?

10. Do you feel that the system of student leadership you have now is adequate, should be enlarged or changed, or done away with? Why?

Utilization of student leaders. Survey conducted by Norman Peck. See answers on facing page.

where the activity will be conducted, and then returned to the storage area. The student leader can help immeasurably in this process and profit from such an experience.

Program planner

Various aspects of the physical education program need to be planned, and students should be involved. Student leaders, because of their special qualifications and interest, are logical choices to participate in such planning. Their knowledge and advice can be utilized to ensure that the program meets the needs and interests of the students who participate in the program. Any curriculum development program should involve such students.

Questions*	Rye	Rye Neck	Mamaroneck	New Rochelle	Valhalla	Hastings	Port Chester	Scarsdale	Bronxville
1	Yes	Yes	Yes	Yes	Yes	Yes	Yes — senior high only	Yes	No
2	Yes	Girls only	Yes	Yes	Yes	Yes	Yes	Yes	—
3	Squad leaders Demonstrators	Squad leaders Demonstrators	Squad leaders Demonstrators Spotters Instructors	Squad leaders	Squad leaders to set up equipment	Squad leaders Demonstrators	Squad leaders	Leaders in various physical education activities	—
4	Yes — varsity club members	Yes — varsity club members	Yes — "M" club members	Yes — varsity club members	Yes — varsity club members	Yes — varsity club members	No	Yes — varsity club members	Yes — leaders club (girls) and varsity club (boys)
5	No	No	Yes — through suggestion to teacher	No	No	Yes — through G.O. council	No	To very limited extent — not important part of program	No
6	Yes	No	Yes	Yes — strategy	Yes — sportsmanship and training	Yes — strategy	Yes	Yes	Yes
7	Yes	Yes — in school service functions	Yes — in all areas and functions	Yes — very much	Yes — in most cases	Yes — in all cases	Doubtful — sometimes good and sometimes poor	Yes	Yes — very much
8	Class — teacher appointed Athletics — appointed by teacher	Class — teacher appointed Athletics — elected by team	Class — high school teacher appointed Athletics — elected by team	Class — teacher appointed Athletics — elected by team	Class — teacher appointed Athletics — elected by team	Class — teacher appointed Athletics — elected by team	Class — teacher appointed Athletics — elected	Class varies with age groups and instructors Athletics — elected by lettermen	Leaders club Teachers selected Varsity club elected by team
9	Class — rotating basis Captain — elected for season	Class — rotating — equal chance for all Captain — elected for season	Class — usually for unit of instruction Captain — elected for season	Class — rotating basis, day — week unit Captain — elected for season	Class — one period all must serve Captain — elected for season	Class — unit Captain — elected for season	Class — rotating basis Captain — elected for season	Class varies — depends on ability and athletics — elected for season	Leaders club Varsity club for all year Captain — elected for season
10	Increasing	Expand to include boys' physical education classes	Change in curriculum will allow for more student leadership	Enlarge program and include safety techniques	Adequate	Increasing	Increasing	Adequate	Needs improvement

*See opposite page.

Record keeper and office manager

Attendance records and inventories must be taken, filing and recording done, bulletin boards kept up to date, visitors met, and other responsibilities attended to. These necessary functions provide worthwhile experiences for the student leader and benefit the program.

Special events coordinator

There are always a multitude of details to attend to when play days, sports days, demonstrations, and exhibitions are planned and conducted. Student leaders should be involved in the planning of these events and also in their actual conduct.

EVALUATION OF THE PROGRAM

An evaluation of the student leadership program should take place periodically to determine the degree to which the program is achieving its stated goals. Students should be involved in this evaluation. Such questions as the following might be asked. "Are the experiences that are provided worth while?" "Are the students developing leadership qualities?" "Is the teacher providing the necessary leadership to make the program effective?" "Are any of the assigned tasks incompatible with the objectives sought?" "If a Leaders' Club exists, is it helping to make for a better leaders' program?"

Questions and exercises

1. What are some of the qualities needed by student leaders?
2. Do a job analysis of a student leader in each of three different schools and evaluate the responsibilities assigned in terms of the development of leadership traits.
3. What are the disadvantages and advantages of being a student leader?
4. Develop a constitution for a Leaders' Club, including those requirements that you feel are most necessary for a sound educational leadership program.
5. Interview three experienced physical educators who were student leaders during their high school days and draw up a list of guidelines for a student leadership program based on their experiences and their evaluation of their own experience.

Selected references

Bell, M. M.: Are we exploiting high school girl athletes? Journal of Health, Physical Education, and Recreation 41:53, 1970.

Bookwalter, K.: Physical education in the secondary schools, New York, 1964, The Center for Applied Research in Education, Inc. (The Library of Education).

Jaeger, E., and Bockstruck, E.: Effective student leadership, Journal of Health, Physical Education, and Recreation 30:52, 1959.

Physical education for girls in high school, Curriculum Bulletin No. 6, Board of Education of the City of New York, 1965-1966.

PART

two

ADMINISTRATION OF PHYSICAL EDUCATION PROGRAMS

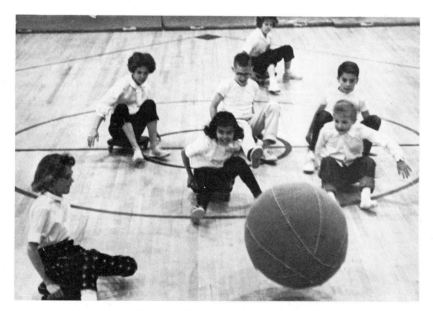

Colorado Springs Public Schools, Colorado Springs, Colo.

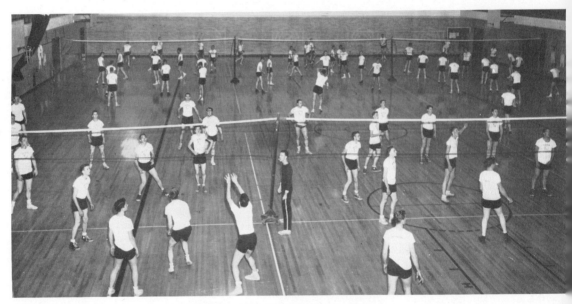

Washington State College, Pullman, Wash.

CHAPTER 7 THE BASIC INSTRUCTIONAL PHYSICAL EDUCATION PROGRAM*

The basic instructional physical education program should provide students with the opportunity to receive instruction, develop essential physical skills, and have enjoyable educational experiences. It is here that opinions are formed and attitudes developed in respect to the physical education program and profession. The fact that some individuals grow into adulthood with an indifferent or unfavorable attitude toward physical education can often be traced back to the physical education they were exposed to in school and college. To some individuals it was something that was jammed down their throats. To others it was presented in an uninteresting manner and seemed unimportant—something to "skip" as often as possible. To still others it was an experience where they were ignored because they had little skill.

Physical education should be presented in a scientific and interesting manner. Students should receive joy and satisfaction from participating in the various activities. Physical education carries its own drive and the teacher should attempt to preserve this natural drive throughout childhood years and into adulthood. It

has been said that if children are exposed to good physical education programs during their formative years there would be no necessity for required physical education programs in later school and college years. The individual would develop skills and attitudes toward physical education that would result in joy and satisfaction from participation. The individual on his or her own initiative would then want to continue such enjoyable experiences.

ENCOURAGING NEW DEVELOPMENTS IN THE TEACHING OF PHYSICAL EDUCATION

There have been several new developments that have emerged in recent years and that augur well for the teaching of physical education in the future. These are (1) getting at the "why" of physical activity, (2) movement education, (3) perceptual-motor programs, (4) the Broadfront Program, and (5) the Battle Creek Physical Education Project.

Getting at the "why" of physical activity

An encouraging new development in physical education is the progress being made toward incorporating the "why" of physical activity into physical education programs, particularly at the high school level. Traditionally, physical education has consisted entirely of physical activity with very little explanation being given to students as to *why* they should be active. Physical education appears to have operated under the assumption that participa-

*School and college physical education programs will be discussed in the next four chapters. This chapter is concerned with the basic instructional physical educational class or service program. Chapter 8 concerns itself with the adapted physical education program. Chapter 9 deals with the intramural and extramural athletic programs, and Chapter 10 is concerned with interscholastic and intercollegiate varsity athletic programs.

tion in games, sports, and other activities alone will develop an understanding of the potential values of these activities, although it is widely accepted that students will function more positively if they know, understand, and appreciate the reasons for participating in various forms of physical activity. Today, it is being increasingly recognized that students need to understand basic concepts about health and fitness in order to be truly physically educated.

The American Association for Health, Physical Education, and Recreation has had a committee working for several years identifying the knowledge and understanding needed in physical education.* This report has been prepared by an outstanding group of leaders and is divided into an introduction and four parts: Introduction, Why Teach A Body of Knowledge in Physical Education?; Part I, Activity Performance (covers such items as basic sport skills, body mechanics, concepts fundamental to movement, skills in strategies and activity patterns, rules and procedures, and protective requirements); Part II, Effects of Activity, Immediate and Long Term; Part III, Factors Modifying Participation in Activities and the Effects of Participation; and Part IV, Standardized Tests.

In keeping with the trend toward getting at the "why" of physical activity, a few textbooks have been published that outline the material that is essential for boys and girls to know in order to be physically educated. I recently published a text entitled *Physical Education for Life*,† which is specifically designed for this purpose and for the use of high school boys and girls. The material included in this text is outlined here in order to give the reader some idea as to what material might be included regarding the "why" of physical activity.

Physical Education for Life includes a full coverage of sports and activities appropriate for both sexes, for boys only, and for girls only. Part One concentrates on such topics as the organic systems of the body related to and affected by physical activity, the requirements for good body mechanics, exercises to correct some atypical posture conditions, how physical movement takes place and the laws of physics that apply to such movement, how skills are learned based on the latest scientific principles of motor learning, the requirements for and the ingredients of a personal regimen for achieving and maintaining physical fitness, and isometric and isotonic exercises for high school students. Furthermore, a chapter is devoted to safety guidelines and first aid procedures common to participation in physical education activities. Each chapter concludes with a series of questions and answers covering additional information pertinent to the subject of the chapter.

Part Two consists of twenty chapters. Each chapter presents a different physical education activity, ranging from archery, badminton, and basketball to dancing, gymnastics, and wrestling. Each chapter includes the history of the activity, terminology, rules of the game, and recommendations for attire, equipment, etiquette, and safety precautions. There is a progressive treatment of the basic skills involved in the beginning, intermediate, and advanced ability levels of each activity. Each chapter ends with a discussion of strategy and activities for improving skill.

When a high school student appreciates and understands the "why" of physical education as well as the physical activity in which he participates, there is a better assurance that he will develop the neces-

*American Association for Health, Physical Education, and Recreation: Knowledge and understanding in physical education, Washington, D. C., 1969, The Association.

†Bucher, C. A.: Physical education for life, St. Louis, 1969, Webster Division, McGraw-Hill Book Co.

sary attitudes and habits and remain physically active all of his life.

Movement education

Movement education is a significant new approach to teaching physical education. It frees the individual student to work and progress at his own pace while it offers opportunities for creative expression and exploration. It helps the student to better understand the physical laws that govern human movement. Physical skills are developed through an individualized problem-solving technique.

Movement education is being introduced into many elementary schools throughout the nation, and various aspects of movement education are taking root in secondary schools and colleges as well.

What is movement education? Experts do not agree on a single definition. They do agree, however, that movement education is dependent on physical factors in the environment and on the individual's ability to intellectually and physically react to these factors. Movement education attempts to help the student to become mentally as well as physically aware of his bodily movements. It is based on a conceptual approach to human movement. Through movement education, the individual develops his own techniques for dealing with the environmental factors of force,

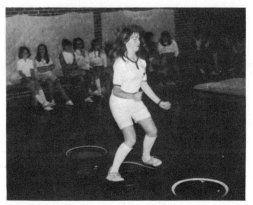

Elementary school physical education. (Henderson County Schools, Hendersonville, N. C.)

time, space, and flow as they relate to various movement problems.

Movement education employs the problem-solving approach. Each skill that is to be explored presents a challenge to the student. Learning results as the student accepts and solves increasingly more difficult problems. For this reason, the natural movements of childhood are considered to be the first challenges that should be presented to the student.

Traditional physical education emphasizes the learning of specific skills through demonstration, drill, and practice. Movement education emphasizes the learning of skill patterns through individual exploration of the body's movement potential. Traditional physical education stresses the teacher's standard of performance. Movement education stresses the individual child's standard of performance.

Perceptual-motor foundations

Another development in physical education that should be noted is the increased recognition of perceptual-motor foundations. For some time there has been an increased recognition of the importance of meaningful perceptual-motor programs for underachievers in the elementary schools. Research conducted by psychologists, physical educators, and others has shown that motor activity, when properly presented, can enhance perceptual development.

One of the most significant developments of this interest has been the publication of the report of a task force of the AAHPER, which studied such subjects as the evolution of perceptual-motor behavior with implications for the teaching-learning process. It also explored interdisciplinary implications and identified areas for future study and research.[*] This study indicates there is a relationship between physical

[*] American Association for Health, Physical Education, and Recreation: Perceptual-motor foundations: a multidisciplinary concern, Washington, D. C., 1969, The Association.

education and the development of perceptual-motor skills and that perceptual-motor skills are essential to learning and scholastic achievement. Therefore the conclusion is drawn that physical education, through the contribution that can be made in this area, has the potential for contributing to and facilitating the educational and academic achievement of certain children in our schools.

The Broadfront Program

Ellensburg, Washington, has developed a comprehensive program in physical education, health, and recreation. The project was started as a result of a Title III grant from the national government. It is designed to help each boy and girl in elementary, junior high, and senior high school develop physical skills, desirable attitudes, and knowledge about physical education, health, and recreation. It not only focuses attention on the normal boy and girl but also the handicapped and the retarded student. Furthermore, it is concerned with linking the school and community together in a program with both student and adult participation. Specifically, the Broadfront Program has five major aspects: (1) the acquisition of skills on the part of the student in individual sports, (2) health education, (3) a community-school program, (4) outdoor education and school camping, and (5) an adapted health and physical education program.

Broadfront is designed to accomplish such goals as ensuring that students develop skill competency in at least two lifetime sports, providing inservice education for classroom teachers both elementary and secondary, utilizing professors and major students from nearby colleges, instructing the adult population of Ellensburg, Washington, in lifetime sports, utilizing all facilities in both the school and community, and providing for the orientation of student teachers who are

majors in physical education, as well as elementary school education majors, so that they will understand and appreciate the program.

The Battle Creek Physical Education Curriculum Project

The Battle Creek Curriculum Project represents an effort on the part of a public school system working with a university to develop and implement a model curriculum for physical education at both the elementary and secondary educational levels. The project team consists of specialists in physical education, curriculum development, child growth and development, sociology, physiology, and educational measurement. The major objectives of the project are to first identify a body of knowledge that can form the framework for a curriculum model. This was accomplished by an intensive search of the literature to find out such things as the influence of physical activity on man's biologic, sociologic, and psychologic development and the relationship of man's various activity patterns to culture and environment. The second objective was to take the findings of this intensive search of the literature and organize it in terms of such things as a philosophy that would act as a guide for the curriculum model and also as a guide for general and behavioral objectives and outcomes. Finally, the development of a model program in physical education will be derived from the previous two steps. The Battle Creek Project has national implications for physical education programs.

THE BASIC INSTRUCTIONAL PROGRAM—INSTRUCTIONAL IN NATURE

The basic instructional program of physical education is the place to teach, not a setting for free play and intramurals or an opportunity for the varsity team to practice. The entire period should be used to teach skills, strategies, understandings, and essential knowledge concerning the relation of physical activity to physical, mental, emotional, and social development.

Skills should be taught from a scientific approach so that the various kinesiologic factors that affect movement are understood clearly by the student. Utilization of demonstrations, super-8 films, loop films, models, slide films, posters, and other visual aids and materials can help in clarifying instruction. Team teaching enables the master teacher of specific skills to be utilized more extensively than in the past.

The material presented throughout the school life of the child should be sequential in development and progressive in application. Just as a student advances in mathematics from simple arithmetic to algebra, geometry, and calculus, so in physical education the pupil should progress from basic skills and materials to more complex and involved skills and strategies.

Standards should be established for student achievement. When boys and girls advance from one grade to another they should have achieved certain standards in various physical education activities, just as they master various levels of skills and understandings in subject matter areas of instruction.

The physical education class should involve more than physical activity itself. As the student understands more fully the importance of sports and activities in life, what happens to the body during exercise, the relation of physical activity to man's biologic, psychologic, and sociologic development, the history of various activities, and the role of physical activity in the cultures of the world, the class takes on more intellectual respectability and meaning for the student and the profession in general.

Just as textbooks are used in other courses in the educational system, so should physical education use a textbook, with regular assignments being given. Textbooks should contain not only material on physi-

cal skills but should also get at the subject matter with which physical education is concerned.

Records that follow a child from grade to grade should be kept throughout his school life. These records will indicate the degree to which the objectives have been achieved by the student, his physical status, his skill achievement, his knowledge about the field, his social conduct, and other aspects that will help to interpret in a meaningful manner what physical education has done for the student and what still needs to be done.

There should also be homework in physical education. The subject matter needs to be mastered, the skills acquired, and standard of physical fitness achieved. Much of this information, skill, and various standards can be met at least partially through homework assignments.

Guidelines

The basic instructional physical education period cannot be conducted in a "hit-and-miss" fashion. It must be planned in accordance with the needs and interests of the individuals it serves.

Some of the initial considerations in planning and developing a physical education program are suggested[*]:

1. The basic instructional physical education program, adapted program, and intramural, extramural, and varsity interscholastic and intercollegiate athletic programs all represent important components of the total physical education program. They must remain in proper balance at all school and college levels and be geared to the needs and interests of the student.

2. A sound philosophy is essential as a basis for the construction of any physical education program.

3. The needs of the individual and of society, as reflected in the objectives of

---

[*]Also see Chapter 11 on Administering School and College Physical Fitness Programs.

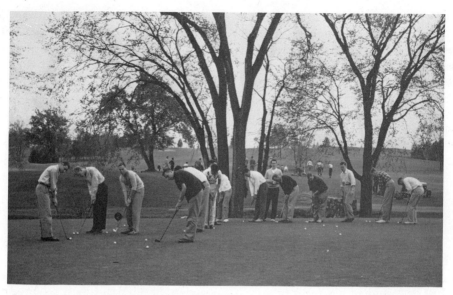

A golf class in the required physical education class program for men. (Department of Physical Education and Athletics, University of Michigan.)

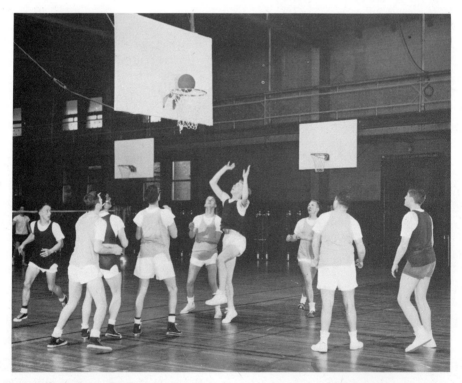

The maxim that physical education carries its own drive should be preserved for every individual who comes in contact with the program. A basketball class in the required physical education class program for men. (Department of Physical Education and Athletics, University of Michigan.)

physical education, represent a main consideration in the establishment of a program of physical education.

4. The fact that physical education contributes to the social, mental, emotional, and physical needs of the individual should be kept in mind.

5. The physical education instructional program should get at the why of the activity as well as the physical activity itself. Provisions should be made for studying, discussing, and assimilating knowledge regarding the subject matter of physical education.

6. The health and recreational aspects of the program must be emphasized. This can best be done by close coordination with the school and college health and recreation programs.

7. Physical education should recognize the importance of coeducational activities for social growth and provide for them in the program.

8. Provisions should be made so that *all* individuals may participate in and benefit from the physical education program.

9. The maxim that "physical education carries its own drive" should be preserved in every individual who comes in contact with the program. Joy and satisfaction should be outcomes from physical education that are guarded jealously.

10. Physical education should receive equal consideration with other subjects in the school and college offerings in respect to necessary supplies, facilities, and administrative support.

11. Qualified leadership is an essential in all phases of the physical education program.

12. Physical education should be planned, organized, and conducted in a manner that will exploit the educational possibilities to the fullest.

13. The program should include a wide variety of activities that can be engaged in by all individuals, indoors and outdoors, and that meet safety, hygienic, and social standards.

14. Instruction in activities should be on a progressive basis and organized in a way that is systematic and most meaningful to the student.

15. Physical education should contribute to the democratic way of life.

16. A program of measurement and evaluation should be developed so that progress toward goals may be noted and weaknesses detected.

The next step in considering the basic instructional program is to examine some of the administrative problems surrounding its organization and administration. These include scheduling, time allotment, size of classes, teaching loads, and grouping; administrative policies concerned with the advisability of having physical education on a required or elective basis, substitutions, credit allowances, class attendance, and excuses; separation of boys and girls in grades one to six; physical education specialist or classroom teacher in the elementary school and the question of self-defense courses; items of class management concerned with planning, dressing and showering, costume, roll taking, grading, and records; matters relating to activities, such as criteria for their selection, classification, and coeducational aspects; and program considerations at the elementary, junior high school, senior high school, and college levels.

SCHEDULING

The manner in which physical education classes are scheduled reflects the physical education leadership in the school or college and the attitude of the central administration. The physical education class will be more meaningful for students if it is scheduled in a manner that is linked to their interests, rather than in the interest of administrative convenience.

Scheduling should be done according to a definite plan. Physical education should not be inserted in the overall master scheduling plan wherever there is time left over after all the other subjects have been provided for. This important responsibility cannot be handled on a hit-and-miss basis, since that disregards the interests and needs of the students. Instead, at the secondary educational level, for example, physical education classes should be scheduled first on the master plan, along with such subjects as English and science that are required of all students most of the time they are in school. This allows for progression and for grouping according to the interests and needs of the individual participants. The three important items to take into consideration in scheduling classes are (1) the number of teachers available, (2) the number of teaching stations available, and (3) the number of students who must be scheduled. This is a formula that should be applied to all subjects in the school offering. Physical education will be scheduled correctly, as will other subjects, if this formula is followed.

All students should be scheduled. There should be no exceptions. If the student can go to school or college he should be enrolled in physical education. Special attention should be given, however, to the exceptional individual to ensure that he is placed in a program suited to his needs. Also, special attention should be given to the so-called "dub" who needs extra help in the development of physical skills.

At the elementary and secondary levels, but especially at the elementary, scheduling should be done on 1-year basis. Special attention should be given to the needs and interests of students in respect to such items as the availability of facilities, equipment, and supplies and the weather. Planned units of work will usually become increasingly longer as the student progresses in grades, because of his longer interest span, greater maturity, and the increased complexity of the acitivities.

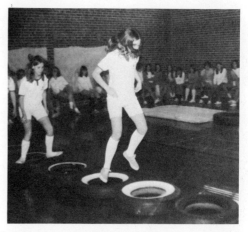

All students should be scheduled for physical education. (Henderson County Schools, Hendersonville, N. C.)

Every physical educator should make a point of presenting to the central administration his or her plans for scheduling physical education classes. The need for special consideration in this area should be discussed with the principal, scheduling committee, and others involved. Through persistent action along this line, progress will be made. The logic and reasoning behind the formula of scheduling classes according to the number of teachers and teaching stations available and the number of students who must be scheduled cannot be denied. It must be planned in this way if there is to be progression in instruction and if a meaningful program is to result.

The innovation of flexible scheduling into school programs has implications for the administration of school physical education programs. Flexible scheduling assumes that the traditional system of having all subjects meet the same number of times each week for the same amount of time each period is passé. Flexible scheduling provides that class periods be of varying lengths, depending on the type of work being covered by the students, methods of instruction, and other factors pertinent to such a system. Whereas the master plan makes it difficult, if not impossible in many

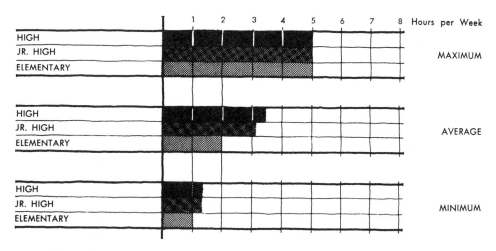

Time spent by students in the physical education program. (From Partial shelter for physical education: a study of the feasibility of the use of limited shelters for physical education, College Station, Texas, 1961, Texas Engineering Experiment Station, Texas A & M University.)

cases, to have flexible scheduling, the advent of the computer has made such an innovation practical and common.

Flexible scheduling also makes it possible to schedule activities for students of differing abilities in a different manner so that all are not required to have a similar schedule based on a standard format of the school day. Under the traditional system all students who were the slowest, for example, took as many courses as the brightest. Under flexible scheduling, some students may take as few as four courses and some as many as eight.

Part of the student's school day will not be scheduled. However, this time is not wasted. Individual study, homework time, skill practice session, conferences with teachers, library study, and many other activities may be scheduled as needed. Such flexible scheduling makes better use of human and physical resources within the school and also offers the student an opportunity to accept responsibility and to make decisions on his own.

Physical educators must give considerable thought as to what type of scheduling should be utilized in physical education classes, what length of periods is best, and

what allocations of time should be fed to the computer. Some schools are experimenting with this problem.

Time allotment

Just as scheduling practices vary from school to school, college to college, and state to state, so does the time allotment. In some states there are laws that are mandatory in nature and require that a certain amount of time each day or week be devoted to physical education, whereas in others permissive legislation exists. For grades one to twelve the requirement varies in different states from none, or very little, to a daily 1-hour program. Some require 20 minutes daily and others 30 minutes daily. Other states specify the time by the week, ranging from 50 minutes to 300 minutes. The college and university level does not usually require as much physical education as grades one to twelve. The usual practice in higher education is to require physical education two times a week for 2 years.

The general consensus among physical education leaders is that in order for physical education to be of value it must be given with regularity. For most individuals this means daily periods. There is also agreement among experts in the field of health that exercise is essential to everyone from the cradle to the grave. Smiley and Gould point out the exercise needs of individuals at various ages:

Ages 1 through 4
  Free play during hours not occupied by sleeping

Ages 5 through 8
  Four hours a day of free play (running, jumping, dancing, climbing, teetering, etc.) and of loosely organized group games (tag, nine pins, hoops, beanbags, etc.)

Ages 9 through 11
  At least three hours a day of outdoor active play (hiking, swimming, gymnastics, group games and relays, soccer, volleyball, broad-and-high jump, 25- and 50-yard dashes, folk dancing, etc.)

Ages 12 through 14
  At least two hours a day of outdoor active play (hiking, swimming, gymnastics, group games, relays, soccer, volleyball, indoor baseball, basketball, baseball, tennis, 60-yard dash, the jumps, shot-put, low hurdles, short relays, folk and gymnastic dancing). Still no endurance contests

Ages 15 through 17
  At least one and one-half hours a day of outdoor active play (hiking, swimming, apparatus work, group games and relays, soccer, volleyball, indoor baseball, basketball, baseball, tennis, football, golf, ice hockey, 60-yard dash, the jumps, shot-put, low hurdles, short relays, folk and gymnastic dancing). Still no endurance contests

Ages 18 through 30
  At least one hour a day of active outdoor exercise (all the types listed in the preceding paragraph and, if examined and found physically fit, in addition, cross-country running, crew, wrestling, boxing, fencing, and polo)

Ages 31 through 50
  At least one hour a day of moderate outdoor exercise (golf, tennis, riding, swimming, handball, volleyball, etc.)

Ages 51 through 70
  At least one hour a day of light outdoor exercise (golf, walking, bowling, gardening, fishing, croquet, etc.)*

---

*Smiley, D. F., and Gould, A. G.: A college textbook of hygiene, New York, 1940, The Macmillan Co., pp. 346-347.

Daily physical education period at elementary and secondary school levels

The time-allotment recommendation usually considered adequate is a daily physical education period for each student. This should represent the minimum requirement. Some individuals feel that, especially in the elementary schools, a program cannot be adapted to a fixed time schedule. However, as a standard, there seems to be agreement that a daily experience in such a program is needed. Such a recommendation is made and should always be justified on the basis of value and contribution to the student and his needs. There should be provision for regular, instructional class periods and, in addition, laboratory periods where the skills may be put to use.

On the secondary level especially, there is a feeling that a full 60-minute period is needed. Since time for dressing and showering is required, this leaves only approximately 45 minutes on the floor or playground. Some have suggested a double period every other day rather than a single period each day. This might be feasible if the daily class periods are too short. However, the importance of daily periods should be recognized and achieved wher-

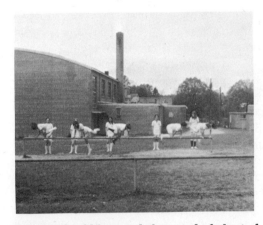

Students should have a daily period of physical education. (Henderson County Schools, Hendersonville, N. C.)

ever possible. Administrators should work toward providing adequate staff and facilities to allow for a daily period.

One of the most intensive and enlightening public interpretation programs ever carried on in modern times in support of a daily program of physical education was conducted in California. The California Association for Health, Physical Education, and Recreation rendered an outstanding service to the profession in cataloguing, describing, and interpreting the values inherent in the daily program of physical education in their state. They incorporated their scientific evidence and research findings in a special issue of the *Journal of the California Association for Health, Physical Education, and Recreation.*

This special issue included supporting statements from such people and organizations as the President of the United States, citizens' committees, American Medical Association, California Heart Association,

---

*Values inherent in the daily program of physical education: fitness for California children and youth, Journal of the California Association for Health, Physical Education, and Recreation, special issue, March, 1965.

physiologists and psychologists, educators, and parent-teachers' associations. As a result of this intensive and aggressive campaign, the public became much better informed regarding the need for daily physical education.

The President's Council on Physical Fitness and Sports has made this statement in regard to the daily physical education period:

> The unanimous support for recommendations of the President's Council on Physical Fitness by a national jury of eminent medical leaders accompanying similar support by the American Medical Association and its committee on Exercise and Physical Fitness, Medical Aspects of Sports, and the Joint Committee of the AMA and its National Education Association indicate the sound position the President's Council has taken in recommending daily physical education instruction involving vigorous exercise in grades 1 to 12.*

Size of classes

Some school and college administrators feel that physical education classes can accommodate more students than the so-

---

*President's Council on Physical Fitness, Washington, D. C., distributed in 1965 (mimeographed).

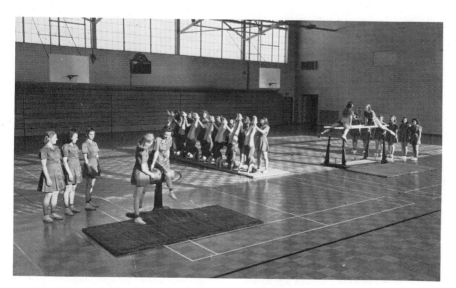

Girls' physical education. (State Teachers College, East Stroudsburg, Pa.)

called academic classes, such as English or social studies. This is a misconception that has developed over the years and is in need of correction. Physical educators themselves are in many cases at fault for such a practice. Some have failed to interpret their field of endeavor adequately to the central administration. Others have followed the practice of throwing a ball to a class and utilizing free play, with little or no organization. This has led some administrators to feel that the same type of teaching job would be done with a small class, and therefore they see no reason to incur the administrative problems and extra expense of more staff and smaller classes.

The problem of class size seems to be more pertinent at the secondary than at other educational levels. At the elementary levels, for example, the classroom situation represents a unit for activity and the size of this teaching unit is usually reasonable. However, there are some schools that combine various classrooms for physical education, resulting in large classes that are not desirable.

Classes in physical education should be approximately the same size as is prevalent for the other subjects in the school or college offering. This is just as essential for effective teaching, individualized instruction, and progression in physical education as it is in other subjects. Physical education contributes to educational objectives on at least an equal basis with other subjects in the curriculum. Therefore, the size of the class should be comparable so that an effective teaching job can be accomplished and the objectives of education attained.

The standard established by LaPorte's committee* after considerable research points up the acceptable size of physical

education classes. It recommends not more than thirty-five students as the suitable size for activity classes. Normal classes should never exceed forty-five for one instructor. Of course, if there is a lecture scheduled it may be possible to have a larger number of students in the class. For remedial and corrective classes the suitable class size is from twenty to twenty-five and should never exceed thirty. With flexible scheduling, the size of classes can be varied to meet the needs of the teacher, facilities, and type of activity being offered.

The American Association for Health, Physical Education, and Recreation* points out that class size should not exceed thirty-five.

Teaching loads

The load of the physical education teacher should be of prime concern to the administrator. In order to maintain a top level of enthusiasm, strength, and other essential characteristics, it is important that the teaching load be adjusted so that the physical educator is not overworked.

The New York State Physical Fitness Conference† recommended that one full-time physical education teacher should be provided for every 240 elementary pupils and one for every 190 secondary pupils enrolled. If such a requirement became universal it would aid considerably in providing adequate staff members in this field and avoid an overload for so many of the teachers.

LaPorte's national study‡ made recommendations in respect to teaching load at precollege educational levels that should

---

*LaPorte, W. R.: The physical education curriculum (a national program), ed. 6, Los Angeles, 1955, University of Southern California Press, pp. 50-51.

*American Association for Health, Physical Education, and Recreation: Administrative problems in health education, physical education, and recreation, Washington, D. C., 1953, The Association, p. 70.
†Report to the Commissioner of Education on the State Fitness Conference, Albany, N. Y., 1952, State Education Department, p. 7.
‡LaPorte, W. R., op. cit., p. 51.

be considered carefully by any teacher or administrator striving to meet acceptable standards. It recommends that class instruction per teacher not exceed 5 clock hours or the equivalent in class periods per day, or 1,500 minutes a week. It never should exceed 6 clock hours per day or 1,800 minutes a week. This maximum should include afterschool responsibilities. A daily load of 200 students per teacher is recommended and never more than 250. Finally, each teacher should have at least one free period daily for consultation and conferences with students.

It is generally agreed that the normal teaching load in colleges and universities should not exceed 15 hours per week.

Grouping

Homogeneous grouping in physical education classes is very desirable. To render the most valuable contribution to students, factors influencing performance must be taken into consideration in organizing groups for physical education instructional work or competition. The lack of scientific knowledge and measuring techniques to obtain such information and the administrative problems of scheduling have handicapped the achievement of this goal in most schools and colleges.

The reasons for grouping are sound. Placing individuals with similar capacities and characteristics in the same class will make it possible to better meet the needs of each individual. Grouping individuals with similar skill, ability, and other factors aids in equalizing competition. This helps the student to realize more satisfaction and benefit from playing. Grouping makes for more effective teaching. Instruction can be better organized and adapted to the level of the student. Grouping facilitates progression and continuity in the program. Furthermore, grouping makes for a better learning situation for the student. Being in a group with persons of similar physical characteristics and skills ensures some suc-

cess, a chance to excel, recognition, a feeling of belonging, and security. Consequently this helps the social and personality development of the individual. Finally, homogeneous grouping helps protect the child. It ensures his participation with individuals who are similar in physical characteristics. This protects the child physically, emotionally, and socially.

The problem of grouping is not as pertinent in the elementary school, especially in the lower grades, as it is in the junior high school and upper levels. At the lower levels the grade classification appears to serve the needs of children. As children grow older, the complexity of the program increases, social growth becomes more diversified, competition becomes more intense, and consequently, there is a greater need for having similar individuals in the same group.

At the present time students are homogeneously classified on such bases as grade, sex, health, physical fitness, multiples of age-height-weight, ability, physical capacity, motor ability, interests, educability, speed, skill, and previous experience. Such techniques as health examinations; tests of motor ability, physical capacity, achievement, and social efficiency; conferences with students; and determination of physiologic age are utilized to obtain such information.

The Sacramento, California, public schools have outlined the various aspects of their physical education program from the elementary grades through the junior college level. Their course of study for the senior high school girls lists the following procedure for grouping in physical education.

I. Basis of classification
   A. Physical examination
     1. Personal history
     2. Menstrual history
     3. Posture test
     4. Feet
     5. Other findings

B. Medical examination
   1. Teeth
   2. Nose, throat
   3. Heart
   4. Nutrition
   5. Blood pressure
   6. Review of findings in physical examinations
II. Classification of physical education activities based upon the above findings
   A. Active or unrestricted physical education
      1. Team sports
      2. Individual sports
      3. Dancing
      4. Gymnastics and unorganized games
      5. Drill
   B. Restricted or modified physical education
      1. Modified games
      2. Posture exercises
      3. Relaxation
   C. Remedial physical education
      1. Exercises for general muscle tone
      2. Menstrual exercises
      3. Posture exercises
      4. Feet exercises
      5. Special, individual exercises
      6. Relaxing
   D. Rest
      This activity includes girls who are under a physician's care and have organic or functional handicaps sufficiently serious to recommend a period of complete rest during their physical education period.

The suggestions of the American Association for Health, Physical Education, and Recreation* are appropriate when considering recommendations for grouping:

1. The need for grouping students homogeneously for instruction and competition has long been recognized, but the inability to scientifically measure such important factors as ability, maturity, interest, and capacity has served as a deterrent from accomplishing this goal.

2. The most common procedure for grouping today is by grade or class.

3. The ideal grouping organization

would take into consideration all factors that affect performance—intelligence, capacity, interest, knowledge, age, height, weight, and so on. To utilize all these factors, however, is not administratively feasible at the present time.

4. Some form of grouping is essential to provide the type of program that will promote educational objectives and protect the student.

5. On the secondary and college levels, the most feasible procedure appears to be to organize subgroups within the regular physical education class proper.

6. Classification within the physical education class should be based on such factors as age, height, and weight statistics and other factors, such as interest and skill, that are developed as a result of observation of the activity.

7. For those individuals who desire greater refinement in respect to grouping, utilization of motor capacity, motor ability, attitude, appreciation, and sports-skills tests may be used.

ADMINISTRATIVE POLICIES

The administrator of any physical education program is perennially confronted with such questions as: Should physical education be required or elective? How much credit should be given? Is it possible to substitute some other activity for physical education? What should be the policy on class attendance? How should one deal with excuses? What provision should be made for sex differences? Should there be courses in self-defense? These and other questions are answered in the following paragraphs.

Should physical education be required or elective?

There is general agreement that physical education should be required at the elementary level. However, there are many advocates on both sides of the question as to whether it should be required or

---

*American Association for Health, Physical Education, and Recreation: Administrative problems in health education, physical education, and recreation, Washington, D. C., 1953, The Association, pp. 71-72.

elective on the secondary and college levels. Both groups are sincere and feel that their beliefs represent what is best for the student. Probably most specialists feel that the program should be required. Some school administrators feel it should be elective. Following are some of the arguments presented by each.

Required

1. Physical education represents a basic need of every student just as English, social studies, and other experiences do. It became part of the school or college offering as a required subject to satisfy such needs and therefore should be continued on the same basis.

2. The student is compelled to take so many required courses that the use of electives is limited, if not entirely eliminated, in some cases. Therefore, unless physical education is a required course, many students will not have the opportunity to partake of this program because of the pressures placed on them by the required courses.

3. The student looks upon those subjects that are required as being the most important and the most necessary for success. Therefore, unless physical education is on the required list, it becomes a subject of second-rate importance in the eyes of the students.

4. Various subjects in the curriculum would not be provided for unless they were required. This is probably true of physical education. Until state legislatures passed laws requiring physical education, this subject was ignored by many school administrators. If physical education were on an elective basis the course of some administrative action would be obvious. Either the subject would not be offered at all or the administrative philosophy would so dampen its value that it would have to be eliminated because of low enrollment.

5. Even under a required program, physical education is not fulfilling its potentialities for meeting the physical, social, and mental needs of students. If an elective program were instituted, deficiencies and shortages would increase, thus further handicapping the attempt to meet the needs of the student.

Elective

1. Physical education "carries its own drive." If a good basic program is developed in the elementary school, with students acquiring the necessary skills and attitudes, the drive for such activity will carry through in the secondary school and college. There will be no need to require such a course, because students will want to take it voluntarily.

2. Objectives of physical education are focused on developing skills and learning activities that have carryover value, living a healthful life, and recognizing the importance of developing and maintaining one's body in its best possible condition. These are goals that cannot be legislated. They must become a part of each individual's attitudes and desires if they are to be realized. A person is more or less "master of his own fate" in regard to his body. He can do with it what he chooses. This is characteristic of life. The student should be guided in setting up his standard of values. However, he makes the final choice as to how he will achieve those values.

3. Many children and young adults do not like physical education. This is indicated in their manner, attitude, and desire to get excused from the program and to substitute something else for the course. Under such circumstances the values that accrue to these individuals are not great. Therefore, it would be best to place physical education on an elective basis where only those students participate who actually desire to.

The question of whether a program should be required or elective will not be decided within a few months or years. It will require considerable study. There are good points on both sides of the issue. A compromise may be possible. The present setup of our educational systems that places some subjects on a pedestal, making them required and focusing attention on them because they have been offered traditionally, may be the reason for the difficulty. Perhaps if a reevaluation of the entire educational system were to take place with each subject evaluated on its contribution to the enriched living of the individual, its value throughout life, and the contributions it can make to an interesting, vigorous, and active life, it would be found that some of the so-called academic subjects might go the way that Latin, for example, has gone. It might be found that many of them are not practical and functional in present-day living. Sometimes the social pressures of the times and the emphasis on material values and false standards govern individuals' choices to too great an extent. When a true set of standards can be established in the mind of every individual so that wise choices can be made, many subjects can be placed on an elective basis. Until then, it is important to make them a requirement.

Should substitutions be allowed for physical education?

A practice exists in some school and college systems that allows students to substitute some other activity for their physical education requirement. This practice should be scrutinized very carefully and resisted aggressively by every administrator.

Some of the activities that are used as substitutions for physical education are athletic participation, Reserve Officers' Training Corps, war service, and band.

There is no substitute for a good program of physical education. In addition to healthful physical activity it is concerned also with developing an individual socially, emotionally, and mentally. It develops in the individual many skills that can be utilized throughout life for worthy use of leisure time. These essentials are lost if a student is permitted to take some other activity in place of physical education. Professional persons who condone substitutions for their physical education classes are not clear as to the goals of their profession. It is important that physical educators recognize that there is no adequate substitute for a well-planned, well-organized, and well-conducted physical education class.

Should credit be given for physical education?

Whether or not credit should be given for physical education is another controversial problem with which the profession is continually confronted. Here again can be found advocates on both sides. There are those who feel the joy of the activity and the values derived from participation are sufficient in themselves without giving credit. On the other hand, there are those who feel that physical education is the same as any other subject in the curriculum and should also be granted credit.

The general consensus among physical education leaders is that if physical education is required for graduation and if it contributes to educational outcomes, credit should be given, just as in other subjects. The credit given should be justified by the contribution physical education makes to the achievement of outcomes toward which all of education is working.

What policy should be established on class attendance?

It is important for every department of physical education to have a definite policy on class attendance that covers absenteeism and tardiness. Since it is felt that students should attend school and colleges regularly, it follows that they should also attend classes regularly, including physical education.

Regular attendance in physical education is essential in order to derive the values and outcomes that accrue from participation. Since attendance is necessary in order to achieve such outcomes, every physical education department should have a clear-cut policy on attendance regulations. These regulations should be few in number and clearly stated in writing so that they are recognized, understood, and strictly enforced by teachers and students. They should allow for a reasonable number of absences and tardinesses, which can always occur in emergency situations over which the student has no control. Perfect attendance at school or college should not be stressed. Many harmful results can develop if students feel obligated to attend classes when they are ill and should be home in bed. There should probably be some provision for makeup work when important experiences are missed. However, makeup work should be planned and conducted so that the student derives essential values from such participation, rather than enduring it as a disciplinary measure. There should also be provision for the readmission of students who have been ill. A procedure should be established so that the program is adapted to these individuals.

A final point to remember is the importance of keeping accurate, up-to-date attendance records. Unless meaningful records are kept, administrative problems will increase.

What about excuses?

The principal, nurse, or physical educator frequently receives a note from a parent or family physician asking that a student be excused from physical education. Many abuses develop if all such requests are granted. Many times for minor reasons the student does not want to participate and obtains the parent's or family physician's support.

Tom Peiffer, a physical educator in the

PHYSICAL EDUCATION EXCUSE

NAME ....

GRADE .... ADVISOR .... GYM PERIOD ....

DATES—EXCUSED FROM .... TO ....

DOCTOR ....

REASON ....

....

NO PHYS. ED. ....

MODIFIED PROGRAM

      FULL PROGRAM EXCEPT COMPETITIVE SPORTS ....

      PARTICIPATION EXCEPT ....

SCHOOL SCHEDULE ADJUSTMENT, IF ANY ....

....

Physical education excuse form. (From Bucher, C. A., Koenig, C. R., and Barnhard, M.: Methods and materials for secondary school physical education, ed. 3, St. Louis, 1970, The C. V. Mosby Co).

New York State public schools, conducted a survey to determine both the extent of required physical education and practices in regard to physical education excuses in secondary schools, colleges, and universities. The questionnaire used in the survey was sent to schools selected at random from fifteen states situated in various sections of the United States. The questionnaire was sent to the high school in the largest city, to a suburban school of that city, to one city in the state with a population of 20,000 to 25,000, to one city in the state with a population of 10,000 to 15,000, and to one community with a population of 3,000 to 5,000. On the college level, questionnaires were sent to one state university, one private institution, and one teacher training institution. Questionnaires were sent to seventy-five secondary schools and sixty-seven colleges and universities. Replies were received from forty-five secondary schools and forty colleges and universities. Among the secondary schools, 37.9% required 4 years of physical education, 28.8% required 3 years, 20% required 2 years, and 13.3% required 1 year. In higher education, 60% of the colleges required 2 years, 25% required 1 year, 10% required 3 years, and 5% did not have a requirement. The number of days per week devoted to physical education is also shown in diagram on p. 145.

Peiffer's survey showed that high schools permitted a student to be excused on the basis of a parental note, a memorandum from the family physician, or the discretion of the physical education teacher. While some schools would accept the recommendation of any of these three persons, other schools would accept only an excuse from the school physician. At the college level most programs accept the college physician's excuse or permit the instructor of each class to use his own discretion in granting excuses to his students.

The reasons listed as to why excuses in physical education were granted were an interesting part of the preceding survey.

Secondary schools grant most of their excuses for participation in athletics and for being in the school band. Some schools permit their athletes to be excused only on the day of the game, while others grant a blanket excuse for the entire sports season. Other reasons for excuses on the secondary level, in addition to athletics, included makeup tests, driver training, counseling, a too-heavy extracurricular load, and medical reasons. At the college level, excuses were granted to athletes, veterans, students who could pass physical fitness tests, honor students, older students, for medical reasons, in "hardship cases," and so on.

Another part of the questionnaire on excuses attempted to discover what was done with the students who were excused. Students in secondary schools were sent to study halls; required to score, officiate, or help around the physical education department; write reports; remain on the sidelines; or report after school. At the college level most colleges did nothing except follow a pattern of failing a student in some cases if he exceeded the legal number of excused absences per semester. A few either required the student to observe the class, substitute a health class, or study in the gymnasium or left it up to the instructor's discretion.

Some school systems have exercised control over the indiscriminate granting of requests for excuses from physical education. Policies have been established, sometimes through conferences and rulings of the board of education, requiring that all excuses must be reviewed and approved by the school physician before they will be granted. Furthermore, family physicians have been asked to state specific reasons for requesting excuse from physical education. This procedure has worked out very satisfactorily in some communities. In other places physical educators have taken particular pains to work very closely with medical doctors. They have established a physical education program in collabora-

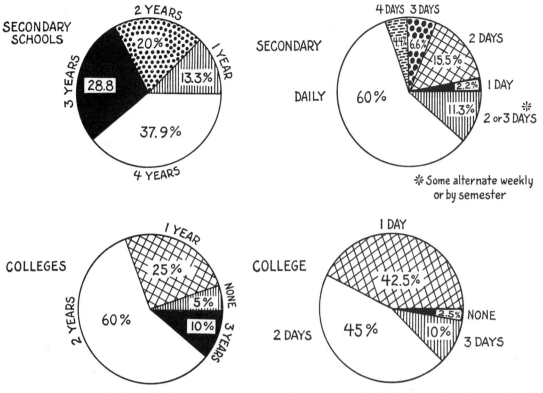

Extent of required physical education in schools surveyed.

Days per week of physical education in schools surveyed.

FORM 860-D   DSP   11-57-500 BKS.   U-857-44603

DENVER PUBLIC SCHOOLS
Department of Health Service

HEALTH EXCUSE FROM SCHOOL

Date..

To the parents or guardian of:..

We consider it best that your child return home today because of the following

health reasons:...

....

....

If the illness continues or becomes worse, please have the child seen by your own

physician; and be sure he/she is well before returning to school.

School Physician or Nurse

School Principal

tion with the school physician so that the needs of each individual are met, regardless of his or her physical condition. They have met with the local medical society in an attempt to clear up misunderstandings in regard to the purpose and conduct of the program. Family physicians have been brought into the planning. As a result of such planning, problems in regard to excuses from physical education have been considerably reduced.

There probably is a correlation between the respect, prestige, and degree to which physical education is understood in any community and the number of excuses that are requested. Furthermore, respect, prestige, and understanding are reflected in the type of leadership that exists. It has been found that in those communities where parents, family physicians, and the lay public in general understand physical education, the number of requests for excuses is relatively small. In such communities, the values that can be derived from participation in the program are clearly recognized, and since most parents and physicians want children to have worthwhile experiences, they encourage rather than attempt to limit such participation. The leadership of any program can eliminate many of the administrative problems in regard to excuses, provided physical education is properly interpreted to the public at large.

A few years ago, a conference concerned with close cooperation between physical education and medical doctors drew up a list of statements in respect to the problem under discussion. These are as follows:

1. Orient the student, parent, and physician at an early date in regard to the objectives of the physical education program.
2. Route all requests for excuse through the school physician. In the absence of the physician the school nurse should have this responsibility. The sympathetic and informed nurse can be a real asset to the physical education program.
3. Discard permanent and blanket excuses. The

school physician should share in planning certain areas of the individual physical education program. Instead of being categorically excused, boys and girls can be given an activity in keeping with their special needs.
4. Students involved in the excuse request should have a periodic recheck as to need for excuse (this tends to reduce requests up to 50%).
5. Conferences between the school physicians and the head of the physical education department on the local level need to be emphasized.
6. The problem of excuse from physical education should be tied up with the total guidance program of the school. It helps also if the administrator and classroom teachers are familiar with the general physical education aims.

Should boys and girls be separated for physical education in grades one to six?

There is disagreement as to whether or not boys and girls should be separated for physical education classes in the elementary school.

Those persons who advocate keeping the pupils together list such reasons as the following to support their position:

1. Separation hinders the social objective.
2. Separation causes unnecessary curiosity on the part of both boys and girls.
3. Schools cannot provide the resources and teachers needed to conduct separate programs.
4. Interests of both boys and girls prior to the adolescent period are much the same.
5. Playing together can carry over to later years, resulting in a happy, shared recreational life.

Those persons who advocate separating the sexes, at least during some of the elementary school years, list such reasons as the following to support their position:

1. Girls are too emotional.
2. Boys are interested in feats requiring strength, endurance, and skill, whereas girls are primarily interested in grace and moderate amounts of skill.
3. Girls and boys shy away from each other and want to be separated in physical activities.

4. Physical activities that the boys like, placing heavy demands on organic vitality, are not appropriate for girls.

5. A segregated program can do more to accomplish the separate objectives of both boys and girls.

6. A program that brings boys and girls together results in boys taking over key positions. Also, boys are more demanding, resulting in less time for girls to practice skills and have fun.

An analysis of the characteristics of boys and girls at the various grade levels shows that in the first and second grades the boys and girls have no preference as to sex, and, at the third grade, boys and girls are just beginning to become conscious of the distinctions between them. Interests and abilities of boys and girls during the first three grades are not significant. Therefore, it is recommended that through the third grade, boys and girls might well take their physical education classes together.

At the fourth-, fifth-, and sixth-grade levels the physical education classes for boys and girls might well be separated, at least for many of the activities that are offered in the program. The reasons that undergird such a statement are well founded. Starting with the fourth grade, open antagonisms become apparent; boys like to rough it up and are more aggressive, girls are more subdued and do not like loud, boisterous action. Girls are nearing puberty at this level and developing at a very rapid rate. During the fifth and sixth grades interests are entirely different, with girls liking rhythmic movement and boys liking tests of strength and endurance. Each sex teases the other continuously. Boys are farther ahead than girls in skill, rules, knowledge, and strategy in many activities.

There should be opportunities, however, for boys and girls to get together periodically in activities that lend themselves to an integrated situation, such as some form of rhythmic activity.

Should the physical education specialist or the classroom teacher conduct the physical education class in the elementary school?

This question has been discussed on a perennial basis for many years. There are educators who advocate the classroom teacher handling physical education classes and also many supporters who want a specialist to take over this responsibility. The issue is quite involved and limited space does not permit taking up in depth each side of the issue. These facts, however, should be pointed out. The classroom teacher has limited professional education in physical education. Some classroom teachers are not interested in teaching physical education. Furthermore, there is increased interest in physical education today, which implies that qualified and interested persons should handle these classes. There is a trend toward more emphasis on movement education, physical fitness, skills, and other aspects of education with which physical education is concerned. There is a need for more research on physical education programs as they relate to the learning and growth of children. There is an increased emphasis upon looking to the specialist in physical education for help and advice in planning and conducting the elementary school program. These developments have implications for a sound inservice program to help the classroom teacher do a better job in physical education.

In light of the present status of physical education in the elementary schools of this country, such recommendations as the following should be very carefully considered. Each elementary school should be staffed with a man or woman specialist in physical education. The classroom teacher may find her best contribution to physical education programs in kindergarten to grade three, but to do her best job she needs preparation in this special field and the advice and help of a physical education specialist in her school. Although the classroom teacher can contribute much to the physical education program in grades four to six, factors such as the growth changes and interests taking place in boys and girls and the more specialized program that exists at this level make it imperative to seek the help of a specialist. A specialist possesses the ability, experience, and training required to meet the needs of growing boys and girls as well as gain their respect and interest. Another statement should be made in regard to the elementary school physical education program. The specialist and the classroom teacher should pool and share their experiences so that the most desirable learning experience may be provided children in the physical education program. Each teacher has much to contribute and should be encouraged to do so.

What about self-defense courses?

There are many arguments pro and con concerning self-defense courses for both men and women. On the affirmative side, the arguments include the need to be prepared in case of attack from a robber, assailant, rapist, and molester. The advocates further stress that knowing the various tricks of dirty fighting and self-defense will enable one to defend himself in various kinds of emergency situations. The increase in crime on our streets and in our homes, others say, makes it necessary to know how to deal with such situations if they arise.

Those persons who oppose self-defense courses argue that a little knowledge is a bad thing; a gangster or criminal always has the advantage with weapons he may carry, the surprise of his attack, and his greater strength and experience. Those opposed also indicate that the tricks learned in such courses may be used to the detriment of friends and associates in playful situations. They also stress that the number of instances of attack do not warrant devoting time to such a course.

Furthermore, some persons stress that such courses are entirely opposed to the values that physical education stresses, namely, social effectiveness and sportsmanship. Finally, some educators indicate that the majority of the students exposed to such courses would find such instruction ineffective in warding off assailants. One further objection of some physical educators is that such courses for women should be opposed because they are not feminine in nature.

CLASS MANAGEMENT

Good class management requires planning. Forethought is needed in order to have a group of students act in an orderly manner, accomplish the tasks that have been established, and have an enjoyable, satisfying, and worthwhile experience. The leader who is in charge of a class where these optimum conditions exist has spent considerable time in planning the details of the class from start to finish. Good class management does not just happen. It requires considerable thought, good judgment, and the making of many plans before the class begins.

There are many reasons for good organization. These should be recognized by every teacher and administrator. Some of these are listed below:

1. It gives meaning and purpose to instruction and to the activities.

2. It results in efficiency, the right emphasis, and the best use of the time that is available.

3. It more fully ensures that the needs and interests of the students will be satisfied.

4. It more fully ensures progression and continuity in the program.

5. It provides for measurement and progress toward objectives.

6. It ensures provision for child health and safety.

7. It encourages program adaptations to each individual's needs and interests.

8. It reduces errors and omissions to a minimum.

9. It helps to conserve the instructor's time and strength and aids in giving her or him a sense of accomplishment.

Some guides with which the teacher and administrator should concern themselves are as follows:

1. There should be long-term planning —for the semester and the year, as well as daily, weekly, and seasonal.

2. A definite time schedule should be planned for each period, taking into consideration time to be devoted to showering and dressing, taking roll, class activity, and other essentials.

3. The activity should be carefully planned so that it proceeds with precision and dispatch, with a minimum amount of standing around and a maximum amount of activity for each student.

4. The physical education class period should be regarded primarily as an instructional period. It is not one for free play. However, in order to have sustained interest and as much satisfaction and joy result from the class as possible, there should be provision for using the instruction received in actual activity.

5. There should be a definite system established for such essentials as taking roll, keeping essential records, grading, adhering to policy on uniform, and dressing and showering.

6. Attention should be given to the preparation of materials to be used in class. The teacher should know beforehand the materials to be used, and they should be ready when the class begins.

7. The setting for the class should be safe and healthful. The equipment should be safe and line markings, arrangements for activities, and other essential details attended to.

8. Procedures to be followed in locker room should be established, to provide for traffic, valuables, clothes, and dressing and showering.

9. A procedure should be established for falling in, taking attendance, organizing for activity, and dismissal.

10. The instructor should always use good English and explain things in a simple, clear, and informative manner. During explanations the class should be attentive.

11. The instructor should always be prompt and punctual for class meetings.

12. The instructor should be tactful and considerate of every pupil. Pupils should not be condemned for making mistakes. It should be remembered that an educational situation is a normal and natural setting for mistakes.

13. Pupils should be encouraged and motivated to do their best.

14. All pupils should be treated in the same manner. There should be no favorites.

15. A planned program of measurement and evaluation should be provided to determine progress being made by pupils and the effectiveness of teaching.

16. The instructor and the class should dress in suitable costume.

17. There should be as few rules of behavior as possible, making sure that those that are established are adhered to. Pupils should participate in the establishment of such rules.

18. The instructor should circulate among the entire class, giving help to those who are in need of it. Individual differences should be adequately provided for.

19. The instructor should have a good command of his subject. The values of demonstrations, visual aids, and other techniques to promote learning should be recognized.

20. Desirable attitudes and understandings toward physical fitness, skill learning, good sportsmanship, and other concepts inherent in physical education should be stressed at all times.

21. Standards of achievement and specific goals that are attainable should be established. Pupils' progress should be

recorded so that they know how they are advancing toward these goals.

Some of the factors concerned with class management that deserve special attention are dressing and showering, costume, taking roll, grading, and records. Each of these will be discussed in more detail.

Dressing and showering

Such factors as the age of the student, time allowed, grade participating, and type of activity should be considered in a discussion of dressing and showering for physical education classes.

The problem of showering and dressing is not so pertinent at the lower elementary level where the age of the participants and type of activities as a general rule do not require special costumes and showering. Also the time allotted is too short in many cases. In the upper elementary and at the junior and senior high school and college levels, however, it is a problem.

Physical education, by its very nature, embodies activities that result in considerable running, jumping, throwing, and other vigorous movements. Participation also frequently results in perspiration. In the interests of comfort and good hygiene practices, provisions should be made for special clothing and showering. The unpleasant features of a student's returning to class after participating in physical education activity, with clothes dripping from perspiration and with the accompanying odors, are not in conformance with establishing good habits of personal cleanliness and grooming. Therefore, all schools should make special provisions for places to dress in comfortable uniforms and for showering. Such places should be convenient to the physical education areas, be comfortable, and afford privacy. Although girls are increasingly becoming accustomed to using a gang shower, there are still many who prefer the private cubicles. In the interests of these individuals, such facilities should be

provided. There should also be some type of towel service. In many schools there are facilities for laundering towels that have worked out very satisfactorily.

In order to ensure that a maximum number of pupils take advantage of the facilities for showering and dressing, it is important that proper attitudes and understanding be developed. The right attitudes toward cleanliness, personal grooming, and sanitation should be developed in each individual. If this is done, the right health practices will be followed and the question of whether or not to establish a rigid rule requiring showers will not be necessary. It should be a matter of education rather than one of coercion. In addition, there should be a reasonable time allotted for showering and dressing. This should be kept at a minimum in order to allow a maximum of time for activity, but at the same time adequate time should be allowed to dress and shower.

Costume

There are many reasons for the use of special costumes in physical education classes above the elementary level:

1. It makes for better appearance if an individual is dressed in a costume that fits the activity in which he is engaging.
2. It provides for more comfort and allows for freedom of movement.
3. It is more economical, since it saves on street clothes. If purchased in lots by the school there can be a considerable saving to the student. Those students who cannot afford uniforms should have them provided free of charge.
4. If all students have the same uniform, it aids morale and promotes equality.
5. It is safer without dangling sleeves or wide skirts to cause accidents.

The costumes do not have to be elaborate. For girls they can be simple, washable shorts and blouse or one-piece suits. For boys white cotton jerseys and trunks will suffice. Of course, suitable shoes should also be worn. An important con-

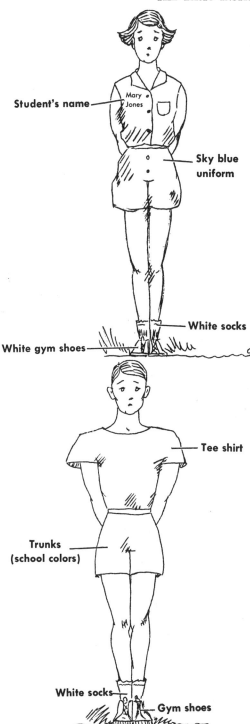

Student's name

Mary Jones

Sky blue uniform

White socks

White gym shoes

Tee shirt

Trunks (school colors)

White socks

Gym shoes

Physical education uniforms for high school girls and boys. (Courtesy Division of Health and Physical Education, Chicago Public Schools, Chicago, Ill.)

sideration is to keep the uniform clean. The instructor should establish a policy on clean uniforms and work diligently toward seeing that hygienic standards are met by all.

Taking roll

There are many methods of taking roll. If a method satisfies the following three criteria, it is usually satisfactory. (1) It is economical of time—roll taking should not consume too much time. It is essential to get into activity as soon as possible, and routine details should be kept to a minimum. (2) It should guarantee accuracy—it is important to know accurately after the class has been held who was present and who was not. This means taking into consideration those who might come to class late or leave early. (3) It should not be complicated. Any system that is used should be very simple and easy to administer.

A number of questions arise in respect to roll taking: Should it be taken on the gymnasium floor or playground or in the swimming pool, shower, or locker room? Or should it be taken on the way to or from the gymnasium or place where the physical education activity is held? When should it be taken? Should it be taken at the beginning of the period; after the class has started, in order to ensure the inclusion of tardy students; or at the end of the period? Who should take it? Should it be taken by the instructor, an assistant instructor, the shower or locker attendant, or squad leader? These questions are pertinent and must be answered by the physical educator in each local situation and in accordance with the influences that play upon the physical education class.

Some of the methods for roll taking that may be used are as follows:

1. *Having numbers on the floor*—each member of the class is assigned a number that he must stand on at the time the signal for "fall in" is given. The person

taking attendance records the numbers that are not covered.

2. *Reciting numbers orally*—each member of the class is assigned a number that he must say out loud at the time the signal for "fall in" is given. The person taking attendance then records the numbers that are not given.

3. *Tag board*—each member of the class has a number that is recorded on a cardboard or metal tag that hangs on a

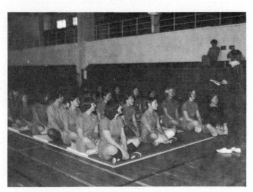

Courtesy Mrs. C. Eaton.

Squad form of attendance taking. (Glastonbury High School, Glastonbury, Conn.)

peg on a board in a central place. Each member of the class who is present removes his tag from the board and places it in a box. The person taking attendance records the absentees from the board.

4. *Delaney system*—a special system developed by Delaney involves using a folder with cards that are turned over when a person is absent. It is a cumulative system that records the attendance of pupils over a period of time. There are adaptations of this system that are used elsewhere.

5. *Squad system*—the class is divided into squads and the squad leader takes the roll for his squad and in turn reports to the instructor.

6. *Issuing towels and equipment*—the roll is taken when a towel is issued to each student or when it is turned in, or when a basket with uniform is issued or returned.

7. *Signing a book or register*—students are required to write their names in a book or register at the beginning of the class. Some systems require the writing of a name at the beginning of a period and crossing it out at the end of a period. The

Attendance record.

Squad #_____

Physical Education Department
Class Data

Dental Note_____

Class_____

NAME (LAST) FIRST	SEPTEMBER	OCTOBER	NOVEMBER	DECEMBER	JANUARY	MID TERM	FEBRUARY	MARCH	APRIL	MAY	JUNE	FINAL
1												
2												
3												
4												
5												
6												
7												
8												
9												
10												

Cumulative class record.

person taking attendance records the names not entered.

Records

Records are essential in keeping valuable information in regard to pupils' welfare. They also are essential to efficient program planning and administration. They should, however, be kept to a minimum and should be practical and functional. They should not be maintained just as "busy" work and for the sake of filling the files. Instead they should have "use" and a place in the program.

Some of the records should be concerned directly with the welfare of the pupil and others with certain administrative factors.

Those records that concern the welfare of the student are the health records, the cumulative physical education form, anecdotal accounts, attendance reports, grades, and accident reports.

Health records are essential. They contain information on the health examination and other appraisal techniques, health counseling, and any other data pertaining to the student's health.

The cumulative physical education record should start when the student first attends school and contain information about activities engaged in, afterschool play, test, anecdotal accounts, interests, needs, and any other pertinent information that should be known in respect to the student and his participation in the physical education programs.

There should be special records for attendance and grades and any special occurrences that have a bearing on the child and that are not recorded in other records.

If a student is involved in an accident, a full account of the circumstances surrounding the accident should be recorded. Usually special forms are provided for such purposes.*

---
*See Chapters 10 and 14 for more information on accidents.

The records dealing with administrative factors are concerned with general administrative information and equipment records. These would include a list of the year's events: activities; records of teams; play days, sports days, intramurals; events of special interest; techniques utilized that have been helpful; budget information; and any other data that would be helpful in planning for succeeding years. The memory of the human being often fails over a period of time, with the result that many good ideas are lost and many activities and techniques of special value not utilized because they are forgotten.

There should be records in regard to equipment, facilities, and supplies. Such records should show the material needing repair, new materials needed, and also the location of various materials, so that they can easily be found.

There is also a need for records in regard to such items as locker or basket assignments and any other pertinent information that is essential to the efficient running of a physical education program.

PHYSICAL EDUCATION ACTIVITIES

Physical education activities represent the heart of the program. They are the means for accomplishing objectives. They represent the media that attract the attention of the student and through participation aid him in the achievement of life's goals. Because they are so important to the physical education profession, they must be selected with considerable care.

Criteria for selection

1. Activities should be selected in terms of the values they have in achieving the objectives of physical education. This means they would not only possess potentialities for developing physical fitness but also would have implications for developing the intellectual, emotional, and social makeup of the individual.

2. Activities should be interesting and

challenging. They should appeal to the students and present them with situations that challenge their skill and ability. For example, golf always presents the challenge of getting a lower score.

3. They should be adaptable to the growth and developmental needs and interests of children and youth. The needs of individuals vary from age to age. Consequently, activities and the pattern of organization must also change if these needs are to be met. The activity must be suited to the child, not the child to the activity. Wherever possible, students should be allowed some choice in the activities in which they participate.

4. Activities should be modifications of racially old, fundamental movements such as running, jumping, throwing, walking, and climbing.

5. Activities, of course, must be selected in the light of the facilities, supplies, equipment, and other resources available in the school, college, or community. One cannot plan an extensive tennis program if only one court is available.

6. Activities should be selected not only with a view to their present value while the child is in school but also with a view to postschool and adult living. Skills learned during school and college days have potentialities for use throughout life, thus contributing in great measure to enriched living. Patterns for many skills utilized in adult leisure hours are developed while the individual is in the formative years of childhood.

7. Activities must be selected for health and safety values. Such an activity as boxing has been in question as to its effect on the health and the safety of individuals.

8. The local education philosophy, policies, and school or college organization must be taken into consideration.

9. School activities should provide situations that are similar to those children experience in natural play situations outside the school environment.

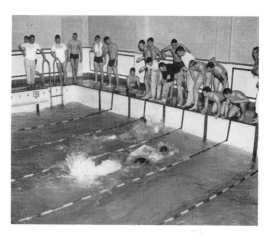

Washington State College, Pullman, Wash.

10. Activities should provide the student with opportunities for creative self-expression.

11. Activities should be selected which have potentialities to elicit the correct social and moral responses through high-quality leadership.

12. Activities should reflect the democratic way of life.

Classification

One survey* produced a list of physical education activities offered throughout the country, here classified into various categories. These do not necessarily meet criteria that have been listed. They merely indicate current offerings in physical education programs in the United States:

Team games

Baseball	Soccer
Basketball	Softball
Code ball	Speedball
Field hockey (women only)	Touch football
Flag football (men only)	Volleyball
Football (men only)	

Outdoor winter sports

Ice hockey	
Roller skating	Snow games
Skating	Snowshoeing
Skiing	Tobogganing

---

*Bucher, C. A.: Foundations of physical education, ed. 5, St. Louis, 1968, The C. V. Mosby Co.

Other activities
  Camping and outdoor activities
  Combatives
  Correctives
  Fly-tying
  Games of low organization
  Movement education
  Relays
  Self-testing activities
Rhythms and dancing
  Folk dancing   Square dancing
  Gymnastic dancing   Social dancing
  Modern dancing   Tap dancing
  Rhythms
Formal activities
  Calisthenics
  Marching
Water activities
  Canoeing   Swimming
  Diving   Sailing
  Lifesaving   Water games
  Rowing
Gymnastics
  Acrobatics   Rope climbing
  Apparatus   Stunts
  Obstacle course   Trampoline
  Pyramid building   Tumbling
Dual and individual sports
  Archery   Darts (women only)
  Badminton   Deck tennis
  Bait and fly casting Fencing
  Bowling   Fishing
  Checkers (women only) Golf

Dual and individual sports—cont'd.
  Handball   Skish
  Horseback riding   Table tennis
  Horseshoes   Tennis
  Paddle tennis   Tether ball
  Rifle   Track and field
  Rope skipping   Wrestling (men only)
  Shuffleboard

LaPorte* has compiled a list of physical education activities, together with time allotments, that meet acceptable criteria (Table 7-1).

The state of California lists the following types of activities:

1. Aquatics, where facilities are available
2. Gymnastics and tumbling
3. Individual and dual sports
4. Mechanics of body movement and health aspects of physical activity
5. Rhythms and dance
6. Team sports
7. Combatives for boys†

---

*LaPorte, op. cit., pp. 28-33.
†California State Department of Education, Bureau of Health Education, Physical Education, and Recreation. Letter dated August 14, 1964, from C. Carson Conrad, Chief, Bureau of Health Education, Physical Education, and Recreation, Sacramento, Calif.

Table 7-1. List of physical education activities*

A. Primary level (grades 1 to 3)	
1. Rhythmical activities	25%
2. Fundamental rhythms	20%
3. Hunting games	20%
4. Relays	15%
5. Stunts and self-testing activities	10%
6. Athletic games of low organization	10%
	100%
B. Elementary level (grades 4 to 6)	
1. Athletic games of low organization	25%
2. Rhythmical activities	30%
3. Hunting games	15%
4. Individual athletic event (self-testing)	10%
5. Relays	10%
6. Tumbling stunts	10%
	100%

*From LaPorte, W. R.: The physical education curriculum (a national program), ed. 6, Los Angeles, 1955, University of Southern California Press, pp. 28-33.

Table 7-1. List of physical education activities—cont'd

C. Junior high school (grades 7 to 9) and senior high school (grades 10 to 12)

	Junior high school (elementary)		Senior high school (advanced)	
	Boys (weeks)	Girls (weeks)	Boys (weeks)	Girls (weeks)
1. Aquatics				
Swimming, diving, lifesaving	18	18	18	18
2. Dancing				
Folk, square, tap, modern (girls)	12	18	12	18
3. Team sports				
A. Court and diamond games Volleyball, softball, basketball, nine-court basketball (junior high school girls)	18	18	18	18
B. Field sports				
Soccer, speedball, touch football (boys), field ball (junior high girls), field hockey (senior high girls)	18	12	18	12
4. Gymnastics				
Tumbling, pyramids, apparatus, relays, stunts, body mechanics, and posture exercises	12	12	12	12
5. Individual and dual sports				
Tennis, badminton, handball, golf, or archery	18	18	18	18
Additional sports from following: boating and canoeing, bowling, hiking and camping, horseshoes, fencing, fly and bait casting, paddle tennis, riding, skating, snowshoeing, squash, table tennis, trampoline, wrestling	12	12	12	12
	Total of 108 weeks		Total of 108 weeks	

D. College (grades 13 to 16) (Each activity is a one-semester course of an advanced type.)

1. Apparatus
2. Archery
3. Badminton
4. Diving
5. Fencing
6. Folk dancing
7. Golf
8. Handball
9. Lifesaving
10. Modern dance (creative, interpretive)
11. Social dancing
12. Social (recreational) games
13. Squash (or squash racquets)
14. Swimming
15. Tap and clog dancing
16. Tennis
17. Tumbling
18. Wrestling
19. Team games (when needed)
20. Specialties (winter activities, etc., when needed)
21. Restricted and remedial for subnormal cases

Coeducational activities

The need for more coeducational activity is being recognized. Past history shows that activities for boys and girls have been combined at the lower elementary levels but at the upper elementary, secondary, and college levels they have been separated. A common sight on college campuses and even at the secondary level is separate sets of facilities for the men and women or boys and girls. In the light of education objectives, this does not seem to be in the interests of what the profession is striving to attain in the schools.

Men and women are continually together in work, home, social, and other situations throughout life. If they are to adjust properly in such situations, it is essential that attention be given to this matter in their childhood and youth years. Our country is faced with the problems of increased divorce rates and disintegration of family life. Individuals who have not had the opportunity to play, work, and socialize with the opposite sex in childhood and youth often find it difficult to adjust satisfactorily when they become adults. Furthermore, if family life is to be a happy experience, the various members of the families should be attuned to such items as the others' interests, temperaments, likes, dislikes, and habits. Such adjustment is obtained only through constant association in a variety of situations. The physical education program should encourage and provide for such associations, rather than be indifferent or oppose such a natural phenomenon. The contributions this specialized field can make to such an objective are very great and should be utilized to the fullest.

PROGRAMS

Many aspects of the elementary, junior high, senior high, and college physical education basic instructional programs have already been discussed. This information will not be repeated. Instead, certain administrative guides are suggested for each level to aid the administrator, teacher, or

Coeducational physical education. (From Bucher, C. A., Koenig, C. R., and Barnhard, M.: Methods and materials for secondary school physical education, ed. 3, St. Louis, 1970, The C. V. Mosby Co.)

other interested person in the conduct of a physical education program.

Program for kindergarten through grade six

The various aspects of the physical education program for elementary school, including characteristics of children at various ages, opportunities they need, and activities that meet these needs and characteristics, were developed by a group of experts at the National Conference on Physical Education for Children of Elementary School Age. The following information has been taken from their report because of its value to all persons interested in elementary school physical education. *Of course, the discussion of movement education recorded earlier in this chapter indicates a vital and important emphasis on elementary school physical education programs.*

PROGRAM*

Growth is a continuous process—an emerging—an unfolding. At no time does a child abruptly

*Report of National Conference of Physical Education for Children of Elementary School Age: Physical education for children of elementary school age, Chicago, 1951, The Athletic Institute, Inc.

complete a particular stage of development and begin the next. Neither is there a time when all children in a group are at exactly the same stage of growth.

Any classification into groups along the route of growth is artificial. The following chart [Tables 7-2 and 7-3 on pp. 160 and 161] is merely a device to help give a picture of activities that seem to suit the changing needs of children. The subdivision and classifications used serve as convenient labels for periods of growth through which children gradually move, each child holding to a path that is his alone.

Program for grades seven and eight

Facilities, time, pupils, and teacher load are some of the factors that will determine the basic physical education instructional program for grades seven and eight. The absence or presence of a swimming pool, for example, would influence the type of program offered.

Boys and girls in grades seven and eight are in a period of rapid physical growth with awkwardness and lack of coordination frequently in evidence. Muscles, bones, heart, and lungs are experiencing the growth spurt. Boys surpass girls in strength and speed, and interests in different types of physical activities are common. There is keen interest in competitive activities, and this motivating factor may create the desire to want to continue par-

Text continued on p. 166.

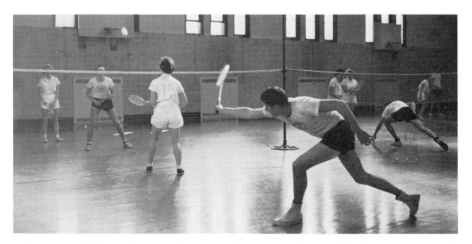

There is need for coeducational activity. (Wisconsin State College, La Crosse, Wis.)

Table 7-2. Early childhood—5 to 8 years of age—kindergarten through third grade*

What they are like	What they need OPPORTUNITIES	What to do
Their large muscles (trunk, legs, and arms) are more developed than the smaller muscles (hands and feet)	To experience many kinds of vigorous activities that involve many parts of the body. To engage in many developmental activities for small muscles	Activities such as hanging, running, jumping, climbing, dodging, or throwing at an object. Beanbag Toss, Jacks, Bouncing Balls, Hopscotch, O'Leary
They have a short attention span	To engage in many activities of short duration	Choice of activity where a child can change frequently, and activities that can be started quickly, such as Magic Carpet, Pincho, Hill Dill, and stunts
They are individualistic and possessive	To play alone and with small groups. To play as an individual in larger groups	Individual activities, such as throwing, catching, bouncing, kicking, climbing, stunts, running, hopping, skipping, building blocks, jumping. Dance activities which allow for expression of self, such as clowns, aviators, firemen, tops, aeroplanes. Activities that may use small numbers of children, such as Stride Ball, Cat and Rat, Hill Dill, Cowboys and Indians, Tag. Singing games such as Looby Loo, Bluebird, Sing a Song of Sixpence
They are dramatic, imaginative, and imitative	To create and explore. To identify themselves with people and things	Invent dance and game activities, such as Cowboys, Circus, Christmas toys; work activities such as pounding, sawing, raking, and hauling. Other play activities: farmers, postmen, grocers, elevators, bicycles, leaves, scarecrows
They are active, energetic, and responsive to rhythmic sounds	To respond to rhythmic sounds such as drums, rattles, voice and nursery rhythms, songs, and music	Running, skipping, walking, jumping, galloping, dodging, swimming. Singing and folk games such as Oats, Peas, Beans, and Barley Grow; Farmer in the Dell; Dixie Polka
They are curious and want to find out things	To explore and handle materials with many types of play	Using materials such as balls, ropes, stilts, beanbags, bars, ladders, trees, blocks. Games and activities such as hiking, Run-Sheep-Run, Huckle-Buckle, Bean-stalk
They want chances to act on their own and are annoyed at conformity	To make choices, to help make rules, to share and evaluate group experiences	Variety of activities with minimum of rules, such as Center Base, Exchange, Midnight, and Red Light. Make-up activities, dances, and games
They are continuing to broaden social contacts or relationships	To cooperate in play and dance, to organize many of their own groups	Group games, such as simple forms of Dodge Ball, Kickball. Dance and rhythmic activities, such as Gustaf's Skoal, Dance of Greeting, Bow Balinda
They seem to be in perpetual motion	To play many types of vigorous activities	Running, jumping, skipping, galloping, rolling

*From Report of National Conference on Physical Education for Children of Elementary School Age: Physical education for children of elementary school age, Chicago, 1951, The Athletic Institute, Inc.

Table 7-3. Middle childhood—9 to 11 years of age—fourth through sixth grades*

What they are like	What they need OPPORTUNITIES	What to do
They grow steadily in muscles, bone, heart, and lungs	To engage in strenuous activity that regularly taxes these organs to the limits of healthy fatigue	Running, jumping, climbing, and hard play
They enjoy rough and tumble activities	To participate in activities that use the elements of roughness	Bumping, pushing, contact activities such as King of the Ring, Poison Pen, Indian Wrestle, Hand Wrestle, Beater Goes 'Round
Sex differences begin to appear with girls taller and more mature than boys. Sex antagonisms may appear	To enjoy their roles as boys and girls, to have wholesome boy-girl relationships in activities and to participate separately for some activities	Activities such as folk dances, mixers, squares, modern Brothers and Sisters, Last Couple Out. Group games such as Volleyball type games, Newcomb or Fist Ball, Softball. Others may be enjoyed separately or together
They respond differently in varying situations	To participate in wide range of activities and organizations using many kinds of materials	Individual, dual, or small and large group activities such as swimming, tumbling, stilts, track, catch, handball, relays, Crows and Cranes, Crackers, Bombardment; folk dances, mixers, and simple square dances such as Csebogar, Captain Jinks, Life on the Ocean Wave
They have a strong sense of rivalry and crave recognition	To succeed in activities that stress cooperative play along with activities that give individual satisfaction	Self-testing activities such as track events, stunts, chinning, sit-ups, push-ups, ball-throwing, for distance and accuracy. Group and team play such as Newcomb, Kickball, Circle or Square Soccer, End Ball, Club Snatch, Progressive Dodge Ball
They may show increasing independence and desire to help	To plan, lead, and check progress	Assist with officiating, serve as squad leaders, act as scorers, help with equipment, elect captains, help with younger children and each other
They want to be liked by their own classmates, to belong. They have a strong loyalty to teams, groups, or "gangs"	To belong to groups, to be on many kinds of teams To engage in a wide range of activities	Group games such as Bounce Volleyball, Line Soccer, Keep Away, Hit Pin Kickball, Net Ball. Partner play such as Deck Tennis (Ring Toss), Tennis, Aerial Darts, Horseshoes
They want approval, but not at the expense of their group relationships	To gain respect and approval of others	Participate in activities in which they achieve in the eyes of their group

*From Report of National Conference on Physical Education for Children of Elementary School Age. Physical education for children of elementary school age, Chicago, 1951, The Athletic Institute, Inc.

Table 7-4. Later childhood—early adolescence—12 to 13 years of age—seventh and eighth grades*

What they are like	What they need OPPORTUNITIES	What to do
This is a period of rapid physical growth that is frequently uneven in various parts of the body. Awkwardness and inability to coordinate sometimes occur	To develop skill and coordination and to take part in activities that do not call attention to their awkwardness or put them in embarrassing situations	Skills in various activities such at batting, throwing, catching, kicking, dribbling, and serving, as used in—Softball, Soccer, Volleyball, Basketball. Skills in body controls as—how to walk, to run, to stand, to sit, to relax. Individual activities as—rope jumping, horseshoes, target throw, jumping, skating, hiking, skiing, and swimming
Muscles, heart, lungs, and bones share liberally in the growth spurt	Vigorous activity to stimulate each of these organs to attain its fullest development	Activities conducted as vigorously as possible with respect for individual reaction
Boys and girls are showing differences in interests and in abilities. Boys tend to surpass girls in strength and speed; girls are usually more interested in dance forms than boys are	To participate in some activities in separate groups and some together. For girls to have more dance in program than boys have	Activities recommended in groupings as follows:

	Boys alone	Girls alone	Both together
Group sports			
Soccer	Yes	Yes	No
Touch football	Yes	No	No
Softball	Yes	Yes	Yes
Basketball	Yes	Yes	No
Volleyball	Yes	Yes	Yes
Individual, dual, and group sports			
Track	Yes	Yes	No
Badminton	Yes	Yes	Yes
Tennis	Yes	Yes	Yes
Swimming	Yes	Yes	Yes
Outing activities	Yes	Yes	Yes
Formal dancing			
Square	Yes	Yes	Yes, preferably
Social	Yes	Yes	Yes, preferably
Creative	Yes	Yes	Yes, preferably
Folk	Yes	Yes	Yes, preferably

What they are like	What they need OPPORTUNITIES	What to do
Interest in members of one's own sex broadens to include an interest in members of the opposite sex	To have coeducational activities in small and large groups	Activities such as Square, Social, and Creative Dance, Tennis, Swimming, and Outing Activities, Volleyball, Table Tennis, Badminton
Great loyalty to groups as clubs, gangs, and teams, and there is a keen desire for group acceptance	To belong to various teams and to plan and develop their own groups	Many teams in all team games such as class teams, homeroom, club, counting off for teams and voting for captains who choose teams

*From Report of National Conference on Physical Education for Children of Elementary School Age: Physical education for children of elementary school age, Chicago, 1951, The Athletic Institute, Inc.

Table 7-4. Later childhood—early adolescence—12 to 13 years of age—seventh and eighth grades—cont'd

What they are like	What they need OPPORTUNITIES	What to do
Strong desire for individual recognition and the urge to be free of adult restrictions	To take part in activities of their own choosing, to be leaders and captains of groups, to create and modify games, and to evaluate progress	Squad-leader directed activities as: a. Testing skills—sit up, push-up b. Officiating in games c. Assigning positions on teams
Emotions are easily aroused and swayed	To be frequently in situations requiring practice of fair play, when winning or losing	Wide variety of activities requiring individual decisions and scoring as in: a. High and broad jumps (boys only) b. Ball-throwing events c. Running against time d. Stunts and tumbling, as jump stick, Indian wrestle, pull-up, sit-up Officiating at games as umpiring in Softball, timing in races and relays
The interest span lengthens. They may want to continue in activities beyond fatigue to exhaustion	To participate in activities that are modified to overcome fatiguing factors as time, speed, distance, and pressures to win. To learn when to stop	Games that involve skills of major sports as: Line Soccer (Soccer), Keep Away (Basketball), End Ball (Basketball), Touch Football (Football), Newcomb (Volleyball), Long Base (Softball) Modifications of standard games involve changing fatiguing factors, as: a. Shortening playing periods in vigorous sports: shorter halves in soccer, shorter quarters in basketball b. Frequent time-outs c. Restricting space: Three-Court Soccer, Six-Court Basketball, One-Basket Basketball
There is a keen interest in competitive activities	To compete in a variety of activities that involve a wide range of skills and organization	Self-testing types with competition against self as tumbling, track events. Skill tests as throwing for baskets, pitching at a target. Games not highly organized as Bombardment, End Ball, Ten Trips, Kick Over, Fist Ball
The enjoyment of organized team sports is keen	To give every boy and girl an opportunity to be a participating member on the types of teams that challenge his interest and ability	Wide variety of team sports such as Soccer, Volleyball, Softball, Basketball, Field Ball. Many teams in each sport organized on such bases as skill and ability, age-height-weight, squads

Table 7-5. Suggested time allotment for a physical program, grade seven*†

	Periods per year	
	Boys	Girls
Conditioning and body mechanics		
Calisthenics, fundamental movement, and posture training	3	5
Aquatics		
Swimming, diving, and water safety	35	35
Lifesaving, skin and scuba diving		
Self-testing activities		
Gymnastics		
Tumbling, stunts, and apparatus	10	15
Track and field	10	15
Weight training	10	
Games		
Group games	4	8
Individual and dual sports		
Archery, horseshoes, fly and bait casting	10	10
Badminton, table tennis, shuffleboard, and quoits	10	10
Tennis and golf	10	10
Bowling, deck tennis, and fencing	4	4
Ice skating and skiing	2	2
Wrestling	8	
Team sports		
Soccer	5	5
Speedaway or speedball	5	5
Softball	7	7
Touch football	10	
Basketball	10	10
Volleyball	5	7
Rhythms, marching, and dancing	10	20
Evaluation, skill, and knowledge tests	7	7
Physical fitness tests	5	5
Total	180	180

*From University of the State of New York, The State Education Department, Bureau of Secondary Curriculum Development: Physical education in the secondary schools, Curriculum Guide, Albany, 1964, State Department of Education, pp. 50-51.

†The suggested number of periods assume a daily schedule. If less than a daily period or fewer facilities are available, appropriate adjustments in the schedule will be necessary.

Table 7-6. Suggested time allotment for a physical education program, grade eight*†

	Periods per year	
	Boys	Girls
Conditioning and body mechanics		
Calisthenics, fundamental movement, and posture training	3	5
Aquatics		
Swimming, diving, and water safety	35	35
Lifesaving, skin and scuba diving		
Self-testing activities		
Gymnastics		
Tumbling, stunts, and apparatus	10	20
Track and field	15	10
Weight training	10	
Games		
Group games	2	4
Individual and dual sports		
Archery, horseshoes, fly and bait casting	10	5
Tennis and golf		5
Bowling and deck tennis		5
Ice skating and skiing		5
Wrestling	15	
Team sports		
Soccer	9	10
Speedaway	5	10
Softball	5	10
Touch football	15	
Basketball	15	10
Volleyball	10	15
Rhythms, marching, and dancing	10	20
Evaluation, skill, and knowledge tests	6	6
Physical fitness tests	5	5
Total	180	180

*From University of the State of New York, The State Education Department, Bureau of Secondary Curriculum Development: Physical education in the secondary schools, Curriculum Guide, Albany, 1964, State Department of Education, pp. 50-51.

†The suggested number of periods assume a daily schedule. If less than a daily period or fewer facilities are available, appropriate adjustments in the schedule will be necessary.

ticipating beyond fatigue to exhaustion. The enjoyment of organized sports is common. The students develop loyalty to groups, have a desire for peer-group approval, and a strong desire for recognition. Emotions are easily aroused.

Boys and girls in the seventh and eighth grades need to have opportunities to participate in activities in which they can experience success—activities that do not emphasize their awkwardness, that provide vigorous activity, that provide for group participation, and that challenge their interest and physical capabilities.

A description of children's characteristics and needs at the seventh and eighth grade levels together with physical education activities suited to these needs is taken from the report of the National Conference on Physical Education (Table 7-4).

The State Department of Education for New York State* has suggested programs for grades seven and eight together with suggested time allotments (Tables 7-5 and 7-6).

Program for grades nine through twelve

A discussion of characteristics and the physical education program for youth 14 through 17 years of age, or grades nine through twelve, is included here.

During this period students display marked characteristics in regard to physical growth and development. In respect to skeletal growth, the girls are about 2 years ahead of the boys. Some girls reach adult height at about 14 years, whereas others continue to grow for several years beyond this age. In the case of boys, some attain adult height at about 16 years and others continue their growth to 20 years or later.

*From University of the State of New York, The State Education Department, Bureau of Secondary Curriculum Development: Physical education in the secondary schools, Curriculum Guide, Albany, 1964, State Department of Education, pp. 50-51.

Bone growth is completed with sexual maturity.

In regard to muscular development, the "awkward age" is ending and there is a definite improvement in coordination. The muscles of boys are becoming hard and firm whereas those of girls remain softer. Posture is improving and control and grace are in evidence, especially by those who have participated in rhythmic activities such as dancing, swimming, and sports.

In respect to organic development, the heart increases in size, with a question being raised as to strenuous competitive sports, since the heart and arteries may be disproportionate in size. The puberty cycle is completed in the majority of cases. There may be a period of glandular instability with fluctuations in respect to energy level. Some characteristic ailments at this age would include headache, nosebleed, nervousness, palpitation, and acne.

The characteristics of the secondary school students are many. The boy or girl of 14 through 17 may have reached physiologic adulthood but needs many new experiences for fuller development. He is emotional and is seeking a feeling of belonging in the life around him. This attempt to adjust may result in some emotional instability. The desire to conform to the standards of the "gang" or group with whom he is closely associated is often greater than the desire to conform to adult standards. However, there are cases of "hero worship," and in such cases adults have considerable influence on youth. This age group is capable of competing in more highly organized games. Groups and "cliques" evolve in accordance with interests and physical maturation. Boys as a rule like to be regarded as big, strong, and healthy, whereas girls desire to be attractive. In both sexes there is interest and an attempt to be physically attractive. As a result, good grooming increases. Appetite is good at this age. Various sexual manifestations during this age may cause undue self-consciousness. Since girls mature before boys, girls are, as a rule, more interested in boys than boys are in girls.

The needs of youth at these ages are many. There is a need for adult guidance, which should allow for considerable freedom and choice on the part of youth. Family life is important and plays a steadying influence on the child at a time when life is becoming more and more complex. There is a need for wholesome activity and experiences where excess emotions and energy can be properly channeled. Certain physical education activities require separate participation on the part of boys and girls. However, there is a need for many experiences where boys and girls play together. Coeducational activities should be adapted to both sexes so that no physiologic or other harm results. Social dancing is very important at this level. Also, at this age students are interested and receive much satisfaction from sports. Although individual differences determine the amount of sleep needed, most can profit from 8 to 10 hours. There is need for a planned after-school program that is adapted to the needs of youth and that includes active recreation as well as the manipulative or contemplative activities.

The types of activities that will best meet the needs of the secondary school student should be wide and varied. Team games of high organization occupy an increasingly important place at the junior high and even more at the senior high school level. The junior high and early senior high school programs should be mainly exploratory in nature, offering a wide variety of activities with the team games modified in nature and presented in the form of lead-up activities. Toward the end of the senior high school period there should be opportunity to select and specialize in certain activities that will have a carryover value after formal education ceases. Furthermore, many of the team games and other activities are offered in a more intensive manner

and in larger blocks of time as one approaches the terminal point of the secondary school. This allows for greater acquisition of skill in selected activities.

As a general rule, boys and girls at the secondary level, including both junior and senior high, can profit greatly from rhythmic activities such as square, folk, and social dancing; team sports such as soccer, field hockey, softball, baseball, touch football, volleyball, and speedball; individual activities such as track and field, tennis, paddle tennis, badminton, hiking, handball, bowling, archery, and fly casting; many forms of gymnastics such as tumbling, stunts, and apparatus activities; and various forms of games and relays. These activities will comprise the major portion of the program at the secondary level. Of course the activities would be adapted to boys and to girls as they are played separately or on a coeducational basis.

A sample physical education program[*] for ninth-grade girls meeting twice weekly is presented in Table 7-7. The program indicates the types of activities that help to meet the objectives sought.

Program for colleges and universities

A recent survey of 406 colleges and universities indicated the following statistics in regard to the required physical education program in these institutions:

1. Of the 406 colleges and universities, 89.6% have required men's physical education programs.
2. A uniform requirement was maintained in physical education for all departments within the college or university in 90.2% of the institutions surveyed.
3. Most colleges and universities require 2 years of physical education.
4. Credit for physical education, which is applied toward graduation, is given in 81% of the institutions surveyed.

---

[*]Bucher, C. A., Koenig, C., and Barnhard, M.: Methods and materials for secondary school physical education, ed. 3, St. Louis, 1970, The C. V. Mosby Co.

Table 7-7. Physical education program for girls in grade nine*

Month and number of weeks		Physical fitness	Physical skills	Knowledge and appreciation	Social development
Sept.	3	Posture Strength	Archery Stance	Archery Etiquette	Individual responsibilities in class
Oct.	4	Endurance Speed	Technique Hockey	Safety Hockey	Program planning Group cooperation
Nov.	1	Agility Accuracy Balance	Dribble Drive Dodge Lunge Tackle	History Rules Offensive and defensive strategies	Teamwork
Total	8		Test	Test	
Nov.	3	Posture Balance	Badminton Serve	Badminton Etiquette	Partnership etiquette
Dec.	3	Agility Accuracy	Forehand Backhand Volleyball Single tap Serve Smash Test	Doubles rules Volleyball History Etiquette Offensive and defensive strategies Rules Rotation	Improved group relationships and teamwork
Total	6			Test	
Jan.	4	Endurance Speed	Basketball Passes	Basketball History	Teamwork New groups
Feb.	2	Accuracy Balance Agility	Dribble Pivot Foul-shooting Goal-shooting Test	Offensive and defensive strategies Rules Notebook	Leadership
Total	6			Test	
Feb.	2	Strength Endurance	Modern dance Types of movement	Modern dance History	Group planning Creativity
Mar.	3	Balance Agility Posture Poise Grace	Axial Swing Sustained Percussive Locomotor Leaps Skips	Noted performers Values Purposes Test	Cooperation Leadership
Total	5		Turns		
Apr.	4	Strength Endurance Balance Agility Posture	Stunts Tumbling Apparatus Parallel bars High bar Ladder Rings	Values of training Olympic performers Safety procedures Spotting	Safety consciousness Leadership Group planning Cooperation
Total	4		Test		

*From Bucher, C. A., Koenig, C., and Barnhard, M.: Methods and materials for secondary school physical education, ed. 3, St. Louis, 1970, The C. V. Mosby Co.

Table 7-7. Physical education program for girls in grade nine—cont'd

Month and number of weeks		Physical fitness	Physical skills	Knowledge and appreciation	Social development
May	4	Strength	Tennis	Tennis	Partnership
		Endurance	Forehand	History	etiquette
June	3	Agility	Backhand	Etiquette	New groups
		Speed	Serve	Doubles rules	Teamwork
		Accuracy	Volley		Leadership
			Softball	Softball	Cooperation
			Base-playing	History	
			Base-running	Rules	
			Batting	Scoring	
			Bunting	Base-playing	
			Catching	Test	
			Throwing		
			Fielding		
Total	7		Test		

5. Most colleges and universities permit the election of physical education courses for credit over and above the institution requirement.
6. The most common formula applied in these colleges and universities is to give one-half credit for each hour of participation in physical education.
7. Physical education grades were averaged together with the student's point-hour grade ration in 71.8% of the institutions surveyed.
8. Students are excused from participation in physical education for such reasons as medical, varsity athletics, ROTC, and marching band.
9. Swimming was the activity most frequently required of all students.
10. Of the 406 colleges and universities, 87.5% administer skill tests or physical performance tests.
11. In the last 5 years the requirement for physical education remained the same in 70.7% of the colleges, increased in 18.2%, and decreased in 10.9%.
12. In the last 5 years the physical education program increased its emphasis on physical fitness activities in 33% of the institutions, on leisure time activities in 15.2% of the institutions, and remained about the same in 51.1% of the institutions.*

Oxendine* conducted a more recent survey on the status of required physical education in 723 colleges and universities in the United States. His survey indicated that 87% of these institutions require physical education for all students, with another 7% having a requirement for students in certain departments or schools. Two-thirds of the institutions that require physical education indicate that the requirement is for a 2-year period. Oxendine's survey also indicated that programs of physical education are on a sounder academic basis in large institutions than in small ones, in public compared to private institutions, and in coeducational as compared to noncoeducational institutions. Finally, Oxendine's survey indicated the trends toward more emphasis on "recreation" and "fitness" activities and on coeducational classes. There is less emphasis on team sports and all-male or all-female classes.

The college and university physical education program is the terminal point for

---

*Carra, L. D., Kent State University, letter dated Nov. 25, 1964.

*Oxendine, J. B.: Status of required physical education programs in colleges and universities, Journal of Health, Physical Education, and Recreation **40**:32, 1969.

formal physical education in the lives of many students. The age range of individuals in colleges and universities is very wide, incorporating those as young as 16 and as old as 60. However, most college students are in their late teens or early twenties. These individuals have matured in many ways. They are entering the period of greatest physical efficiency. They have developed the various organic systems of the body. They possess a high degree of strength, stamina, and coordination. In this respect the program does not have to be restricted for the average college population. College and university students have many interests. They want to prepare themselves adequately for certain vocations. They desire to be a success in their chosen fields of work. Such an objective offers potentialities for the physical education teacher who can show how the outcomes derived from the physical education program can contribute to success in their work. College students are interested in the opposite sex and are beginning to look for a marital partner. They want to develop socially. This has implications for a broad coeducational program. They are interested in developing skills that they can use throughout life and from which they will obtain a great deal of enjoyment.

The physical education program at the college and university level should ensure that these students leave school with skills in their possession for future participation in many enjoyable and worthwhile sports activities. The emphasis should be on leisure-time or recreational skills. If a student possesses sufficient skill in swimming, badminton, golf, or tennis, for example, when he or she leaves school, the chances are that he will engage in such activities throughout adult years. If the physical education program does not see that such skills are developed, the individual may never have another opportunity to acquire them. This responsibility rests heavily upon the physical educator's shoulders.

In formulating a program at the college and university level one needs to remember that many students enter with limited activity backgrounds. Therefore, the program should be broad and varied at the start, with opportunities to elect activities later. There should be considerable opportunity for instruction and practice in those activities in which a student desires to specialize. As much individual attention as possible should be given to ensure the necessary development of skill.

Most colleges offer physical education twice a week for 2 years. There are others, however, where the requirement is for 1, 3, or 4 years' duration. It would seem that the longer the requirement, the greater would be the assurance that the individual would leave school with the necessary skills. Some colleges and universities require only that the allotted time be put in, while others state that certain standards of achievement must be met. Both requirements are important if the objectives of physical education are to be realized. It would seem that sports skills are as important to the development of the "whole" individual as being able to compute some mathematical problem, operate a typewriter, or use a slide rule.

The program of activities should be based on the interests and needs of students and the facilities and staff available. There is an important place for coeducation at the college level in such activities as tennis, dancing, swimming, badminton, volleyball, and golf. Some of the experiences that might be included in the women's program are as follows: team activities —field hockey, soccer, speedball, basketball, softball, and fieldball; aquatics in all forms; dancing—folk, square, social, and modern; individual activities—bowling, table tennis, skating, badminton, archery, tennis, deck tennis, horseback riding, and hiking; formal activities—tumbling and stunts; and camping activities. Some of the activities that have been popular in men's programs are

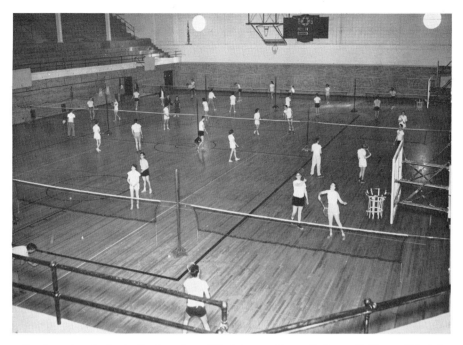

Coeducational physical education. (Washington State College, Pullman, Wash.)

team activities—basketball, touch football, softball, volleyball, soccer, and speedball; aquatics in all forms; dancing—folk, square, and social; individual activities—skating, fishing, squash, badminton, tennis, golf, bowling, archery, hiking, horseshoes, handball, fencing, and wrestling; formal activities—tumbling and apparatus work; and camping activities.

A publication of the President's Council on Physical Fitness and Sports entitled *Fitness for Leadership** contains many suggestions for college and university programs in physical education.

Some of the pertinent suggestions for physical education programs in this report include the recommendation that physical achievement tests should be utilized to assess student needs and assure progress. Special help and prescribed programs should be offered to help physically under-

developed students. Another suggestion is to institute a requirement that would make it necessary for all students to demonstrate and develop proficiency in swimming, conditioning exercises, and several other physical activities.

Special considerations for junior college physical education programs

The growth of the 2-year college in recent years has been phenomenal. Approximately one and one-half million students are enrolled in about 900 junior colleges from coast to coast. In many respects the activities for the 2-year college are the same as those for the 4-year institution. However, since approximately 70% of community college students will terminate their education after 2 years of study, there is a need to provide skills and interests to enrich their leisure and stimulate a desire to keep themselves fit throughout their lifetimes.

Most of the 2-year colleges require students to take physical education both

---

*President's Council on Physical Fitness and Sports: Fitness for leadership, Washington, D. C., 1964, U. S. Government Printing Office.

Table 7-8. Coeducational carryover physical activities offered in California junior colleges*

Activity	Number of schools in which taught	Rank	Offered	Rank
Aquatics	16	4	109	3
Archery	20	2	87	4
Badminton	15	5-6-7	74	5
Bowling	10	8	38	8
Fencing	4	12	10	12
Folk and square dance	9	9-10	17	10
Golf	21	1	132	2
Ice skating	1	13-14	6	13
Modern dance	8	11	15	11
Sailing	1	13-14	3	14
Social dance	15	5-6-7	44	7
Tennis	18	3	157	1
Tumbling, gymnastics, and trampo-line	9	9-10	22	9
Volleyball	15	5-6-7	73	6

*Eiland, H. J.: Emphasis in junior college physical education programs should be on carryover physical recreation activities, Journal of Health, Physical Education, and Recreation 36:35, 1965.

years. Most of the programs require 2 hours each week and stress the successful completion of the service program as a requirement for graduation.

The California 2-year colleges take into consideration their responsibility for a wide variety of coeducational carryover physical activities. Table 7-8 shows information accumulated from the spring schedules of twenty-two junior colleges in California.

INTERRELATIONSHIPS OF ELEMENTARY, SECONDARY, AND COLLEGE AND UNIVERSITY PROGRAMS

Provision should be made for close interrelationships of the physical education programs at the elementary, secondary, and college levels. Continuity and progression should mark the program from the time the student enters school until he or she graduates. Overall planning is essential to guarantee that duplication of effort, waste of time, omissions, and shortages do not occur in respect to the goal of ensuring

that each student become physically educated.

Continuity and progress do not exist today in many of the school systems of the United States. To a great degree each institutional level is autonomous, setting up its own program irrespective of the other levels and with little regard as to what has preceded and what will follow. Many are concerned only with their own little niche and not with the overall program. If the focus of attention is on the student—the consumer of the product—then it would seem that program planning would provide the student with a continuous program, developed in the light of his needs and interests, from the time he starts school until the time he finishes. There should also be consideration given to adult years. Directors of physical education for the entire community should shoulder this responsibility and ensure that such a program exists. Some communities like Great Neck, Long Island, and Long Beach, California, have directors over all the school and community physical education and recreation programs. This offers many possibilities for ensuring a continuous program for community residents "from the cradle to the grave."

A system of standardized and meaningful record keeping is essential to ensure continuity and progression. Regardless of which elementary or secondary school the student attends, his records should follow him when he passes on to the next level. These records would show the activities engaged in by the student, progress made, weaknesses, measurement and evaluation results, notations on conferences and counseling, and any other pertinent information that would be helpful in planning a purposeful physical education program.

Good interrelationships among the various institutional levels are a must if physical education is to provide the best type of program possible in the light of the needs and interests of those they serve.

PROVIDING FOR THE HEALTH OF THE STUDENT

Every effort must be put forth by the physical education staff to safeguard the health of all individuals in the program. To accomplish this objective satisfactorily there must be a close working relationship with staff members in the school health program. Every child should have periodic health examinations with the results of these examinations scrutinized very carefully by the physical educator. Frequent conferences should be held with the school physician. A physical education program must be adapted to the needs and interests of each student. The physical educator must assume responsibility for health guidance and health supervision in the activities over which he is responsible. The school physician should be consulted when students return after periods of illness, when accidents occur, when students want excuses from the program, and at any other time that qualified advice is needed.

Special precautions must be taken to make activity safe for the student. The desire to win in sports competition must not be used to exploit a student's health. If a disagreement arises, the physician's decision should be final. These and many other phases of the physical education department's interrelationship with the school health program must be carefully attended to.

CRITERIA FOR EVALUATING PHYSICAL EDUCATION ACTIVITY CLASSES

Piscopo has developed the accompanying checklist for evaluating physical education activity classes. It should help in better understanding the essentials of this phase of the physical education program.

CRITERIA FOR EVALUATING PHYSICAL EDUCATION ACTIVITY CLASSES*

	Poor (1)	Fair (2)	Good (3)	Very good (4)	Excellent (5)
Meeting physical education objectives					
1. Does the class actively contribute to the development of physical fitness?	☐	☐	☐	☐	☐
2. Does the class activity foster the growth of ethical character, desirable emotional and social characteristics?	☐	☐	☐	☐	☐
3. Does the class activity contain recreational value?	☐	☐	☐	☐	☐

*From Piscopo, J.: Quality instruction: first priority, The Physical Educator **21**:162, 1964.

Continued.

CRITERIA FOR EVALUATING PHYSICAL EDUCATION ACTIVITY CLASSES—cont'd

	Poor (1)	Fair (2)	Good (3)	Very good (4)	Excellent (5)
Meeting physical education objectives–cont'd					
4. Does the class activity contain carryover value for later life?	☐	☐	☐	☐	☐
5. Is the class activity accepted as a regular part of the school curriculum?	☐	☐	☐	☐	☐
6. Does the class activity meet the needs of *all* students in the group?	☐	☐	☐	☐	☐
7. Does the class activity encourage the development of leadership among students?	☐	☐	☐	☐	☐
8. Does the class activity fulfill the safety objective in physical education?	☐	☐	☐	☐	☐
9. Does the class activity and conduct foster a better understanding of democratic living?	☐	☐	☐	☐	☐
10. Does the class activity and conduct cultivate a better understanding and appreciation for exercise and sports?	☐	☐	☐	☐	☐

Perfect score: 50   *Actual score:*_____

	Poor (1)	Fair (2)	Good (3)	Very good (4)	Excellent (5)
Leadership (teacher conduct)					
1. Is the teacher appropriately and neatly dressed for the class activity?	☐	☐	☐	☐	☐
2. Does the teacher know the activity thoroughly?	☐	☐	☐	☐	☐
3. Does the teacher possess an audible and pleasing voice?	☐	☐	☐	☐	☐
4. Does the teacher project an enthusiastic and dynamic attitude in class presentation?	☐	☐	☐	☐	☐
5. Does the teacher maintain discipline?	☐	☐	☐	☐	☐
6. Does the teacher identify, analyze, and correct faulty performance in guiding pupils?	☐	☐	☐	☐	☐
7. Does the teacher present a sound, logical method of teaching motor skills, for example, explanation, demonstration, participation, and testing?	☐	☐	☐	☐	☐
8. Does the teacher avoid the use of destructive criticism, sarcasm, and ridicule with students?	☐	☐	☐	☐	☐
9. Does the teacher maintain emotional stability and poise?	☐	☐	☐	☐	☐
10. Does the teacher possess high standards and ideals of work?	☐	☐	☐	☐	☐

Perfect score: 50   *Actual score:*_____

	Poor (1)	Fair (2)	Good (3)	Very good (4)	Excellent (5)
General class procedures, methods, and techniques					
1. Does class conduct yield evidence of preplanning?	☐	☐	☐	☐	☐
2. Does the organization of the class allow for individual differences?	☐	☐	☐	☐	☐

CRITERIA FOR EVALUATING PHYSICAL EDUCATION ACTIVITY CLASSES—cont'd

	Poor (1)	Fair (2)	Good (3)	Very good (4)	Excellent (5)
General class procedures, methods, and techniques–cont'd					
3. Does the class exhibit maximum pupil activity and minimum teacher participation? e.g., overemphasis on explanation and/or demonstration?	☐	☐	☐	☐	☐
4. Are adequate motivational devices such as teaching aids and audiovisual techniques effectively utilized?	☐	☐	☐	☐	☐
5. Are student or squad leaders effectively employed where appropriate?	☐	☐	☐	☐	☐
6. Does the class start promptly at the scheduled time?	☐	☐	☐	☐	☐
7. Are students with medical excuses from the regular class supervised and channelled into appropriate activities?	☐	☐	☐	☐	☐
8. Is the class roll taken quickly and accurately?	☐	☐	☐	☐	☐
9. Are accurate records of pupil progress and achievements maintained?	☐	☐	☐	☐	☐
10. Are supplies and equipment quickly issued and stored?	☐	☐	☐	☐	☐

Perfect score: 50   Actual score:____

Pupil conduct

	Poor (1)	Fair (2)	Good (3)	Very good (4)	Excellent (5)
1. Are the objectives of the activity or sport clearly known to the learner?	☐	☐	☐	☐	☐
2. Are the students interested in the class activities?	☐	☐	☐	☐	☐
3. Do the students really enjoy their physical education class?	☐	☐	☐	☐	☐
4. Are the students thoroughly familiar with routine regulations of class roll, excuses, and dismissals?	☐	☐	☐	☐	☐
5. Are the students appropriately uniformed for the class activity?	☐	☐	☐	☐	☐
6. Does the class exhibit a spirit of friendly rivalry in learning new skills?	☐	☐	☐	☐	☐
7. Do students avoid mischief or "horseplay"?	☐	☐	☐	☐	☐
8. Do students take showers where facilities and nature of activity permit?	☐	☐	☐	☐	☐
9. Do slow learners participate as much as fast learners?	☐	☐	☐	☐	☐
10. Do students show respect for the teacher?	☐	☐	☐	☐	☐

Perfect score: 50   Actual score:____

Continued.

CRITERIA FOR EVALUATING PHYSICAL EDUCATION ACTIVITY CLASSES—cont'd

	Poor (1)	Fair (2)	Good (3)	Very good (4)	Excellent (5)
Safe and healthful environment					
1. Is the area large enough for the activity and number of students in the class?	☐	☐	☐	☐	☐
2. Does the class possess adequate equipment and/or supplies?	☐	☐	☐	☐	☐
3. Are adequate shower and locker facilities available and readily accessible?	☐	☐	☐	☐	☐
4. Is the equipment and/or apparatus clean and in good working order?	☐	☐	☐	☐	☐
5. Does the activity area contain good lighting and ventilation?	☐	☐	☐	☐	☐
6. Are all safety hazards eliminated or reduced where possible?	☐	☐	☐	☐	☐
7. Is first aid and safety equipment readily accessible?	☐	☐	☐	☐	☐
8. Is the storage area adequate for supplies and equipment?	☐	☐	☐	☐	☐
9. Does the activity area contain a properly equipped rest room for use in injury, illness, or rest periods?	☐	☐	☐	☐	☐
10. Does the activity area contain adequate toilet facilities?	☐	☐	☐	☐	☐

Perfect score: 50   Actual score:_____

Criteria	Perfect score	Actual score
Meeting physical education objectives	50	_____
Leadership (teacher conduct)	50	_____
General class procedures, methods, and techniques	50	_____
Pupil conduct	50	_____
Safe and healthful environment	50	_____
Total points	250	_____

Questions and exercises

1. Write a 300-word essay on the total physical education program, bringing out the three main components and the contributions that each phase makes to the education of the individual.
2. Outline a physical education program for one of the educational levels. Show how the experiences that you include in your program contribute to the goals of physical education.
3. Select a school or college and evaluate its entire program in the light of the findings disclosed in this chapter.
4. What are some initial considerations that must be brought about before a program can be planned?
5. Develop a set of standards that could be used to evaluate a physical education program.
6. Develop a list of principles that would serve as guides in the scheduling of physical education activities.
7. What part does each of the following play in scheduling: (a) time allotment, (b) size of classes, (c) teaching stations, (d) teaching loads, (e) grouping, and (f) administrative philosophy?

8. Have a class discussion on each of the following:
   (a) Physical education should be elective in school.
   (b) The Reserve Officers' Training Corps is not a substitute for physical education.
   (c) Credit should be given for physical education.
   (d) Attendance should be voluntary in physical education.
   (e) All excuses should be accepted in physical education.
9. What are some essential points to keep in mind in regard to good class management?
10. Outline what you consider to be a desirable grading procedure in physical education.
11. Prepare a list of principles to guide the selection of activities in physical education.
12. What place do coeducational activities have in the physical education program? Justify your stand.
13. Develop a plan to ensure continuity in physical education from the elementary through the college level.
14. How can physical education and health education work together to help promote the health of each individual?
15. Why is an adapted program needed in physical education?

Reading assignment in *Administrative Dimensions of Health and Physical Education Programs, Including Athletics:* Chapter 5, Selections 21 to 27.

Selected references

American Association for Health, Physical Education, and Recreation: Children in focus, 1954 Yearbook, Washington, D. C., 1954, The Association.

American Association for Health, Physical Education, and Recreation: Broadfront, Journal of Health, Physical Education, and Recreation **38:10**, 1967.

American Association for Health, Physical Education, and Recreation: Knowledge and understanding in physical education, Washington, D. C., 1969, The Association.

American Association for Health, Physical Education, and Recreation: Perceptual-motor foundations: a multidisciplinary concern, Washington, D. C., 1969, The Association.

Association for Childhood Education International: Physical education for children's healthful living, Washington, D. C., 1968, The Association.

Baker, G. M.: Survey of the administration of physical education in public schools in the United States, Research Quarterly **33:632**, 1962.

Battle Creek Physical Education Curriculum Project Team: Battle Creek Physical Education Curriculum Project, Journal of Health, Physical Education, and Recreation **40:25**, 1969.

Bookwalter, K. W.: Physical education in the secondary schools, New York, 1964, The Center for Applied Research in Education, Inc. (The Library of Education).

Bucher, C. A., editor: Methods and materials in physical education and recreation, St. Louis, 1954, The C. V. Mosby Co.

Bucher, C. A.: Foundations of physical education, ed. 5, St. Louis, 1968, The C. V. Mosby Co.

Bucher, C. A.: Physical education for life, St. Louis, 1969, McGraw-Hill Book Co. (A textbook in physical education for high school boys and girls.)

Bucher, C. A., Koenig, C., and Barnhard, M.: Methods and materials for secondary school physical education, ed. 3, St. Louis, 1970, The C. V. Mosby Co.

Bucher, C. A., and Reade, E. M.: Health and physical education in the modern elementary school, New York, 1971, The Macmillan Co.

Espenschade, A. S.: Physical education in the elementary schools—what research says to the teacher, Washington, D. C., March, 1963, Department of Classroom Teachers, American Educational Research Association of the National Education Association.

Fitness for California Children and Youth: Values inherent in the daily program of physical education, Journal of the California Association for Health, Physical Education and Recreation, March, 1965 (special issue).

LaPorte, W. R.: The physical education curriculum (a national program), ed. 6, Los Angeles, 1955, University of Southern California Press.

Oxendine, J. B.: Status of required physical education programs in colleges and universities, Journal of Health, Physical Education, and Recreation **40:32**, 1969.

Physical education in the junior college, Journal of Health, Physical Education, and Recreation **36:33**, 1965.

President's Council on Physical Fitness: Fitness for leadership, Washington D. C., 1964, Superintendent of Documents.

Reams, D., and Bleier, T. J.: Developing team teaching for ability grouping, Journal of Health, Physical Education, and Recreation **39:50**, 1968.

Report of the National Conference on Physical Education for Children of Elementary School Age: Physical education for children of elementary school age, Chicago, 1951, The Athletic Institute, Inc.

The University of the State of New York, The State Education Department, Bureau of Secondary Curriculum Development: Physical education in the secondary schools, Curriculum Guide, Albany, 1964, State Department of Education.

Von Bergen, E.: Flexible scheduling for physical education, Journal of Health, Physical Education, and Recreation 38:29, 1967.

Wisconsin State Department of Education: Standards for physical education: grades one through twelve, Madison, Wis., May, 1964, State Department of Education.

CHAPTER 8   THE ADAPTED PROGRAM*

The term *adapted* is used here, although in many books and programs other terms, such as *corrective, individual, modified, therapeutic, remedial, special, restricted,* and *atypical* are used. The adapted program refers to that phase of physical education that meets the needs of the individual who, because of some physical inadequacy, functional defect capable of being improved through physical activity, or other deficiency, is temporarily or permanently unable to take part in the regular physical education program. It also refers to a significant segment of a school or college student population that does not fall into the classification "average" or "normal" for their age or grade. These students deviate from their peers on a physical, mental, emotional, or social measure or on a combination of these traits.

Many times health examinations such as medical, physical fitness, or other type indicate that some pupils are not able to participate in regular physical activity programs. For example, those students with organic weakness and functional or growth abnormalities need special attention. Other students who are atypical include the culturally disadvantaged, mentally retarded, emotionally disturbed, poorly coordinated, and gifted or creative. Special adaptations also need to be made for these students.

The principle of individual differences is being recognized increasingly by educators. Education is for each and every individual in a democracy. The observance of this principle has resulted in special provisions in the schools for backward as well as for superior children, for those with heart disturbances, defective sight, physical disabilities, and other deviations from the normal, and for those who are culturally deprived or emotionally disturbed.

The principle of individual differences that applies to education as a whole should also apply to physical education. Most administrators believe that as long as a student can come to school or college, he should be required to participate in physical education. If this tenet is adhered to, it means that programs must be adapted to individual needs. Many children and young adults who are recuperating from long illnesses or operations or who are suffering from other abnormal conditions require special consideration in their program of activities.

It cannot be assumed that all individuals in physical education classes are normal. Unfortunately, many programs are administered on this basis. One estimate has been made that one out of every eight students in our schools is handicapped to the extent that special provision should be made in the educational program.

Schools and colleges will always have students who, because of many factors such as heredity, environment, disease, accident, or other reason, will have physical or other

---

*A detailed discussion of the care and education of exceptional children is given in Chapter 13 on school health services. Much of this material is pertinent to the adapted program but will not be repeated here. However, the reader may wish to read that important section.

This chapter is designed to outline briefly the adapted program as a component of total school and college physical education programs.

form 86C 3000 3-46

PHYSICAL EXAMINATION RECORD

NEW TRIER TOWNSHIP HIGH SCHOOL
WINNETKA, ILLINOIS

NAME _____ LAST _____ FIRST _____

PARENT OR GUARDIAN _____

ADVISER _____ TELEPHONE _____

ADDRESS _____

PHYSICIAN _____

DENTIST _____

PLEASE CHECK IF YOU HAVE HAD THE FOLLOWING DISEASES

Chickenpox | Whooping Cough | Mumps | Scarlet Fever | Typhoid Fever | Diphtheria | Rheumatism | Tonsillitis | Vaccination for Smallpox | Diphtheria Immunization | Measles

What operations have you had? _____

Give type of operation and dates _____

What serious injuries have you had? _____

Specify injury and date _____

Remarks _____

	Date			
	Age			
	Weight	Height	Weight	Height
Development				
Nourishment				
SKIN	Acne			
	Ringworm			
	Plantar Warts			
EYES	Vision R L		R L	
	Exophthalmos			
	Conjunctiva			
EARS	Hearing R L		R L	
	Discharge R L		R L	
	Cerumen R L		R L	
NOSE	Obstruction			
SINUSES				
MOUTH				
THROAT	Tonsils			
	Advise Removal			
	Removed			
NECK	Thyroid			
	Pulsation of Vessels			
CHEST				
LUNGS	Palpation			
	Percussion			
	Auscultation			

(Continued Below)

HEART	Murmurs		
PULSE	At Rest		
	After Exercise, 20 hops		
	After 2 Min. Rest		
SPINE AND POSTURE			
ABDOMEN			
HERNIA			
GENITALS	Varicocele		
	Hydrocele		
	Speech Defect		
NERVOUS SYSTEM	Coordination		
	Tremor		
FEET			
SUMMARY	Classification		
	Reason		
	Length of Time		
	Comments and Suggestions		
	Excused from Swimming		
	How Long?		
	Excused from Showers		
	How Long?		
REMARKS			

Class "A"—Unrestricted physical education activity.
Class "B"—Regular physical education but no intramural competition.
Class "C"—Restricted physical education activity (special classes).
Class "D"—Supervised rest.

X—Means defect present.
XX—Means defect needs attention—parents notified.
XXX—Means defect needs immediate attention—parents notified.

Physical examination record. This record is an aid in adapted program. (New Trier Township High School, Winnetka, Ill.)

LOS ANGELES CITY SCHOOL DISTRICTS
Health Education and Health Services Branch—Auxiliary Services Division
Corrective Physical Education‹Section

CORRECTIVE PHYSICAL EDUCATION ACTIVITY GUIDE
A Guide for the Teacher and Physician
In Planning a Restricted Program of Physical Education

Pupil _____ Date _____

School _____ Corrective Phys. Ed. Teacher _____

I. TYPES OF MOVEMENTS	OMIT	*MILD	**MODERATE	UNLIMITED	REMARKS
Bending					
Climbing					
Hanging					
Jumping					
Kicking					
Lifting					
Pulling					
Pushing					
Running					
Stretching					
Throwing					
Twisting					

II. TYPES OF EXERCISES	OMIT	*MILD	**MODERATE	UNLIMITED	REMARKS
Abdominal					
Arm					
Breathing					
Foot					
Head					
Knee					
Leg					
Trunk					
Relaxation					

III. TYPES OF POSITIONS	LIMITED	UNLIMITED
Lying supine		
Lying prone		
Sitting		
Standing		

IV. TYPES OF ACTIVITIES	YES	NO
Competitive sports		
Games——Sitting		
Games requiring standing but no running or jumping		
Officiating		
Swimming		
Coeducational activities		
Social dancing		
Square dancing		
Sports and games		

Recommended until _____ 196_

Remarks:

_____
Signature of Physician

*Very little activity.
**Half as much as the unlimited program.

impairment. Many of these students have difficulty in adjusting to the demands that society places upon them. It is the responsibility of physical education programs to help each and every individual who comes into class. Even though a person may be atypical, this is not cause for neglect. In fact, it should represent an even greater challenge to see that he enjoys the benefits of participating in physical activities adapted to his needs. Provision for a sound adapted program has been a shortcoming of physical education throughout the nation because of a lack of properly trained teachers, the financial cost of remedial instruction, and the fact that many administrators and teachers are not aware of their responsibility and the contribution they can make in this phase of physical education. These obstacles should be overcome as the public becomes aware of the need of educating *all* individuals in *all* phases of the total education program.

Parker has grasped the importance of

providing for the exceptional person in these words:

The exceptional person needs an opportunity to become a responsible citizen; to become an economically efficient producer and consumer of goods, or services; to develop an understanding of human relationships of home, neighborhood, and wider social groups; and to realize whatever personal potentialities the Creator has bestowed. For an exceptional child it means a well-planned curriculum of many rich experiences of the kinds he is capable of having, which brings to him some measure of ability to make and keep friends, to share with others some if not all of the common social experience, to care for himself personally and for his home, perhaps even to earn his living or a reasonable part of it, and to enjoy life as he must live it.*

Stone and Deyton frame the value of adapted physical education in these terms:

These children receive health and vocational guidance from interested teachers, who have discovered the value of rehabilitation through corrective physical education. Through these cooperative efforts, physically and psychologically atypical children are trained to face and accept their handicaps, to realize their limitations, and to adapt to them. The aims of the corrective programs for these children are to meet the physical and emotional needs of each one, to prove to each individually that there is a place for him which he alone can fill best, to help fit himself for that place, and within his handicap to allow him to "play, too."†

EXTENT OF ATYPICAL CONDITIONS AMONG STUDENTS

Although records are insufficient, there have been several estimates as to the number of children with handicapping conditions in the nation's schools. One estimate indicates that 8% to 10% of school-age children are handicapped, emotionally disturbed, brain injured, or auditorily impaired or have chronic health problems.

*Parker, R.: Physical education for the handicapped, Journal of Health and Physical Education 17:254, 1946.
†Stone, E. B., and Deyton, J. W.: Corrective therapy for the handicapped child, New York, 1951, Prentice-Hall, Inc., pp. 1-2.

It has been conservatively estimated that at least 3 million children in the United States between the ages of 4 and 19 years are physically handicapped. The great majority of these boys and girls, approximately 83%, are in the elementary schools.

Some specific figures in regard to handicapping conditions have been given. One source states that there are approximately 10,000 children who are totally blind and 58,000 children of school age who have partial sight. There are more than 500,000 in each of the following classifications: crippled, deaf, or hard of hearing. There are approximately 700,000 speech-handicapped children, and a similar number of children are considered socially maladjusted. Each year in the United States more than 126,000 babies are born with some degree of mental retardation. At present there are more than 7 million mentally retarded children and adults in the United States. According to the Director of Programs for the Handicapped of the AAHPER, 4 million children of school age in the United States have physical, mental, or emotional handicaps. In addition to the handicapped, there are those students with poor motor ability, low physical fitness, and weight problems who represent 20% to 25% of the total school population. The Ford Foundation indicates at least 50% of the children living in cities are culturally disadvantaged. There are also over 500,000 children with special health problems.

OBJECTIVES OF THE ADAPTED PROGRAM

Physical education can be of great value to the atypical individual in many ways. It can help in identifying deviations from normal and in referring students to proper individuals or agencies, when necessary. It can help the atypical person to have a happy, wholesome play experience. It can help the student to achieve, within his limitations, physical skill and exercise. It can provide many opportunities for the learning of skills that are appropriate for the handicapped person to achieve success. Finally, physical education can help to contribute to a more productive life on the part of the handicapped individual by developing those physical qualities that are needed to meet the demands of day-to-day living.

Some of the objectives that have been set forth for the adapted program are listed here. The first list for the physically handicapped was established by the University of the State of New York:

1. To correct faulty body mechanics for the purpose of giving the vital organs better opportunity to perform their functions.
2. To build up positive physical fitness by improving muscle tone and by developing functional harmony and poise.
3. To correct and develop habits of and attitudes toward health and physical activity.
4. To improve and develop habits of *individually* correct body mechanics in motor activities.*

Daniels and Davies developed a very comprehensive list of objectives for the adapted physical education program, which represents a worthy guide for administrators everywhere. The list follows:

1. Accomplish needed therapy or correction for conditions which can be improved or removed (pertains particularly to temporary disabilities such as reduced dislocations and post appendectomies).
2. Aid in the adjustment and/or resocialization of the individual when the disability is permanent (permanent disabilities like amputation, cerebral palsy can benefit greatly from adapted physical education programs).
3. Protect the condition from aggravation by acquainting the student with his limitations and capacities and arranging a program within his physiological work capacity or exercise tolerance.

4. Provide students with an opportunity for the development of organic power within the limits of the disability.
5. Provide students with an opportunity to develop skills in recreational sports and games within the limits of the disability.
6. Provide students with an opportunity for normal social development through recreational sports and games appropriate to their age group and interests.
7. Contribute to security through improved function and increased ability to meet the physical demands of daily living.*

An analysis of these objectives indicates that through their accomplishment the needs of every individual will be provided for, regardless of whether he has a temporary or a permanent disability, whether he has a need for organic, mental, emotional, or social adjustment, or whether he needs a broad or limited program. These are excellent goals for physical educators.

PLANNING THE ADAPTED PHYSICAL EDUCATION PROGRAM

To have an effective adapted physical education program requires considerable thought and planning. The Bureau of Health Education, Physical Education, and Recreation of the California State Department of Education has prepared a special publication for distribution to their schools and physical educators.† Among many outstanding features of this publication are suggestions for planning an adapted physical education program. These suggestions presented in adapted form include the following:

1. Instruction and practice in basic skills of locomotion and skills for physical

---

*University of the State of New York: Physical education syllabus, book 4. Secondary schools (grades 7 to 12), boys, Albany, 1944, University of State of New York Press.

*Daniels, A. S., and Davies, E. A.: Adapted physical education, ed. 2, New York, 1965, Harper & Row, Publishers, pp. 82-88.
†Dexter, G.: Special physical education classes for physically handicapped minors, Sacramento, Calif., June, 1964, California State Department of Education, pp. 3-4.

recreation should be provided for all age groups.

2. The regular physical education program in the intermediate grades and secondary schools should provide for a minimum of two units in the mechanics of body movement.

3. Where there is a need for special help by students in overcoming poor body alignment, there should be special classes in those schools in which such classes are possible and by individual assignments in regular classes in other schools.

4. From kindergarten through high school, each teaching unit should be planned to teach motor skills for movement patterns that will, in turn, provide for a successful experience in those physical activities included in the program.

5. Where the pupil's ability is limited he should either be permitted to participate in regular courses if the experience can be successful, or provision should be made for other units of instruction that will provide the special help needed.

6. If a student's condition is such that rest and relaxation are needed, such should be possible.

7. Policies concerned with pupils who are absent from class should take into consideration the welfare of the student.

8. When assigning students with severe physically handicapping conditions to special classes or when following other procedures to provide special instruction for pupils, all experiences should be regarded and operated as integral parts of the total, regular physical education program.

9. A special program should be offered to those pupils who score below the twenty-fifth percentile of the California Physical Performance Tests or a similar battery of tests.

10. Both school and family physicians should understand the nature and scope of the adapted physical education program in order to intelligently recommend a student's participation in physical education.

CONTRIBUTION OF PHYSICAL EDUCATION TO VARIOUS TYPES OF ATYPICAL CONDITIONS

There is no one way to group students in the adapted program. As has been indicated, there are many different types of boys and girls in the program. It would be wise for the physical educator and health educator to sit down with the school physician, school psychologist, and/or nurse and include in their planning the various types of atypical students they have in their institution. The discussion in this section includes the following atypical conditions: (1) physically handicapped, (2) mentally retarded, (3) emotionally disturbed, (4) culturally disadvantaged, (5) poorly coordinated, and (6) physically gifted and creative students.

Physically handicapped students

Various methods have been utilized to classify physically handicapped persons. Three types of classification that have been used are given here.

Hilleboe's* classification includes the following five categories:

1. Orthopedic defectives
   a. Children with posture defects
   b. Crippled children
2. Visual defectives
3. Hearing defectives
4. Speech defectives
5. Respiratory-cardio-nutritional defectives

The University of the State of New York† lists the following specific deficiencies or growth abnormalities that require adapted physical education activities:

1. Heart and lung disturbances
2. Postoperative and convalescent patients

---

*Hilleboe, G. L.: Finding and teaching atypical children, New York, 1930, Bureau of Publications, Teachers College, Columbia University, p. 25.

†University of the State of New York: Physical education syllabus, book 4. Secondary schools (grades 7 to 12 inclusive), boys, Albany, 1944, University of State of New York Press.

3. Faulty body mechanics, including posture
4. Underweight
5. Overweight
6. Nervous instability
7. Functional defects
8. General muscular weakness resulting from lack of exercise, or systemic deficiences
9. Conditions, congenital or acquired, affecting bone or muscle mechanism
10. Certain eye conditions

LaPorte* points to the fact that corrective cases may be classified under the following headings:

1. Nutrition (overweight and underweight)
2. Poor posture
3. Weak and flat feet
4. Functional and organic heart conditions
5. Hernias
6. Infantile paralysis and other crippling conditions
7. Neurasthenia or nervous instability
8. Menstrual and endocrine disorders

Whatever the physical disability, a physical education program must be provided. Some handicapped students will be able to participate in a regular program of physical education with certain minor modifications. A separate adapted program must be provided for those students who cannot participate in the basic instructional program of the school. The physically handicapped student cannot be allowed to sit on the sidelines and become only a spectator. The handicapped student needs to have the opportunity to develop and maintain adequate skill abilities and fitness levels.

Physical handicaps, which may stem from congenital or hereditary causes or may develop later in life through environmental factors, such as malnutrition, disease, or accident, sometimes cause negative psychologic and social traits to develop because of the limitations imposed on the individual. A physically handicapped student is occasionally ignored or rebuffed by

---

*LaPorte, W. R.: The physical education curriculum (a national program), ed. 6, Los Angeles, 1955, University of Southern California Press, p. 59.

classmates who do not understand the nature of the disability or who ostracize the student because his disability prevents him from participating fully in the activities of the school. These attitudes toward the handicapped force them to withdraw in order to avoid becoming hurt and result in their becoming further isolated from the remainder of the student body.

Some experts have noted that the limitations of the handicap often seem more severe to the observer than they are in fact to the handicapped individual. When this misconception occurs, the handicapped student must prove his abilities in order to gain acceptance and a chance to participate and compete on an equal basis with his nonhandicapped classmates.

The blind or deaf student or the student with a severe speech impairment has a different set of problems from the orthopedically handicapped student. The partially sighted, the blind, the deaf, and the speech-impaired student cannot communicate with great facility. The orthopedically handicapped student is limited in the physical education class but not necessarily in the academic classroom. The student with vision, hearing, or speech problems may be limited in both physical education and the academic classroom.

There is a lack of physical educators who are specially trained to teach physically handicapped students. School systems find that the cost of providing special classes taught by specially trained physical educators is sometimes prohibitive. Where there are no special classes, the physical educator must provide, within the regular instructional program, those activities that will meet the needs of the handicapped student. Further, placing the physically handicapped student in a regular physical education class will help give him a feeling of belonging. This advantage is not always possible where separate adapted classes are provided.

Some handicapped students will be able

Name of child_____ Date_____
Birthday of child_____ School attended (if any)_____
Address_____ Phone_____
Parent, guardian, or other informant_____
Reason for examination:_____

Name of clinics, hospitals, or doctors serving child	Clinic_____	Date Last Seen _____
	Private M.D._____	_____
	Specialist_____	_____

PAST AND FAMILY HISTORY: (Parent present ☐ or if not, nurse obtains data from home)

Birth: (type, weight, trauma, etc.)_____ Convulsions_____
Mother's health during this pregnancy_____
Health, age, sex of siblings_____
Child stat up_____ Talked_____ Walked_____ Child's difficulty first noted_____
Diseases_____ Accidents_____
Operations: T&A_____ Others_____

PHYSICAL EXAMINATION: Height_____ Weight_____
Vision test (current) Rt._____ Lt._____ Comments_____
Hearing test (current) Rt._____ Lt._____ Comments_____
Check below (o) if essentially negative or (x) if abnormal and describe on back of sheet.

Mouth____	Glands____	Heart____	Genitalia____	Skin____	Coordination____
Teeth____	Eyes____	Abdomen____	Hernia____	Gait____	Skel. deform.____
Tonsils____	Ears____	Extremities____	Nutrition____	Allergies____	Toilet habits____

IMPRESSION OF CHILD AND MEDICAL RECOMMENDATIONS FOR EDUCATIONAL PROGRAM:

1. General physical condition is_____
2. Health practices seem to be_____
3. Family attitudes apparently are_____
   _____
   _____

4. Specific health problems include: Vision ☐   Hearing ☐   Motor Incoordination ☐   Hyperactivity ☐
   Convulsive Disorder ☐ (on medication ☐   no medication ☐) Frequency of Episodes_____
   Date of last episode, etc._____
   Other:_____
   _____
   _____
   _____

5. Recommendations:
   Further attention to_____
   Placement in limited P.E. ☐   Regular P.E. ☐   Swimming ☐
   Other:_____
   _____

_____   _____
Date of Evaluation   Signature of Physician

FORM 808   DSP   8-64-500   8-621-54560

Health evaluation of pupils for placement in special education programs. (Health Services Department, Denver Public Schools, Denver, Colo.)

to participate in almost all of the activities that nonhandicapped students enjoy. Blind students, for example, have successfully engaged in team sports where they can receive aural cues from their sighted teammates. Some athletic equipment manufacturers have placed bells inside game balls; the blind student is then able to rely on this sound as well as the supplementary aural cues. Ropes or covered wires acting as hand guides also enable the blind student to participate in track and field events. Still other activities such as swimming, dance, calisthenics, and tum-

DENVER PUBLIC SCHOOLS
HEALTH SERVICE DEPARTMENT

_____
(Date)

REFERRAL OF PUPIL FOR HEALTH REASONS

I am sending_____   _____
(Name)   (Rm. or Sect.)

to the office or nurse at _____ for:
(Time)

Cold symptons ... ☐   Nausea................ ☐   Stomach-ache....... ☐

Headache............. ☐   Skin Rash............ ☐   Toothache.......... ☐

Injury_____

Other reason_____

_____
(Teacher)

Office or nurse reply:

Will remain in clinic ☐   Will return to class ☐

Home contacted, pupil going home ☐

Comments_____

Signature_____
(Office Personnel or Nurse)

STOCK NO. 10704
FORM 804   DSP   8-68-3500 PADS   G-123-60627

Referral of pupil for health reasons. (Health Services Department, Denver Public Schools, Denver, Colo.)

bling require little adaptation or none at all, except in regard to heightened safety precautions.

In general, deaf students will not be restricted in any way from participating in a full physical education program. Some deaf students experience difficulty in those activities requiring precise balance, such as balance-beam walking, and may require some remedial work in this area. The physical educator should be prepared to offer any extra help that is needed.

Other physically handicapped students will have a variety of limitations and a variety of skill abilities. Appropriate program adaptations and modifications must be made in order to meet this range of individual needs. The physician is the individual most knowledgeable about the history and limitations of a student's handicap. He is therefore in the best position to recommend a physical activity program for the student. The student's abilities and levels of fitness should be tested in those areas where medical permission for participation has been granted. This will insure

not only a proper program for the individual but will also help in placing the student in the proper class or section of a class. Careful records should be kept showing the student's test scores, activity recommendations, activities, and progress through the program.

The adapted and the regular physical education programs should be as similar as possible. Where the programs are totally divergent, the physically handicapped student is isolated from his classmates. When the programs are as similar as possible, the handicapped student can be made to feel a part of the larger group and will gain self-confidence and self-respect. Physically handicapped students need the challenge of a progressive program. They welcome the opportunity to test their abilities, and they should experience the fun of a challenge and the success of meeting it. The handicapped should be given an opportunity to seek extra help and extra practice after school hours. During this time they can benefit from more individualized instruction than is possible during the class period. The fitness level of each student, his ability, recreational needs, sex, age, and interest will help to determine the activities the student will engage in pleasurably. Safe facilities and safe equipment are essential. Intramural and club programs should be provided, but they should be of such a nature that physically handicapped students can enjoy them in a safe and controlled atmosphere that precludes the danger of injury.

Mentally retarded students

In some schools, special physical education classes are offered for mentally retarded students, while in still other schools the mentally retarded participate in the regularly scheduled physical education classes.

Mental retardation can be a result of hereditary abnormalities, a birth injury, or an accident or illness that leads to impairment of brain function. There are degrees of mental retardation ranging from the severely mentally retarded, who require custodial care, to the educable mentally retarded, who function with only a moderate degree of impairment.

Many agencies are conducting research in the field of mental retardation in an attempt to discover the causes of mental retardation, the nature of mental retardation, and the methods through which retardation may be prevented. Some agencies are operating innovative training schools for the mentally retarded. The Joseph P. Kennedy, Jr., Foundation is spearheading much of the research concerned with mental retardation and is also a leader in providing camping and recreational programs for the mentally retarded. The Kennedy Foundation has also sponsored training programs for teachers of the mentally retarded. The United States government is sponsoring experimental physical education programs for mentally retarded persons staffed by special education teachers, specially trained physical edu-

cators, vocational rehabilitation technicians, and architectural engineers. Special programs and special equipment have been designed especially for use by the mentally retarded. Climbing devices, obstacle courses, and unique running areas, as well as a swimming pool, are part of the special facilities. The objectives of this program include social and personal adjustment and development of physical fitness, sports skills, and general motor ability.

Mentally retarded students show a wide range of intellectual and physical ability. Experts seem to agree that a mentally retarded child is usually closer to the norm

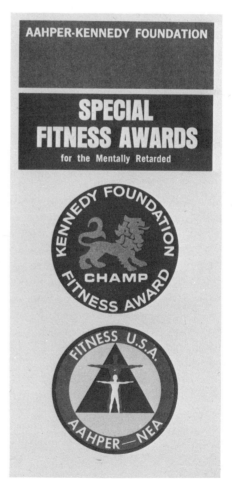

Special fitness awards for the mentally retarded, AAHPER–Kennedy Foundation.

for his chronologic age in physical development than he is in mental development. Some mentally retarded students are capable of participating in a regular physical education class, while others have been able to develop only minimal amounts of motor ability. In general, most mentally retarded students are 2 to 4 years behind their normal peers in motor development alone.

Despite a slower development of motor ability, mentally retarded students seem to reach physical maturity faster than do normal boys and girls of the same chronologic age. The mentally retarded tend to be overweight and to lack physical strength and endurance. Their posture is generally poor, and they lack adequate levels of physical fitness and motor coordination. Some of these physical problems develop because the mentally retarded have had little of the play and physical activity experiences of normal children. The problems of some mentally retarded youngsters are further multiplied by attendant physical handicaps and personality disturbances.

The mentally retarded require a physical educator with special training, special skills, and a special brand of patience. The mentally retarded lack confidence and pride and need a physical educator who will help them to change their negative self-image. The physical educator must be able to provide a program designed to give each student a chance for success. The physical educator must be ready to praise and reinforce each minor success. The physical educator must be capable of demonstrating each skill, give simple and concise directions, and be willing to participate in physical education activities with the students. Discipline must be enforced and standards adhered to, but the disciplinary approach must be a kind and gentle one.

The physical educator must be especially mindful of the individual characteristics of each mentally retarded student. Those students who need remedial work should be afforded this opportunity, while those students who can succeed in a regular physical education program should be placed in such a class or section.

Most mentally retarded students need to be taught how to play. They are frequently unfamiliar with even the simplest of childhood games, and they lack facility in the natural movements of childhood, such as skipping, hopping, and leaping. The mentally retarded are often seriously deficient in physical fitness and need work in postural improvement. Further, the mentally retarded find it difficult to understand and remember game strategy such as the importance of staying in the right position, and cannot relate well to the rules of sports and games.

The majority of mentally retarded students need a specially tailored physical education experience. For those who can participate in a regular physical education class, care must be taken so that these students are not placed in a situation where they will meet failure. In a special physical education class, the mentally retarded student can be exposed to a variety of physical education experiences. Physical fitness and posture improvement, along with self-testing activities and games organized and designed according to the ability and interests of the group, will make up a vital part of the special program. In such a class, activities can be easily modified and new experiences introduced before interest wanes. Research has indicated that specially tailored physical education classes can help mentally retarded students to progress very rapidly in their physical skill development. Movement education is especially suited to the mentally retarded. These students have often not engaged in the natural play activities of childhood and need to develop their gross motor skill abilities in order to be able to find success in some of the more sophisticated motor skills.

Emotionally disturbed students

The emotionally disturbed student presents special problems for the physical educator, who must be concerned not only with teaching but also with the safety of the students in the class.

A single emotionally disturbed student can have a disastrous effect on a class and can affect the behavior of the rest of the students in that class. Effective teaching cannot take place when discipline deteriorates.

Emotionally unstable students have difficulty maintaining good relationships with their classmates and teachers. Some of their abnormal behavior patterns stem from a need and craving for attention. Sometimes the disruptive student exhibits gross patterns of aggressiveness and destructiveness. Other emotionally unstable students may be so withdrawn from the group that they refuse to participate in the activities of the class, even to the extent of refusing to report for class. In the case of physical education, the emotionally disturbed student may refuse to dress for the activity when he does report. These measures draw both student and teacher reaction and focus attention on the nonconforming student.

Emotionally unstable students are often restless and unable to pay attention. In a physical education class they may poke and prod other students, refuse to line up with the rest of the class, or insist on bouncing a game ball while a lesson is in progress. These are also ploys to gain attention. The student behaves in the same manner in the academic classroom for the same reason.

Some emotionally disturbed students may have physical or mental handicaps that contribute to their behavior. Others may be concerned about what they consider to be poor personal appearance such as extremes of height or weight or physical maturity not in keeping with their chronologic age. Still other emotionally disturbed students may simply be in the process of growing up and are finding it difficult to handle their adolescence.

If negative student behavior stems from some aspect of a student's personality, then the physical educator must take positive steps to resolve the problem so that teaching can take place. The physical educator must deal with each behavioral problem on an individual basis and seek help from those school personnel who are best equipped to give aid. The school psychologist and the student's guidance counselor will have information that will be of help to the physical educator. A conference with these individuals may reveal methods that have proved effective with the student in the past. Further, the observations made by the physical educator will be of value to the continuing study of the student.

The physical educator will find that not all emotionally disturbed students are continual and serious behavior problems. The physical educator should have a private conference with the student whose behavior suddenly becomes negative and try to understand why the student has reacted in a way unusual for him. Such a conference will lead to mutual understanding and often help to allay future problems with the same student.

Much of the physical educator's task is student guidance. In individual cases of disruptive behavior, the physical educator should exhaust all of his personal resources to alleviate the problem before enlisting aid from other sources. Any case of disruptive behavior demands immediate action on the part of the physical educator to prevent minor problems from becoming major ones.

The majority of school pupils enjoy physical activity and physical education. They look forward to the physical education class as one part of the school day in which they can express themselves and gain a release of tension in an atmosphere that encourages this. For this reason, the student who is disruptive in the classroom is often one of the best citizens in the physical education class.

Physical education is in a unique position to help the emotionally disturbed student. Most students profit from the activities of physical education, and through their actions in this phase of the school curriculum teaching personnel can gain many insights into understanding student behavior. Individual knowledge of each student is of utmost importance in physical education and in understanding individual behavior patterns. Recognizing a student's needs and problems early in the school year will help in offsetting future behavior problems.

While physical education classes are conducted in a less formal manner than are classroom subjects, this does not mean that lower standards of behavior are acceptable. Students should know what the standards are on the first day of class and should be expected to adhere to these standards in all future classes.

Respect for the individual student is a necessity. No student likes to be criticized or embarrassed in front of his peers. When a student is singled out from a group and used as a disciplinary example, the atmosphere in the class will deteriorate. Respect for the student means maintenance of respect for the teacher. If disciplinary matters are handled on a one-to-one basis, rapport is enhanced. If the disruptive student knows that the physical educator expects him to behave in a bizarre manner, he will react in just this way. Good behavior should be expected until the student acts otherwise. Constant failure only abets disruptive behavior. If a student is known to be hostile and disruptive, an attempt should be made to avoid placing him in situations where he feels inadequate and shows this in his behavior. If, for example, a disruptive student does not run well, he may still make a superior goalie in soccer, a position that

would not require him to run. If the emotionally disturbed student has a special skill talent, he might be asked to demonstrate for the class. This will give him the recognition and attention he needs. Praise should be given for a skill that is well performed.

No student is going to participate in extra class activities unless he really wants to. Therefore, behavioral standards should be set for each activity, and it should be available to all students in the school who meet the standards. Acceptance into a club or participation on an intramural team may help the disruptive student gain self-respect and peer recognition and approval.

Culturally disadvantaged students

Recently, culturally disadvantaged students have become a real concern to various communities and to the schools serving these communities. It is a common error for the public to associate only the black child with cultural deprivation. Professional educators especially must realize that cultural deprivation crosses all color lines and ignores none of them. The culture of poverty is especially apparent in the large urban centers. Culturally disadvantaged persons may be found in Appalachia, suburbia, and isolated small towns and rural villages all across the United States.

The culturally disadvantaged student feels isolated from the mainstream of life. His home and neighborhood environments serve as negative influences, destroying his confidence, robbing him of a chance for success, and defeating any aspirations he may have. A culturally disadvantaged student does not achieve success in school because the cultural standards of the school and the home environment are usually inconsistent. Even schools in ghetto or slum areas are staffed by teachers who represent the middle-class segment of society. Continual failure in the classroom negatively affects the school behavior of the culturally disadvantaged student. His short attention span, emotional instability, excitability, and restlessness often contribute to disruptive behavior patterns.

In physical education the culturally disadvantaged student can be given an opportunity to meet success. Physical activity has a strong appeal for these youngsters whether they are students in a school in their neighborhood or community or part of the student body in a school in an affluent area.

The physical educator is the most important single factor in a school physical education program for the disadvantaged. The physical educator should have a sincere interest in these students and must be willing to assume the responsibility for physically educating them. He should have an adequate background and special training in general education and physical education courses concerned with teaching the disadvantaged. These courses will help him come to a fuller understanding of the culturally disadvantaged student and the educational problems he faces. The physical educator should have the ability to develop rapport with the culturally disadvantaged so that he can better respect, understand, and help these students. The physical educator should be able to provide an enriched program that will help to motivate the culturally disadvantaged student to make the best use of his physical, intellectual, and creative abilities.

Through physical education activities many general educational knowledges, skills, and abilities can be enhanced. Through folk dances, for example, it is possible to acquaint the student with the dress and customs of various cultures. This knowledge will help a class in history to become more interesting to the student and will help him to develop pride in his own culture. Through a sport such as baseball, mathematics can be brought to life. The students will be able to see the rela-

tionship between mathematics and its uses in determining baseball batting averages, computing team won-lost percentages, and the importance of understanding angles as applied to laying out a baseball diamond.

The school physical education program frequently is the only supervised physical activity program for the culturally disadvantaged student. These students usually do not have a neighborhood recreational facility available and must conduct their sports and games on unsupervised streets or in dangerously littered lots. The school physical education experience must be designed to afford this student the physical education and recreational activities that are denied him elsewhere. There must be a wide choice of physical education activities offered so that these students can select not only those experiences they find pleasurable but also those in which they can find success.

The program should include activities that will help these students to increase their physical fitness and optimum skill levels. Lack of structured programs outside the school denies culturally disadvantaged students the opportunity to participate in a regular program of physical activity. This often prevents these students from maintaining even minimal fitness levels. Competitive sports and games must be a part of the class program, but time must also be alloted for the individual to compete with himself to raise a physical fitness test score or to improve in a skill performance.

Culturally disadvantaged students need to develop a background in the lifetime sports. Swimming, dancing and tennis, as well as other recreational activities such as bowling, should be included in the program. There should be records, a phonograph, and a variety of rhythm instruments. The culturally disadvantaged enjoy rhythmic activities and find that they are successful in such areas as dance, gymnastics, and tumbling, where they can demonstrate their creativity and express their individuality. Many warm-up activities, as well as many games, can be done to a musical accompaniment.

The culturally disadvantaged are especially conscious of their individuality, and the program must allow ample opportunity for self-expression and creativity. Teacher recognition and praise for the most minor accomplishment is of utmost importance to the continued success of these students. If possible, culturally disadvantaged students should not be in a large class because little teaching takes place and because the individual student becomes lost in the mass.

Poorly coordinated students

The student with low motor ability is often ignored by the physical educator. He may be unpopular with his classmates because he is considered a detriment in a team sport. He may be undesirable as a partner in a dual sport and may wind up paired with an equally uncoordinated and awkward partner. The student with low motor ability needs special attention so that he can improve his physical skill performances, derive pleasure from success in physical activity, and gain a background in lifetime sports.

Poorly coordinated students are frequently placed in regular physical education classes when they have no mental or physical handicaps. The only concession made to their problem is through ability grouping in schools where facilities and personnel are adequate. Even then, ability grouping sometimes is used only to separate the "duds" from the "stars," thus increasing the poorly coordinated student's feelings of inadequacy. The poorly coordinated student may be held up to ridicule by fellow students as well as by physical education teachers, who use him as an example of how not to perform a physical skill.

The poorly coordinated student will resist learning new activities because the challenge this presents offers little chance for success. The challenge of a new skill or activity to be learned may create such tension within the student that he becomes physically ill. In other instances this tension may result in negative behavior.

Poor coordination may be the result of several factors. The student may not be physically fit, or he may have poor reflexes, or he may not have the ability to use mental imagery. For some reason such as a lengthy childhood illness, the poorly coordinated student may not have been normally physically active. Other poorly coordinated students may enter the secondary school physical education program from an elementary school that lacked a trained physical educator, had no facilities for physical education, or had a poor program of physical education.

In working with poorly coordinated students the physical educator must exercise the utmost patience. He must know why the student is poorly coordinated and be able to devise an individual program for each student that will help him to move and perform more effectively. The physical educator must be sure that the student understands the need for special help and try to motivate him to succeed. When a skill is performed with even a modicum of improvement, the effort must be praised and the achievement reinforced.

With a large class and only one instructor, there can be relatively little time spent with each individual. Buddy systems—that is, pairing a poorly coordinated student with a well-coordinated partner—often enables both students to progress faster. The physical educator must be careful not to push the student beyond his limits. A too difficult challenge coupled with the fatigue that results from trying too hard may result in retardation, rather than acceleration, of improvement. Any goal set for the poorly coordinated student must be a reasonable one.

The objectives of the program for poorly coordinated students will not differ from the objectives of any physical education program.

Before a program is devised, the status of the students will need to be known so that their individual abilities and needs can be identified. Physical fitness and motor ability testing should be on-going phases of the program. Through the physical education program the students should come to realize that their special needs are being met because they are as important as the well-skilled students in the eyes of the physical educator.

Separating students into ability groups may cause poorly coordinated students to feel that they are being pushed out of the way. If ability grouping is used, the poorly coordinated must receive adequate instruction, a meaningful program, and have equal access to good equipment and facilities.

If a student has poor eye-hand or eye-foot coordination, he will not succeed in such activities as tennis or soccer. Activities should be chosen that suit the abilities of the students and at the same time help them to develop the needed coordinations. Work on improving fitness and self-testing activities should form only a part of the program. Appropriate games, rhythmics and dance, and such activities as swimming and archery will help to stimulate and maintain interest. Physical fitness clubs, swimming clubs, and other clubs open to all students will also benefit the poorly coordinated.

With carefully arranged teams and schedules in an intramural program, the poorly coordinated can be given a chance to compete with other students on their own level of ability. Preparation for intramural competition should be a part of the class program.

Dancing lends itself to coeducational instruction. When classes can be combined and coeducational instruction offered, the poorly coordinated will have an opportunity to develop social skills. Different groupings for different activities will stimulate interest and provide students with a variety of partners.

The student's progress should be evaluated periodically. When an adequate level of success has been attained in a particular activity, the student should be assigned to a faster moving and more highly skilled group. A selection of activities should be offered that will appeal to the poorly coordinated and guide their selections in relation to their abilities.

Physically gifted and creative students

Gifted and creative students in physical education also need a specially tailored physical education experience.

The physically gifted student has superior motor skill abilities in many activities and maintains a high level of physical fitness. This student may be a star athlete, but in general he is simply a good all-around performer. In a game situation, he always seems to be in the right place at the right time. The physically gifted student learns quickly and requires a minimum of individual instruction. He is usually enthusiastic about physical activity and practices his skills of his own volition. Any individual instruction he does require is in the form of coaching rather than remedial correction. The physically gifted student has a strong sense of kinesthetic awareness and understands the principles of human movement. The student may not be able to articulate these latter two qualities, but observation by the physical educator will reveal that the student has discovered how to exploit his body as a tool for movement.

The creative student also has a well-developed sense of kinesthetic awareness and knows how to use his body properly. This student is the girl who dances with ease and grace or who is highly skilled in free exercise. It is the boy who is the lithe

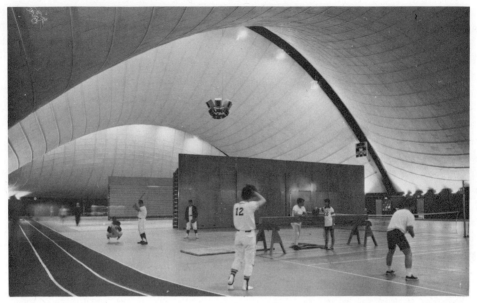

Shaver & Company, Salina, Kan.

The creative and gifted student has developed a kinesthetic awareness. (Graceland Fieldhouse, La Moni, Iowa.)

tumbler or gymnast. These students develop their own sophisticated routines in dance, tumbling, gymnastics, apparatus, and synchronized swimming. They may or may not be extraordinarily adept in other physical education activities, but they are as highly teachable as are the physically gifted.

The beginning physical educator may find it especially difficult to teach a student who possesses many more physical abilities than the teacher does. However, there is no student in school who knows all there is to know about an activity. Many experiences will still be new to them.

The physically gifted and creative students may not have attempted a wide range of activities, but they may have experienced all the activities offered in the school physical education program. Both the physically gifted and the creative student as well as the average student will be stimulated and challenged by the introduction of new activities. The creative student in dance may be introduced to a

new kind of music, or the boy skilled on apparatus may enjoy adding new moves to his routines. The athlete may be a good performer, but perhaps he needs to become a better team player. Or he may rely on his superior skills rather than on a complete knowledge of the rules and strategies of sports and games.

A well-planned physical education program will be adaptable to the needs of all the students it serves. But before the program can be definitively developed, the specific needs, limitations, and abilities of the students in the program must be defined. The activities offered must be adapted to the needs of the students, since the students cannot be adapted to the program.

The exceptional student needs a structured program of physical activity, since this is a vital part of his mental, social, emotional, and physical development. Some schools have made it a policy to excuse athletes from the activity program when their varsity sport is in season. This is a disservice to the student, especially when the varsity sport and the unit being taught in class are different. A student benefits from physical activity in a regular program. The physical educator can keep the interest of the exceptional student high by adopting some tested methods.

A leader's program has proved valuable in many schools. Leaders can assist the physical educator in innumerable ways, and they develop a sense of responsibility for the program because they are directly involved. Members of Leaders' Clubs have served as gymnastics and tumbling spotters in classes other than their own and can assist as officials in both the class program and during intramural contests. Members of Leaders' Clubs thus still participate in the activities of their own class, but at the same time receive the benefit of extra exposure to activities. Movies, film strips, loop films, and slides interest and benefit all students. The exceptional student can compare his performance with those of experts and can gain new insights into skills.

Textbooks in physical education are not in wide use in secondary school physical education programs. Students can benefit from the use of a textbook, special outside readings, assignments, and research problems, and these provide an additional challenge for the exceptional student.

Many highly skilled or creative students will be able to assist those students who have low motor skill abilities. By working on a one-to-one basis, the amount of individualized instruction will be increased. The student with low motor ability will receive the special assistance he needs, and the gifted student will be helped to realize that not all students possess high levels of ability.

The exceptional student can assist in the intramural program by acting as a coach on a day when his team is not playing. Coaching a team will help the student to become more cognizant of the importance of team play, sportsmanship, and the need for rules.

A skilled gymnast may not benefit from a beginning unit in tumbling. If his class is on this unit, the exceptional student can be assigned to work on advanced skills or on an advanced routine. A girl who shows great creativity in dance can be assigned to design a new dance or to devise some new steps.

SCHEDULING THE ADAPTED PROGRAM

Before scheduling a student in the adapted program, a thorough understanding should be gained of the boy's or girl's atypical condition and the type of procedure that will best meet his or her total development.

Because of the shortage of funds, space, and staff, many scheduling difficulties arise in respect to the adapted program. Many times equipment has to be improvised, special groups must be scheduled within the regular class period, and staff members have to devote out-of-school time to this important phase of the total physical education program. Unfortunately, some teachers solve the problem by sending the exceptional student to study hall or letting him observe from the bleachers, thus failing to provide for a modified program.

There is a feeling among physical education leaders that scheduling atypical children and youth in separate groups is not always satisfactory. Many educators who have studied this problem feel that the atypical student should take his physical education along with the normal students and, to provide for the handicapped condition, the program be modified and special methods of teaching used. In such cases, the administrator should make sure that the modification of the program for the student is physically and psychologically sound. Sometimes mental and emotional defects can be minimized if the teacher acquaints other students with the general

ANNUAL PHYSICAL ACTIVITY FORM

Junior and Senior High School

Sponsored by Bureau of School Health Service, Division of Pupil Personnel Services, New York State Department of Education and New York State Heart Assembly, Inc.

Date _____

To Dr. _____

From Dr. _____ School Physician

_____ School

_____
Address

Re:_____   _____
   Name of pupil   Grade in school

     All pupils registered in the schools of New York State are required by the education law to attend courses of instruction in physical education   These courses are required to be adapted to meet individual needs. This means that a pupil who is unable to participate in the entire program should have his activities modified to meet and/or improve his condition. The physical education classes are approximately _____ minutes in length and are held __ times a week.

     The final responsibility for the determination of a student participation rests with the school physician. Your recommendation will assist him in making a decision. If further clarification is needed, the school physician will arrange a conference with you.

     This child may participate in all physical education class activities and in competitive sports, intramural and interscholastic.   Yes_____ No_____

DIAGNOSIS: _____

     If activity is limited, please check what he may do, in the following list:

PHYSICAL EDUCATION CLASS ACTIVITIES

( ) Basketball	( ) Trampoline	( ) Square dancing
( ) Baseball	( ) Tumbling	( ) Social dancing
( ) Football	( ) Volleyball	( ) Apparatus
( ) Soccer	( ) Wrestling	( ) Archery
( ) Softball	( ) Track	( ) Field hockey
		( ) Swimming

INTRAMURAL AND INTERSCHOLASTIC SPORTS

( ) Basketball	( ) Wrestling	( ) Golf
( ) Baseball	( ) Track and field	( ) Swimming
( ) Football	( ) Cross country	( ) Cheerleading
( ) Soccer	( ) Bowling	

1. Does this child require a rest period during school hours?   Yes_____ No_____
2. Duration of restrictions: weeks_____ months_____ school year_____
3. Do you wish the patient to return to you for reevaluation?   Yes_____ No ___Date___

_____ _____ M. D. _____
Date   Address
Prepared and pretested by: Nassau TB, Heart and Public Health Association, Inc.

Adapted physical education record. (Bureau of School Health Service, Division of Pupil Personnel Services, New York State Department of Education and New York State Heart Assembly, Inc.)

LAST NAME   FIRST NAME   MIDDLE NAME   SCHOOL   GRADE

CHANGE IN PHYSICAL EDUCATION ASSIGNMENT

The physical education assignment of the above student may be changed as indicated on this form when approved by the committee members appearing below.

ASSIGNMENT TO SPECIAL PHYSICAL EDUCATION CLASS   WITHDRAWAL FROM SPECIAL PHYSICAL EDUCATION CLASS

Person Originating Recommendation   Title   Person Originating Recommendation   Title

Reason for Recommendation: Reason for Recommendation:

Recommended for   Recommended for withdrawal from

Rest_____ Modified_____ Orthopedic _____   Rest_____ Modified_____ Orthopedic _____

Recommended by Committee   ### Recommended by Committee

School Physician   Date   School Physician   Date

School Nurse   Date   School Nurse   Date

School Counselor   Date   School Counselor   Date

Special Physical Education Teacher   Date   Special Physical Education Teacher   Date

Chairman, Physical Education Dept.   Date   Chairman, Physical Education Dept.   Date

Approved by   Date   **Approved by**   Date

Date admitted to class_____   Date withdrawn from class_____

                                                   Number weeks in special class_____

Return to P.E. Department Chairman   Return to P.E. Department Chairman

7500 5-56 - 9881   LONG BEACH PUBLIC SCHOOLS
                            SPECIAL PHYSICAL EDUCATION TRANSFER

INDIVIDUAL REMEDIAL PHYSICAL EDUCATION
PUPIL PASS   DATE..........................

BK. NO.
OR SEC......................   NAME ....

ASSIGNED TO:

DAY	PERIOD	ROOM NO.	SUBJECT	TEACHER'S SIGNATURE
MON.				
TUE.				
WED.				
THU.				
FRI.				

RELEASED FROM:

DAY	PERIOD	ROOM NO.	SUBJECT	TEACHER'S SIGNATURE
MON.				
TUE.				
WED.				
THU.				
FRI.				

TEACHER ....

THIS CARD MUST BE RETURNED TO THE TEACHER OF INDIVIDUAL REMEDIAL PHYSICAL EDUCATION WHEN COMPLETELY SIGNED.

FORM PEH 95—REMEDIAL CLASSES, PUPIL PASS—SCHOOL DISTRICT OF PHILADELPHIA (JAN. 1961)

Please Admit _____   _____   _____   _____
                                                    (Name)   (Adviser)   (Period)   (Group or Class)

New Trier Township High School—Winnetka, Illinois

PHYSICAL EDUCATION CLASS ADJUSTMENT DUE TO SICKNESS OR INJURY

East Gymnasium ___( )	Athletic Field _____( )	Free Throwing _____( )	Badminton _____( )
Main Gymnasium ___( )	Field House _____( )	Horseshoes ____ ____( )	Hand Ball _____( )
North Gymnasium __( )	Natatorium _____( )	Playing Catch _____( )	Running _____( )
South Gymnasium __( )	Nurse's Office _____( )	Special Exercise ____( )	Tennis _____( )
Stage Gymnasium __( )	Training Room _____( )	Table Tennis _____( )	Walking _____( )
Locker Room _____( )	Remarks:		

Monday	Tuesday	Wednesday	Thursday	Friday

NOTE: Instructor should initial proper date if student reports and does satisfactory work. If assignment is for more than one day, the card should be left in attendance book. If assignment is of long duration, the books will be changed to check attendance.

problems of the handicapped person and encourages their cooperation in helping the student to make the right adjustment and maintain his self-esteem and social acceptance. There also seems to be a trend, at least in secondary schools, to follow an adapted sports program rather than to have a corrective type of program.

In the larger schools it sometimes has been possible to schedule special classes for students with some types of abnormalities. There also have been special schools established for the severely handicapped. These two types of procedures have not always proved satisfactory, however, because of the financial cost and the feeling that boys and girls should be scheduled with normal students for social and psychologic reasons.

In some smaller schools and colleges where there is a staff problem, those students needing an adapted program have been scheduled as a separate section within the regular physical education class period. In some cases group exercises have been devised together, with the practice of encouraging pupils to assist one another in the alleviation of their difficulties. These methods are not always satisfactory but, according to the schools and colleges concerned, are much better than not doing anything about the problem. In other schools and colleges, atypical pupils have been scheduled during special periods, where individual attention can be given to them.

The procedure that any particular school or college follows in scheduling students for the adapted program will depend upon its educational philosophy, finances, facilities and staff available, and the needs of the students.

SELECTION OF ACTIVITIES FOR ADAPTED PHYSICAL EDUCATION

The activities should be selected for the adapted physical education program with the needs of the atypical student in mind. It must usually be done on an individual basis after consultation with proper medical authorities. The activities should be selected in light of the objectives so that worthwhile skills are developed, a proper state of organic fitness is maintained, and the social and emotional needs of the student are considered. In no case should an activity ever aggravate an existing injury or atypical condition. Of course, all activities should be appropriate to the age level of the student and be ones in which he can find success. As far as possible and practical, activities should reflect the regular program of physical education offered at the school or college. The fewer changes made in the original activity, the more the atypical person feels that he is being successful and not different from the other students. Activities should contribute to the development of basic movements and skills. There should be as much group activity as possible since the socializing benefits of participation are important in providing students with a feeling of belonging and being a part of a group.

THE TEACHER IN THE ADAPTED PROGRAM

The physical education teacher who works with children and youth in the adapted program needs special training in order to do the job effectively. It requires more than a knowledge of sports and routine physical education.

In discussing the qualifications of health and physical educators, much has been said about the training needed by physical education teachers. These qualifications are very important and necessary for the teacher in the adapted program. However, in addition to these qualifications, the teacher should understand the student with the atypical condition—the various atypical conditions, their causes, and treatment. The teacher should like to work with students who need special help and be able to establish a good rapport so as to instill confidence and faith in the work that needs to be done. The teacher should appreciate

the various mental and emotional problems that confront an atypical person and the methods and procedures that can be followed to cope with these problems. The teacher must in some ways be a psychologist, creating interest and stimulating motivation toward physical activity for the purpose of hastening improvement. The teacher should be sympathetic to the advice of medical personnel. She or he should be willing to give corrective exercise under the guidance of physicians and to plan the program with their help. In addition, it is necessary to know the implications of medical and other findings for the adapted physical education program, to be familiar with the medical, psychologic, or other examinations of each student, and, with the help of the physician, psychologist, social worker, or other specialist, to work out a program that best meets the needs of the student.

Since some of the most effective work with children in the adapted program can be done at the elementary level, this has implications for the classroom teacher as well as the physical education specialist. In many elementary schools across the country there exists the "self-contained" classroom where the same teacher has the children for all subjects. The classroom teacher should therefore have sufficient knowledge, understanding, and training in the adapted program to provide adequately for her children's needs in this area.

THE ADAPTED PROGRAM IN SCHOOLS AND COLLEGES

The administrator of physical education should understand the components that make up a well-rounded adapted program and should strive toward including these essential phases in his particular school or college system.

One of the best descriptions that has been developed to point out the broad outlines of an adapted program primarily for the physically handicapped was published

Physical Inspection

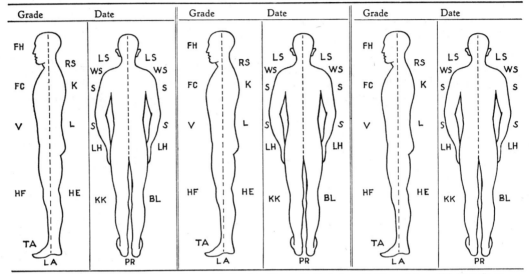

CODE — FH—Forward head   FC—Flat Chest   RS—Round shoulders   K—Kyphosis   V—Visceroptosis   HF—Hyper-flexion
HE—Hyper-extension   TA—Transverse arch   LA—Longitudinal arch   LS—Low shoulder   WS—Winged scaula   S—Scoliosis
LH—Low hip   KK—Knock knee   BL—Bow leg   PR—Pronation   Circle letters and indicate degree with 1, 2, 3 EXAMPLE (FH2)

Physical inspection. (Long Beach, Calif., Public Schools.)

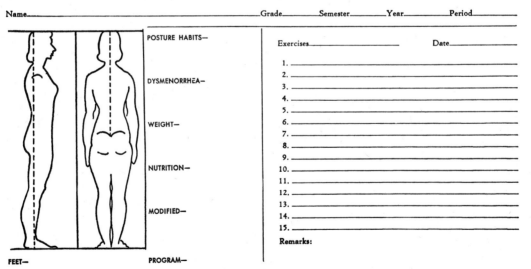

PE 27 3M 7-56 9912

LONG BEACH UNIFIED SCHOOL DISTRICT
PERMANENT INDIVIDUAL EXERCISE CARD — DEPARTMENT OF PHYSICAL EDUCATION

Name_____Grade_____Semester_____Year_____Period_____

POSTURE HABITS—

DYSMENORRHEA—

WEIGHT—

NUTRITION—

MODIFIED—

FEET—

PROGRAM—

BODY ALIGNMENT—

Exercises_____   Date_____

1. _____
2. _____
3. _____
4. _____
5. _____
6. _____
7. _____
8. _____
9. _____
10. _____
11. _____
12. _____
13. _____
14. _____
15. _____

Remarks:

Permanent individual exercise card. (Long Beach, Calif., Public Schools.)

in the Yearbook of the American Association for Health, Physical Education, and Recreation entitled *Children in Focus.** It will be valuable for any administrator to have the main points of this program reproduced here in slightly adapted form:

1. **Health examinations.** A thorough examination should be given to all students by either the school or the family physician.
2. **Classification for physical education based on the examination.** The results of the health examination will determine the type of handicap, if any, and whether the student should be in the regular or adapted program.
3. **Conference with students needing special consideration.** Conference can uncover student's needs, interests, limitations, and capabilities in the area of adapted physical education.
4. **Scheduling accomplished in accordance with school policy or size of school.** A suggested plan is as follows:
    (a) Large schools—separate classes.
    (b) Medium-sized schools—student spends some time in special class and also in regular class; suggest one day a week in special class and the other days in regular class.
    (c) Smaller schools—both handicapped and nonhandicapped in same class but program is modified and adapted to meet the needs of the handicapped within the regular group of normal students.
5. **Phases of the adapted program.** The program may involve three areas:
    (a) Special conditioning—includes developmental exercises to meet student needs such as to increase muscle power, help postural deviations, or improve range of motion.
    (b) Aquatics—aquatic activities to meet student needs, such as those concerned with remedial, recreational, and adjustment factors.
    (c) Recreational sports—sports are considered the best type of physical activity. Students should be transferred from exercise therapy to active sports therapy or placed directly in adapted sports program in preference to exercises. Recreational sports may contribute in such areas of development as adjustment and socialization.
6. **Evaluation of progress.** Evaluation can be accomplished through the utilization of such techniques as tests, conferences, standards of behavior, etc. Objective measures, if available, should receive first consideration.
7. **Records.** A record that contains data on the handicapped condition, physician's recommendations, program objectives for the student, recommended activities, record of special treatments, consultations, progress rating, and other pertinent information should be kept.
8. **Relationships.** An effective adapted program recognizes the importance of harmonious working relationships between medical and nursing personnel, the home, the school administrators, and other teachers.

ADMINISTRATIVE PRINCIPLES

The following statement was prepared for general use in schools and colleges rather than for special schools for handicapped children. It was approved by the Board of Directors, American Association for Health, Physical Education, and Recreation, and endorsed in principle by the Joint Committee on Health Problems in Education, American Medical Association and National Education Association:

It is the responsibility of the school to contribute to the fullest possible development of the potentialities of each individual entrusted to its care. This is a basic tenet of our democratic faith.

1. *There is need for common understanding regarding the nature of "adapted physical education."*

Adapted physical education is a diversified program of developmental activities, games, and sports suited to the interests, capacities, and limitations of students with disabilities who may not safely or successfully engage in unrestricted participation in the vigorous activities of the general program.

2. *There is a need for "adapted physical education" in schools and colleges.*

The number of children of school age in the United States with physical handicaps is alarmingly high. Of the 33,500,000 in the age groups five to nineteen, approximately 4,000,000 children have physical handicaps which need some kind of special educational consideration. (Of these, 65,-000 are blind or partially seeing; 335,000, orthopedic disabilities; and 500,000 each, deaf or hard of hearing, organic heart disease, and delicate or undeveloped.) The major disabling conditions each affecting thousands of children are cerebral palsy, poliomyelitis, tuberculosis, traumatic injuries,

---

*Daniels, A.: What provision for the handicapped? In American Association for Health, Physical Education, and Recreation: Children in focus, 1954 Yearbook, Washington, D. C., 1954, The Association.

and heart disease. Further evidence indicates that, on the college level, there is a significant percentage of students who require special consideration for either temporary or permanent disabilities.

3. *"Adapted physical education" has much to offer the individual who faces the combined problem of seeking an education and overcoming a handicap.*

"Adapted physical education" should serve the individual by:

(a) Aiding in discovering deviations from the normal and making appropriate referrals where such conditions are noted.

(b) Guiding students in the avoidance of situations which would aggravate their conditions or subject them to undue risks of injury.

(c) Improving general strength and endurance of individuals who are poorly developed and of those returning to school following illness or injury.

(d) Providing opportunities for needed social and psychological adjustment.

4. *The direct and related services essential for the proper conduct of adapted physical education should be available in our schools.*

These services should include:

(a) Adequate and periodic health examinations.

(b) Classification for physical education based on the health examination and other pertinent tests and observations.

(c) Guidance of individuals needing special consideration with respect to physical activity, general health practices, recreational pursuits, and vocational planning.

(d) Arrangement of appropriate physical education programs.

(e) Evaluation of progress through observations, appropriate measurements, and consultations.

(f) Integrated relationships with other school personnel, medical and its auxiliary services, and the family to assure continuous guidance and supervisory services.

(g) A cumulative record for each individual, which should be transferred from school to school.

5. *It is essential that adequate medical guidance be available for teachers of adapted physical education.*

Programs of adapted physical education should not be attempted without the diagnosis, written recommendation, and supervision of a physician. Problems of correction may be very profound. Where corrective measures are deemed necessary, they must be predicated upon medical findings and accomplished by competent teachers working with medical supervision and guidance. There should be an effective referral service between physicians, physical education, and parents, aimed at proper safeguards and maximum student benefits.

6. *Teachers of adapted physical education have a great responsibility as well as unusual opportunity.*

Physical educators engaged in teaching adapted physical education should have adequate professional education fitting them for this work. They must be motivated by the highest ideals with respect to the importance of total student development and satisfactory human relationships. They must have the ability to establish rapport with students who may exhibit social maladjustment as a disability. It is essential that they be professionally prepared to implement the recommendations provided by medical personnel for the adapted physical education program.

7. *Adapted physical education is necessary at all school levels.*

The student with a disability faces the dual problem of overcoming a handicap and acquiring an education which will enable him to take his place in society as a respected citizen. Failure to assist a student with his problems may sharply curtail the growth and development process. Offering adapted physical education in the elementary grades, and continuing through the secondary school and college, will assist the individual to improve function and make adequate psychological and social adjustments. It will prevent attitudes of defeat and fears of insecurity. It will be a factor in his attaining maximum growth and development within the limits of the disability. It will help him face the future with confidence.*

ADAPTED PHYSICAL EDUCATION— AN ESSENTIAL

Physical education programs should give increasing attention to the educational needs of individual children and youth, including those who are physically handicapped or who otherwise deviate from the normal. Physical education programs can offer remedial work as well as modify the program so that each boy and girl receives maximum benefit from participation. Furthermore, by providing an adapted program, students can be expected to be

*Committee on Adapted Physical Education, American Association for Health, Physical Education, and Recreation.

present for each class period and not excused or allowed to observe from the sidelines because of some atypical condition.

In order to have an effective adapted program, the physical education administrator and his staff must work harmoniously with the school and college medical staff, parents, and community agencies. Through cooperative effort each student can learn to live at his highest level of health.

Questions and exercises

1. What is meant by the term *adapted physical education?*
2. What are the objectives of the adapted physical education program?
3. What is the relationship between the principle of individual differences and the adapted physical education program?
4. How should students be classified for the adapted program?
5. What are the various methods of scheduling students for the adapted program? List the advantages and disadvantages of each.
6. What qualifications does the teacher of physical education need to work in the adapted program?
7. Outline an adapted physical education program for a high school or college.
8. Read three references on adapted physical education and give a report to the class on these readings.
9. How can the physical educator best adapt his program to the needs of the mentally retarded student?
10. What special physical education needs does the creative student have?
11. To what other resources can the physical educator turn when he needs assistance in understanding and working with the atypical student?

Reading assignment in *Administrative Dimensions of Health and Physical Education Programs, Including Athletics:* Chapter 6, Selections 28 to 33.

Selected references

Activity programs for the mentally retarded, Journal of Health, Physical Education, and Recreation 37:24, 1966.

Adapted physical education, Journal of Health, Physical Education, and Recreation 40:45, 1969.

American Association for Health, Physical Education, and Recreation: Project on recreation and fitness for the mentally retarded, Challenge, May, 1968.

Clarke, H. H., and Clarke, D. H.: Developmental and adapted physical education, Englewood Cliffs, N. J., 1963, Prentice-Hall, Inc.

Conant, J. B.: Slums and suburbs, New York, 1964, New American Library.

Cratty, B. J.: Social dimensions of physical activity, Englewood Cliffs, N. J., 1967, Prentice-Hall, Inc.

Daniels, A. S., and Davies, E. A.: Adapted physical education, ed. 2, New York, 1965, Harper & Row, Publishers.

Dexter, G.: Special physical education classes for physically handicapped minors, Sacramento, Calif., June, 1964, State Department of Education.

Duggar, M. P.: Dance for the blind, Journal of Health, Physical Education, and Recreation 39:28, 1968.

Fantani, M. D., and Weinstein, G.: The disadvantaged: challenge to education, New York, 1968, Harper & Row, Publishers.

Frankel, E. C.: Toward a rebirth of creativity, Journal of Health, Physical Education, and Recreation 38:65, 1967.

Hein, F. V.: Health classification vs. medical excuses from physical education, Journal of School Health 32:14, 1962.

Kretchmar, R. T.: The forgotten student in physical education, Journal of Health, Physical Education, and Recreation 31:21, 1960.

Mathews, D. K., Kruse, R., and Shaw, V.: The science of physical education handicapped children, New York, 1962, Harper & Row, Publishers.

National Society for the Study of Exceptional Children: The education of exceptional children, forty-ninth yearbook, National Society for the Study of Education, Chicago, 1950, University of Chicago Press.

Ratchick, I., and Koenig, F. G.: Guidance and the physically handicapped child, Chicago, 1963, Science Research Associates, Inc.

Riessman, F.: The culturally deprived child, New York, 1962, Harper & Row, Publishers.

Schoon, J. R.: Some psychological factors in motivating handicapped students in adapted physical education, The Physical Educator 19: 138, 1962.

Stein, J. U.: A practical guide to adapted physical education for the educable mentally handicapped, Journal of Health, Physical Education, and Recreation 33:30, 1962.

Wienke, P.: Blind children in an integrated physical education program, The New Outlook for the Blind 60:73, 1966.

Intramurals and *extramurals* refer to that phase of the school or college physical education program that is geared to the abilities and skills of the entire student body and consists of voluntary participation in games, sports, and other activities. It offers intramural activities within a single school or college and such extramural activities as "play" and "sports" days that bring together participants from several institutions. It is a laboratory period for sports and other activities, whose fundamentals have been taught in the basic instructional program. It affords competition for all types of individuals, the strong and the weak, the skilled and the unskilled, the big and the small. It also includes both sexes, separately and in corecreational programs. It is not characterized by the highly organized features of varsity sports, including commercialization, many spectators, considerable publicity, and stress on winning. It is a phase of the total physical education program, however, that should receive considerable emphasis.

OBJECTIVES

The objectives of intramural and extramural activities are compatible with the overall objectives of physical education and also with those of education in general. The objectives as listed by the University of Connecticut men's *Intramural Sports Handbook* are presented here in adapted form:

1. To provide the students at the institution with opportunities for fun, enjoyment, and fellowship through participation in sports.
2. To provide the students at the institution

with opportunities that will be conducive to their health and physical fitness.
3. To provide the students at the institution with opportunities for release from tensions and aggressions and to provide for a feeling of achievement through sports participation, all of which are conducive to mental and emotional health.

The objectives of the intramural and extramural programs may be classified under four headings: (1) health, (2) skill, (3) social development, and (4) recreation. Each objective will be discussed briefly.

Health

Intramural and extramural activities contribute to the physical, mental, social, and spiritual health of the individual. They contribute to physical health through participation in activity that affords healthful exercise. Such characteristics as strength, agility, speed, body control, and other factors that prove their worth in day-to-day living are developed. They contribute to mental health by providing opportunities for interpretive thinking, making decisions under highly charged emotional situations, and keeping one's mind occupied in worthwhile pursuits. They contribute to social health through group participation and working toward the achievement of group goals. They contribute to spiritual health through practical applications of the "golden rule," fair play, sportsmanship, and high standards of conduct.

Skill

Intramural and extramural activities offer the opportunity for every individual to display and develop his or her skill in var-

BOYS' INTRAMURAL STAFF APPLICATION
New Trier Township High School - Winnetka, Illinois

The Boys Intramural Sports Staff is dedicated to the task of providing sports competition and recreation for all New Trier boys. Most of the organization and administration of this program is done by students. If you are interested in becoming a member of the I.M. Sports Staff, fill out this application and return it to the I.M. Office.

Important: This application must be completely filled out to be considered.

Name _____ Adviser_____ Phone_____
    first (nickname)   last

Address _____ Class of 19____ Grade average

to date _____

Do you (or will you) have a job that will interfer with your probable assignment in I.M. Sports? _____

In which of the following areas would you like to work?

Supervising games and tournaments	Point Staff	Publicity
____ team sports	____ recorder	____ writing
____ individual sports	____ participation and awards	____ display
		____ radio

In what interscholastic sports have you participated (indicate year)? _____

In what other extracurricular activities do you participate and what offices do you hold?_____

Approximately what is your I.M. point total as of the date below? _____

READ THE FOLLOWING ITEMS CAREFULLY BEFORE YOU SIGN AND RETURN THIS APPLICATION

When I sign this application I understand that:

1. I am offering my service gratis, with no expectation of receiving special privileges or awards of any kind, except that of serving the students of New Trier High School.

2. I am willing to work one afternoon per week (3:40 until about 5:15 P.M.) and occasionally two. (This does not always apply to the point and publicity staffs.)

3. I am to conduct myself with the dignity and leadership necessary for a student leader at New Trier High School.

_____   _____
date of application   student's signature

(Do not write below this line.)
_____

_____ Date received   _____ Date rating sheet was sent

_____ Date of interview   _____ I.M. point total

_____ Accepted   _____ rejected

Boys' intramural staff application. (From Intramurals for senior high schools, The Athletic Institute, Chicago, Ill.)

ious physical education activities. Through specialization and voluntary participation they offer an opportunity to excel and to experience the thrill of competition. It is generally agreed that an individual enjoys those activities in which he has developed skill. Participation in athletics offers the opportunity to develop proficiency in various activities in group situations where individuals are equated according to their skill, thus providing for equality of competition. This helps to guarantee greater success and more enjoyment of participation. In turn there will be a carryover into adult living of skills that will enable many to spend leisure moments in a profitable and enjoyable manner.

Social development

Opportunities for social development are numerous in intramural and extramural activities. Through many social contacts, co-educational experiences, playing on teams, and other situations desirable qualities are developed. Individuals learn to subordinate their desires to the will of the group, develop sportsmanship, fair play, courage, group loyalty, social poise, and other desirable traits. Voluntary participation exists in such a program, and students who desire to play under such conditions will live by group codes of conduct. These experiences offer good training for citizenship, adult living, and human relations that are so essential in present-day living.

Recreation

Intramural and extramural programs help to establish a permanent interest in many sports and physical education activities. This interest and enthusiasm will carry over into adult living and provide the basis for many happy leisure hours. These programs also provide the basis for recreation during school days, when idle moments can have potentialities for fostering antisocial as well as constructive social behavior.

RELATION TO INTERSCHOLASTIC AND INTERCOLLEGIATE VARSITY ACTIVITIES

Both intramural and extramural activities and interscholastic and intercollegiate varsity athletics are integral phases of the total physical education program. As has been pointed out, the total physical education program is made up of the basic instructional class program, the adapted program, the intramural and extramural program, and the interscholastic and intercollegiate varsity athletic programs. Each has an important contribution to make to the achievement of physical education objectives. The important thing is to maintain a proper balance so that each phase enhances and does not restrict the other phases of the total program.

Whereas intramurals and extramurals are for the entire student body, interscholastic and intercollegiate varsity athletics are for those individuals who are skilled in various physical activities. Intramurals and extramurals are conducted primarily on a school and college basis, while interscholastic and intercollegiate varsity athletics are conducted, as the name implies, on an interschool or intercollege basis.

There is no conflict between these two phases of the program if the facilities, time, personnel, money, and other factors are apportioned according to the degree to which each phase achieves the educational outcomes desired, rather than the degree of public appeal and interest stimulated. One should not be designed as a training ground or farm system for the other. It should be possible for a student to move from one to the other, but this should be incidental in nature, rather than planned.

If conducted properly, each phase of the program can contribute to the other, and through an overall, well-balanced program the entire student body will come to respect sports and the great potentials they have for improving physical, mental, social, and emotional growth. When a physical education program is initially developed, it would seem logical to first provide an intramural program for the majority of the students, with the interscholastic or inter-

collegiate varsity athletic program coming as an outgrowth of the former. The first concern should be for the many or majority, and the second for the few or minority. This is characteristic of the democratic way of life. Although the intramural and extramural athletic programs are designed for every student, in practice they generally attract the poor and moderately skilled individuals. The skilled person finds his niche in the program for those of exceptional skill. This has its benefits in that it is an equalizer for competition.

PLAY, SPORTS, AND INVITATION DAYS

Play, sports, and invitation days are rapidly growing in popularity and deserve a prominent place in the extramural athletic program of any school or college. Although they have been utilized mainly by girls' and women's physical education programs, they are equally important for boys and men at the elementary, junior high school, senior high school, and college levels. They have received the endorsement of the American Association for Health, Physical Education, and Recreation, the Division for Girls' and Women's Sports, and many other prominent associations concerned with physical education. They are an innovation that should receive more and more stress in those places where overemphasis on athletics, highly competitive sports for children of elementary and junior high school ages, and the desire to win at any cost are threatening the accomplishment of the goals of physical education programs.

Sports days refer to that phase of the program where one or several schools or colleges participate in physical education activities. Schools or colleges may enter several teams in various sports. When organized in this manner, each team is identified with the institution it represents. Sports days may also be used to culminate a season of activity for participants within

PLAYER'S PERMIT

Name ----------------- Address ---------------- School -------------- Date ----

is physically fit and has our permission to participate in the play day to be held on

---------------------------------- at --------------------------------.

Physician -------------------------------

Parent or Guardian ----------------------

High School Principal --------------------

the same school or college. When several schools or colleges particpate in a sports day, the number of activities may range anywhere from one to eight, although it is generally agreed that having too many activities sometimes works to a disadvantage rather than an advantage. There are no significant awards for the various events and the publicity is not of a nature that builds up the desire to win.

Play days usually refer to a day or part of a day that is set aside for participation in physical education activities. It may be for students from the same school or college, from several institutions in the same community, or from many schools and colleges in various communities. In the play day each team is composed of individuals from different educational organizations. Here the organization loses it identity, whereas it was maintained in the sports day. The teams usually are labeled by distinctive colored uniforms, arm bands, numbers, or some other device. The activities can be individual as well as team in nature and competitive or noncompetitive. It would be noncompetitive, for example, if several students desired to engage in an activity like riding, not for the purpose of competing against one another but simply for the sociability of the occasion.

An *invitation day* is informal in nature, as are the sports and play days. In this event two schools or colleges usually meet for competition in an activity. This practice

has worked out successfully at the end of a seasonal activity, when the winning intramural team or representatives from several teams compete against a similar group from another school or college. The emphasis, however, is not on placing selected, highly skilled players on one team in order to enhance the chances of winning but on the social benefits and fun that can be gained from the occasion.

The advantages of play, sports, and invitation days are very much in evidence. They offer opportunities for the entire student body to participate in wholesome competition, regardless of skill. They offer the student an opportunity to participate in many and varied activities in a spirit of friendly rivalry. They stress both social and physical values. They eliminate the pressures and undesirable practices associated with highly competitive athletics. They are available to the entire student body. They are especially adaptable for immature youngsters who should not be exposed to the practices and pressures of high-level competition. They add interest to student participation and offer innumerable opportunities for leadership.

ACTIVITIES

The activities that comprise the intramural and extramural programs represent the substance that will either attract or divert attention. Therefore, it is important that the right activities be selected. Some ad-

INTRAMURAL EQUIPMENT

The following Intramural supplies are available to you. List items desired.

You are responsible for each item.

Please leave your I.D. card.

_____ Bow
_____ Arrows
_____ Badminton bird
_____ Badminton racket
_____ Basketball
_____ Football
_____ Golf balls
_____ Golf clubs
_____ Handball ball
_____ Handball glove, pr.
_____ Horseshoes
_____ Paddleball ball
_____ Paddleball paddle
_____ Ping Pong ball
_____ Ping Pong paddle
_____ Smashball ball
_____ Smashball paddle
_____ Soccer ball
_____ Softball ball
_____ Softball bat
_____ Softball glove
_____ Softball mask
_____ Squash ball
_____ Squash racquet
_____ Tennis balls
_____ Tennis racket
_____ Volleyball ball
_____ Volleyball net

O-2879   **You will be fined for equipment kept overnight.**

Intramural equipment. (From Intramurals for senior high schools, The Athletic Institute, Chicago, Ill.)

ministrative guides that may be listed to help in the selection of these activities are as follows:

1. Activities should be selected in accordance with the season of the year and the conditions and influences that prevail locally.
2. Activities should be presented in a progressive manner from the elementary through the college level.
3. Activities should be selected in accordance with the needs and interests of the students.
4. Activities that have implications for adult living should be given a prominent place in the program.

5. Corecreational activities should be provided.
6. The activities that are included in the physical education class program should have a bearing on the activities that are included in the intramural and extramural programs. The latter should act as a laboratory for the former.
7. Many desirable activities require little special equipment and do not require long periods of training in order to get the participant in physical condition.
8. Consideration should be given to such activities as field trips, story-telling, dramatics, hiking, handicraft, and others of a more recreational nature.
9. Activities in the elementary school should be selected with special attention to the ability of the child.

The following lists of activities are identified in a publication of The Athletic Institute*:

Individual and dual sports

Achievement tests	Physical fitness
Archery	Rope climbing (boys)
Badminton	Scuba diving
Basketball goal	Shooting
and foul	Shuffleboard
Billiards	Skiing
Bowling	Swimming
Deck tennis	Table tennis
Golf	Tennis
Gymnastics	Track and field
Handball	Tumbling
Horseshoes	Weight training
Paddle tennis	Wrestling (boys)

NOTE: Boxing is not approved as an activity.

Club or group activities

Camping and cookouts	Hosteling
Canoeing	Ice skating
Cycling	Marching tactics
Dance—social, folk,	Outdoor skills
square, and modern	Rifle
Figure skating	Roller skating
Fishing	Rowing
Fly or bait casting	Sailing
Hiking	Tumbling
Horseback riding	

*Matthews, D. O., editor: Intramurals for the senior high school, Chicago, 1964, The Athletic Institute.

Team sports

Baseball (boys)	Speedball
Basketball	Soccer
Blooper ball	Softball
Field hockey	Swimming
Gymnastics	Touch (or flag) football
Ice hockey	Track and field
Kick ball	Volleyball
Lacrosse	Water games (water polo,
Speed-a-way	water basketball)

NOTE: Tackle football for boys may be included in team sports only if the proper conditioning and training, instruction, coaching, officiating, and supervision are provided and the recommended protective equipment is used.

Corecreational activities

Badminton	Ice skating
Bowling	Picnics and outings
Canoeing	Roller skating
Curling	Shuffleboard
Cycling	Skiing
Dance—social, folk,	Softball
square, and modern	Swimming
Deck tennis	Table tennis
Golf	Tennis
Horseback riding	Volleyball

UNITS AND TYPES OF COMPETITION FOR INTRAMURAL AND EXTRAMURAL ACTIVITIES

The careful selection of appropriate units and types of competition will help to enhance the values that accrue from intramural and extramural activities.

Units of competition

There are many ways of organizing competition for the intramural and extramural programs. The units of competition should be such as to lend interest, create enthusiasm, and allow for identity with some group where an esprit de corps can be developed and where a healthy flavor is added to the competition.

At the elementary level, the classroom provides a basis for such activity. It may be desirable in some cases to organize on some other basis, but the basic structure of the homeroom lends itself readily to this purpose.

At the junior and senior high school levels, several units of organization are possible. Organization may be by grades or classes, homerooms, age, height, weight, clubs, societies, residential districts, physical education classes, study groups, or the arbitrary establishment of groups by staff members. The type of unit organization will vary from school to school and from community to community. The staff member in charge of the program should try to determine the method of organization best suited to the local situation.

At the college or university level there are also several possible units for organization. It can be on the basis of fraternities or sororities, classes, colleges within a university, departments, clubs, societies, physical education classes, boarding clubs, churches, residential districts, geographic units or zones of the campus, dormitories, marital status, social organizations, assignment by lot, honorary societies, or groups set up in an arbitrary manner. Again, the best type of organization will vary from situation to situation.

Types of competition

There are several different ways of organizing competition. Three of the most common are on the bases of leagues, tournaments, and meets. These methods of organization take many forms, with league play popular in the major sports, elimination tournaments utilized to great extent after league play has terminated, and meets held to culminate a season or year of sports activity.

Individual and group competition may be provided. Individual competition is adaptable to such activities as tennis, wrestling, and skiing, whereas group competition is adaptable to such team activities as basketball, softball, and field hockey.

Various types of tournament competition have been widely written up in books specializing in intramurals and other aspects of sports. For this reason only a brief discussion of these items will be included here.

The round robin tournament is probably one of the most widely used and one of the best types of competition, since it allows for maximum play. It is frequently utilized in leagues, where it works best when there are not more than eight teams. Each team plays every other team at least once during the tournament. Each team continues to play to the completion of the tournament and the winner is the one who has the highest percentage, based on wins and losses, at the end of scheduled play.

The elimination type of tournament does not allow for maximum play; the winners continue to play, while the losers drop out. A team or individual is automatically out when it or he loses. However, this does represent the most economical form of organization from the standpoint of time in determining the winning player or team.

The single or straight elimination type of tournament is set up so that one defeat eliminates a player or team. Usually there is a drawing for positions, with provisions for the seeding of the better players or teams on the basis of past experience. Such seeding provides for more intense competition as the tournament moves toward the finals. Under such an organization, byes are

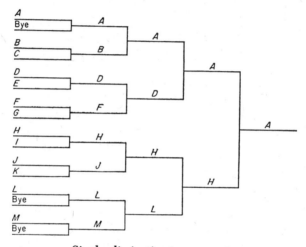

Single-elimination tournament.

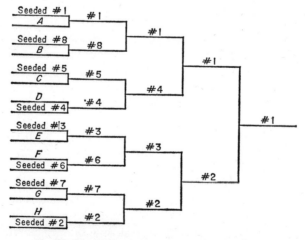

Single-elimination tournament with seedings.

I. 1 vs. 5
   2 vs. 6
   3 vs. 7
   4 vs. 8

II. 1 vs. 2
    3 vs. 5
    4 vs. 6
    8 vs. 7

III. 1 vs. 3
     4 vs. 2
     8 vs. 5
     7 vs. 6

IV. 1 vs. 4
    8 vs. 3
    7 vs. 2
    6 vs. 5

V. 1 vs. 8
   7 vs. 4
   6 vs. 3
   5 vs. 2

VI. 1 vs. 7
    6 vs. 8
    5 vs. 4
    2 vs. 3

VII. 1 vs. 6   Round-robin rotation for an eight-team league.
     5 vs. 7
     2 vs. 8
     3 vs. 4

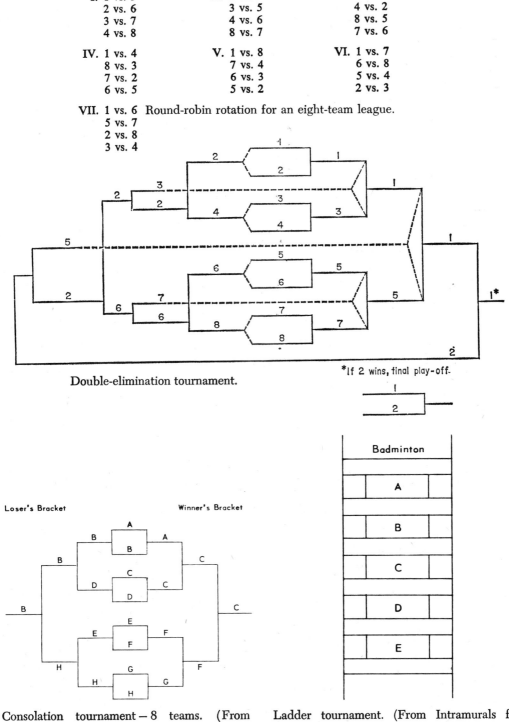

Double-elimination tournament.

*If 2 wins, final play-off.

Loser's Bracket   Winner's Bracket

Badminton

Consolation tournament — 8 teams. (From Intramurals for senior high schools, The Athletic Institute, Chicago, Ill.)

Ladder tournament. (From Intramurals for senior high schools, The Athletic Institute, Chicago, Ill.)

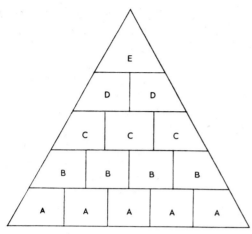

Any A may challenge any B.
Any B may challenge any C.
Any C may challenge any D.
Either D may challenge E.

Pyramid tournament. (From Intramurals for senior high schools, The Athletic Institute, Chicago, Ill.)

awarded in the first round of play whenever the number of entrants does not equal a multiple of two. Although such a tournament is a timesaver and is quick, it is weak in the respect that it does not adequately select the second- and third-place winners. The actual winner may achieve the championship because another player who is better has a bad day. Another weakness is that the majority of participants play only once or twice in the tournament.

The double elimination tournament does not have some of the weaknesses of the single elimination because it is necessary for a team or individual to have two de-

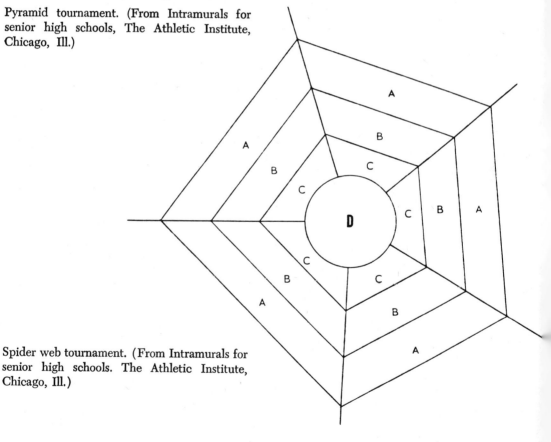

Spider web tournament. (From Intramurals for senior high schools. The Athletic Institute, Chicago, Ill.)

Note: Any A may challenge any B.
       Any B may challenge any C.
       Any C may challenge D.

feats before being eliminated. This principle is also characteristic of various types of consolation elimination tournaments that permit the player or team to play more than once.

In some consolation tournaments all the players who lose in the first round and those who, because they received a bye, did not lose until the second round get to play again to determine a consolation winner. In other similar tournaments they permit any player or team who loses once, irrespective of the round in which the loss occurs, to play again. There are also other tournaments such as the Bagnall-Wild Elimination Tournament that place emphasis on second and third places.

The ladder type of tournament adapts well to individual competition. Here the contestants are arranged in ladder or vertical formation with rankings established arbitrarily or on the basis of previous performance. Each contestant may challenge the one directly above or in some cases two above, and if he wins the names change places on the ladder. This is a continuous type of tournament that does not eliminate any participants. However, it is weak from the standpoint that it may drag and interest may wane.

The pyramid type of tournament is similar to the ladder variety. Here, instead of having one name on a rung or step, there are several names on the lower steps, gradually pyramiding to the top-ranking individual. A player may challenge anyone in the same horizontal row and then the winner may challenge anyone in the row above him.

The spider web tournament takes its name from the bracket design, which is the shape of a spider's web. The championship position is at the center of the web. The bracket consists of five (or any other selected number) lines drawn radially from the center and the participant's names are placed on concentric lines crossing these radial lines. Challenges may be made by persons on any concentric line to any person on the next line closer to the center. This type of tournament provides more opportunity for activity.

The type of tournament organization adopted should be the one that is best for the group, activity, and local interests. The goal should be to have as much participation as possible for the facilities and time available. Tournaments make for more student interest and enthusiasm and are an important part of intramural and extramural athletic programs.

AWARDS, POINT SYSTEMS, RECORDS, AND ELIGIBILITY

Awards, point systems, records, and eligibility requirements may present problems in the organization and administration of intramural and extramural competition.

Awards

There are arguments pro and con in respect to awards for intramural and extramural competition. Some of the arguments for awards are that they stimulate interest, serve as an incentive for participation, and recognize achievement. Some of the arguments against awards are that they make for a more expensive program, a few individuals win most of the awards, and they are unnecessary, since individuals would participate even if no awards were given. Leaders who oppose awards also stress the ideas that there should be no expectation of awards for voluntary, leisure-time participation; it is difficult to make awards on the basis of all factors that should be considered; the incentive is artificial; and the joy and satisfaction received are enough reward in themselves.

One study indicates that approximately four out of five intramural directors give awards. Letters, numerals and similar awards are used most frequently in the junior high schools. Medals and trophies are given more extensively on the junior college and college levels.

NORFOLK CITY PUBLIC SCHOOLS

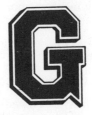

INTRAMURAL   CERTIFICATE

This is to certify that ✍

_____

HAS COMPLETED THE REQUIREMENTS OF THE PHYSICAL EDUCATION

DEPARTMENT AND IS AWARDED THIS CERTIFICATE FOR

PARTICIPATION IN_____FOR THE YEAR_____

ASSISTANT DIRECTOR _____   PRINCIPAL _____

TEACHER _____   TEACHER _____

When awards are given, they should be inexpensive. They can take the form of medals, ribbons, certificates, plaques, cups, or letters.

Point systems

Most intramural programs have some type of point system that is cumulative in nature and many times figured on an all-year basis. The keeping of such points makes for continued interest and enthusiasm over the course of the school year. It also encourages greater participation.

A system of keeping points should be developed that takes into consideration those factors that stimulate wholesome competition over a period of time, maintains continued interest, and is in conformance with the objectives sought in the total program. The system should be readily understood by all and easy to administer. Under such conditions points should be awarded on the basis of such considerations as contests won, championships gained, standing in a league or order of finish, participation, sportsmanship, and contribution to the objectives of the program.

A point system used by one school system is based on the following items:

Each entry: 10 points
Each win: 2 points
Each loss: 1 point
Forfeits: 0 points
Each team championship: 10 points
Second-place team championship: 6 points
Third-place team championship: 3 points
Each individual championship: 6 points
Second-place individual championship: 4 points
Third-place individual championship: 3 points
Each game an official works: 3 points
Being homeroom representative: 10 points
Each meeting attended by homeroom representative: 2 points

Records

Efficient administration of the program will necessitate the keeping of records. These should not be extensive in nature but should contain the information needed to determine the worth of the program and the progress being made.

Such records allow for comparison with other schools of a similar nature. They show the degree to which the program is providing for the needs of the entire student body and the extent to which students are participating. They show the activities that are popular and the ones that are not as popular. They focus attention on the best units of competition, needs of the program, administrative procedures that are effective, and leadership strengths and

DATE	COURT				TIME		

vs

(Team)   (Team)

Referee _____   Umpire _____   Scorer _____

AM _____

| | | | FIRST HALF | | SECOND HALF | | |
| | | | Time out | Time out | Time out | Time out | Over |
PLAYERS	NO.	FOULS	1st Quarter	2nd Quarter	3rd Quarter	4th Quarter	Time
		1 2 3 4 5					
		1 2 3 4 5					
		1 2 3 4 5					
		1 2 3 4 5					
		1 2 3 4 5					
		1 2 3 4 5					
		1 2 3 4 5					
		1 2 3 4 5					
		1 2 3 4 5					
		1 2 3 4 5					
		1 2 3 4 5					
		1 2 3 4 5					
		1 2 3 4 5					
		1 2 3 4 5					
		1 2 3 4 5					

TEAM	1 2 3 4 5 6 7 8 9 10 11 12 13 14 15 16 17 18 19 20 21 22 23 24 25 26 27 28 29 30
	31 32 33 34 35 36 37 38 39 40 41 42 43 44 45 46 47 48 49 50 51 52 53 54 55 56 57
	58 59 60 61 62 63 64 65 66 67 68 69 70 71 72 73 74 75 76 77 78 79 80 81 82 83 84
TEAM	1 2 3 4 5 6 7 8 9 10 11 12 13 14 15 16 17 18 19 20 21 22 23 24 25 26 27 28 29 30
	31 32 33 34 35 36 37 38 39 40 41 42 43 44 45 46 47 48 49 50 51 52 53 54 55 56 57
	58 59 60 61 62 63 64 65 66 67 68 69 70 71 72 73 74 75 76 77 78 79 80 81 82 83 84

| TEAM | | | FIRST HALF | | SECOND HALF | | |
| | | | | | Time out | Time out | Over |
PLAYERS	NO.	FOULS	1st Quarter	2nd Quarter	3rd Quarter	4th Quarter	Time
		1 2 3 4 5					
		1 2 3 4 5					
		1 2 3 4 5					
		1 2 3 4 5					
		1 2 3 4 5					
		1 2 3 4 5					
		1 2 3 4 5					
		1 2 3 4 5					
		1 2 3 4 5					
		1 2 3 4 5					
		1 2 3 4 5					
		1 2 3 4 5					
		1 2 3 4 5					
		1 2 3 4 5					
		1 2 3 4 5					

Sample intramural basketball score card. (From Intramurals for senior high schools, The Athletic Institute, Chicago, Ill.)

INTRAMURAL ATHLETICS

NAME_____

	1ST SEMESTER				2ND SEMESTER		
SPORTS	SOPH. YR:	JR. YR:	SR. YR:	SPORTS	SOPH. YR:	JR. YR:	SR. YR:
FOOTBALL	7	7	7	BASKETBALL	7	7	7
VOLLEYBALL	7	7	7	WRESTLING	2	2	2
TUG-OF-WAR	2	2	2	BOWLING	10	10	10
SHUFFLEBOARD S	3	3	3	GYMNASTICS	2	2	2
HORSESHOES-S	3	3	3	TRACK	2	2	2
BADMINTON-S	3	3	3	SOFTBALL	3	3	3
FUNGO HITTING	1	1	1	HANDBALL-S	3	3	3
FOOTBALL KICK	1	1	1	HORSESHOES-D	2	2	2
HANDBALL-D	2	2	2	BADMINTON-D	2	2	2
SHUFFLEBOARD D	2	2	2	TABLE SHUFFLEBOARD			
TABLE SHUFFLEBOARD				LONG-S	3	3	3
LONG-D	2	2	2	SHORT-S	3	3	3
SHORT-D	2	2	2	PING PONG - S	3	3	3
GOLF	1	1	1	PING PONG - D	2	2	2
TENNIS	1	1	1	FREE THROWS	1	1	1
INDOOR SHOT	1	1	1	ROPE CLIMB	1	1	1
MINATURE GOLF	1	1	1	BONGO	1	1	1

1 2 3 4 5 6 7 8 9 10 11 12 13			
14 15 16 17 18 19 20 21 22 23 24 25 26 27		=	1 CREDIT
28 29 30 31 32 33 34 35 36 37 38 39 40 41		=	2 CREDITS
42 43 44 45 46 47 48 49 50 51 52 53 54 55		=	3 CREDITS
56 57 58 59 60 61 62 63 64 65 66 67 68 69		=	4 CREDITS
		70 OR MORE =	5 CREDITS
HOME ROOM		CREDIT	

Intramural athletics. (From Intramurals for senior high schools, The Athletic Institute, Chicago, Ill.)

INTRAMURAL SOFTBALL SCORE CARD

DATE _____   TIME _____   DIAMOND _____

UMPIRE _____   SCORE KEEPER _____

TEAM:			INNING									SYMBOLS
NAME: First Last		1	2	3	4	5	6	7	8	9		Walk - W
1.												Single-1B
												Double-2B
2.												Triple-3B
												Home run-HR
												Fly out-F.O.
3.												Ground out-G.O.
												Pop out-P.O.
4.												Strike out-K
												Sacrifice-Sac.
5.												Fielders Choice-F.C.
												For Error-
6.												1BE,2BE, etc.
												Fill in bottom
7.												half of diag. if runner scores.
8.												Write "O" in bottom half of diag. if run-
9.												ner is picked off, out steal-
												ing, etc.
TOTALS	Runs Hits											Final Score

Sample Intramural softball score sheet. (From Intramurals for senior high schools, The Athletic Institute, Chicago, Ill.)

PROTEST FORM

Protesting Team _____

Quarter and Time Remaining _____

Score At Time Of Protest _____

Ball Possession At Time Of Protest _____

Situation: (Be Specific)

_____

                                                      Head Official

Protest form for intramural officials. (From Intramurals for senior high schools, The Athletic Institute, Chicago, Ill.)

weaknesses. Record keeping is an important phase of the program that should not be overlooked.

Eligibility

There is a need for a few simple eligibility rules. These should be kept to a minimum, since the intramural and extramural programs should render a contribution to the vast majority of the student body.

It is generally agreed that there should be no scholarship rules. There should be rules that forbid varsity players from participating in activities when they are on the varsity team or squad. Professionals should be barred from those activities in which they are professional. A student should be allowed to participate on only one team in a given activity during the season. Students, of course, should be regularly enrolled in the school and carrying what the institution rules is a normal load. Unsportsmanlike conduct should be dealt with in a manner that is in the best interests of the individual concerned, the program, and the established goals. Certain activities by their very nature should not be engaged in by individuals with certain health defects. Therefore, such individuals should be cleared by the health department of the school before participation is allowed in such activities.

The eligibility rules established by one college that have implications for high schools as well as colleges are as follows:

1. All men students of the college in good standing shall be eligible to compete in any activity promoted by the Intramural Department, except as provided later in these articles.
2. A varsity man is one who is retained by the coach after the final cut has been made.
3. The varsity and freshman coaches are requested to pass on the list of their respective squads. Participation on these squads will automatically make a man ineligible for intramural athletics in that particular sport.
4. A man may represent but one team in a given sport in a given season.

5. A team shall forfeit any contest in which an ineligible player was used. The director shall eliminate any points made by an ineligible man in meets. These infractions of the rules must be discovered within forty-eight hours after the contest.
6. Members of the freshman or varsity squads who become scholastically ineligible in any particular sport shall be ineligible to participate in any allied intramural activity.
7. The director may declare a man ineligible to participate in intramural athletics for unsportsmanlike conduct toward officials or opponents.
8. A man receiving a varsity award is ineligible to participate in that particular intramural sport until one complete season has passed since earning his letter.*

INTRAMURAL AND EXTRAMURAL PROGRAMS IN THE ELEMENTARY SCHOOL

The intramural and extramural programs in the elementary school should be outgrowths of the instructional program. They should consist of a broad variety of activities including stunts, rhythmic activities, relays, and tumbling. They should be suited to the age and sex differences of children at this level. They should be carefully supervised. The younger children in the primary grades probably will benefit most from free play. In the upper elementary grades, recess periods and afterschool activity can take place on both intragrade and intergrade bases. The programs should be broad, varied, and progressive in nature, with participants similar in maturity and ability.

A committee of the American Association for Health, Physical Education, and Recreation adopted the following policy statement with respect to elementary school boys and girls:

The kind of competitive sports planned for children in the elementary school must be based on what is best for the growth and de-

---

*From the Handbook of intramural athletics, Michigan State College.

```
                                        RES.
Team Name_____League:  HALL, FRAT., IND.  Sport _____
                                        (Circle One)
REGISTER THE DAYS AND HOURS YOUR TEAM PREFERS NOT TO PARTICIPATE.  BE SPECIFIC.  IF POSSIBLE,
THIS TIME WILL BE AVOIDED.  YOU MAY BE SCHEDULED ON THESE DAYS _____
_____

Manager's Name_____Telephone Number _____
Address_____Room Number _____
- - - - - - - - - - - - - - - - - - - - - - - - - - - - - - - - - - - - - - - - - -
This certifies that I understand the Intra-  | This certifies that I have read and understand
mural Eligibility Rules and have completely  | the Intramural Eligibility Rules, and will
checked all the players on my team.  If there | comply with them.  Also, that I have not, and
is any discrepancy, I will assume full re-    | will not play with any team, other than the
sponsibility.  If there is any question about | one listed above.  (Rule 6, Sec. D., I.M.
rules or eligibility, I will contact the      | Handbook).  Failure to comply with this rule
Intramural Office.                            | will result in my suspension from I.M. compe-
                                              | tition.
         Manager's Signature
                          TEAM  | ROSTER
_____
         MANAGER'S COLUMN        |            PLAYER'S SIGNATURE
_____
 1.
 2.
 3.
 4.
 5.
 6.
 7.
 8.
 9.
10.
11.
12.
13.
14.
15.
16.
17.
18.
19.
20.
21.
22.
23.
24.
```

Michigan State intramural sports roster. (From Intramurals for senior high schools, The Athletic Institute, Chicago, Ill.)

velopment of boys and girls at this level of maturity.

In the elementary school, children grow at variable rates, and at the same chronological age there are many differences in maturity. In children who are growing rapidly growth demands much of their energy. Emotional pressures may drive the child past the stage of healthful participation. Bone ossification and development are incomplete.

In consideration of these factors, the kinds of competition indicated in the following program outline are recommended as best meeting the physical activity needs of elementary school boys and girls:

1. First, as a foundation, all children should have broad, varied, and graded physical education under competent instruction through all grades. In many of the activities in this program, the competitive element is an important factor. The element of competition provides enjoyment and, under good leadership, leads to desirable social and emotional as well as physical growth.

2. Based upon a sound, comprehensive instructional program in grades five through eight, children should have opportunity to play in supervised intramural games and contests with others who are of corresponding maturity and ability within their own school. In grades below the fifth, the competitive elements found in the usual activities will satisfy the needs of children.

3. As a further opportunity to play with others, beyond the confines of their own school or neighborhood, play or sports day programs may be planned with emphasis on constructive social, emotional, and health outcomes. Teams may be formed of participants coming from more than a single school or agency, thus making playing together important.

Tackle football and boxing should not be included in the program because of common agreement among educational and medical authorities that these activities are undesirable for children of elementary school age.

Schools should plan with parents and community agencies to insure the kind of program outlined above is part of the educational experiences of every child.

It should be kept in mind that the child is important in this setting and not the teacher, parent, school, or agency.[*]

INTRAMURAL AND ENTRAMURAL PROGRAMS IN THE JUNIOR HIGH SCHOOL

In the junior high school the main concentration in athletics should be on intramurals and extramurals. It is at this particular level that students are taking a

special interest in sports, but at the same time their immaturity makes it unwise to allow them to engage in a highly organized interscholastic program. The program at this level should provide for both boys and girls, appeal to the entire student body, have good supervision by a trained physical education person, and be adapted to the needs and interests of the pupils.

Many authoritative and professional groups have gone on record in favor of broad intramural and extramural programs and against a varsity interscholastic, competitive program. They feel this is in the best interests of youth at this age level.

The junior high school provides a setting for giving students fundamental skills in many sports and activities. It is a time of limitless energy when physiologic changes and rapid growth are taking place. Youth in junior high schools should have proper outlets to develop themselves in a healthful manner.

INTRAMURAL AND EXTRAMURAL PROGRAMS IN THE SENIOR HIGH SCHOOL, COLLEGE, AND UNIVERSITY

At both the high school and college levels the intramural and extramural programs should receive a major emphasis. At this time the interests and needs of boys and girls require such a program. These students want and need to experience the joy and satisfaction that are a part of playing on a team, excelling in an activity with one's own peers, and developing skill. Every high school, college, and university should see to it that a broad and varied program is part of the total physical education plan.

The intramural and extramural programs for boys and girls should receive more emphasis than they are now getting at the senior high school and college levels. They are basic to sound education. They are settings where the skills learned and developed in the instructional program can

---

[*]National Conference on Physical Education for Children of Elementary School Age: Physical education for children of elementary school age, Chicago, 1951, The Athletic Institute, Inc., p. 22.

be put to use in a practical situation, with all the fun that comes from such competition. They should form a basis for the utilization of skills that will be used during leisure time, both in the present and in the future.

There should be adequate personnel for such programs. Good leadership is needed if the programs are to prosper. Each school should be concerned with developing a plan where proper supervision and leadership are available for afterschool hours. Qualified officials are also a necessity in order to ensure equal and sound competi-

---

NEW TRIER TOWNSHIP HIGH SCHOOL

Winnetka, Illinois

Boys' Intramural Sports

MATCH NOTICE
(for individual or doubles matches)

Adviser _____

Name _____

REMINDER: You are scheduled to play a _____

match tomorrow _____.

If you wish, you may play any time BEFORE the scheduled date and time by making arrangements with your opponent.

The winner must turn in the score by 8:45 the morning following the scheduled time.

Matches may not be postponed without the consent of the I. M. Office, G211.
        I. M. 65

New Trier Township High School boys' intramural sports match notice. (From Intramurals for senior high schools, The Athletic Institute, Chicago, Ill.)

tion. Facilities, equipment, and supplies should be apportioned on an equitable basis for the entire physical education program. There should be no monopoly on the part of any group or any program.

The college and university level offers an ideal setting for play and sports days for both boys and girls.

Sports clubs should be encouraged in those activities having special appeal to groups of students. Through such clubs greater skill is developed in the activity and the social experiences are well worthwhile.

Corecreational activities should play a prominent part in the programs. Girls and boys need to participate more together. Many of the activities in the high school and college programs adapt themselves well to both sexes. Such activities include volleyball, softball, tennis, badminton, table tennis, folk and square dancing, bowling, swimming, and skating. In some cases the rules of the games will need to be modified. The play and sports days that are conducted also offer a setting where both sexes can participate and enjoy worthwhile competition together.

INTRAMURAL AND EXTRAMURAL PROGRAMS FOR GIRLS AND WOMEN*

Most of what has been discussed thus far is applicable to girls and women as well as to boys and men. The objectives, play and sports days, activities, units of competition, and programs at the various institutional levels have been discussed with both sexes in mind. At the same time, women have progressed so rapidly in the intramural and extramural phases of the physical education program that it seems wise to make special reference to them.

According to many leaders in the field, intramurals and extramurals are preferred and emphasized for women as against var-

---

*See also Chapter 10.

sity interscholastic athletics. They point out that certain biologic, social, and psychologic characteristics of girls and women adapt better to this type of organization and program. The Division for Girls' and Women's Sports of the American Association for Health, Physical Education, and Recreation has pointed out that sports, when conducted in the right manner, contribute to such desirable outcomes as fitness for living and to the development of the most desirable and attractive qualities for womanhood. These include many physical, mental, and social qualities.

The program should be composed of a wide variety of team and individual sports and other activities that may be played among the girls themselves or in mixed groups. Girls have spearheaded the drive for sports and play days and so these deserve special emphasis. There should be qualified women leaders directing all phases of the program, although men should work very closely with them and lend support and help at every opportunity. Women should officiate in their own activities. Every safeguard should be taken to protect girls from harmful practices. There should be no commercial exploitation or harmful publicity attached to the program.

GENERAL ADMINISTRATIVE POLICIES FOR ORGANIZATION AND ADMINISTRATION OF INTRAMURAL AND EXTRAMURAL PROGRAMS

Some general administrative policies for the organization and administration of the intramural and extramural programs follow.

General administration

Intramural and extramural activities should be centered in the physical education program. However, they should be separate divisions of the overall program, receiving equal consideration with the instructional and interscholastic or intercol-

HEALTH AND PHYSICAL EDUCATION DEPARTMENT

GIRLS' INTRAMURAL ATHLETIC REPORT

Season_____

Activity	Number of teams	Number of pupils participating	Pupils participating in at least 80% of games
Apparatus and tumbling			
Archery			
Badminton			
Basketball			
Bowling			
Camping			
Croquet			
Deck tennis			
Fencing			
Field hockey			
Folk dancing			
Golf			
Handball			
Horseshoes			
Ice skating			
Lacrosse			
Modern dance			
Paddle tennis			
Shuffleboard			
Skiing			
Soccer			
Social dancing			
Softball			
Speedball			
Swimming and water safety			
Table tennis			
Tap dancing			
Tennis			
Volleyball			
Other			

Number of different girls in intramural program _____ (Do not count any girl more than once even though she participates in two or more activities)

GIRLS' INTERSCHOOL ACTIVITIES

How many interschool activities were held for girls: sports days_____;
     invitation games_____; other invitation activities_____.
Total number of girls who participated in these activities _____.
How many different girls are represented by these figures?_____

School _____
Date _____   Teacher's name _____

Girls' intramural athletic report.

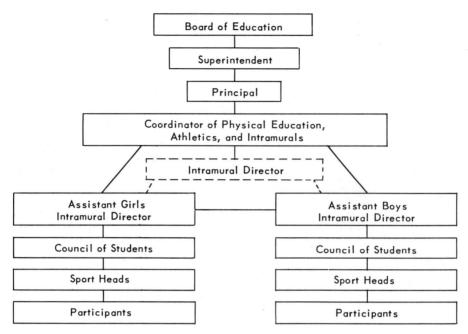

Suggested organization chart for intramurals. (From Intramurals for senior high schools, The Athletic Institute, Chicago, Ill.)

legiate athletics divisions in respect to staff, finances, facilities, equipment, supplies, and other essentials. There should be one staff member who has direct responsibility for this program. Such an individual should be one who is well trained in physical education and whose chief interest is intramural and extramural activities. This may not be possible in some smaller schools or colleges. However, it is necessary that the person in charge have adequate time and a sincere interest to do a commendable job in this area. Along with the director there should be assistant directors, supervisors, student managers, and other staff members as needed, depending upon the size of the school or college. There should also be adequate provision for officials. These should be selected and trained with care because of their importance to the program. Varsity players when carefully selected make good officials. Also, varsity coaches, staff members, and student managers should be considered for this work. A list of policies governing the various

features of the program should be prepared in written form and well publicized. Sometimes these are effectively publicized through a handbook.

An important feature of the overall administration of an intramural or extramural program is the establishment of a council. This usually is an elected council with representatives from the students, central administration, intramural staff, health department, and faculty. This body could be most influential in the establishment of policy and practices for a broad program of athletics for all students.

A significant development on the national scene was the establishment of the National Intramural Sports Council as a joint project of the Division of Men's Athletics and the Division of Girls' and Women's Sports of the American Association for Health, Physical Education, and Recreation. The purpose of creating the organization was to provide national leadership for intramural programs across the country.

Matthews has developed a set of intra-

G. A. A. POINT RECORD

School_____

Name_____   Letter, Yr._____All City Yr._____

SCHOOL YEAR	Total brought forward	Archery	Basketball	Badminton	Bicycling	Dancing	Deck Tennis	Demonstration	Executive Board	Field Ball	Golf	Hiking	Horseback Riding	Kittenball	Refereeing	Scholarship	Shuffle Board	Shooting	Ice Skating	Roller Skating	Swimming	Table Tennis	Tennis	Tobogganing	Tumbling	Volley Ball		TOTAL	Verifications of earned points in transferred cases will be complete, with instructors signature on this card.
12th																													
11th																													
10th																													
9th																													

5M 8-57

Girls' Athletic Association record.

mural administration principles that will be helpful to schools and colleges alike in establishing and administering sound intramural and extramural programs. These principles in adapted form are as follows:

1. Policies relative to intramurals should have rapport with the total welfare of the educational institution. Example: they should complement and supplement the academic program. Units of competition should not reflect racial or religious groupings.
2. Good human relationships and attitudes should be stressed. Example: rating plans, supervision, officiating, meetings, rules, etc. should stress sportsmanship.
3. Student planning and management should be encouraged. Example: the administrative council represents an opportunity for student involvement. Team manager, captains, scorers, etc. offer such opportunities as well.
4. The health and welfare of all participants should be protected. Example: periodic physical examinations are mandatory, and constant and close inspection of facilities and equipment is a must.
5. Competition should be equalized so that all participants experience success. Example: a constant loser will soon drop from intramurals and for this as well as other reasons

competition should enable all participants to be successful in this phase of the educational program.
6. A variety of activities should be offered. Example: students should be consulted and activities should reflect strenuous and nonstrenuous, team and individual, and also corecreational activities. At least five different sports should be offered.
7. The officiating should be carefully selected and supervised. Example: a program that involves training and orientation for the officials as well as testing and observation is important.
8. Grievances and protests should receive fair and equal treatment. Example: channels for grievances should be established, thus helping to assure some degree of satisfaction and success for all concerned.
9. Rules of eligibility and procedures should be established and publicized. Example: committees and/or the council should carefully establish the rules and see that all concerned are provided with copies of the same.
10. The program should be financed in a manner consistent with school policy. Example: the intramural program is an important part of total educational program and therefore should be subsidized financially through monies allocated by the

SUGGESTED PHYSICAL EXAMINATION FORM

(Cooperatively prepared by the National Federation of State High School Athletic Associations
and the Committee on Medical Aspects of Sports of the American Medical Association)
Physical examination for athletes cannot be rendered before August 1 preceding school year
concerned.

PLEASE LETTER   (Name of Student)   (City and School)
SIGNIFICANT PAST ILLNESS OR INJURY_____HEIGHT_____
_____WEIGHT_____
EYES, EARS, NOSE, AND THROAT 20/   20/   _____ HEARING   /15   /15
LUNGS _____
HEART _____BLOOD PRESSURE_____
ABDOMEN _____
GENITALIA _____ HERNIA _____
MUSCULO-SKELETAL _____
REFLEXES _____
URINALYSIS _____ DATE OF LAST IMMUNIZATIONS
BLOOD COUNT, X-RAY (if indicated)_____ POLIO _____

| File in high school office | TETANUS _____ |
| | OTHERS _____ |

I certify that I have on this date examined the above student and recommend him (or her) as
being physically able to compete in supervised activities NOT CROSSED OUT BELOW:

BASEBALL	FOOTBALL	ROWING	SOFTBALL	TRACK
BASKETBALL	HOCKEY	SKATING	SPEEDBALL	VOLLEYBALL
CROSS COUNTRY	GOLF	SKIING	SWIMMING	WRESTLING
FIELD HOCKEY	GYMNASTICS	SOCCER	TENNIS	OTHERS_____

DATE OF EXAMINATION:_____SIGNED: _____
                                              Examining Physician

Suggested physical examination form. (From Intramurals for senior high schools, The Athletic
Institute, Chicago, Ill.)

MICHIGAN STATE INTRAMURAL INJURY HOSPITAL SLIP

Name_____   Student Number _____   Date of Injury _____ 19___

Age_____
The above named student was injured in { □ Scheduled }
                                        { Informal □ } _____ activity.

| Body location and type of injury |
| |

Time injury reported _____

SUPERVISOR _____

Frank Beeman
Intramurals

R-367   Give detailed report of ACTION causing injury

Basic Cause

Michigan State intramural injury hospital slip. (From Intramurals for senior high schools, The
Athletic Institute, Chicago, Ill.)

```
┌─────────────────────────────────────────────────────────────┐
│              TEAM NOTICE--INTRAMURAL SPORTS                   │
│                                                               │
│      NEW TRIER TOWNSHIP HIGH SCHOOL, Winnetka, Illinois       │
│                                                               │
│              Adviser Room _____                │
│                                                               │
│                                                               │
│      REMINDER:   Your _____ team plays tomorrow.  │
│                                                               │
│      _____ .                          │
│                                                               │
│                                                               │
│      Your opponents are_____ .                    │
│                                                               │
│      Sign up the players below who can play tomorrow.         │
│                                                               │
│      1._____     2._____     3._____      │
│                                                               │
│      4._____     5._____     6._____      │
│                                                               │
│      7._____     8._____     9._____      │
│                                                               │
│      IMPORTANT: If you have enough players, then keep this     │
│      sheet for your own use. If you do not have enough         │
│      players, you MUST RETURN THIS SHEET TO THE I. M.          │
│      OFFICE IMMEDIATELY.                                       │
│            I. M. 60                                            │
└─────────────────────────────────────────────────────────────┘
```

Team notice for intramural sports. (From Intramurals for senior high schools, The Athletic Institute, Chicago, Ill.)

board of education or central administration.[*]

Health examinations

Health examinations should be required of all participants as a safeguard to their health. Sometimes this is taken care of through the annual health examination and at other times through special examinations given before a seasonal activity starts.

Finances

The finances involved in intramural and extramural programs are raised in various ways. Since these programs have as many contributions to make to educational objectives as other parts of the educational program, or more, they should be financed out of board of education and central administration funds, just as other phases of the program are financed. They should be in-

cluded in the regular physical education budget and supported through regularly budgeted school or college income.

There is another method of financing the programs that has proved quite satisfactory in some high schools and colleges. This plan incorporates the cost of running the programs in the regular activity fee that includes such student activities as dramatics, the interscholastic athletic program, musicals, and band concerts. This allows for stable funds that are in proportion to the student enrollment and can be anticipated in advance. Also, this method eliminates any additional charges to the student.

Other methods of financing that are utilized but that are questioned in some quarters are using money taken from athletic gate receipts, charging spectators to see the games, requiring an entry fee, and special fund-raising projects like athletic nights, carnivals, and presentation of talented athletic and other groups. Some of the arguments against such practices are that they

[*]Matthews, D. O.: Intramural administration principles, The Athletic Journal **46**:82, 1966.

create a wrong emphasis on gate receipts and result in many evils, that they discourage spectators from attending and students from participating, and that they require special projects to raise money, which should not be necessary for such a valuable phase of the educational program.

Publicity and promotion

It is essential that the student body, faculty, and public in general understand the intramural and extramural programs, the individuals they serve, the activities offered, and the objectives they attempt to attain. Such information can be disseminated to the right individuals only through a well-planned and organized publicity and promotion program.

The newspapers should be encouraged to give appropriate space to these activities. Brochures, bulletin boards, and the school newspaper can help to focus attention on the program. Notices can be prepared and sent home to parents in the elementary and secondary schools. A handbook can be prepared that explains all the various aspects of the total program and given to all students and others who are interested. Record boards can be constructed and placed in conspicuous settings. Clinics can be held in the various sports. Orientation talks and discussions can be held in school and college assemblies and at other gatherings. Special days can be held with considerable publicity and such catch slogans as "It Pays to Play" can be adopted. Through utilizing several devices and techniques, a good job of publicity and promotion can be done, with consequent greater participation among the student body and better understanding among the public.*

Time of day

The time when intramural and extramural activities should be held will depend upon the school or college level, facilities, season of year, community, and other influences.

One of the most popular and convenient times in many schools is late afternoon. This has proved best for elementary and

---

*See also Chapter 20 on public relations for more information on publicity and promotion.

```
                    INTRAMURAL GAME BLANK

    SPORT _____          DATE _____

    PLAYER _____         H.R. ____ SCORE ____
                         *VS*
    PLAYER _____         H.R. ____ SCORE ____

    _____         _____
        LOSING PLAYER                  POINT FOR GAME
    THIS BLANK MUST BE COMPLETELY FILLED OUT AND RETURNED
    BY WINNER TO INTRAMURAL MANAGER OR ROOM 701 ON DAY OF
    CONTEST OR A FORFEIT WILL RESULT.
```

Intramural game blank. (From Intramurals for senior high schools, The Athletic Institute, Chicago, Ill.)

junior and senior high schools. For some seasons of the year—namely, spring and fall—it has also been popular in college. It is a time that is economical, does not require lights, and has the outdoors available. It also ensures faculty supervision to a greater degree.

Evenings have been used quite extensively at the college level during the winter. This is not recommended at the elementary or junior and senior high school levels.

Some schools utilize hours within the school day. However, it should be remembered that the physical education class is primarily an instructional period, and to use this period for such a program does not seem to be in conformance with the standards set in the profession. However, some schools have satisfactorily utilized free, activity, and club periods for the program where facilities would allow.

Noon hour has been popular in some schools, especially at the elementary and secondary levels, and particularly in rural schools where students do not go home for lunch. Since students will be active anyway, such a period offers possibilities in selected situations, if strenuous activities are not offered.

Recess periods in the elementary school have proved to be a good time for many communities to conduct some of their intramural activities.

Saturdays have also been utilized in some situations. Although the weekend has proved to be a problem in some localities because many individuals have work to do or have planned this time to be with their parents, it has worked successfully in many communities.

The time before school in the morning has also proved satisfactory in a few schools. Getting up early in the morning does not seem to be a handicap to some individuals.

Special days are set aside in some schools for "field days" when classes are abandoned by administrative decree and all the students participate in a day or a half-day devoted entirely to activities that comprise the program.

AN INTRAMURAL PROGRAM EVALUATION CHECKLIST*

A program can be evaluated in terms of the stated principles and objectives or according to prevalent acceptable standards.

How does the intramural program measure up to acceptable minimum standards? By taking a few minutes to check off the items listed below, a quick evaluation can be made of the present status of the excellence of the program.

Yes	No	*Philosophy and objectives*
_____	_____	1. Is a written philosophy or a set of objectives available to the participants?

Yes	No	*Organization and administration*
_____	_____	1. Is the director professionally qualified to administer the program?
_____	_____	2. Does the director devote at least 7.5 hours per week to administering his program?
_____	_____	3. Are students included in the management of the program?
_____	_____	4. Is there an advisory committee composed of students and faculty?

Yes	No	*Units of competition*
_____	_____	1. Are students classified according to ability, age, height, or weight within the competitive unit?
_____	_____	2. Within the basic unit, are students permitted to choose the members of their teams?

*From Matthews, D. O.: Intramural administration principles, The Athletic Journal 46:82, 1966. Reproduced courtesy The Athletic Journal.

Continued.

AN INTRAMURAL PROGRAM EVALUATION CHECKLIST—cont'd

Yes	No	*Program of activities*
___	___	1. Does the director consult with the students to make sure that their interests are of prime consideration in the choice of activities in the program?
___	___	2. Are there both strenuous and nonstrenuous sports in the program?
___	___	3. Are there both team and individual sports in the program?
___	___	4. Are there at least five different sports making up the program?
___	___	5. Does at least one corecreation activity make up part of the program?

Yes	No	*Time periods*
___	___	1. Does the hour immediately after school receive top priority for scheduling?
___	___	2. Is the noon hour utilized as a time period for intramurals?

Yes	No	*Methods of organizing competition*
___	___	1. Is the round robin tournament used whenever possible in preference to others?

Yes	No	*Point system of awards*
___	___	1. Is recognition of any kind given to the participants for their achievements?
___	___	2. Is the award primarily for achievement instead of incentive for participants?

Yes	No	*Rules and regulations*
___	___	1. Are the rules defining such things as eligibility, health, safety, forfeits, postponements, and team membership distributed to all participants?
___	___	2. Is the lack of good sportsmanship regarded as a rule violated?
___	___	3. Is equipment provided for all the activities offered?

Yes	No	*Publicity*
___	___	1. Is there a special bulletin board for intramural information?

Yes	No	*Finances*
___	___	1. Does the board of education through the school budget provide funds for the operation of the program?

Rating scale

A "yes" answer must be given in each category if a program is to be considered *good* or *excellent*.

Excellent	15 to 22
Good	13 to 14
Fair	10 to 12
Poor	9 or below

Questions and exercises

1. What is the place of intramural and extramural programs in the total physical education plan of a school or college? How do they complement and supplement the other phases of the total program?
2. To what extent are the objectives of intramurals and extramurals compatible with those of general education? Give specific evidence to support your answer.
3. Survey at least three schools on either the high school or the college level to determine if there is proper balance between the intramural and extramural and the interschool programs. Prepare a statement of findings.
4. Prepare a plan for a sports or play day that could be held in your school.
5. Why have sports, play, and invitation days increased so much in popularity during the last few years?
6. Develop a set of principles that could be used as guides for the selection of activities in intramural and extramural programs.
7. Draw up a seasonal list of activities that could be offered in a school of your choosing. Take into consideration facilities, climate, leadership, and other essential influences.
8. Identify the following: round robin tournament, unit of competition, straight elimination tournament, and ladder tournament.
9. Prepare a debate on the question: Should awards be given in intramural and extramural programs?
10. Develop what you consider to be ideal intramural and extramural programs at the elementary, junior high school, senior high school, or college level.

11. What are some important considerations in administering athletic programs for girls and women? Discuss in detail.

Reading assignment in *Administrative Dimensions of Health and Physical Education Programs, Including Athletics:* Chapter 7, Selections 34 to 38.

Selected references

American Association for Health, Physical Education, and Recreation: Girls sports organization handbook, Washington, D. C., 1961, The Association.

American Association for Health, Physical Education, and Recreation: Intramural sports for college men and women, Washington, D. C., 1961, The Association.

Anton T., and Toschi, L.: A practical approach to intramural sports, Portland, Me., 1964, J. Weston Walsh.

The Athletic Institute: Intramurals for the senior high school, Chicago, 1964, The Athletic Institute, Inc.

Bucher, C. A.: Field days, The Journal of Health and Physical Education 19:22, 1948.

Bucher, C. A., editor: Methods and materials in physical education and recreation, St. Louis, 1954, The C. V. Mosby Co.

Bucher, C. A.: Foundations of physical education, ed. 5, St. Louis, 1968, The C. V. Mosby Co.

Bucher, C. A., and Cohane T.: Little league baseball can hurt your boy, Look, Aug. 11, 1963, p. 74.

Bucher, C. A., and Dupee, R. K., Jr.: Athletics in schools and colleges, New York, 1965, The Center for Applied Research in Education, Inc. (The Library of Education).

Cummings, P.: The dictionary of sports, New York, 1949, A. S. Barnes & Co.

Division for Girls' and Women's Sports: Special events in the girls' sports program, Washington, D. C., 1961, The American Association for Health, Physical Education, and Recreation.

Educational Policies Commission: School athletics ─problems and policies, Washington, D. C., 1954, National Education Association.

Forsythe, C. E.: The administration of high school athletics, Englewood Cliffs, N. J., 1962, Prentice-Hall, Inc.

Grieve, A. W.: Directing high school athletics, Englewood Cliffs, N. J., 1963, Prentice-Hall, Inc.

Jacobson, R. O.: Intramurals are recreation for all in the high school, School Activities 35:183, 1964.

Mallory, O.: Co-recreational intramurals, School Activities 35:68, 1963.

Matthews, D. O.: Intramural administration principles, The Athletic Journal 46:82, 1966.

Report of the Joint Committee on Athletic Competition for Children of Elementary and Junior High School Age: Desirable athletic competition for children, Washington, D. C., 1952, American Association for Health, Physical Education, and Recreation.

Rule books for all boys' sports. Available from the National Federation of State High School Athletic Associations, 7 S. Dearborn St., Chicago, Ill.

Rule books for all girls' sports. Available from the Division for Girls' and Women's Sports, American Association for Health, Physical Education, and Recreation, 1201 16th St., N. W., Washington, D. C.

Watkins, J. H.: Intramurals in the junior high school, Journal of the American Association for Health, Physical Education, and Recreation 21: 281, 1950.

CHAPTER 10 THE INTERSCHOLASTIC AND INTERCOLLEGIATE
VARSITY ATHLETIC PROGRAMS

Each phase of the educational process must have clear-cut objectives if it is to justify its existence. This is essential in order to know where it is heading, what it is striving for, and what it hopes to accomplish. Interscholastic and intercollegiate varsity athletic programs are no exception to this rule.

The aim of all education is the enrichment of life. This is the ultimate goal upon which attention has been focused. The objectives of athletics as part of the physical education program are more definite and specific than this aim, and through them the ultimate goal is brought nearer to realization. Therefore, it is essential that everyone associated with this work help in the achievement of these goals.

The executive secretary of the Missouri State High School Activities Association[*] indicates that school athletic programs should include the development of the following goals for its youth. They are presented here in adapted form:

1. An appreciation of why the school provides an athletic program
2. A knowledge of the values of athletics to the individual and society
3. An understanding of the rules essential to playing the game
4. The ability to think as an individual and as a team member

5. Faith in and respect for the democratic processes
6. An appreciation of the values of group ideals
7. The development of motor skills
8. Health and physical fitness
9. An understanding and appreciation of what constitutes wholesome recreation and entertainment
10. The desire to be successful and excel
11. Moral and ethical standards
12. Self-discipline, emotional maturity, and self-control
13. Social competence
14. Recognition of the importance of conforming to the rules
15. Respect for the rights of others and those in authority
16. Good human relationships

An era of great expansion in athletics started in the post–World War II period. The physical defects revealed by the draft, the value of sports in building morale, and the emphasis on physical fitness during the war and during the present period of national emergency have combined to encourage athletics to a degree that has never been equaled in the history of this country.

The emphasis on athletics has been the focus of much attention and controversy and consequently the program should be considered carefully by all interested in administration. Interscholastic and intercollegiate athletics have a definite place in senior high school and college programs of physical education. Such competition can help players achieve a higher standard of mental, moral, social, and physical fitness, provided the overall objectives of physical education are kept in mind.

[*]Keller, I. A.: School athletics—its philosophy and objective, American School Board Journal 153:22-23, 1966. Reprinted, with permission, from the American School Board Journal, August, 1966. Copyright assigned 1967 to The National School Boards Association. All rights reserved.

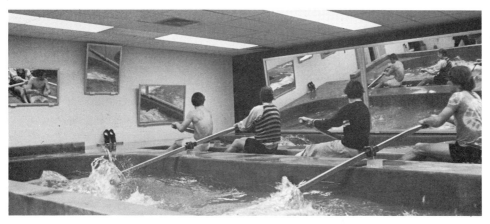

Varsity crew in rowing tank with mirrors. (Trinity College, Hartford, Conn.)

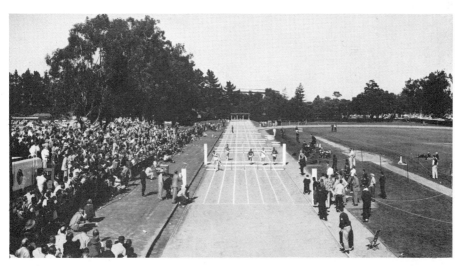

Angell Field, Stanford University, with an intercollegiate dual meet in progress. Note the television coverage of this meet. The rim of Stanford Stadium is visible in the center background.

RELATIONSHIP TO TOTAL PHYSICAL EDUCATION PROGRAM

Varsity interscholastic and intercollegiate athletics represent an integral part of the total physical education program. They should develop out of the intramural and extramural athletic programs.

Athletics, with the appeal they have to youth, should be the heart of physical education and should aid in achieving goals that will help to enrich living for all who participate.

The challenge of providing sound educational programs in varsity interscholastic and intercollegiate athletics is one that all physical education personnel should recognize. The challenge can be met and resolved if physical educators aggressively bring to the attention of administrators, school and college faculties, and the public in general the true purposes of athletics in a physical education program. It is important to stress that there is a need for having an athletic program that meets the needs of all; that such a program is organized and administered with the welfare of the individual in mind; that it is conducted in the light of educational objectives that are not compromised when exposed to pressures from sports writers, alumni, and townspeople; and that it provides leadership trained in physical education.

In actual practice the organization of athletics takes two forms. At times they are organized as an integral part of the physical education structure and at other times as a separate unit apart from physical education. Some departments of athletics that operate as separate units evolved from the nineteenth century, when they were not considered an integral part of education. If athletics are looked upon as intrinsically related to education, they should be a part of the physical education program.

THE ATHLETIC COUNCIL

Most colleges and many schools have some type of athletic council, board, or committee that establishes athletic policies for the institution. It may involve only faculty members or it may also involve students. Such councils, boards, or committees are responsible for giving the athletic program proper direction in the educational program.

The composition of such committees or councils varies widely from school to school and college to college. In a school, the principal may serve as chairman, or this position may be held by the director of physical education or other faculty member. The committee may include coaches, members of the board of education, faculty members, students, or members of the community at large. In a college or university, the composition of the committee may consist of administrators, faculty members, students, athletic director, coaches, and others.

THE ATHLETIC DIRECTOR

The athletic director implements the athletic policies as established by the council, board, or committee. Responsibilities of the athletic director include preparing the budget for the sports program, purchasing equipment and supplies, scheduling athletic contests, arranging for officials, supervising eligibility requirements, making arrangements for transportation, seeing that medical examinations of athletes and proper insurance coverage are adequate, and supervising the program in general.

A rating card was developed by Kelliher for the evaluation of the effectiveness of the athletic director. It is reproduced here for the benefit of the reader.

RATING CARD FOR ATHLETIC DIRECTORS FOR EVALUATING THE ADMINISTRATION OF AN ATHLETIC PROGRAM

A high school rating card has been adapted from Kelliher's college criteria.* These evaluation items assist the athletic director in checking the effectiveness of his program.

The actual rating card includes a column for evaluating each of these thirty-six items. The column is headed "Performance in this Area Is Given: Great Attention; Moderate Attention; Little Attention."

A. Financial soundness
    1. He operates on a sound financial basis.
    2. There is equitable balance in the budget for all sports.

*Kelliher, M. S.: Successful athletic administration, Journal of Health, Physical Education, and Recreation 30:31, 1959.

RATING CARD FOR ATHLETIC DIRECTORS FOR EVALUATING THE ADMINISTRATION OF AN ATHLETIC PROGRAM—cont'd

B. Organization of the department
   3. He handles the business of the department efficiently and promptly.
   4. All members of the department handle their work assignments efficiently.
   5. He operates effectively without waste of time or materials.
   6. He develops close cooperation between all members of his staff.
   7. Policies and procedures are written out and are made clear to both players and staff members.
   8. He cooperates with other departments of the school and maintains good relations with the administration.
   9. He is fair and firmly in control of his staff and never fails to recognize organizational channels.
   10. He is easily available to anyone with an interest in the athletic program.

C. Professional status of the staff
   11. His operations are in harmony with the philosophy and objectives of the school and of the physical education department.
   12. His operations are in harmony with the spirit and rules and regulations of interscholastic athletics as established by the state high school athletic association.
   13. He is able to justify the athletic program as an important phase of education.
   14. The director is an educator. His status in the school is comparable to other department heads and is considered high.
   15. He cooperates with the administration; he works with the faculty and keeps them well informed.

D. Well-being of the staff
   16. He has developed a high degree of esprit de corps among all members of his department.
   17. He cooperates with the administration in the selection of staff members who believe in high standards of competitive athletics.
   18. He develops a staff of men with high professional standards and education.
   19. He is loyal to the administration and to his staff and gets facts before making a move.

E. Well-being of the students
   20. The health protection of athletes is rated high.
   21. He insists that athletes strive to keep up with their class.
   22. The best possible education for the boy is the most important criterion.
   23. He produces a program that appeals to a large number of participants.
   24. He considers the after-graduation success of former athletes a measure of success of the athletic department.
   25. He prefers that athletes carry on a career program.
   26. He has understanding of and cooperates with general student body interests.
   27. Students assigned to work in the department give reasonable service for experience and credit earned.

F. Public relations
   28. There is an efficient program of public relations.
   29. He maintains friendly relations with press and radio.
   30. He conducts athletics in an efficient, crowd-pleasing manner.
   31. He insists that squad members are school representatives at all times and that they conduct themselves accordingly.
   32. The activities of the department are well received by the administration, faculty, and community.
   33. The record of sportsmanship of all competitive teams under his administration is high.

G. Care of property and equipment
   34. Teams are well equipped, neat, and clean.
   35. The equipment of the department is cared for in an excellent manner and according to sound procedures.
   36. The buildings and grounds under the supervision of the director are kept in excellent condition.

THE COACH

One of the most popular phases of physical education professional work is that of coaching. Many students who show exceptional skill in some interscholastic sport such as basketball, baseball, or football feel that they would like to become members of the profession so that they may coach. They feel that since they have proved themselves outstanding athletes in high school, they will be successful in coaching. This, however, is not necessarily true. It may seem paradoxic to the layman, but there is insufficient evidence to show that exceptional skill in any activity necessarily guarantees success in teaching that activity. Many other factors such as personality, interest in youth, knowledge of human growth and development, psychology, intelligence, integrity, leadership, character, and a sympathetic attitude carry great weight in coaching success.

Coaching should be recognized as teaching. Because of the nature of his position, a coach may be in a more favorable position to teach concepts that make for effective daily living than any other member of a school faculty. Youth, with their inherent drive for activity and action and their quest for the excitement and competition found in sports, look up to the coach and in many cases feel that he is the type of individual to be emulated. Therefore, the coach should recognize his influence and see the value of such attributes as character, personality, and integrity. Although a coach must know thoroughly the game he is coaching, these other characteristics are of equal importance.

The coach of an athletic team has within himself the power to build future citizens who possess traits that are desirable and acceptable to society, or citizens who have a false conception as to what is right and proper. The coach is sometimes tempted to seek outcomes not educational in nature by the insecurity of his position, the emphasis on winning teams, student and alumni pressure, the desire for lucrative gate receipts, and the publicity that goes with winning teams. Unless the coach is an individual of strong character and is willing to follow an unswerving course in the direction of what he knows to be right, many evil practices may enter the picture.

Coaching is characterized in some schools and colleges by insecurity of position. Whether a coach feels secure depends to a great extent upon the school, college, community, and the administration. Coaching offers an interesting and profitable career to many individuals. However, one should recognize the possibility of finding himself in a situation where the pressure to produce winning teams may be so great as to cause unhappiness, insecurity, and even the loss of a job.

Coaching is only one phase of the physical education profession; and coaching is teaching. Because of this close relationship with physical education and the education field in general, a coach should be thoroughly qualified as a physical education person. He needs a background in physical and biologic science, skills, behavioral sciences, education, and the humanities. Only in this way can he best serve youth who are interested in athletics.

There are four qualifications that are found in the outstanding coach. First, he has an ability to teach the fundamentals and strategies of his sport; he *must* be a good teacher. Second, he understands the boy or girl who is a player. The coach needs to understand how a youth functions at his particular level of development—with full appreciation of skeletal growth, muscular development, and physical and emotional limitations. Third, he understands the game he coaches. Thorough knowledge of techniques, rules, and similar information is basic. Fourth, he has a desirable personality and character. Patience, understanding, kindness, honesty, sportsmanship, sense of right and wrong, courage, cheerfulness, affection, humor, energy, and

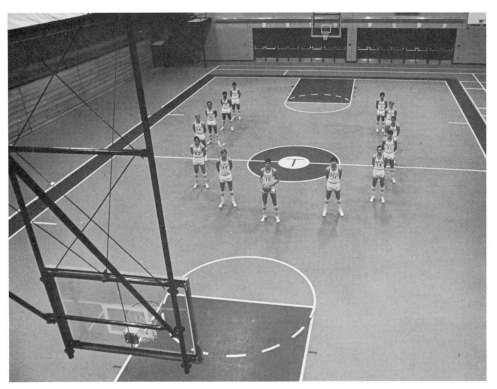

Varsity basketball. (Trinity College, Hartford, Conn.)

enthusiasm are imperative, since the youngsters will be idolizing and emulating his every move.

Too often coaches are chosen because of one qualification—they have played the game. Most principals, superintendents of schools, and college presidents would be flattered to have an All-American coaching their football teams. In terms of the welfare of youth, however, the other qualifications are even more important, and the administration will be most likely to find a coach with these qualifications in a person who has been trained in physical education.

It is just as important to employ a coach who has been trained in his field as it is to employ a science teacher who has been prepared to teach in his subject matter area. Who has heard of an administrator employing a science instructor whose training was in history but who had dabbled in

science on an extracurricular basis and had won the science fair contest in high school? Athletics is one part of the total physical education program, not an end in itself. Basic experiences in sports techniques, first aid, anatomy and physiology, philosophy of physical education, and other courses will make a person a better coach in the educational setting.

School and college administrators, physical educators, coaches, state certificating officers, and others should try to arrive at some common standards for employing a coach rather than having it done on a hit-or-miss basis.

Professional preparation of the coach

About one-fourth of all coaches in the junior and senior high schools in this country have no professional preparation, and the percentage is much higher among college coaches. The only qualification many coaches have is the fact that they have played the game or sport in high school, college, or the professional ranks. It is generally recognized that the best preparation that a coach can have is training in the field of physical education. In light of this fact, several states are attempting to see that coaches, particularly at the precollege level, have at least some training in the field of physical education.

A group of persons has been working as a committee in the American Association for Health, Physical Education, and Recreation to encourage certification of coaches. They feel that a coach should be prepared in each of the following five areas:

Medical aspects of athletic coaching
Principles and problems of coaching
Theory and techniques of coaching
Kinesiologic foundations of coaching
Physiologic foundations of coaching

The Men's Physical Education Department at California State College, Long Beach, has initiated a coaching emphasis minor program that includes the following:

Departmental approval required for admittance to program courses in:
Scientific foundations
Behavioral problems in athletics and
    physical education
Athletic injuries

Field work in coaching or student teaching
    in coaching
Coaching courses
Electives

The preparation of the coach is receiving more and more attention and, in time, at least a minimum of preparation will be required in many states. This is in keeping with the great growth of sports in our society and the need to safeguard the best interests of American youth.

SOME ADMINISTRATIVE CONSIDERATIONS IN VARSITY ATHLETIC PROGRAMS

There are many administrative considerations pertinent to the conduct of an interscholastic or intercollegiate varsity athletic program. Some of the more important of these are: (1) crowd control, (2) health of the players, (3) contracts, (4) officials, (5) protests and forfeitures, (6) game management, (7) schedules and practice periods, (8) awards, (9) records, and (10) transportation. Each will be discussed in the following paragraphs.

Crowd control

Crowd control at athletic contests is becoming of increasing importance in light of recent dissent, riots, and disturbances on both high school and college campuses

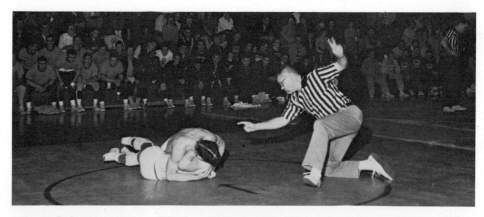

Interscholastic wrestling. (Richwoods Community High School, Peoria Heights, Ill.)

and in public gathering places. The elimination of night athletic activities has been on the increase, particularly in our large cities. School districts and college authorities are taking increased precautions to avoid any disturbances. More police are being brought in to help supervise the crowds at athletic contests, sportsmanship assemblies are being held, townspeople are being informed, administrators are discussing the matter, and careful plans are being developed.

The Sixth National Conference of City and County Directors of the AAHPER, which was held in Washington, D. C., in December, 1968, spent considerable time on the subject of crowd control at athletic contests. A summary of their discussions as reported in their proceedings is reproduced here.

APPROACHES TO CROWD CONTROL*

Summary of reports: small group discussions

The nature and seriousness of the problems in crowd control have recently become more drastic and bizarre as they have occurred in increasing frequency. They take on the collective character of a deliberate attempt either to ignore or confront the system. This social problem may be impossible to eliminate completely, but an attempt must be made to cope with the immediate symptoms. Our only hope is for imaginative and coordinated efforts by the school administration, the majority of students, and community authorities to promote standards of conduct conducive to continuing spectator sports in comparative tranquility. The alternatives are to allow a disruptive element to completely negate the nature of school athletics, to play with no spectators, or to abandon the activity.

The following will present some causes of crowd control problems and some approaches to solutions.

Some causes of problems

Lack of anticipation of, and preventive planning for, possible trouble

Lack of proper facilities

Poor communication resulting in lack of information

Lack of involvement of one or more of the following: school administration, faculty, student body, parents, community, press, and law enforcement agencies

Lack of respect for authority and property

Attendance at games of youth under the influence of narcotics

Increased attitude of permissiveness

School dropouts, recent graduates, and outsiders

Some approaches to solutions

Develop written policy statements, guidelines, and regulations for crowd control.

1. Consult the following before writing policy statements or promulgating regulations: school administration, athletic director, coaches, faculty members involved in the school sports program, school youth organizations, local police departments.
2. Properly and efficiently administer regulations and provide for good communications.
3. Constantly evaluate regulations and guidelines for their relevance and effectiveness.
4. Make guidelines and regulations so effective that the director of athletics who follows them is secure in knowing he has planned with his staff for any eventuality and has sufficient help, appropriately briefed, for any situation that may arise.

Provide adequate facilities.

1. Plan and design stadiums, fieldhouses, and gymnasiums for effective crowd control.
2. Provide for adequate rest room facilities.
3. Establish a smoking area when indoor contests are held.
4. Complete preparation of facilities before game time.

*From Sixth National Conference of City and County Directors, American Association for Health, Physical Education, and Recreation: Crowd control, Washington, D. C., 1968, The Association, pp. 17-22.

Continued.

APPROACHES TO CROWD CONTROL—cont'd

Teach good sportsmanship throughout the school and the community.

1. Begin education in good sportsmanship in the earliest grades and continue it throughout the school life.
2. Make frequent approving references to constructive and commendable behavior.
3. Arrange for program appearances by faculty members and students jointly to discuss the true values of athletic competition including good sportsmanship.
4. Make use of all news media through frequent and effective television, radio, and press presentations and interviews, commentaries, and frequent announcement of good sportsmanship slogans.
5. Distribute a printed Code of Ethics for Good Sportsmanship.
6. Include the good sportsmanship slogan in all printed programs at sports events.
7. Urge the use of athletic events as an example in elementary school citizenship classes, stressing positive values of good conduct at games, during the raising of the flag and singing of the national anthem; courtesy toward visitors.
8. Involve teachers in school athletic associations, provide them with passes to all sports events, and stress the positive values of their setting an example of good sportsmanship.

Intensify communications prior to scheduled games.

1. Arrange for an exchange of speakers at school assembly programs; the principals, coaches, or team captains could visit the opposing school.
2. Discuss with appropriate personnel of the competing school the procedures for the game, including method and location of team entry and departure.
3. Provide superintendent or principal, athletic director, and coach with a copy of written policy statement, guidelines, and regulations.
4. Meet all game officials and request them to stress good sportsmanship on the field.
5. Meet with coaches and instruct them not to question officials during a contest; stress the importance of good sportsmanship and the fact that their conduct sets the tone for spectator reaction to game incidents.
6. Instruct students what to expect and what is expected of them.
7. Schedule preventive planning conferences with local police to be assured of their full cooperation and effectiveness in spectator control.

Inform the community.

1. Request coaches and athletic directors to talk to service groups and other community groups.
2. Stress the need for exemplary conduct of coaches at all times.
3. Invite community leaders (non-school people) to attend athletic events.
4. Post on all available notice boards around town, in factories and other public places, posters showing the Sportsmanship Code of Ethics and Guidelines in brief.
5. Release constructive information and positive statements to news media and request publication of brief guidelines on sports pages.
6. Provide news media with pertinent information as to ways in which the community may directly and indirectly render assistance in the crowd control problem.

Involve law enforcement personnel.

1. Police and other security personnel should be strategically located so as to afford the best possible control.
2. Law enforcement professionals should handle *all* enforcement and disciplining of spectators.
3. Strength in force may be shown by appearance of several policemen, motorcycles, police cruise cars, et cetera, at and near the site of the game.
4. Women police may be stationed in women's rest rooms.
5. Civil Defense organizations could patrol parking areas.
6. A faculty member from the visiting school may be used as a liaison with police and local faculty in identifying visiting students.
7. Attendants, police, county sheriffs, deputies should be in uniform. Uniformed authority figures command greater respect.

Use supervisory personnel other than police.

1. Select carefully teacher supervisors who are attentive and alert to signs of possible trouble.
2. Identify faculty members by arm bands or other means.
3. Provide for communication by means of walkie-talkie systems.

APPROACHES TO CROWD CONTROL—cont'd

4. Assign some faculty members to sit behind the visiting fans; this reduces verbal harassment of visitors.
5. Employ paid ticket takers and paid chaperones to mingle strategically among the crowd and to remain on duty throughout the game, including half-time.
6. Issue passes to junior high physical education teachers to provide more adult supervision.

Plan for ticket sales and concession stands.

1. Arrange for advance sale of student tickets to avoid congestion at the gate.
2. Sell tickets in advance only to students in their own schools, and avoid sale of tickets to outsiders and non-students.
3. Provide for a close check at the gate or entrance.
4. Arrange for concession stands to be open before the game, during half-time, and after the game, but closed during actual play.
5. Channel the flow of traffic to and from concession stands by means of ropes, or other means; keep traffic moving.

Prepare spectators and contestants.

1. Encourage as many students as possible to be in the uniforms of the athletic club, pep club, booster clubs, band, majorettes, cheer leaders.
2. Bus participants to and from the site of the game.
3. Have participants dressed to play before leaving for a game or contest.
4. Adhere to established seating capacity of stadiums and gymnasiums.
5. Request home team fans to remain in their own stands until visiting team fans have left.
6. Try to arrange for a statewide athletic association regulation prohibiting all noise makers including musical instruments except for the school band or orchestra under professional supervision.
7. Request the assistance of visiting clubs.
8. Educate cheerleaders, student leaders, band captains, pep squads, and faculty supervisors by means of a one day conference program.
9. Keep spectators buffered from the playing area as much as practical.
10. Request that elementary school children be accompanied by an adult.

Miscellaneous.

1. Inform and involve school superintendents fully when problems arise in connection with sports events.
2. Impose severe penalties on faculty and student leaders guilty of poor conduct.
3. Publish the identity of offenders at games and notify parents, if possible; any penalties inflicted should also be noted. (Note: If the offense leads to Juvenile Court action, care should be taken not to contravene laws about publishing names of juvenile offenders.)
4. Consistently enforce rules and regulations; this is a necessity.
5. Work toward the assumption of responsibility for strong regulation and enforcement of team behavior on the part of the state athletic associations.
6. Attempt to work with the courts toward greater cooperation.
7. Avoid overstressing the winning of games.
8. Discontinue double headers and triple headers.
9. After-game incidents away from the proximity of the stadium or gymnasium are out of the control of school officials, but cause bad public reaction.

Summary

Sound safety controls and crowd controls at school athletic functions are a must! Greater concentration on treating the causes of the problem is essential. Preliminary groundwork is the key to good crowd control. Coordination and cooperation of school and law enforcement agencies is the key to success.

Youth should be taught to know what to expect and what is expected of them. Consistent enforcement of rules and regulations is a necessity if youth is to respect authority. Adult behavior should be such that it may be advantageously and admirably emulated by youth whose actions hopefully may result in deserving praise instead of negative criticism and disapproval.

The athletic program is a constructive and valuable school activity. It should be permitted to function in a favorable, healthful, and friendly environment.

Health of the players

Interscholastic and intercollegiate athletics should contribute to the health of the players. Through wholesome physical activity the participant should become more physically, mentally, emotionally, and socially fit.

Medical examination. One of the first requirements for every participant in an athletic program should be a medical examination to determine physical fitness and capacity to engage in such a program.

*See also Chapter 13.

HEALTH QUESTIONNAIRE FOR SPORTS CANDIDATES

(To be completed by parents or family physician and returned to team physician or trainer)

Name .... Birth Date ....

Home Address ....

Parent's Name .... Tel. No...............

Family Physician .... Tel. No. ....

1. Has had injuries requiring medical attention	YES	NO
2. Has had illness lasting more than a week	YES	NO
3. Is under physician's care now	YES	NO
4. Takes medication now	YES	NO
5. Wears glasses	YES	NO
Contact lenses	YES	NO
6. Has had surgical operation	YES	NO
7. Has been in hospital (except for tonsillectomy)	YES	NO
8. Do you know of any reason why this individual should not participate in all sports?	YES	NO

Please explain any "YES" answers to above questions:

....

....

....

9. Has had complete poliomyelitis immunization, by inoculations (Salk) or oral vaccine (Sabin)	YES	NO
10. Has had tetanus toxoid, and booster inoculation within past 3 years	YES	NO

....

PARENT OR PHYSICIAN

Health questionnaire.

The strenuous nature of athletics and the demands placed upon the participant make it imperative that a thorough medical examination be required. This should be a practice in all schools and colleges and for all individuals.

The medical examination may be conducted by the family, school, or college physician. The trend appears to be to have the examination given by the family physician. However, the best method of administering the examination should be determined in light of local conditions. The school or college physician should review the examination results and health histories or otherwise determine if there are any defects or other conditions that would be aggravated by participation. No student should be permitted to participate unless a physician can state that he is fit for such competititon.

Safety. Everything possible should be done to ensure that the safety of the participant is provided for. Only well-trained and qualified coaches should be permitted to be on the staff. Such a coach will always conduct his program with the health of the players in mind. He will have a knowledge of first aid. He will be continually alert to stop players from further participation if they are unduly fatigued; have received head, spine, or neck injuries; or are dazed. He will not allow a player who has been unconscious as a result of injury to resume play until a thorough check and approval have been given by a qualified physician. He will work closely with the team or school physician, trying to make every effort possible to guard the health of his players.

Proper conditioning and training should take place before any player is subjected to competition. Such conditioning and training should be progressive in nature and allow for gradual achievement of a state of acceptable physical fitness. There should always be enough players on the squad to allow for substitutions in the event a person is not physically or otherwise fit for play.

Proper facilities and equipment should be available to guard the safety and health of the players. This means that facilities are constructed according to recommended standards in respect to size, surfacing, and various safety features. Protective equipment should be provided as needed in the various sports. If desirable facilities and equipment are not available, such competition should not be provided.

Games should be scheduled that result in equal and safe competition. The desire of small schools to defeat larger schools, where the competition is not equal, often brings disastrous results to the health and welfare of the players. Under such circumstances, one often hears the remark, "They really took a physical beating." Competition should be as equitable as possible.

Prompt attention should be given to all injuries. Injured players should be examined by a physician and given proper treatment. There should be complete medical supervision of the athletic program. The trainer is not a substitute. A medical doctor should be present at all games and practices, if at all possible. The doctor should be the one to determine the extent of an injury. A player after being ill or hurt should not be permitted to participate again until the coach receives an approved statement from the family, school, or college physician.

Proper sanitary measures should be taken. Individual towels and drinking cups should be provided. The day of the "team" towel and the "team" drinking cup has passed. Equipment and uniforms should be cleaned as often as necessary. Locker, dressing, shower, toilet, and other rooms that are used by players should be kept clean and in a sanitary condition. Playing areas should be kept clean and safe. Gymnasia should be properly heated, and every measure taken to ensure as nearly ideal conditions as possible for students engaging in the athletics program.

Injuries and insurance.* The state athletic association in many states sponsors an athletic insurance plan. Such plans pay various medical, x-ray, dental, hospitalization, and other expenses according to the terms of the plan. There are also some private insurance companies that have such plans. The Wisconsin Interscholastic Athletic Association with its Athletic Accident Plan, recognized as one of the better types of athletic insurance, was a pioneer in the field. This plan covers injuries while practicing for or participating in interscholastic athletics. It has a premium rate for "all sports" coverage and also one for all sports except football. As pointed out by this association, the purpose of the plan is to provide enrolled athletes with benefits that will help to meet the costs of medical, dental, and hospital care in the event of accidental injury resulting from participation in physical education or athletics sponsored by a participating school. The amount of any payment for an injury shall be only in the amount of the actual expenses incurred but not in excess of the amounts listed in the schedule of allowance for such injury. In order to collect benefits, plan requirements must be met.

The insurance covered by various state and independent plans usually includes benefits for accidental death or dismemberment, hospital expenses, x-ray fees, physicians' fees, and surgical and dental expenses. Dental benefits may or may not be included in the schedule of surgical benefits. In some plans, catastrophe benefits are also available for injuries requiring extensive medical care and long-term hospitalization. Coverage is normally provided on a deductible basis, with the insurance company paying 75% to 80% of

the total cost over the deductible amount up to a maximum of $2,500 to $5,000.

After the Wisconsin High School Athletic Association inaugurated its school athletic insurance in 1930, several other state high school athletic associations followed suit. The number of such athletic insurance plans reached twenty-five in the 1940's. However, the commercial insurance industry, seeing the promise and need for athletic insurance, gradually came into the market, some of them providing many attractive premiums. Many school administrators were sympathetic to this type of coverage. Increasingly, the commercial insurance people have gained a strong foothold in the school athletic insurance program and today many schools and colleges utilize their policies.

State high school athletic associations in a few states still operate successful benefit plans, primarily by adopting many of the benefits utilized by the insurance industry, namely, nonallocated benefits, catastrophic coverage, and nonduplication of benefits.

California is the only state in this country that by law requires schools to furnish accident insurance for pupils. However, most school districts voluntarily purchase athletic insurance or make it available to parents.

Every school and college should have a written policy in regard to financial and other responsibilities associated with injuries. The administrator, parents, and players should be thoroughly familiar with the responsibilities of each in regard to injuries.

Contracts

Written contracts are usually essential in the administration of interscholastic and intercollegiate athletics. On the college level, in particular, games are scheduled many months or years in advance. Memories and facts tend to fade and become obscure with time. In order to avoid misunderstanding and confusion, it is best to

---

*See also Chapter 18.

have in writing a contract between the schools or colleges concerned.

Contracts should be properly executed and signed by official representatives of both schools and colleges. Many athletic associations provide specially prepared forms for use of member schools or colleges. Such forms usually contain the names of the schools, dates, and circumstances and conditions under which the contest will be held. Furthermore, they usually provide for penalties if the contract is not fulfilled by either party.

Officials

The officials will greatly influence the interscholastic or intercollegiate athletic program and determine whether it is conducted in a manner that will be of most benefit to the players and the schools or colleges concerned. Officials should be well qualified. They should know the rules and be able to interpret them accurately; recognize their responsibility to the players; be good sportsmen; and be courteous, honest, friendly, cooperative, impartial, and able to control the game at all times.

In order to ensure that only the best officials are utilized, machinery should be established to register and determine those who are qualified. Officials should be required to pass examinations on rules and to demonstrate their competency. Rating scales have been developed that aid in

Sec. XI	Officials Rating Card	NYSPHSAA

Sport .... League .... Game Date ....

Varsity ....   Score

Jr. Varsity .... Home Team ....

Jr. High .... Visiting Team ....

NAME OF OFFICIAL .... RATING	CODE	
Referee	EXCELLENT	5
	GOOD	4
Umpire	ACCEPTABLE	3
	POOR	2
Other	UNSATISFACTORY	1
Other	NO SHOW	0

CRITERIA — GAME CONTROL   JUDGEMENT — RULES — SPEED   ACCURACY   APPEARANCE
GAME DIFFICULTY — PERSONALITY

COMMENTS ....

....

....

....

....

Any rating of 0, 1 or 2 must be accompanied by reasons or a letter. This card must be mailed within one week following game.

COACH .... ATH. DIR. ....

Officials rating card of the New York State Public High School Athletic Association.

making such estimates. Most athletic associations have some method of registering and certifying those acceptable officials whom they wish to use. The Division for Girls' and Women's Sports of the AAHPER has a rating committee that certifies officials. In some states the officials who are used, in turn, rate the schools or colleges as to facilities, environment, and circumstances surrounding the game.

Subject to contract differences, officials usually are chosen by the home team with approval of opponents. The practice of the home team selecting officials without any consideration of the wishes of other schools or colleges or regard for impartial officiating has resulted in relations that have not been in the best interests of players or of athletics in general. A growing practice of having the conference or association select officials to be used has many points in its favor.

Officials should be duly notified of such details as the date and time of the contests to which they have been assigned. Officials' fees usually vary from school to school and from college to college, although some associations have set up standard rates. It is usually considered best to pay a flat fee that includes salary and expenses, rather than to list both separately.

Protests and forfeitures

There should be a set procedure for handling protests and forfeitures in connection with athletic contests. Of course, there should be careful preventive action beforehand in order to avoid a situation where such protests and forfeitures will occur. Proper interpretation of the rules, good officiating, elimination of undue pressures, and proper education of schools, colleges, and coaches on the objectives of interscholastic and intercollegiate athletics will act as preventive measures against such action.

However, the essential procedure for filing protests and forfeitures of contests should be established. This procedure should be clearly stated in writing and contain all the details, such as the person

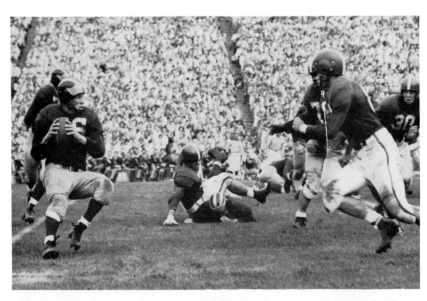

Athletics, with the appeal it has for youth, should be the heart of physical education. Scene from 1950 Michigan–Michigan State game. (Department of Physical Education and Athletics, University of Michigan.)

DEPARTMENT OF PHYSICAL EDUCATION
ATHLETIC REPORT

School_____ Sport_____ Game No._____

Game with_____ Played at_____

Date_____ Score_____ Opponents_____
(your score)

Referee_____ Umpire_____ H. L._____
Rating of officials: (Use numerals: 1-excellent, 2-good, 3-fair, 4-poor)

Attendance_____ Receipts_____ Guarantee (paid)_____
Received _____

Weather conditions_____ Principal's lists were (not) exchanged_____

	Player (full name)	No.	Position	List total participation			Remarks
				Quarters	Innings	Events	
1							
2							
3							
4							
5							
6							
7							
8							
9							
10							
11							
12							
13							
14							
15							
16							
17							
18							
19							
20							
21							
22							
23							
24							
25							

Scorer_____ Record compiled by_____
Time _____ Signature of Coach _____

Athletic report.

HEALTH AND PHYSICAL EDUCATION DEPARTMENT

BOYS' INTERSCHOLASTIC ATHLETIC PROGRAM

Season _____

Activity	Duration of season		Total number of games played						Number of boys participating		
	Date of first practice	Date of last game	Var-sity	Jr. Var-sity	Won		Lost		Varsity	Jr. Var-sity	Total
					Varsity	Jr. Varsity	Varsity	Jr. Varsity			
Baseball											
Basketball											
Cross country											
Football											
Golf											
Ice hockey											
Soccer											
Swimming											
Tennis											
Track and field											
Others											

Number of different boys in interscholastic program _____. (Do not count any boy more than once even though he participated in two or more activities.)

List any school honors or outstanding individual achievements, such as team or individual championships W. I. A. A. selections, etc.:

_____

_____

School _____

Date _____   Teacher's name _____

Boys' interscholastic athletic program.

ATHLETIC PERMIT

ATHLETIC APPLICATION FOR_____
(SPORT)

Name_____
(last)   (first)

I hereby apply for the privilege of trying out for the

_____team in_____
(sport)   (yr.)

I recognize my responsibilities if I try out for the above sport. I will make it a point to so govern myself that my association with the sport will bring honor to it and the school, and expect to be asked to withdraw from the team in case I do not.

If extended the above privilege I will:

A.   Train consistently as advised by the coach.
B.   Abide by all training rules.
C.   Make a serious endeavor to keep up my studies.
D.   Make it a point to abide by the rules and regulations of the student body.
E.   So conduct myself, at all times, that I will bring credit to my team.

I promise on my word of honor to do the above.

SIGNED_____

PARENTS WAIVER

Date_____

This is to certify that

_____
has my permission to train for and compete in

_____
(sport)
I assume for myself full responsibility should any accident occur to him either in training for such competition or in the competition itself, or in traveling to and from various fields where contests are played or practices held.

Signature_____

Athletic permit.

to whom the protest should be sent, time limits involved, person or group responsible for action, and any other information that is necessary. A frequent reason for a protest is the utilization of ineligible players. Most associations require the forfeiture of any game in which ineligible players participate.

Game management

Since there are so many details in connection with game management it is possible to include only a brief statement of the more important items. In order to have an efficiently conducted contest, it is important to have good organization. There must be someone responsible. Attention must be given to details. There must be planning. Many details must be attended to before the game, during the game, and after the game. Forsythe discusses such items. The various ones that he includes are reproduced here as a checklist for the administrator responsible for such management:

Before-game preparation (home contests)
  a. Contracts
  b. Eligibility records
  c. Physical examinations
  d. Parents' permission
  e. Athletic officials
  f. Equipment
  g. Field or court
  h. Publicity
  i. Courtesies to the visiting school
  j. Reserve games
  k. Tickets
  l. Contest programs
  m. Concessions
  n. Ushers
  o. Police protection and parking
  p. Reserved areas
  q. Cheerleaders
  r. Scoreboards
  s. Conditions of stadium, bleacher, or gymnasium
  t. Bands and half-time arrangements
  u. Decorations
  v. Public-address system
  w. Physician at contest
  x. Scorers, timers, judges

Game responsibilities (home contests)
  a. Supplies and equipment
  b. Tickets
  c. Ushers
  d. Contest programs
  e. Officials' quarters
  f. Visiting team quarters and courtesies
  g. Flag raising
  h. Intermission program
  i. Players' benches
  j. Physician
  k. Bands
  l. Contracts
  m. Contract guarantees and payments
  n. Eligibility lists
  o. Scoreboard arrangements
  p. Guards for dressing room
  q. Extra clothing for substitutes
  r. Concessions
  s. Cheerleaders
  t. Police
  u. Public-address system
  v. Rest rooms
  w. Guarding extra equipment

After-game responsibilities (home contests)
  a. Payment of officials
  b. Payment of visiting school
  c. Storage of equipment
  d. Contest receipts
  e. General financial statement
  f. Concessions report
  g. Record of officials
  h. Participation records
  i. Filing of contest data

Preparation for out-of-town games
  a. Transportation
  b. Parents' permits
  c. Finances for trip
  d. Equipment
  e. Game details
  f. Eligibility records
  g. Game contract
  h. Trip personnel
  i. Participation record books[*]

Schedules and practice periods

The trend in athletics is to limit the length of seasons for various sports. If this is not done, overemphasis often results with a particular sport monopolizing the

---

[*]Forsythe, C. E.: The administration of high school athletics, Englewood Cliffs, N. J., 1962, Prentice-Hall, Inc., chap. 7.

time of students and allowing only little time for other activities. Football has often been accused of this with its fall practice before school or college starts, postseason games that run into the new year, spring practice, and summer work in preparation for the fall season. Such a schedule is not in the interests of the students' general welfare.

There should be defined limits in respect to the length of seasons. These should have the approval of school and college authorities. The length of seasons should be so arranged that they interfere

---

STATEMENT OF PHILOSOPHY REGARDING AWARDS

There are arguments pro and con in respect to awards for athletic participation. Some of the arguments for awards are: they stimulate interest, they serve as an incentive for participation, and they recognize achievement. Some of the arguments against awards are: they make for a more expensive program, a few individuals win most of them, they are unnecessary since students would participate even if no awards were given, it is difficult to make awards on the basis of all factors that should be considered, and the incentive is artificial since the joy and satisfaction received are enough reward in themselves.

Although the conferring of awards is overdone in many cases, the practice of giving out valuable awards indiscriminately cannot be justified educationally or financially. The responsibility of the physical education department is to teach boys and girls to play for the "love of playing" without any thought of an award. It is the feeling of this committee that the human desire for recognition is most natural. The receiving of an award for achievement in athletics in the form of a ribbon, emblem, certificate, or simple medal fosters personal pride in accomplishment. Academically, we recognize students with high grades. We select valedictorians and members of local and national honor societies.

Awards are symbols of achievement and should not be recognized as a prize. In Greek times the olive wreath given to a victor was the most coveted award that could be obtained by a Greek athlete. The importance of such an award was not its material value, but what it symbolized. The custom of awarding insignia or letters by school and college authorities to athletic teams in order to foster school spirit and personal pride in accomplishment and set up high ideals of sportsmanship is almost universal. Because of the long tradition of granting awards and because of the fact that this is a common practice in other activities of life, simple awards — mere symbols of achievement with little or no monetary value — seem to be justifiable.

The school should consider such factors as attitude, dependability, school citizenship, scholarship, participation, and improvement, as well as athletic prowess, in establishing a policy for the conferring of awards. Such a practice would make it advisable for many school officials to be involved in the determination of who receives awards. Furthermore, the basis for students receiving awards should be broadened to include as many levels and kinds of achievement as possible while still keeping the award meaningful as a form of recognition.

Principles for administering athletic awards

1. Awards should have little or no monetary value and should serve as a symbol of achievement.
2. Awards should not detract from the primary goal, namely, the enjoyment of the activity for the activity itself.
3. Opportunities should be provided for all students to obtain awards.
4. Good sportsmanship, scholarship, character, attitude, and citizenship should be considered along with participation and achievement in the conferring of awards.
5. Awards should be presented as a culminating activity of the physical education program.
6. Money for awards should come from the budgeted school funds and not be secured through clubs, alumni, and civic organizations.
7. Awards and dinners or other events given in honor of athletes, should be sponsored *only* by school authorities and not by clubs, alumni, or civic organizations.
8. There should be no major and minor distinction in presenting awards.

as little as possible with other school and college work. They should provide for adequate practice before the first game so that the players are in good physical condition. There should be limits as to the total number of games, depending upon the sport, and also upon the number of games played in any 1 week. Postseason games are not considered advisable by many educators. Teams that are as nearly as possible of equal ability and equal skill should be scheduled.

Awards

The basis for awards in interscholastic and intercollegiate athletics is the same as that for intramural and extramural athletics. As pointed out, there are arguments for and against giving awards. Some individuals feel that the values derived from playing a sport—joy and satisfaction, physical, social, and other values—are sufficient in themselves and that no awards should be given. Others point to the fact that awards are symbolic of achievement and are traditional in our culture and should be given.

The policy that will be adopted in respect to awards should be determined locally. A definite policy should be established that cuts across all the affairs of the school or college. At the present time the practice of giving awards in the form of letters, insignia, or some other symbol is almost universal. It is recommended that when awards are given they should be very simple and of very little monetary value. Some state athletic associations, for example, have stated that the award should not cost more than $1.00. Furthermore, it seems wise not to distinguish between so-called major and minor sports when giving awards. They should be treated on an equal basis.

On p. 253 is the statement of the philosophy and principles for administering athletic awards used in one school system.

Records

The good administrator and coach will keep accurate records of all the details concerned with the administration of interscholastic or intercollegiate athletics. There should be records of students' participation, for eligibility purposes and to show the extent of the program; records of the conduct of various sports from year to year so that they can be compared over a period of time and also compared with other schools and colleges; statistical summaries of player and game performance that will help the coach to determine weaknesses in game strategy or identify players' performances and other items essential to well-organized play; records of equipment and supplies; officials' records; financial records, and other items in connection with the conduct of the total program. Good business and good administration demand good record keeping.

Transportation

Transporting athletes to games and contests presents many administrative problems. Such questions arise as; Who should be transported? In what kind of vehicles should athletes be transported? Is athletics part of a regular school or college program? Should private vehicles or school- and college-owned vehicles be used? What are the legal implications involved in transporting athletes in school- and college-sponsored events?

It appears that the present trend is to view athletics as an integral part of the educational program so that public funds may be used for transportation purposes. At the same time, however, statutes vary from state to state, and any person administering athletic programs should examine carefully the statutes in their own state.

The feeling among many administrators in regard to transportation is that athletes and representatives of the school or college concerned, such as band and cheerleaders, should travel only in transportation provided by the educational institution. Where private cars belonging to coaches, students, or other persons are used, the administrator should be sure to determine whether he is in conformity with the state statutes regarding liability. Under no circumstances should students or other representatives be permitted to drive unless they are authorized drivers and recognized as such by the state statutes. Under most circumstances it is recommended that students not be used as drivers.

SOME ADMINISTRATIVE PROBLEMS

There are many problems with which the administration of any interscholastic or intercollegiate athletic program has to contend. Some that are particularly prominent at the present time are those concerned with (1) gate receipts, (2) tournaments and championships, (3) eligibility, (4) scholarships, (5) recruitment, (6) proselyting, and (7) scouting.

Gate receipts

Gate receipts are the source of many evils in athletics. Too often they become the point of emphasis rather than the valuable educational outcomes that can accrue to the participant. When this occurs, athletics cannot justify existence in the educational program. Furthermore, the emphasis on gate receipts results in a vicious cycle—the money increases the desire for winning teams so that there will be greater financial return, which in turn results in greater financial outlays to secure and develop even better teams. This goes on and on, with a false set of standards forming the basis for the program.

Throughout the country interscholastic and intercollegiate athletics are financed through many different sources. These include gate receipts, board of education and central university funds, donations, special projects, students' fees, physical education department funds, magazine subscriptions, and concessions. In high schools a "general organization" quite frequently handles the funds for athletics. Some colleges finance part of the program through endowment funds.

It has long been argued by leaders in the physical education profession that athletics have great educational potentials. They are curricular in nature rather than extracurricular. This means they contribute to the welfare of students like any other subject in the curriculum. Upon this basis, therefore, the finances necessary to support such a program should come from board of education or central university funds. Athletics should not be self-supporting or used as a means to support part or all of the other so-called extracurricular activities of a school or college. They represent an integral part of the educational program and as such deserve to be treated in the same manner as other aspects of the program. This procedure is followed in some schools and colleges with benefits to all concerned and should be an ideal toward which all should strive.

Tournaments and championships

The question frequently arises as to whether postseason tournaments and championship playoffs should be conducted as part of an athletic program. It is generally agreed by physical education leaders that all the educational values that can be derived from athletics can be gained without ever playing a tournament or championship game. The main purposes of such ventures are usually to make money, to entertain the public, and to crown a winner. Furthermore, many evils enter the picture when tournaments and championships are conducted. As a result of such contests the emphasis on winning becomes more pronounced, participation often results in physical and emotional strain on players, spectator pressure increases, gambling often enters the picture, and the emphasis is on a few individuals.

Eligibility

Standards in regard to the eligibility of contestants are essential. These should be in writing, disseminated widely, and clearly understood by all concerned. They should be established well ahead of a season's or year's play so that the student, coaches, and others will not become emotional when they suddenly realize they will lose their chance to win a championship because they cannot use a star player who is ineligible.

Standards of eligibility in interscholastic circles usually include an age limit of not more than 19 or 20 years; a requirement that an athlete be a bona fide student; rules on transfer students that frequently require their being bona fide residents in the community served by the school; satisfactory grades; a limit of three or four on number of seasons of competition allowed (playing in one game usually constitutes a season); regular attendance at school; permission to play on only one team during a season; and a requirement that the participant have a medical examination, anateur status, and parent's consent. These regulations vary from school to school and from state to state.

The National Federation of State High School Athletic Associations considers a student ineligible for amateur standing if (1) he has accepted money or compensation for playing in an athletic contest, (2) he has played under an assumed name, (3) he has competed with a team whose players received pay for their playing, and (4) he has signed a contract to play with a professional team.

Eligibility requirements at the college and university level include rules in respect to such items as residence, undergraduate status, academic average, amateur status, limits of participation, and transfer. In general, most players must have been in residence for at least 1 year (sometimes waived for small colleges); be a bona fide, fully matriculated student carrying on a full program of studies; have a satisfactory grade-point average; and have had only 1 year of freshman competition and 3 years of varsity competition. Also, a student cannot participate after the expiration of four consecutive 12-month periods following the date of his initial enrollment in an institution of higher learning. Amateur status is also a requirement.

Scholarships

Should athletes receive scholarships or special financial assistance in schools and colleges? This subject is argued pro and con and is mainly a problem at the college level. Those in favor of scholarships and financial assistance claim that a student who excels in sports should receive aid just as much as one who excels in music or any other activity. They claim that such inducements are justified in the educational picture. Those opposed point to the fact that scholarships should be awarded on the basis of the need and general academic qualifications of a student, rather than his skill in some sport.

One solution is to have a list of criteria drawn up for the purpose of making such grants and have them handled by an all-school or all-college committee. This plan is based on the premise that scholarships and student aid should not be granted to the athletic or to any other department. Instead, they should be handled on an all-school or all-college basis and given to students who need them most and are best qualified. In this way, those students who are in need of assistance, regardless of the area in which they specialize, will be the ones who will receive aid.

Recruitment

The recruitment of athletes in order to develop star and winning teams is not condoned for any educational institution. The procedure for admittance should be the same for all students, regardless of whether they are athletes, chemistry students, music students, or others. No special consideration should be shown to any particular group. The same standards, academic and otherwise, should prevail. In this respect the statements below apply equally well to high schools and colleges:

> The athletic teams of an institution should be composed of bona fide students who were attracted to the institution by its educational program. Special efforts to recruit students of athletic prowess for the primary purpose of developing winning athletic teams are unworthy of an institution of higher education. . . .
>
> The encouragement or condonation by an institution of outside organizations engaged in the recruitment or subsidization of athletes is symptomatic of an unwholesome athletic situation. Where such an organization exists, the institution affected by the efforts of this organization will be expected to repudiate these efforts and to take effective steps to prevent relationships between its students and the organization.*

Proselyting

Proselyting is a term applied to a high school or college that has so strongly overemphasized athletics that it has stooped to unethical behavior to secure outstanding talent for winning teams. High schools are not troubled with this problem as much as colleges, but in some quarters they also have difficulties. There have been incidents where a father was provided employment so that he would move his family to a particular section of a city or a particular community so that his boy would be eligible to play with the local team. However, thanks to vigilant state athletic associations, such incidents have

been kept to a minimum. The following represent some of the rules in force in many states to eliminate special inducements to attract athletes. These rules have been established by many state high school athletic associations:

1. A student shall not be allowed to receive for participation in athletic contests any sweater, blanket, or trophy of any sort except the unattached letter, monogram, or other insignia of the school.
2. A student shall not receive any award from an individual or an organization other than an educational institution of this Association.
3. No student shall be given any trip or excursion of any kind by any individual, group, or organization outside of this Association.
4. An association school shall not receive any award from any individual, groups, or organization outside of this Association.
5. Local individuals, local organizations, or local groups may give complimentary dinners to local athletes or members of athletic teams, provided such dinners meet with the approval of the local superintendent of schools.*

Scouting

Scouting has become an accepted practice at high school and college levels. By watching another team perform, the formations and plays used will be known and certain weaknesses will be discovered. One coach said that his scouting consisted of watching players to determine little mannerisms they had that would give away the play that was going to be used.

Many schools and colleges are spending considerable money in this manner. Some schools and colleges scout a rival team every game during the season. Some use three or four persons on the same scouting assignment, and such schools and colleges take moving pictures at length so that the

*Commission on Colleges and Universities, North Central Association of Colleges and Secondary Schools: An interpretation of the revised policy on intercollegiate athletics of the North Central Association, Chicago, 1952, The Association, pp. 11-12.

*Joint Committee: Administration problems in health education, physical education, and recreation, Washington, D. C., 1953, American Association for Health, Physical Education, and Recreation, p. 126.

opponent's play can be studied in great detail. Such money, it is felt by some physical educators, could be spent more wisely if used to enhance the value of the game for the participants, rather than to further any all-important effort to win.

Many unethical practices have entered into scouting. Coaches have been known to have scouts observe secret practice sessions and utilize other unethical methods. DeGroot pointed out that the Code of Ethics of the American Football Coaches Association has the following to say on scouting: "It shall be considered unethical under any circumstances to scout any team, by any means whatsoever, except in regularly scheduled games. Any attempt to scout practice sessions shall be considered strictly unethical. The head football coach of each institution shall be held responsible for all scouting. This shall include the use of moving pictures.*

Many coaches feel that the only reason they want to scout is that they themselves are being scouted. Therefore, they feel it will work to their disadvantage unless they follow the same procedure. If something could be done to eliminate or restrict scouting, considerable time and money could be put to much more advantageous use.

INTERSCHOLASTIC ATHLETICS AT THE ELEMENTARY AND JUNIOR HIGH SCHOOL LEVELS

Since athletics was first introduced into the educational picture, there has been a continual pushing downward of these competitive experiences into the lower educational levels. Educational athletics started at the college level with a crew race between Harvard and Yale in 1852. Then other sports were introduced to the

campuses throughout the United States. As higher education athletic programs expanded and gained recognition and popularity, the high schools felt that sports should also be a part of their educational offerings. As a result, most high schools in America today have some form of interscholastic athletics. In recent years, junior high schools have also felt the impact of interscholastic athletic programs. A survey made by the National Association of Secondary-School Principals, and including 2,296 junior high schools, showed that 85.2% had some program of interscholastic athletics while 14.8% did not.

There should not be any interscholastic athletics at the elementary school level. In kindergarten to grade six physical activities should be geared to the developmental level of the child. Starting with grade four it may be possible to initiate an intramural program on an informal basis. However, there should not be undue emphasis on developing skill in a few sports or requiring children to conform to adult standards of competition.

The special nature of grades seven through nine, representing a transition period between the elementary school and the senior high school and between childhood and adolescence, has raised a question in the minds of many educators as to whether an interscholastic athletic program is in the best interests of the students concerned.

Many of the guidelines of the American Academy of Pediatrics listed below apply to the junior high school level, as well as to the elementary school level, and to the type of athletic competition that should be offered:

1. All children should have opportunities to develop skill in a variety of activities.
2. All such activities should take into account the age and developmental level of child.
3. a. Athletic activities of elementary school children should be part of an over-all school program. Competent medical supervision of each child should be ensured.

*DeGroot, D. S.: Code of Ethics of the American Football Coaches Association, The Journal of the American Association for Health, Physical Education, and Recreation 24:51, 1953.

b. Health observation by teachers and others should be encouraged and help given by the physician.

4. Athletic activities outside of the school program should be on an entirely voluntary basis without undue emphasis on any special program or sport, and without undue emphasis upon winning. These programs should also include competent medical supervision.

5. Competitive programs organized on school, neighborhood and community levels will meet the needs of children twelve years of age and under. State, regional and national tournaments; bowl, charity and exhibition games are not recommended for this age group. Commercial exploitation in any form is unequivocally condemned.

6. Body-contact sports, particularly tackle football and boxing, are considered to have no place in programs for children of this age.

7. Competition is an inherent characteristic of growing developing children. Properly guided it is beneficial and not harmful to their development.

8. Schools and communities as a whole must be made aware of the needs for personnel, facilities, equipment and supplies which will assure an adequate program for children in this age group.

9. All competitive athletic programs should be organized with the cooperation of interested medical groups who will ensure adequate medical care before and during such programs. This should include thorough physical examinations at specified intervals, teaching of health observation to teachers and coaches, as well as attention to factors such as: (a) injury; (b) response to fatigue; (c) individual emotional needs; and (d) the risks of undue emotional strains.

10. Muscle testing is not, per se, a valid estimate of physical fitness, or of good health.

11. Participation in group activities is expected of every child. When there is a failure to do so, or lack of interest, underlying physical or emotional causes should be sought.

12. Leadership for young children should be such that highly organized, highly competitive programs would be avoided. The primary consideration should be a diversity of wholesome childhood experiences which will aid in the proper physical and emotional development of the child into a secure and well-integrated adult.

The research in regard to a highly organized athletics at the junior high school level indicates points of substantial agreement, as listed in the following section*:

1. The junior high school educational program should be adapted to the needs of boys and girls in grades seven, eight, and nine. This is a period of transition from elementary school to senior high school and from childhood to adolescence. It is a time when students are trying to understand their bodies, gain independence, achieve adult social status, acquire self-confidence, and establish a system of values. It is a time when a program of education unique to this age group is needed to meet the abilities and broadening interests of the student.

2. The best educational program at the junior high school level is one that provides for program enrichment to meet the needs of students in grades seven through nine, rather than using the senior high school or other educational level as a blueprint to follow.

3. There is need for a distinct and separate educational climate for these grades in order to ensure that the program will not be influenced unduly by either the elementary or the senior high school.

4. There is a need for teachers (including coaches) whose full responsibilities involve working with grades seven, eight, and nine and whose training has included an understanding of the needs of these students and of the educational program required to meet those needs.

5. The junior high school should provide for exploratory experiences with specialization being delayed until senior high school and college.

6. The junior high school should provide for the mental, physical, social, and emotional development of students.

*New York State Education Department: Interscholastic athletics at the junior high school level, Albany, 1965, The Department. (Charles Bucher, consultant, New York State Department of Education.)

7. Out-of-class as well as in-class experiences should be provided.

8. There should be concern for the development of a sound standard of values in each student.

9. The principal and other members of the administration have the responsibility for providing sound educational leadership in all school matters. The type of physical education and athletic programs offered will reflect the type of leadership provided.

10. The physical education program at the junior high school level should consist of a class program, an adapted program, and intramural and extramural programs (the interscholastic athletic program is controversial).

11. The interscholastic athletics program, if offered, should be provided only after the prerequisites of excellent physical education class, adapted, and intramural and extramural programs have been developed, and only as special controls in regard to such items as health, facilities, game adaptations, classification of players, leadership, and officials have been provided.

12. The physical education program should be adapted to the needs of the junior high school student. There is a need for a wide variety of activities, based on physical and neuromuscular maturation, that will contribute to the development of body control, enable each student to experience success, provide for recognition of energy output and fatigue, and take into consideration the "growth spurt" of early adolescence.

13. The physical education program should represent a favorable social and emotional climate for the student. There should be freedom from anxiety and fear, absence of tensions and strains, a feeling of belonging for each student, a social awareness that contributes to the development of such important traits as respect for the rights of others, and an atmosphere that is conducive to growing into social and emotional maturity.

14. Personal health instruction should be closely integrated into the physical education program.

15. Coeducational activities should be provided.

16. All physical activities should be carefully supervised medically and conducted under optimum health and safety conditions.

17. Students who are not physiologically mature should not engage in activities where there is danger of body contact, a high degree of skill is required, great amounts of endurance are necessary, and highly competitive conditions are present.

18. The menstrual cycle and reproductive organs of girls require special consideration in the selection and conduct of activities.

19. Physiologic maturity is the best criterion for determining whether a student is physiologically ready for participation in most interscholastic athletic activities.

20. Competition itself is not the factor that makes athletics dangerous to the physiologically mature student. Instead, such items as the manner in which the program is conducted, type of activity, facilities, leadership, and physical condition of the student are the determining factors.

21. Physiologic fitness can be developed without exposure to an interscholastic athletic program.

22. Competitive athletics, if properly conducted, have the potential for satisfying such basic psychologic needs as recognition, belonging, self-respect, and feeling of achievement, as well as providing a wholesome outlet for the physical activity drive. However, if conducted in the light of adult interests, community pressures, and other questionable influences, they can prove psychologically harmful.

23. Interscholastic athletics, when conducted in accordance with desirable standards of leadership, educational philosophy, activities, and other pertinent factors, have the potential for realizing beneficial social

effects for the student, but when not conducted in accordance with desirable standards they can be socially detrimental to the student.

24. Of all competitive activities, tackle football, ice hockey, and boxing are subject to most criticism as being of questionable value for junior high school students.

INTERSCHOLASTIC ATHLETICS AT THE HIGH SCHOOL LEVEL

The responsibility of the school for the interscholastic athletic program is one that cannot be avoided. Therefore, it is essential that all administrators be aware of the best practices recommended for the various phases of the total program. The Joint Committee on Standards for Interscholastic Athletics of the National Association of Secondary School Principals, the National Federation of State High School Associations, and the American Association for Health, Physical Education, and Recreation have established standards.* These make it possible for every school to examine its athletic program in a critical manner and see how well it meets recommended practices. The preface to the list of standards includes the following statements:

Basic to any consideration of acceptable standards in interscholastic athletics for secondary schools in this statement of the GUIDING POLICIES for the organization, administration, and development of a program of athletics for the youth of our schools:

1. Athletics are to be an integral part of the secondary school program and should receive financial support from tax funds on the same basis as other recognized parts of the total educational program. As part of the curriculum, high school sports are to be conducted by secondary school authorities and all instruction provided by competent, qualified, and accredited teachers so that desirable, definite educational aims may be achieved.

---

*Joint Committee Report: Standards in athletics for boys in secondary schools, The Journal of the American Association for Health, Physical Education, and Recreation 22:16, 1951.

2. Athletics are for the benefit of all youth. The aim is maximum participation, a sport for every boy and every boy in a sport, in a well-balanced intramural interscholastic program with emphasis on safe and healthful standards of competition.

3. Athletics are to be conducted under rules which provide for equitable competition, sportsmanship, fair play, health, and safety. High school sports are for amateurs who are bona fide undergraduate high school students. These youths must be protected from exploitation and the dangers of professionalism. Pre-season, post-schedule, post-season, all-star games, or similar types of promotions are not consistent with this principle. It is necessary to develop a full understanding of the need for observance of local, league, sectional, state, and national standards in athletics.

The Constitution of the California Interscholastic Federation lists the following "Cardinal Athletic Principles" and "Code of Ethics":

CARDINAL ATHLETIC PRINCIPLES

To be of maximum effectiveness, the athletic program will:

1. Be a well-coordinated part of the secondary school curriculum.
2. Justify the use of the tax funds and school facilities because of the educational aims achieved.
3. Be based on the spirit of amateurism.
4. Be conducted by secondary school authorities.
5. Provide opportunities for many students to participate in a wide variety of sports in every sport season.
6. Eliminate professionalism and commercialism.
7. Prevent "All-Star" contests or other promotional events.
8. Foster training in conduct, game ethics, and sportsmanship for participants and spectators.
9. Include a well-balanced program of intramural sports.
10. Engender respect for local, state, and national rules and policies under which the school program is conducted.

CODE OF ETHICS

It is the duty of all concerned with high school athletics:

1. To emphasize the proper ideas of sportsmanship, ethical conduct, and fair play.

2. To eliminate all possibilities which tend to destroy the best values of the game.
3. To stress the values derived from playing the game fairly.
4. To show cordial courtesy to visiting teams and officials.
5. To establish a happy relationship between visitors and hosts.
6. To respect the integrity and judgment of sports officials.
7. To achieve a thorough understanding and acceptance of the rules of the game and the standards of eligibility.
8. To encourage leadership, use of initiative, and good judgment by the players on the team.
9. To recognize that the purpose of athletics is to promote the physical, mental, moral, social, and emotional well-being of the individual players.
10. To remember that an athletic contest is only a game—not a matter of life or death for player, coach, school, officials, fan, community, state, or nation.*

INTERCOLLEGIATE ATHLETICS

It is at the college and university level that overemphasis has taken place to the largest extent in the field of varsity athletics. Commercialization flourishes when 60,000 people gather for a sports spectacle, the cost of tickets ranges from $2.00 to $8.00, and large stadia, long trips, and many scholarships predominate. A few colleges have established "easy courses" in the curriculum so that athletes will not have to meet the usual academic standards. Records have been falsified to enable some to meet entrance requirements. Others have been given tuition, board, spending money, and sometimes even a car to attract them. Players have been recruited from various sections of the country through unethical means. Alumni pressure for winning teams, the firing of coaches, and other undesirable practices have been in evidence in some quarters.

Much of the responsibility for eliminating the abuses from college athletic circles

---

*California Interscholastic Federation: Constitution and by-laws, 1959, The Federation.

has been placed upon the shoulders of the various regional accrediting agencies. One of the largest of these has the following to say in regard to policy:

1. Some of the most serious abuses of athletics really arise from the abuses of instruction. It is not good university and college practice to permit soft spots in the curriculum. Students call these "snap" courses. They are too easy or too frivolous to occupy the time of university or college students. Their presence aids and abets corruption of athletics. The same applies to low standards of entrance and performance in any of the colleges or courses of the university. Sub-college standards of academic work anywhere in the institution afford a hiding place for youths who lack the ability to be university students or young men whose athletic duties prove too exacting to permit them to pass courses of truly university grade.

2. The notion that institutions of higher education have a responsibility for providing public entertainment in the form of athletic spectacles is alien to the true functions of such institutions.

3. The manner in which an institution spends its funds is the best possible evidence of the values it fosters. A college or university will give financial support to programs and activities in proportion to the importance it attaches to them. A first-rate educational institution will in the very nature of things devote as much of its income as possible to functions that bring a high educational return. This applies to all phases of operation, not alone to athletics.

4. The chief administration officer of a college or university is ultimately responsible for the wholesome conduct of the intercollegiate athletics in his institution, and this ultimate responsibility he cannot properly delegate to subordinate officers. It is his duty to be well informed about the athletic policies and practices of his institution and to take the necessary steps to assure that the athletic program is making its full contribution to the attainment of educational objectives.

5. A high quality institution does not resort to athletic renown as a means of securing public support. Rather, it makes its appeal on the basis of its educational merit. If athletic prominence is an indispensable element in the public relations of a college or university, that fact is of itself a reflection on the academic worth of the institution.

6. When the winning of contests per se becomes the major emphasis of an athletic program, this results almost inevitably in practices

that are detrimental to the moral tone and educational seriousness of purpose of the institution. This emphasis can have such far-reaching consequences, sometimes penetrating to the very core of institutional integrity, that the existence of an unsatisfactory athletic situation in an institution will be regarded as a serious enough weakness to justify the denial of accreditation.*

Bucher and Dupee have surveyed the standards for high school and collegiate athletics and have summarized the selected recommended standards for these educational levels. They are presented here for the information and reference of the reader.

Summary of selected recommended standards for varsity interscholastic and intercollegiate athletics†

1. Organization
   (a) The wholesome conduct of the athletic programs should be the ultimate responsibility of the school administration.
   (b) Athletic policy should be adopted, evaluated, and supervised by a faculty committee.
   (c) Athletic policy should be implemented by the director of physical education and the director of athletics.
   (d) Athletics should be organized as an integral part of the department of physical education.
2. Staff
   (a) All members of the coaching staff should be members of the faculty.
   (b) All coaches should be hired on their qualifications to assume educational responsibilities, and not on their ability to produce winning teams.
   (c) All coaches should enjoy the same privileges of tenure, rank, and salary which are accorded other similarly qualified faculty members.
   (d) All public school coaches should be certified in physical education.

---

*Commission on Colleges and Universities, North Central Association of Colleges and Secondary Schools: An interpretation of the revised policy of intercollegiate athletics of the North Central Association, Chicago, 1952, The Association.

†Bucher, C. A., and Dupee, R. K., Jr.: Athletics in schools and colleges, New York, 1965, The Center for Applied Research in Education, Inc. (The Library of Education), pp. 99-101.

3. Finances
   (a) The financing of interscholastic and intercollegiate athletics should be governed by the same policies that control the financing of all other educational activities within an institution.
   (b) Gate receipts should be considered an incidental source of revenue.
4. Health and safety
   (a) An annual physical examination should be required of all participants; a physical examination on a seasonal basis would be preferable.
   (b) Each school should have a written policy for the implementation of an injury-care program.
   (c) Each school should have a written policy concerning the responsibility for athletic injuries and should provide or make available athletic accident insurance.
   (d) All coaches should be well qualified in the care and prevention of athletic injuries.
   (e) A doctor should be present at all contests at which injury is possible.
   (f) Only that equipment offering the best protection should be purchased.
   (g) Proper fitting of all protective equipment should be insured.
   (h) Competition should be scheduled only between teams of comparable ability.
   (i) Games should not be played until players have had a minimum of three weeks of physical conditioning and drill.
   (j) Playing fields should meet standards for size and safety.
5. Eligibility
   (a) All schools should honor and respect the eligibility rules and regulations of respective local, state, and national athletic associations.
   (b) A student who is not making normal progress toward a degree or diploma should not be allowed to participate.
6. Recruiting
   (a) The athletic teams of each school should be composed of bona fide students who live in the school district or who were attracted to the institution by its educational program.
   (b) All candidates for admission to a school should be evaluated according to the same high standards.
   (c) All financial aid should be administered with regard to need and according to the same standards for all students. The recipient of financial aid should be given

a statement of the amount, duration, and conditions of the award.

7. Awards
   (a) The value of athletic awards should be limited.
   (b) There should be no discrimination between awards for different varsity sports.
   (c) The presentation of all-star, most valuable-player, and most-improved-player awards should be discouraged.

GIRLS' AND WOMEN'S ATHLETICS

The question of highly organized athletics for girls is a controversial matter. The questions of how much, how little, and what is a happy medium are frequently raised with enthusiastic supporters on both sides of the issue. There seems to be a general consensus of opinion that athletics can render a valuable service to girls. The question arises as to what type of program can best render this service. Girls can develop a better state of total fitness, skills for worthy use of leisure time, and other desirable qualities and attributes, just as boys and men can. However, it must be recognized that girls and women are not boys and men. There are many biologic, social, and

Student's Name_____ School_____

Entered H.S._____19____ Initiated_____19____ School Group (Check) ☐ 1 ☐ 2

| AWARD REQUIREMENTS (Check when completed.) | | | | POINTS EARNED | AWARDS RECEIVED | APPROVED BY: (Adviser) |

Year in H. S. 1 2 3 4

Scholarship____ Fresh._____ 1st Local_____19____ _____

Sportsmanship____ Soph._____ 2nd Local_____19____ _____

Heart Examination____

Satisfactory P. E. Grade____ Junior_____ 1st State_____19____ _____

Others: (Local)____ Senior_____ 2nd State_____19____ _____

Total (to date) GAA Pin_____19____ _____

PARTICIPATION POINTS (To be given only for participation in the elective sports program; i.e., intramural, after-school, noon-hour, etc.)

Year in H. S. 1 2 3 4 | Year in H. S. 1 2 3 4 | Year in H. S. 1 2 3 4

Archery____ | Brought Forward | Brought Forward
Tests | Rebound Tumbling Stunts____ | Tennis____
Badminton____ | | Tests
Tests | Soccer____ | Tumbling Stunts
Basketball____ | Tests | (Check) 1, 2, 3, 4, 5, 6, 7, 8, 9, 10, 11, 12, 13, 14, 15,
Tests | Softball____ | 16, 17, 18, 19, 20, 21, 22,
Bowling____ | Tests | 23, 24, 25, 26, 27, 28, 29,
Tests | Speedball____ | 30, 31, 32, 33, 34, 35, 36,
Campcraft____ | Swimming____ | 37, 38, 39, 40
Dance____ | Red Cross Tests: | Tumbling ____
Folk Dance Tests | Beginners |
Rhythm Tests | Intermediate | Volley Ball____
Tap Tests | Swimmers | Tests
Hiking____ | Advanced | Other Activities:
Hockey____ | Survival Tests | (Write in)
Tests | Jr. Life Saving |
Leaders Class____ | Sr. Life Saving |
Test | Dives |
Total | Total | Total Activity Pts.

Award Granted_____19____ By_____

Sample record of the Illinois League of High School Girls' Athletic Associations. (From Felshin, J.: Girls' sports organization handbook, Washington, D. C., 1961, The Division for Girls' and Women's Sports.)

other differences that must be taken into consideration. It is impossible to take the boys' program and duplicate it for the girls without any changes.

The girls' program should be concerned especially with the individual sports and activities, as well as the team games. The women in charge and those doing the officiating should be qualified. Official girls' rules should be followed. The girls' games should be separated from the boys', except in coeducational activity, which should occupy a prominent place in the program. The social aspects should be stressed, jumping and body contact should be limited or eliminated altogether. Health safeguards should be observed, limited seasons and restrictions on the amount of competition of any one girl should be enforced. Publicity and commercial aspects should be controlled so that the girls are not exploited.

If athletics for girls are conducted in a sound manner, many benefits can accrue. Some of these benefits have been brought out by the American Association for Health, Physical Education, and Recreation:

The values or purposes may be summarized thus: to satisfy the human desire of belonging to a group which represents the school; to stimulate greater interest in the physical education class program, and wider participation in the intramural program; to develop and maintain physical fitness among players; to provide opportunities for girls to become participants as well as spectators; to strengthen individual qualities, such as initiative, resourcefulness, loyalty, cooperation, and other similar qualities, through game experiences of great importance to the individual; to encourage girls to become skilled in activities as a personal and social asset; to offer challenging competition to the accelerated or gifted student in physical education; to offer opportunities for participation in activities that may be continued throughout life.*

---

*Joint Committee: Administration problems in health education, physical education, and recreation, Washington, D. C., 1953, American Association for Health, Physical Education, and Recreation, p. 117.

Procedures and practices in respect to interscholastic and intercollegiate athletic competition for girls vary from state to state. Some schools and colleges have broad programs of interscholastic athletics, others do not have any, and some have modified programs. In those having modified programs, play days, sports days, invitation games, and telegraphic meets are increasingly playing a more prominent part. Most states do not set up specific requirements for girls' athletics but feel that their established regulations apply to both girls and boys. A few states have athletic associations for girls that are similar to those for boys.

The Division for Girls' and Women's Sports of the American Association for Health, Physical Education, and Recreation is the most influential organization affecting athletics for girls and women. This organization is comprised of leaders in the field of physical education and recreation. The purpose of the organization is to develop, promote, and supervise desirable sports programs for girls and women. In order to accomplish this purpose, guiding principles and standards have been developed and publicized. The DGWS also publishes many official guides in various sports, scorebooks, pamphlets on desirable practices, and special publications concerned with such matters as menstruation, teaching materials, audiovisual resource list, and special events for girls' and women's programs.

Guiding principles and standards established by the DGWS are concerned with the sports program, leader, and participant. The organization feels that the program should be developed on the basis of such factors as individual differences among girls and women and the environment in which the activity is conducted. The leaders of these programs should have a full understanding of the needs and interests of girls and women and be exemplary in their conduct. The participant should develop skill and other characteristics in accordance with her potential, and the activities in which she engages should contribute to her health and welfare. Competition should be so designed as to enable each player to participate and at the level of her ability. Officials should understand the role of girls and women and sports, and the rules of the DGWS should be the official rules of all contests.

Recommendations of Division of Girls' and Women's Sports

The recommendations of the Division of Girls' and Women's Sports of the American Association for Health, Physical Education, and Recreation with regard to competitive sports for various age level groupings represent a definitive statement of standards for girls' and women's athletics:

In junior high school, it is desirable that intramural programs of competitive activities be closely

integrated with the basic physical education program. Appropriate competition at this level should be comprised of intramural and informal extramural events consistent with social needs and recreational interests. A well-organized and well-conducted sports program should take into account the various skill levels and thus meet the needs of the more highly skilled.

In senior high school, a program of intramural-extramural participation should be arranged to augment a sound and inclusive instructional program in physical education. It should be recognized that an interscholastic program will require professional leadership, time, and funds in addition to those provided for the intramural programs. Facilities should be such that the intramural and instructional programs need not be eliminated or seriously curtailed if an interscholastic program is offered.

Specifically, the following standards should prevail:

1. The medical status of the player is ascertained by a physician and the health of the players is carefully supervised.

2. Activities for girls and women are planned

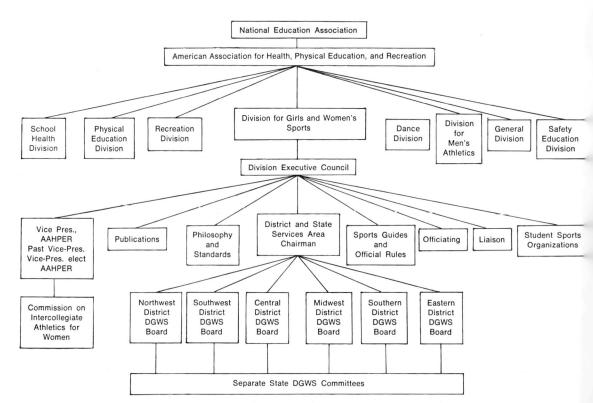

DGWS organizational chart. (From Philosophy & standards for girls' and women's sports, American Association for Health, Physical Education, and Recreation, 1969, p. 50.)

to meet their needs, not for the personal glorification of coaches and/or sponsoring organizations.

3. The salary, retention, and promotion of an instructor are not dependent upon the outcome of the games.

4. Qualified women teach, coach, and officiate

wherever and whenever possible, and in all cases the professional background and experience of the leader meet established standards.

5. Rules approved by DGWS are used.

6. Schedules do not exceed the ability and endurance relative to the maturity and

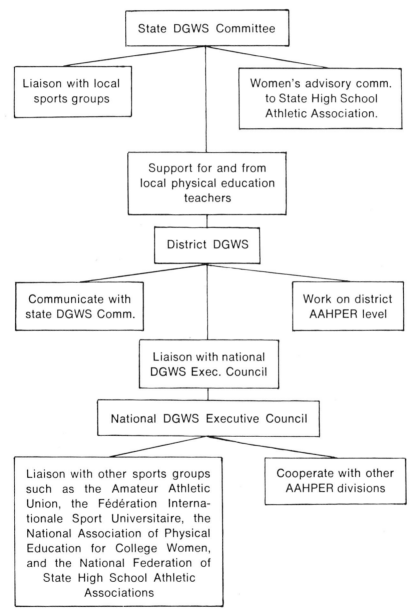

Relations of DGWS to other sports and policy-making groups. (From Philosophy and standards for girls' and women's sports, American Association for Health, Physical Education, and Recreation, 1969, p. 51.)

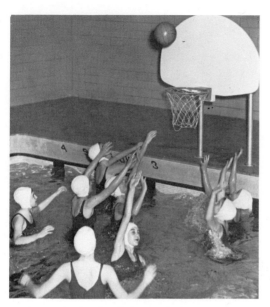

Junior high school. (Waterloo, Iowa.)

physiological conditioning of the participants. Standards for specific sports are defined by DGWS and appear in sports guides, published by the American Association for Health, Physical Education, and Recreation, 1201 16th St. N. W., Washington, D. C.

7. Sports activities for girls and women are scheduled independently from boys' and men's sports. Exceptions will occur when the activities and/or time and facilities are appropriate for both.

8. Girls and women may participate in appropriate corecreational activities or teams. Girls and women may not participate as members of boys and men's teams.

9. The program, including health insurance for players, is financed by budgeted school or organization funds rather than entirely by admission charges.

10. Provision is made by the school or organization for safe transportation by bonded carriers, with chaperones who are responsible to the sponsoring group.

In colleges and universities it is desirable that opportunities be provided for the highly skilled beyond the intramural program. Regulations for the conduct of collegiate competition have been developed by the National Joint Committee on Extramural Sports for College Women and are available from the committee for any specific sport activity. While the statements of NJCESCW

apply to approval for state-wide or wider geographical tournaments, the principles may also be applicable to or guide the conduct of local and district tournaments.

In addition to the standards previously listed, other standards pertinent to the colleges are:

1. The amount and kind of intercollegiate competition should be determined by the women's physical education department.

2. The financial arrangements relative to all intercollegiate sport events should be administered with the approval of the women's physical education department.

3. The time involved in relation to intercollegiate competition should not interfere with the academic program of the institution sponsoring the event and should not make excessive demands upon the participants' academic schedules.

4. All housing arrangements relative to visiting participants should be approved by the women's physical education department.*

The DGWS cooperates with many national sports organizations. This is becoming increasingly common as the desire for more desirable competitive sports experiences for girls and women becomes a part of our culture. A few of the cooperative relationships are Council for National Cooperation in Aquatics, Women's National Aquatics Forum, United States Field Hockey Association, United States Women's Lacrosse Association, United States Volleyball Association, International Joint Softball Rules Committee, National Federation of State High School Athletic Associations, Amateur Athletic Union, United States Track and Field Federation, United States Gymnastics Federation, United States Olympic Development Committee, Athletic and Recreation Federation for College Women, and the National Association for Physical Education of College Women.†

---

*Division for Girls' and Women's Sports: Philosophy and standards for girls and women's sports. Washington, D. C., 1969, AAHPER, pp. 34-35.

†Crawford, E.: DGWS cooperates with national sports organizations, Journal of Health, Physical Education, and Recreation 36:25, 1965.

Girls' and women's athletics are occupying an increasingly prominent role in the nation's schools and colleges. The programs appear to be well supervised and controlled and free of many of the abuses and problems associated with boys' and men's athletics. A large measure of the credit for developing such a sound program is due to the Division for Girls' and Women's Sports of the American Association for Health, Physical Education, and Recreation.

Criteria for the evaluation of programs in girls' and women's sports

The accompanying criteria have been established by the Division for Girls' and Women's Sports to assist administrators and others in determining if their program meets acceptable standards.

ATHLETIC ASSOCIATIONS

An individual school or college, by itself, finds it difficult to develop standards and

---

CRITERIA FOR EVALUATION*

Standards and guidelines established by the Division for Girls and Women's Sports should be used to evaluate program on local, regional, and national levels.

The sports program should be evaluated frequently according to criteria based on sound educational philosophy and scientific research.

Frequent evaluation of the program is necessary to ascertain if the objectives are being realized. The following list of criteria may be of help in this evaluation:

1. The administrator assumes responsibility for the realization of the values and objectives of the sports program.
2. Professionally qualified teachers and leaders are selected and delegated appropriate responsibility and authority to administer the program.
3. The objectives and policies which govern the sports program are determined by competent professional leaders.
4. The objectives of the program are concerned with the total growth and development of the individual.
5. Educational objectives take precedence over matters of expediency.
6. The educational and recreational aims of the school or sponsoring agency are realized through the sports program.
7. In all situations the spirit of fair play predominates.
8. The program is planned using knowledge based on current research.
9. The program is planned and conducted with primary concern for the welfare of the individual player.
10. The program is considered to be both worthwhile and enjoyable by the players and the leaders alike.
11. Sports experiences are so conducted that maximum values are realized by the participant.
12. Participants in sports activities have a voice in the planning and execution of the program.
13. The diversity within the program meets the needs of all age and skill levels.
14. Qualified women direct, coach, and officiate the program.
15. Trained officials are used in the program.
16. The most recent DGWS rules, standards, skills, and tactics of specific sports are used; where these are not specified, the leader employs professional judgment.
17. The participant meets her responsibility in perpetuating the spirit of good sportsmanship.
18. The total sports program includes instruction, intramurals, and extramurals.
19. Established DGWS standards and guidelines are used in frequent evaluations of the program.
20. Financing of the total sports program is included in the school recreational budget.

*From Division for Girls' and Women's Sports: Philosophy and standards of girls' and women's sports, Washington, D. C., 1969, American Association of Health, Physical Education, and Recreation, pp. 26-27.

control athletics in a sound educational manner. However, by uniting with other schools and colleges such a project is possible. This has been done on local, state, and national levels in the interest of better athletics for high schools and colleges. By establishing rules and procedures well in advance of playing seasons, the necessary control for conducting a sound athletic program is provided educators, coaches, and others. It aids them in resisting pressures of alumni, students, spectators, townspeople, and others who do not always have the best interests of the program in mind.

There are various types of athletic associations. The ones that are most prevalent in high schools and colleges are student athletic associations, local conferences or leagues, state high school athletic associations, National Federation of State High School Athletic Associations, National Collegiate Athletic Association, and various college conferences.

The student athletic association is an organization within a school that is designed to promote and participate in the conduct of the athletic program of that school. It is usually open to all students in attendance. Through the payment of fees it often helps to support the athletics program. Such associations are found in many of the high schools throughout the country. They can be very helpful in the development of a sound athletic program.

There are various associations, conferences, or leagues that bind together athletically several high schools within a particular geographic area. These are designed in the main to regulate and promote wholesome competition among the member schools. They usually draw up schedules, approve officials, handle disputes, and have general supervision over the athletic programs of the member schools.

The state high school athletic association that now exists in almost every state is a major influence in high school athletics. It

is open to all professionally accredited high schools within the state. It has a constitution, administrative officers to conduct the business, and a board of control. The number of members on the board of control varies usually from six to nine. Fees are usually paid to the association on a flat basis or according to the size of the school. In some states there are no fees, since the necessary revenue is derived from the gate receipts of tournament competition. State associations are interested in a sound program of athletic competition within the confines of the state. They concern themselves with the usual problems that have to do with athletics, such as rules of eligibility, officials, disputes, and similar items. They are interested in promoting good high school athletics, equalizing athletic competition, protecting participants, and guarding the health of players. They are an influence for good and have won the respect of educators in the various states.

The National Council of Secondary School Athletic Directors

The American Association for Health, Physical Education, and Recreation recently established the National Council of Secondary School Athletic Directors. The increased emphasis in sports and the important position of athletic directors in the nation's secondary schools seemed to warrant an association where increased services could be rendered to enhance the services given to the nation's youth. The membership in the National Council is open to members of the AAHPER who have primary responsibility in directing, administering, or coordinating interscholastic athletic programs. The purposes of the Council are as follows:

To improve the educational aspects of interscholastic athletics and their articulation in the total educational program

To foster high standards of professional proficiency and ethics

To improve understanding of athletics throughout the nation

To establish closer working relationships with related professional groups

To promote greater unity, good will, and fellowship among all members

To provide for an exchange of ideas

To assist and cooperate with existing state athletic directors' organizations

To make available to members special resource materials through publications, conferences, and consultant services

The National Federation of State High School Athletic Associations

The National Federation of State High School Athletic Associations was established in 1920 with five states participating. At the present time nearly all the states are members. The National Federation is particularly concerned with the control of interstate athletics. Its constitution states this purpose:

The object of this Federation shall be to protect and supervise the interstate athletic interests of the high schools belonging to the state associations, to assist in those activities of state associations which can best be operated on a nationwide scale, to sponsor meetings, publications and activities which will permit each state association to profit by the experience of all other member associations, and to coordinate the work so that waste effort and unnecessary duplication will be avoided.

The National Federation has been responsible for many improvements in athletics on a national basis, such as doing away with national tournaments and working toward a uniformity of standards.

The National Collegiate Athletic Association

The National Collegiate Athletic Association began in the early 1900's. The alarming number of football injuries and the fact that there was no national control of the game of football led to a conference of representatives of universities and colleges, primarily from the eastern section of the United States, on December 12, 1905. Preliminary plans were made for a national body to assist in the formulation of sound requirements for intercollegiate athletics, particularly football, and

the name Intercollegiate Athletic Association was suggested. At a meeting March 31, 1906, a constitution and bylaws were adopted and issued. On December 29, 1910, the name of the association was changed to National Collegiate Athletic Association. The purposes of the NCAA are to uphold the principle of institutional control of all collegiate sports; to maintain a uniform code of amateurism in conjunction with sound eligibility rules, scholarship requirements, and good sportsmanship; to promote and assist in the expansion of intercollegiate and intramural sports; to formulate, copyright, and publish the official rules of play (in eleven sports); to sponsor and supervise regional and national meets and tournaments for member institutions; to preserve athletic records; and to serve as headquarters for collegiate athletic matters of national import.

National Association of Intercollegiate Athletics

Also on the college and university levels is the National Association of Intercollegiate Athletics, which has a large membership, especially among the smaller schools. This organization has recently become affiliated with the American Association for Health, Physical Education, and Recreation.

The National Junior College Athletic Association

The National Junior College Athletic Association is an organization of junior colleges who sponsor athletic programs. It has nineteen regional offices with an elected regional director for each. Regional business matters are carried on within the framework of the constitution and bylaws of the parent organization. The regional directors hold an annual legislative assembly in Hutchinson, Kansas, are run by an executive committee, and determine the policies, program, and procedures for the organization. The *Juco Review* is the official publication of the organization.

Standing and special committees are appointed each year to cover special items and problems that develop. Membership, which costs $75.00 annually, entitles each member to the services provided by the NJCAA.

National championships are conducted in such sports as basketball, cross country, football, wrestling, baseball, track and field, golf, and tennis. National invitation events are also conducted in such activities as soccer, swimming, and gymnastics.

The NJCAA is affiliated with the National Federation of State High School Athletic Associations and the National Association of Intercollegiate Athletics. It is also a member of the United States Track and Field Federation, Basketball Federation, the United States Collegiate Sports Council, United States Olympic Committee, United States Gymnastics Federation, National Basketball Committee, and American Association for Health, Physical Education, and Recreation.

Some of the services offered by the NJCAA to its members include an insurance plan for athletics, recognition in official records, publications, film library, and participation in events sponsored by the association.

Other organizations

In higher education, there are in addition many leagues, conferences, and associations formed by a limited number of schools for athletic competition. Examples are the "Ivy League" and the "Big Ten Conference." These associations regulate athletic competition among their members and settle problems that may arise in connection with such competition.

EXTRA PAY FOR EXTRA SERVICES*

One of the most popular topics for discussion at school meetings in recent years

*National Congress of Parents and Teachers: PTA guide to what's happening in education, New York, 1965, Scholastic Book Services, pp. 203-210.

is: Should teachers receive extra pay for extra services? Parents, taxpayers, and school boards have been trying to decide whether or not athletics, coaches, band leaders, dramatics supervisors, publication consultants, and others who do work in addition to their teaching load should receive additional compensation for such services.

A sensible solution to this problem is essential to the good morale of a school staff. Besides, since school systems are demanding more and more services, some policy must be formulated to cover the extra duties that are being heaped on the shoulders of our teachers.

To help solve the extra-pay dilemma, many surveys, studies, and conferences have been conducted during recent years. The National Education Association, the American Association for Health, Physical Education, and Recreation, several state organizations, local boards of education, and other groups have been busy gathering data on the problem. They have found that many communities give extra pay for extra services. However, this is by no means standard procedure.

My own study has shown that practices in selected school systems across the country generally fall into five groups:

Extra pay is provided for all school activities that require work beyond the normal school day.

Extra pay is given only in the area of athletics.

Release time is provided for extra work.

Supplemental teachers are hired.

All school activities are considered part of the normal teaching load, and no additional pay is given.

Practices across the country

The public schools in one school system in South Dakota pay for all extra activities. The assistant football coach receives $250 a year and the ticket manager, $150. Intramural activities pay $50 per sport. The band director gets $600; the supervisor of school publications, $250; the staff member in charge of the school radio program, $175; and the printing instructor, $250. In a school system in Tennessee extra pay is given at varied rates, ranging all the way from $15 a month for a special teacher of spastic children to $75 a month for a senior high school coach.

In a community on Long Island, New York, extra pay for extra work is based on five criteria: the time required for the activity, the number of students involved, the pressure to which a teacher may be subjected by public performances, the closeness with which the activity is related to the curriculum, and the extent to which the activity is a teaching rather than a supervisory or an advisory function. On the basis of these criteria, each extracurricular activity is placed in one of five categories, each carrying its own rate of pay. The pay ranges from $360 to $880 a year for the various kinds of activity.

The salary policies for coaching selected sports in Class AA schools in the state of Iowa are reported as follows*:

1. All but one of the assigned coaches was given monetary compensation for coaching.
2. Eleven schools reported that they gave an extra free period to some of the head coaches during the season in which they coached.
3. Sixty-nine out of the seventy-one schools have a salary schedule for coaching.
4. Of the schools reporting, 73% indicated they used the lock-step method of payment, 13%, the percentage method of payment, and 11%, the annual increment method of payment.
5. Eight schools permit coaches to come into their system on advance coaching salary steps as a result of past experience.
6. Coaches' salaries vary from school to school and sport to sport.
7. Five schools reported payments to coaches on a merit basis.
8. Most schools pay assistant coaches.

---

*Mauro, D. R.: Salary policies for teaching of selected sports in class AA schools of Iowa, Iowa Journal of Health, Physical Education, and Recreation, May, 1969.

The State College Area School District in Pennsylvania has established a rating method for extra pay for extra duty that involves nine criteria. An illustrated version of this rating method is seen in Table 10-1.

Many schools faced with the extra-pay problem pay for coaching duties only. A city in Utah follows this practice. There the annual pay for senior high school athletic coaches is $474 more than that of other teachers with similar training and experience, except for teachers of special education, who receive the same rate as coaches. In a Kentucky city some athletic coaches receive as much as $800 in extra compensation, but the board of education has not supplemented the salaries of teachers in charge of band, dramatics, and other activities. A few individual schools give some of these teachers part of the proceeds from plays and other activities that they supervise. A city in New York pays its athletic instructors supplementary salaries ranging from $600 for the football coach to $3.00 an hour for athletic league coaches in grade schools.

Some schools throughout the country do not give extra pay. Instead, release time is provided. As Benjamin C. Willis, former superintendent of schools in Chicago, pointed out: "In our salary schedule we do not provide extra pay for extra services. We make an exception for teachers who work beyond the normal school day—that is, those who have additional classes because of the shortage of space. We pay extra compensation for this extra time. In regard to the coaching of athletics, we adjust the teaching schedule to compensate for this work."

In one city in California, junior college supplemental teachers are hired to take on certain activities. The supervisor of personnel research reports that the supplemental teachers are assigned to an afterschool activity that is not part of the full day's program and that requires up to 40 hours a month. The activity may be in drama, music, stagecraft, journalism, yearbook,

Table 10-1. Rating method — extra pay for extra duty*†

I. All athletics and nonclass-related activities

Criteria	A	B	C	D	E	F	G	H	I		
Possible rating scores	1-10	1-10	1-5	1-5	1-5	1-20	1-20	1-5	1-5		
Weighted value	4	4	3	2	2	3	2	1	2		
Example	5	3	2	2	0	0	2	0	0	Raw rating	
Activity xx (rating X value)	20	12	6	4	0	0	4	0	0	Weighted rating 46	Final rounded 45

CRITERIA			
	A&B: Hours—550-600	rating 10	C: Students
	500-549	9	150 pupils or more 5
A *Hours*—total out of school	450-499	8	100-149 4
B *Weekend*—vacation hours—Friday 3—Sunday	400-449	7	50- 99 3
C *Students*—directly involved	350-399	6	25- 49 2
D *Experience*—training necessary	300-349	5	under 25 1
E *Injury risk*—to pupil (other than normal classroom risk)	250-299	4	
F *Pressures*—crowd, spectator, community, faculty, administration	200-249	3	
G *Responsibility*—equipment, facilities, funds	150-199	2	
H *Environmental influence*—outdoor, indoor weather conditions	100-149	1	
I *Travel supervision*—bus trips, etc.	under 100	.5	

II. Rating method—class-related activities

Criteria	A	B	C	D	E	F	G	H	I
Possible ratings	1-10	1-10	1-5	1-5	1-5	1-20	1-20	1-5	1-5
Weighted value	4	4	1	1	2	1	1	1	2

*From Solley, P. M.: Extra pay for extra duty, Today's Education, **58:**54, 1969.
†State College Area School District guide, "Extra Pay for Extra Duty."

speech, or other areas. Such teachers receive $6.16 an hour.

Finally, there is the great mass of schools where coaching, band, orchestra, and similar activities are considered part of the normal teaching load and no additional pay is provided. The school system of a community in Missouri is typical of this group. These schools "believe in paying all teachers well," writes a member of the school administration. "In turn, they expect teachers to do the work for which they are hired. No . . . teacher has been paid above schedule. . . . A full explanation of the situation is given at the time of employment." In a town in Connecticut, pressure for extra pay has been exerted by coaches and other groups. The board of

education has held, however, that their duties are part of their regular job.

Roundup of suggestions

The many-faceted problem of extra pay and extra services concerns a large number of educators, administrators, and laymen. Various ideas of solving it have been advanced, of which the following are perhaps the most pertinent.

The educational program in all school systems should rest on a sound financial base. Teachers' salaries should be sufficient to provide a comfortable living. Faculty members should not have to seek extra work in school or elsewhere to make ends meet.

If possible, there should be enough staff

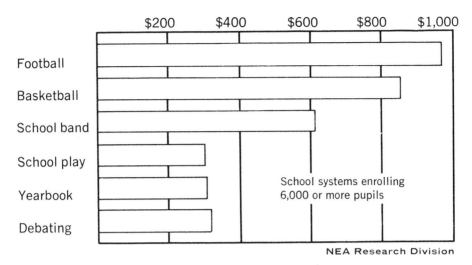

Average maximum annual supplements 1967-1968 for selected pupil-participating activities. (From NEA Research Bulletin **46**:79, 1968.)

members in every school to make it unnecessary for anyone to take on an extra load.

Extra work means loss of efficiency. A teacher can perform at his best for only a certain number of hours a day, then the law of diminishing returns sets in.

All teachers work beyond the school day. They prepare teaching assignments, grade papers, keep records, and take on other professional responsibilities. It is difficult, therefore, to determine what is "extra work."

Extra work in education is not comparable to extra work in business or industry. Professional ethics dictate that positions in public service cannot be categorized in the same way as can those involving only personal gain.

Teaching loads should be equalized as far as possible. If inequalities exist that cannot be corrected through extra staff, extra pay is justified.

Where extra pay is provided, it should be distributed equitably for all who work beyond a normal school day. Teachers should perform extra work only in areas where they are qualified.

The most acceptable form of compensation for additional duties appears to be extra salary. The practice of release time does not seem to meet the wishes of most teachers.

The problem of extra pay for extra service is not an easy one to resolve. Convincing arguments can be given for or against the views that have been presented. Since local needs differ, a nationwide solution cannot be prescribed. However, any community that is wrestling with this problem may well be guided by the foregoing points. They represent the thinking of many teachers and administrators throughout the country.

Educators state their views

Thurston, a consultant on teacher salaries and negotiations of the Office of Professional Development and Welfare of the National Education Association, proposes an index relationship in respect to extra pay for extra services. This reflects the time spent in the activity as a ratio to the basic schedule. The formula, shown on p. 276 shows how this would work.

EXTRA PAY FOR EXTRA SERVICES*

$$\frac{\text{Number of hours spent in activity per day}}{\text{Number of hours in school day}} \times \frac{\text{Length of activity per school year (days, weeks, months)}}{\text{Length of normal school year}} = \text{Basic time index}$$

Example 1.   High school basketball coach who spends 2 hours per day with his squad. Season lasts 5 months in 10-month year with an 8-hour day.

$$2/8 \times 5/10 = \text{basic index} = .125$$

Example 2.   High school chemistry teacher spends 1 hour, twice a month with science club. School operates on 8-hour day and 200-day year.

$$1/8 \times 20/200 = \text{basic index} = .0125$$

These time indices may be applied on a B.A. base, base of degree held, step on B.A. scale, or step on teacher's basic salary scale.

*From Thurston, J. P.: Secondary school athletic administration: a new look, Report of the Second National Conference on Secondary School Athletic Administration, Washington, D. C., January 12-15, 1969, pp. 82-83.

A dean of the School of Education, Syracuse University, believes that ideally the teacher should be released from teaching duties to offset extraschool services, "thus maintaining a balanced load and a uniform salary schedule. In many school situations the administration is not in a position to do this and must load certain teachers . . . with extra duties, including dramatics, band, athletics, supervision of school paper, and so on. Where teachers are assigned such responsibilities over and above the regular teaching load, certainly extra compensation should be provided. This is only fair to those who are called upon to carry added responsibilities."

A professor of elementary education, Graduate School of Education, Indiana University, thinks that "the services would be part of the regular load of the people directing them. If these activities are added to an already full load the teacher ought to be paid extra at a rate comparable to his regular salary. This is an area where people can be easily exploited unless a definite policy exists to protect them."

And from an executive secretary emeritus of the American Association of School Administrators comes this statement: "Under ordinary circumstances the assignment of any teacher should be a full load, but not an extra one. In general, then, there should be no extra pay for extra work. When the situation, manpower-wise, is such that members of the regular staff must temporarily accept an unreasonable load, they should be compensated for this assignment. . . . Regular overtime assignments reflect a condition of understaffing, and the best answer is not that of overloading and extra pay but of additional staff."

The answer to the important question—Should teachers receive extra pay for extra services?—must be resolved in each community. A satisfactory solution, however, requires these essentials:

The educational program must rest on a sound financial foundation.

Salaries should compensate adequately for the work performed.

As far as possible, normal loads should be assigned to all teachers. Whenever teaching loads cannot be held to a desirable level, the teacher should be provided with extra compensation.

CONCLUDING STATEMENT ON ATHLETICS

The standards for athletics at school and college levels have been clearly stated. There should be no doubt in any individual's mind as to the types of interscholastic and intercollegiate programs that are sound educationally and in the best interests of students who will participate in them. It is the responsibility of administrators and others concerned with such programs to implement the various standards that have been established. *In every case, it is not a question of deemphasis but a question of reemphasis along educational lines. Good leadership will make the interscholastic program a force for good in education that has no equal.*

Athletics are a part of the total physical education program. The objectives that have been stated earlier in this book for physical education also apply to inter-school and intercollegiate athletics. The administrator can evaluate his or her program in terms of the extent to which the listed objectives are being achieved. There should be no question as to where a school stands.

The Educational Policies Commission Report on School Athletics* provides guidelines for physical educators, coaches, administrators, and other individuals interested in a sound school athletic program. This report contains 100 questions that can be used to evaluate any school athletic program. *The information in this report represents the ideals toward which all educators should be striving.*

Questions and exercises

1. Develop a set of standards that could be used to appraise an athletic program at the high school or college level.
2. Have a debate on the question: Resolved: that all gate receipts for interscholastic athletic contests should be abolished.
3. Write a profile of what you consider to be the ideal coach.
4. As a Director of Athletics what plans would you have to make for a season of play in basketball? Outline in detail.
5. What are some essential points to keep in mind in respect to each of the following: (a) contracts, (b) officials, (c) protests and forfeitures, (d) game management, (e) schedules, (f) awards, (g) records, and (h) medical examinations?
6. Describe in detail how athletic insurance works.
7. As a Director of Athletics, what administrative policy would you recommend in respect to each of the following: (a) gate receipts, (b) tournaments and championships, (c) eligibility, (d) scholarships, (e) recruiting, (f) proselyting, and (g) scouting?
8. What is the role of the Athletic Association in the conduct of athletics?
9. Develop a set of guiding administrative principles for girls' athletics.
10. Write an essay of 500 words on the topic: Desirable sports competition for children.
11. Debate the following question: Do national playoffs in sports constitute a desirable activity for children under 12 years of age?
12. What practical suggestions can you make for eliminating the "big business" aspects of intercollegiate athletics?
13. Read the Educational Policies Commission report on "School Athletics" and give a report to the class.

Reading assignment in *Administrative Dimensions of Health and Physical Education Programs, Including Athletics:* Chapter 8, Selections 39 to 47.

Selected references

American Association for Health, Physical Education, and Recreation: Administrative problems in health education, physical education, and recreation, Washington, D. C., 1953, The Association, Area V.

American Association for Health, Physical Education, and Recreation: Coaches handbook—a practical guide for high school coaches, Washington, D. C., 1960, The Association.

American Association for Health, Physical Education, and Recreation: Approaches to problems of public school administration in health, physical education and recreation, Proceedings of the Sixth National Conference of City and

---

*Educational Policies Commission: School athletics — problems and policies, Washington, D. C., 1954, National Education Association.

County Directors, Washington, D. C., 1968, The Association.

American Association for Health, Physical Education, and Recreation: Secondary school athletic administration, Washington, D. C., 1969, The Association.

Bucher, C. A., editor: Methods and materials in physical education and recreation, St. Louis, 1954, The C. V. Mosby Co.

Bucher, C. A.: Foundations of physical education, ed. 5, St. Louis, 1968, The C. V. Mosby Co.

Bucher, C. A., and Cohane, T.: Little league baseball can hurt your boy, Look, Aug. 11, 1953, p. 74.

Bucher, C. A., and Dupee, R. K., Jr.: Athletics schools and colleges, New York, 1965, The Center for Applied Research in Education, Inc. (The Library of Education).

Bucher, C. A., Koenig, C., and Barnhard, M.: Methods and materials for secondary school physical education, ed. 3, St. Louis, 1970, The C. V. Mosby Co.

Division for Girls' and Women's Sports: Philosophy and standards for girls and women's sports, Washington, D. C., 1969, American Association for Health, Physical Education, and Recreation.

Educational Policies Commission: School athletics —problems and policies, Washington, D. C., 1954, National Education Association.

Forsythe, C. E.: The administration of high school athletics, Englewood Cliffs, N. J., 1962, Prentice-Hall, Inc.

George, J. F., and Lehmann, H. A.: School athletic administration, New York, 1966, Harper and Row, Publishers.

Grieve, A. W.: Directing high school athletics, Englewood Cliffs, N. J., 1963, Prentice-Hall, Inc.

Healey, W. A.: The administration of high school athletic events, Danville, Ill., 1961, The Interstate Printers & Publishers, Inc.

Hixson, C. G.: The administration of interscholastic athletics, New York, 1967, J. Lowell Pratt and Co.

Joint Committee on Athletic Competition for Children of Elementary and Junior High School Age: Desirable athletic competition for children, Washington, D. C., 1952, American Association for Health, Physical Education, and Recreation.

Ray, R. F.: Trends in intercollegiate athletics, Journal of Health, Physical Education, and Recreation 36:21, 1965.

Reed, W. R.: Big time athletics' commitment to education, Journal of Health, Physical Education, and Recreation 34:29, 1963.

Rogers, F. R.: The future of interscholastic athletics, New York, 1929, Bureau of Publications, Teachers College, Columbia University.

Rule books for all boys' sports. Available from the National Federation of State High School Athletic Associations, 7 S. Dearborn St., Chicago, Ill.

Rule books for all girls' sports. Available from the Division for Girls' and Women's Sports, American Association for Health, Physical Education, and Recreation, 1201 16th St. N.W., Washington, D. C. 20036.

The administration of physical fitness programs requires an understanding of the nature and scope of fitness and also of some of the historical background responsible for the current physical fitness emphasis. School and college physical educators and health educators will render a greater service to their students when they become more knowledgeable about physical fitness.

Fitness is the ability of the individual to live a full and balanced life. It involves physical, mental, emotional, social, and spiritual factors and the capacity for their wholesome expression. All are closely interwoven into the fabric of the whole person.

The totally fit person has a healthy and happy outlook on life. He satisfies such basic needs as physical well-being, love, affection, security, and self-respect. He likes people and lives happily with them. As he grows older, he develops a maturity that is characterized by submersion of self and an interest in serving humanity. He makes peace with his God and believes in and exemplifies high ethical standards.

A fit person is one who (1) *physically* has a strong organic base, exhibits vigor, is active, is skilled in some physical activities, and enjoys a sense of well-being; (2) *socially* recognizes the principle once stated by Justice Stone that "no man can live unto himself alone" and, therefore, understands and respects the rights of others, likes people, practices service above self, and makes satisfactory group adjustments; (3) *mentally* has a healthy outlook on life, thinks independently and constructively, has good judgment, is resourceful, and wants to be fit; and (4) *emotionally* has stability and self-control, faces reality in an honest manner, and has high ethical standards.

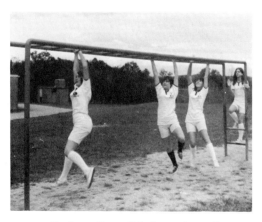

Henderson County Schools, Hendersonville, N. C.

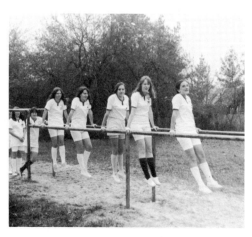

Henderson County Schools, Hendersonville, N. C.

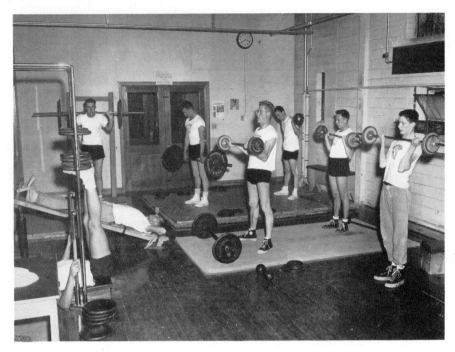

Weight lifting in the required physical education program at Washington State College helps to build physical fitness.

PHYSICAL FITNESS

Physical fitness, as one aspect of total fitness, involves three important concepts. It is related to the tasks the person must perform, his potential for physical effort, and the relationship of his physical fitness to his total self. The same degree of physical fitness is not necessary for everyone. It should be sufficient to meet the requirements of the job, plus a little extra as a reserve for emergencies. A football player or a foot soldier in the Army needs a different type of physical fitness from that required by a train conductor or a stenographer. The question of "fitness for what" must always be asked. Furthermore, discussion of the physical fitness of a person must be within the context of his own human resources and not to those of others. It depends on his potentialities in the light of his own physical makeup. Finally, physical fitness cannot be considered by itself but, instead, as it is affected by mental, emotional, and spiritual factors as well. Human beings function as a whole and not in segmented parts.

COMPONENTS OF PHYSICAL FITNESS

The attempt to define and break down the term *physical fitness* has led to the identification of certain specific components that collectively make up physical fitness. Such factors as resistance to disease, or the ability of the body to keep its disease-fighting equipment in good shape; muscular strength, or the ability to exert force against a resistance; muscular endurance, or the ability to repeat activities involving resistance; and cardiorespiratory endurance, or the ability of the circulatory and respiratory systems to support activities requiring sustained effort, such as distance running or swimming—these make up the components of physical fitness set forth by most authorities.

Larson and Yocom[*] list ten components of physical fitness—namely, resistance to disease, muscular strength and endurance, cardiovascular-respiratory endurance, muscular power, flexibility, speed, agility, coordination, balance, and accuracy. McCloy and Young[†] list components such as the speed of muscular contraction, dynamic energy, ability to change direction, agility, dead weight, and flexibility. Cureton[‡] appraises physical fitness in terms of physique and organic efficiency, which he says implies anatomic and physiologic soundness, and adds a component that he calls "motor fitness." This motor fitness, according to Cureton, includes endurance, power, strength, agility, flexibility, and balance.

Morehouse and Miller[§] include a psychologic component that to them implies possession of necessary emotional stability, drive or motivation, intelligence, and educability.

As can be seen from these statements of leaders in the field of physical education, there is not complete agreement as to what physical fitness is and what its components are. Research is needed to obtain more valid evidence about this important aspect of health and physical education work.

DEVELOPING PHYSICAL FITNESS

The question of how to obtain physical fitness is a controversial point. Since we do not know exactly what it is and what its components may be, the answer as to how one obtains it is also somewhat nebulous. We do know, however, that heredity plays an important role. The form and structure of the body is determined largely by parents. Heredity sets certain direction and limitations to development. Good nutrition is essential. Good health habits—such as having proper rest, relaxation, and sleep and otherwise providing good care for the body—are necessary. The important contributions of mental, emotional, spiritual, and social health must be considered. In addition, there is increasing recognition of the importance of physical activity. The value of exercise in developing many of the components of physical fitness and, in addition, in contributing to mental, social, and emotional well-being is an important factor.

Up to now there has been a reserved caution in regard to the benefits of exercise, with many persons feeling that it is unimportant as a contributor to the fit individual. However, research is proving the value of physical activity in physical fitness. A statement from Steinhaus[*] is a fitting conclusion to this section:

The muscles are by weight about 43 percent of the average adult male human body. They expend a large portion of all the kinetic energy of the adult body. The cortical centers for the voluntary muscles extend over most of the lateral psychic zones of the brain, so that their culture (the culture of muscles) is brain building. They are in a most intimate and peculiar sense organs of the will. They have built all the roads, cities, and machines in the world, written all of the books, spoken all the words, and, in fact, done everything that man has accomplished with matter. If they are undeveloped or grow flabby, the dreadful chasm between good intentions and their execution is liable to appear and widen. Character might be in a sense defined as a plexus of motor habits.

Methods of developing physical fitness

Some of the methods of utilizing physical activity in the development of physical

[*]Larson, L. A., and Yocom, R.: Measurement and evaluation in physical, health and recreation education, St. Louis, 1951, The C. V. Mosby Co., p. 162.

[†]McCloy, C. H., and Young, N. D.: Tests and measurements in health and physical education, ed. 3, New York, 1954, Appleton-Century-Crofts, pp. 4-5.

[‡]Cureton, T. K.: Physical fitness appraisal and guidance, St. Louis, 1947, The C. V. Mosby Co., p. 21.

[§]Morehouse, L. E., and Miller, A. T., Jr.: Physiology of exercise, ed. 5, St. Louis, 1967, The C. V. Mosby Co., p. 268.

[*]Steinhaus, A. H.: Health and physical fitness from the standpoint of the physiologist, Journal of Health and Physical Education 7:225, 1936.

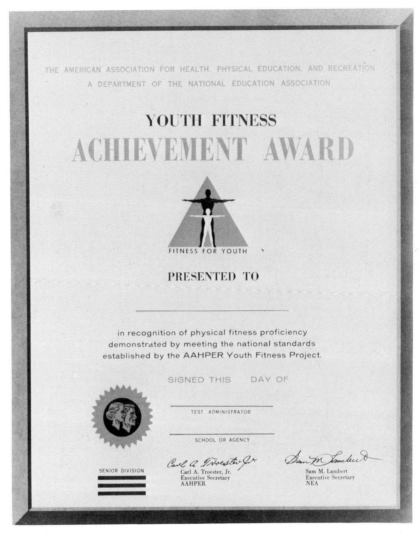

Youth Fitness Achievement Award. (Courtesy American Association for Health, Physical Education, and Recreation.)

fitness include circuit training, interval training, weight training, weight lifting, isometric exercises, and the Exer-Genie.

Circuit training involves a series of exercises, usually around ten, that are performed in a progressive manner. Physical activity is performed at each of the ten stations. The training is done on a time basis and progress is checked against the clock. The length and nature of activities performed can be changed as the performer becomes stronger.

Interval training requires physical activity involving distance to build endurance, an increase of speed, an increase in the number of repetitions, and the rest or recovery period. As the performer becomes stronger the recovery interval is reduced. Its main contribution is in the area of cardiovascular endurance development.

Weight training utilizes resistance exercises, taking into consideration the number of repetitions of resistance exercises and also the duration and intensity of the exercises being performed.

Weight lifting involves the lifting of

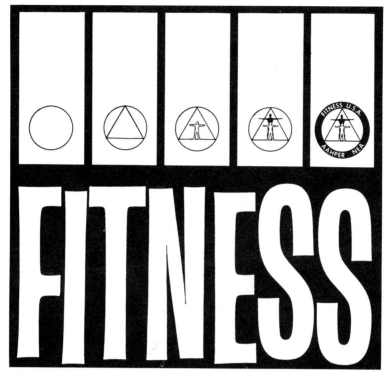

Fitness. (Courtesy American Association for Health, Physical Education, and Recreation.)

weights and usually involves only a few repetitions.

Isometric exercises are exercises whereby muscles contract and build up tension and hold without any shortening or lengthening. (*Static* or *isometric* is derived from the words *iso*, meaning same, and *metric*, meaning length.) They are valuable in developing strength.

In *calisthenic exercises* the muscles contract so that they shorten and the ends are brought together (concentric), or the muscles lengthen and the ends go away from the center, as in the beginning of a pull-up when one lowers himself into a hanging position (eccentric) (isotonic).

The *Exer-Genie* can utilize either isometric or isotonic exercises. It is an instrument sold commercially that involves rope and handles. The amount of strength required to pull the ropes in various positions can be adjusted, thus enabling a progressive development of strength and endurance.

HISTORICAL BACKGROUND OF CURRENT PHYSICAL FITNESS EMPHASIS

The subject of fitness is not new to the American educational system. There have been numerous times during the educational history of this country when educators have been called upon to upgrade the fitness of American youth. World Wars I and II both caused the pendulum to swing toward more emphasis in this direction.

During the past few years there has been a renewed stress on the subject of fitness. Results of some physical fitness tests have revealed the softness of American children and youth as compared to children and youth in other countries. Although some of these tests have been criticized by many physical education leaders as not possessing validity, they have stirred up considerable interest in the area of physical fitness. The information forthcoming from these tests caught the ears of the President of

NAME _____

SCHOOL _____ / _____ Entrance Date

SCHOOL _____ / _____ Entrance Date

SCHOOL _____ / _____ Entrance Date

PRIMARY WASHINGTON MOTOR FITNESS TEST: KEY: S = Score; P = Points; R = Rating

RATING: S = Superior; G = Good; A = Average; BA = Below Average; NI = Needs Improvement

AGE	POWER Standing Broadjump			STRENGTH & ENDURANCE									SPEED 30 Yard Dash			PHYSICAL FITNESS		
				Bench Push Ups			Curl Up			Squat Jump								
	S	P	R	S	P	R	S	P	R	S	P	R	S	P	R	P		R
GRADE I																		
Fall																		
Repeat																		
Spring																		
GRADE II																		
Fall																		
Repeat																		
Spring																		
GRADE III																		
Fall																		
Repeat																		
Spring																		

PFI (OREGON SIMPLIFICATION)   AAHPER FITNESS TEST KEY S = Score; % = Percentile

	Age	Hgt.	Wgt.	Leg Lift	Back Lift	Push Up	Pull Up	PFI	Stdg. BJ.		50 yd. Dash		40 yard Shuttle Run		Softball Throw		Wall Volley	
									S	%	S	%	S	%	S	%	S	%
GRADE IV																		
Fall																		
Repeat																		
Spring																		
GRADE V																		
Fall																		
Repeat																		
Spring																		
GRADE VI																		
Fall																		
Repeat																		
Spring																		

-2-

PFI (OREGON SIMPLIFICATION)

AAHPER FITNESS TEST Key: S = Score; % = Percentile

	Age	Hgt.	Wgt.	Leg Lift	Back Lift	Push Up	Pull Up	PFI	Stdg. BJ. S	%	50 Yard Dash S	%	40 Yard Shuttle Run S	%	600 Yard Run S	%	Pull Ups S	%	Sit Ups S	%
GRADE VII																				
Fall																				
Repeat																				
Spring																				
GRADE VIII																				
Fall																				
Repeat																				
Spring																				
GRADE IX																				
Fall																				
Repeat																				
Spring																				
GRADE X																				
2nd Test																				
3rd Test																				
GRADE XI																				
Follow Up																				
GRADE XII																				
Follow Up																				

LIFETIME SPORTS PROFICIENCY

Sport	Date Listed	Signature of Instructor

DEVELOPMENTAL CLASSES

Grade Level _____ Date _____ PFI _____

Grade Level _____ Date _____ PFI _____

Grade Level _____ Date _____ PFI _____

Grade Level _____ Date _____ PFI _____

Grade Level _____ Date _____ PFI _____

Cumulative physical fitness record, Broadfront Program, used at Ellensburg Public Schools, Ellensburg, Wash.

the United States, with the result that a program of action was established in high government circles.

A President's Conference on Fitness of American Youth, held at the United States Naval Academy, Annapolis, Maryland, June 18-19, 1956, initiated a government-sponsored program in fitness that was destined to influence considerably the fields of health education and physical education. It was attended by 150 leaders in sports, education, medicine, public relations, government, and other areas. Most of the conferees were presidents, directors, or other top officials of organizations interested in the fitness of American youth. At the closing session of the conference the Vice-President announced that a President's Council on Physical Fitness, composed of members of the Cabinet, would be established to help improve the mental and physical health of the nation's young people. The President also announced that a President's Citizens' Advisory Committee on the Fitness of American Youth would be established. These committees have been functioning since their formation. The Advisory Committee, according to the President, "is to examine and explore the facts and, thereafter, to alert America on what can and should be done to reach the much-desired goal of a happier, healthier, and more totally fit youth in America."

A summary of some of the recommendations resulting from group discussions at this conference shows the challenge that fitness has for the schools:

1. There is a need for more research.
2. An agency or commission on fitness for American youth should be created.
3. Much is being done at the present time for the fitness of American youth. However, it is not enough and what is being done is very poorly coordinated.
4. Youth must be involved in much of the planning.
5. Programs must be fitted to the needs of the individual child and they must reach *all* the children.
6. Better school health examinations are needed.
7. The fitness of this nation is based on the fitness of its people. If there is something we need and know we need—this nation should have it!
8. There should be more and better leadership.
9. Leaders should themselves believe in fitness and provide a fitting example for the youth of this country.
10. Community leadership should be drawn from schools, recreation agencies, parents, law enforcement agencies, labor, management, youth groups, and the whole gamut of community life.
11. Higher salaries and other inducements for attracting qualified leadership into this work should be provided.
12. Families should make the best possible use of their own resources. Home space should be provided for children's play.
13. School facilities should receive maximum use. Other facilities, such as camps, fairgrounds, parks, etc., should also be used.
14. Foundations should be urged to contribute to the support of fitness endeavors.
15. Colleges and universities and mass communication media can help gain public support.
16. Parents must be impressed with the importance of taking an active interest in fitness of children—spending time with them, teach sportsmanship, loyalty, spirit, etc.
17. Youth must be sold on importance of being physically fit.
18. Fitness programs should begin in the home, and all members of the family should engage in these activities.
19. The schools do not represent the only facet of community life that should have a role in building fitness—churches, social agencies, veterans groups, government agencies, sports groups, and others can play an important part.
20. Girls should receive as much attention as boys.
21. Greater financial support is needed for better and larger programs.

The present administration has emphasized the role of the schools and colleges in physical fitness. The recommendations of the President's Council on Physical Fitness and Sports are discussed later in this chapter.

PHYSICAL ACHIEVEMENT AND THE SCHOOLS

According to the President's Council on Physical Fitness and Sports much progress has been made during the 1960's in improving the physical achievement standards of American youth—for example: 9.2 million children are participating in school physical activity programs; four out of every five pupils now successfully pass standardized physical fitness tests (only two out of three passed in 1961); 68% of all schools have strengthened their physical activity programs; the number of parochial schools providing physical education instruction has doubled; seventeen states have raised their school physical education requirements; and teaching positions for health and physical education have increased by 27%—school enrollments have increased 11%.

Although much progress has been made in recent years, there is much left to be done—for example: 14% of children in school today do not participate in any physical activity program, and an additional 27% participate only 1 or 2 days per week; only four schools in ten provide physical education programs 5 days per week; and 23% of the schools have administered the American Association of Health, Physical Education, and Recreation seven-item physical achievement test, but on this test only 57% of the boys and 51% of the girls were reported to have scored "satisfactory" on all items.

The charts on pp. 290 and 292 reflect a comparison of American youngsters tested in 1958 and their counterparts tested in 1965. The statistics reflect a general improvement over the years.

WHAT SCHOOLS AND COLLEGES CAN DO

Education in its broadest sense means preparation for life. It should help each in-

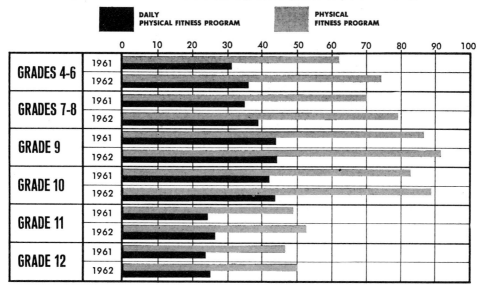

U. S. OFFICE OF EDUCATION SURVEY

The following findings are based on a scientific sampling of the public, private and church-related schools. Every effort was exerted to maintain a proper balance between these various types of schools, between schools of various sizes and between the various instructional levels (elementary, secondary and combined).

Pupil participation on physical fitness programs. (Courtesy The Advertising Council, Inc., New York, N. Y.)

dividual to become all he is capable of being. Therefore, it is inexorably tied in with fitness. Education must be concerned with developing in each individual optimum health, vitality, emotional stability, social consciousness, knowledge, wholesome attitudes, and spiritual and moral qualities. Only as it accomplishes this task will it achieve its destiny in the American way of life.

Schools and colleges have the responsibility for providing many opportunities for understanding and developing fitness. Of all the agencies involved in carrying out the President's fitness program, the schools and colleges are the focal point. The fact that some 60 million children and youth can be reached through them is an important reason for recognizing their worth. The schools and colleges also have the needed facilities and their teachers are trained for carrying out such a program. The school and college can instill children and youth with a desire for fitness. Education can likewise equip youngsters with the necessary tools to attain and maintain fitness throughout life. Their qualified teachers can also provide leadership in community programs that have valuable contributions to make.

The schools and colleges should be fitness conscious. Programs must be so constituted that experiences and services contribute to fitness. This means that health knowledge, attitudes, and practices are stressed; that protective health services are provided; that physical activities are available to and engaged in by *all*—not just the few who are skilled; that necessary facilities are provided; that the environment is conducive to proper growth and development; that experiences in every area stress proper social and ethical behavior.

Leadership in the schools and colleges should exemplify fitness—fitness is the responsibility of all disciplines and all teachers and staff. It should permeate the entire program and all persons connected with it.

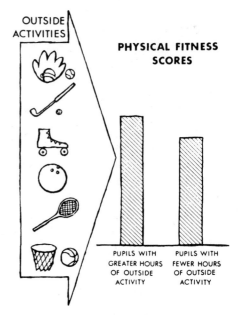

Those students who participated more in activities outside the school had higher fitness scores than those pupils with fewer hours of physical activity outside the school. (Physical fitness achievement in selected physical education programs, Albany, 1965, The University of the State of New York.)

It is not the responsibility of only one area and just a few people.

The schools and colleges represent only one force for developing a fit populace. The home, church, recreational agency, volunteer groups, and other persons and organizations also have major contributions to make. Schools and colleges should work closely with and play a leading role in mobilizing the entire resources of each community to do the job.

Children and youth must want to be fit. Unless the desire to be fit is resident in each child, the way of life that results in fitness will not be achieved. By the time they leave school and college behind and enter into adult life, the importance of fitness in achieving personal ambitions and desires, in feeling well and happy, in living most and serving best, and in contributing to a strong nation must be inculcated

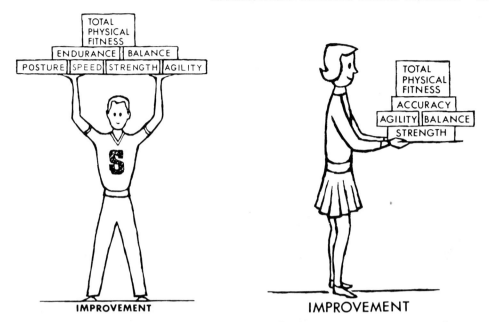

Boys and girls who participated in high quality physical education programs improved more in physical fitness than did those pupils participating in minimum programs. (Physical fitness achievement in selected physical education programs, Albany, 1965, The University of the State of New York.)

in every boy and girl who attends our schools and colleges.

There is a responsible role for the schools and colleges to pursue, but a very necessary one. It is a challenge we must take up if we are not to become a nation of "softies" and unfit individuals.

Health education and physical education can contribute much to the development of total fitness. Many benefits accrue to those persons who have experiences in these specialized fields. They possess an understanding of the human body—its needs and its limitations—the ability to discriminate fad from scientific fact, the interest and desire to be physically fit, the resources to spend leisure hours in a manner that contributes to fitness, and the skill in activities that provide release from strains and tension associated with modern living. They are also provided with experiences that contribute to wholesome personal and group adjustments and opportunities for creative expression. These

are only a few of the many benefits that can be listed. These values, however, do not automatically accrue. Leadership is the key to their fulfillment.

Leaders in health, physical education, and recreation must never lose sight of the fact they are working with the "whole" individual. Programs should make provision for the selected activities that best develop all aspects of self. They should also be concerned with the contributions their respective fields can make, individually and collectively, to this "whole" development.

More specifically, some essential points that school and college health and physical education and recreation programs must consider if they are to adequately promote the health and well-being of boys and girls who attend our schools are listed here:

1. School and college health and physical education programs must be available to *all* children and youth and based on their individual differences.

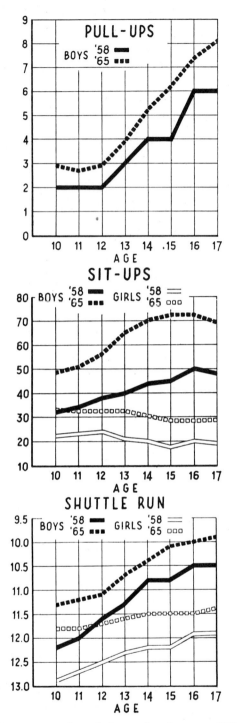

PULL-UPS

BOYS '58 ▬ '65 ▪▪▪

SIT-UPS

BOYS '58 ▬ GIRLS '58 ═ '65 ▪▪▪ '65 □□□

SHUTTLE RUN

BOYS '58 ▬ GIRLS '58 ═ '65 ▪▪▪ '65 □□□

Comparison of youth fitness data between 1958 and 1965. (From Hunsicker, P. N., and Reiff, G.: A survey and comparison of youth fitness, 1958 to 1965, Ann Arbor, 1965, University of Michigan, Cooperative Research Project No. 2418.)

2. Every student should have one period of each school day devoted to the physical education program. College youth should have a required and a voluntary program to meet their needs. Anything less is inadequate.

3. Sports and games should not be limited to only the varsity squads in football, basketball, or baseball. Every student should get into the act, whether he is a dub or skilled, weak or strong, boy or girl.

4. Boys and girls need professionally trained teachers in the fields of health and physical education. Furthermore, the ratio of teachers to students in such classes should be the same as for English, mathematics, or geography.

5. Children and youth should participate in physical education programs that include class periods, intramurals, play, sports, and field days, adapted activities, and scholastic and collegiate sports.

6. Physical activities contribute to physical fitness as they are planned around the following three essentials: *Frequency*—regular daily workouts are needed to develop and maintain a state of optimum health. *Intensity*—big muscles must be vigorously used, with resulting stimulation of the heart and breathing rates. As many muscles should be put into action as possible. *Duration*—1 hour a day, with frequent rest periods, should be devoted to physical activity.

7. In addition to the benefits received from the physical activity program, young people should also understand the importance of being in good health and the factors that build fitness. There should be a comprehensive program of health instruction for all pupils based on their interests and needs.

8. Many health services are essential to promoting physical fitness in the schools and colleges. Most important is a good medical examination in which health defects can be uncovered and steps taken to ensure their correction.

A PHYSICAL FITNESS CHECKLIST*

Medical aspects   Yes   No

1. Thorough dental and health examination each year
   (a) Fit heart and circulatory system, digestive system, nervous system, etc.
   (b) Proper body development, according to age and sex (height and weight, etc.)
2. Correction of remedial health defects, i.e., vision, hearing, overweight etc.

Physical activity

1. At least 1½ to 2 hours a day spent in vigorous physical activity, preferably outdoors
2. Adequate muscular strength and endurance
3. After running 50 yards, heart and breathing return to normal rates within 10 minutes
4. Average skill in running, jumping, climbing, and throwing
5. Control of body in activities involving balance, agility, speed, rhythm, accuracy

Posture

1. When standing upright, string dropped from tip of ear passes through shoulder and hip joints and middle of ankle
2. When sitting in a chair, trunk and head are erect, weight balanced over pelvis, or trunk slightly bent forward
3. When walking, slumping is avoided, body is in proper balance, and excessively wasteful motions of arms and legs are eliminated

Health habits

1. Rest: at least 8 hours of sleep each night
2. Diet: consists of four servings daily from each of the four basic food groups
   (a) Meat, poultry, fish, and eggs
   (b) Dairy products
   (c) Vegetables and fruits
   (d) Bread and cereals
3. Cleanliness:
   (a) Daily bath
   (b) Teeth brushed after every meal
   (c) Clean hair, nails, and clothing
4. Abstain from use of tobacco and alcohol

*From Bucher, C. A., Koenig, C., and Barnhard, M.: Methods and materials for secondary school education, ed. 3, St. Louis, 1970, The C. V. Mosby Co.

---

9. There should be coordination between school, college, and community programs to ensure the conduct of sound out-of-school and college programs of recreation, sports, and athletics. Efforts to expand public and private facilities such as YMCA's, Boys' Clubs, and playgrounds must be continued. Present facilities meet only about 15% of our public needs.

10. A healthful environment is essential to fitness. Safe, sanitary, and attractive facilities and equipment, plus an atmosphere that is conducive to optimum mental and emotional health, are necessary.

11. Motivation for fitness must be developed. Students and the public must be oriented as to the importance of fitness for living. People will change only if sufficiently motivated.

12. There should be homework in physi-

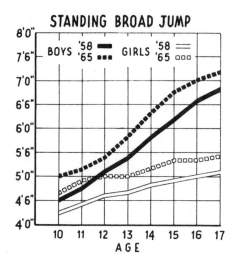

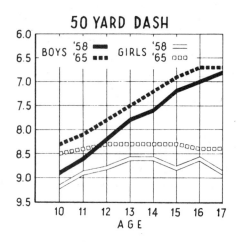

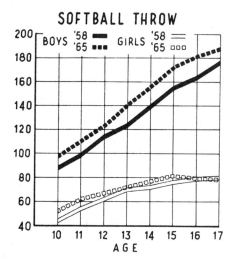

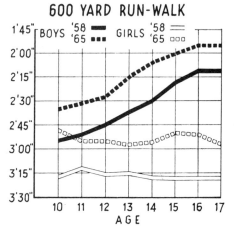

Comparison of youth fitness data between 1958 and 1965. (From Hunsicker, P. N., and Reiff, G.: A survey and comparison of youth fitness, 1958 to 1965, Ann Arbor, 1965, University of Michigan, Cooperative Research Project No. 2418.)

cal activities. It cannot all be done in the gymnasium, swimming pool, or playground. Activities must be taught that may be enjoyed away from the conventional gymnasium and athletic fields. The program should include many kinds of home activities that can be conducted in backyards or basements.

13. If the schools and colleges are going to build strong bodies, they need the necessary equipment and facilities. Taxpayers and administrators must recognize the importance of this work and supply the necessary funds.

14. Health and physical education should receive equal recognition with other subjects in the curriculum. This means credit and other considerations should be

given. Participation in musical organizations, military training, driver education, or other activities should not be permitted to serve as a substitute for physical education.

15. Health and physical education classes should be scheduled early in the program if the needs of students are to be met. In many cases this means they will be scheduled before other subjects. Other things being equal, the school subjects that have the greatest number of pupils enrolled should receive first consideration. The number of staff members and teaching stations are also considerations.

16. Utilization of valid techniques to determine which students are below par in physical fitness is needed, so that special programs may be provided.

17. A progressive program should be provided in health and physical education from kindergarten through college.

THE PRESIDENT'S COUNCIL AND PHYSICAL FITNESS*

The President's Council on Physical Fitness and Sports continues to be active in promoting the cause of physical fitness throughout the United States. In a recent year it attracted more than 10,000 persons to physical fitness clinics that were conducted by Council staff members and outstanding sports and physical education experts. It continues to award the Presidential Physical Fitness Awards to boys and girls who qualify. The number of young people receiving the award exceeds 100,000 in a year. It has established over 130 schools throughout the nation as physical fitness demonstration centers. It has been active in poverty areas in organizing programs of swimming, basketball, and other sports. These are only a few of the projects the Council is undertaking.

*President's Council on Physical Fitness: Youth physical fitness—suggested elements of a school-centered program, parts 1 and 2, Washington, D. C., July, 1961, The Council.

The President's Council on Physical Fitness and Sports, an extension of the President's Council on Youth Fitness established in 1956, came into being by Executive Order on March 4, 1968. Its purpose is to "expand opportunities to engage in exercise, active recreation and sports."

The President of the United States has urged the adoption of the recommendations of his Physical Fitness Council by the schools in order to ensure a basic program of physical developmental activity. A summary of these recommendations and the suggestions for implementing them follow.

Recommendations

1. Identify pupils who have a low level of muscular strength, agility, and flexibility through appropriate testing and require them to participate in a prescribed developmental activity and exercise program.

2. Devote a minimum of 15 minutes a day in the physical education period to vigorous exercises and developmental activities.

3. Use valid tests to determine the physical fitness level of students.

4. Provide a comprehensive program of health education and physical education.

Implementation

1. Utilize three simple tests (pull-ups, sit-ups, and squat-thrusts) to determine pupils who are physically below par.

2. Arrange for all pupils to have a minimum of 15 minutes each day of vigorous physical activity.

3. Test physically underdeveloped boys and girls every 6 weeks until they reach the minimum level.

4. Utilize a validated physical fitness test.

5. Utilize the physical fitness test results for diagnosis and motivation.

6. Provide for testing at least twice yearly.

7. Continually improve and upgrade

total programs of health and physical education.

8. Provide for a qualified person to coordinate the total program.

FURTHER RECOMMENDATIONS OF PRESIDENT'S COUNCIL FOR EMPHASIZING PHYSICAL FITNESS IN HEALTH AND PHYSICAL EDUCATION PROGRAMS

Programs of health education and physical education recommended by the President's Council should include the following items.

Health and safety education

Direct instruction relating to specific health concepts and problems should be provided at every grade level. The topics treated should be in keeping with the interests, needs, and maturational level of the children as they progress grade by grade. Such direct instruction would be augmented by the teaching of healthful and safe behavior through the health appraisal procedures, by capitalizing on interest-arousing events, by correlating health and safety with other subjects, and by other means.

Grades 1 to 3; Ages 6 to 8. At this level, much of the child's health learning relates to developing good practices in daily living at home, in the school, and in the community. Health needs include attention to cleanliness; nutrition; sleep, rest, and relaxation; healthful physical activities; acquaintance with the dentist, nurse, and physician; learning about community health agencies; care of the eyes, ears, and teeth; and elementary concepts of prevention and control of disease.

Grades 4 to 6; Ages 9 to 11. Increasing attention is given to the understanding of *why* health practices should be followed. Elementary treatment of the scientific bases of healthful and safety behavior is carried forward. New units are introduced on the body structure and function, simple first-aid procedures, elementary principles of mental and emotional health, and other topics.

Grades 7 to 9; Ages 12 to 14. Direct instruction in health and safety should amount to at least one semester of five regular periods per week during the 3 years. At this level, heavier emphasis should be given to the physiological and other scientific bases and to the use of scientific methods in solving health and safety problems. The focus should be on problems of adolescence and should include units on: growth and develop-

ment; differences in rate of growth; physical maturation; acne and skin disorders; effects of maintaining an adequate diet; use of tobacco, alcohol, and other drugs; getting along with parents; establishing friendships; desirable relationships with the opposite sex; introduction to vocations, including health careers; importance of exercise and physical forms of recreation; and other related topics.

Grades 10 to 12; Ages 15 to 18. Instruction centers around problems of adult living and of family and community health. Important topics include: emotional health; chronic disease, such as heart disease, cancer, diabetes, and mental illness; instruction concerning consumer health (intelligent utilization of health services and products); national and international health organizations; health careers; health and safety aspects of civil defense; safety in the home, in transportation, recreation; more advanced first aid; the role of exercise in developing and maintaining health and fitness; exercise and weight control; health problems relating to alcohol, tobacco, and narcotics.

Adequate coverage of these topics requires, at a minimum, the equivalent of a full semester of daily periods of regular length. Two full semesters are recommended.

Physical education

The physical education curriculum should include a core of physical fitness activities designed to develop strength, speed, agility, balance, coordination, flexibility, muscular endurance, good posture and body mechanics, and organic efficiency. Activities and exercises should affect all parts and systems. The curriculum should also include a broad scope and balance of physical activities that promote well-rounded physical, social, and intellectual development. Activities should become progressively more complex in organization and skills, and more demanding of physical development and control grade by grade.

The programs should be adapted to the needs, interests, and capacities of each child and youth, including those pupils who, for physical and other reasons, are unable to participate safely and successfully in the general program. All pupils should be motivated to achieve high levels of physical fitness, compatible with their capabilities.

Grades 1 to 3; Ages 6 to 8. Emphasis should be placed upon learning the fundamentals of movement and building a foundation of physical fitness.

Walking, running, hopping, skipping, balancing, jumping, sliding, catching, climbing, hanging, throwing; elementary rhythmical activities, creative movement experience, and simple games which set the stage for later, more complicated activity skills; activities on the jungle gym and other types of playground equipment; simple stunts and tumbling; elementary swimming wherever possible—all of these activities and more should be included. Active participation and vigorous movement should be highlighted.

Grades 4 to 6; Ages 9 to 11. The "fitness core" should have continued emphasis, giving particular attention to development of the back, chest, shoulders, and arms. This age group is ready for elementary calisthenics. Class instruction should include fundamentals of sports skills in several team sports, track and field, and simple forms of individual and dual sports. Opportunity to practice the skills and to gain knowledge in organized games should be provided.

Folk dances and other rhythmical activities are important as are relays, simple games involving running, tumbling, and simple gymnastics. Vigorous outdoor activities such as skating and cycling should be encouraged.

Screening for physical capacity as well as physical achievement testing should begin at this level and continue periodically thereafter. Simple tests of skills and knowledge should also be used.

Grades 7 to 9; Ages 12 to 14. The physical fitness core should include advanced conditioning and developmental activities, e.g., weight-resistance exercises, and the activities should increase in intensity, frequency, and distance. The wide range of individual differences among these youngsters in prepubertal and pubertal stages of development should be noted and programs adjusted accordingly.

The curriculum should include a broad range of offerings in sports and other activities. Emphasis should be given to skillful participation in team sports and increasing attention to individual and dual sports that carry over to recreation hours. Intramural and extramural sports programs should be conducted.

Folk, square, and social dancing are important activities for this age group. Also to be highlighted are stunts, tumbling, gymnastics, and trampolining; aquatics (whenever feasible), with emphasis on survival tactics; combative activities, e.g., wrestling (for boys); and outing activities, e.g., hiking, camping, and hunting.

Grades 10 to 12; Ages 15 to 18. The fitness core continues to be stressed with more opportunities for individual leadership provided.

The broad program is carried forward with particular emphasis on sports, rhythmics, and other activities that carry over into recreation hours throughout life. Specialization in such activities should be encouraged. Ways of maintaining physical fitness at various age levels under varying circumstances should be taught. Additional attention should also be given to outing activities and recreational activities for the family unit, particularly those that promote physical aspects of fitness.*

PHYSICAL FITNESS TESTING

The history of physical fitness testing goes back many years. It probably started as part of the physical education profession at the time when anthropometry was utilized. Anthropometry involved the measuring of the body and its parts, since size seemed to be related to strength. Then there was the emphasis on strength testing, often through use of dynamometers. The work of Dudley A. Sargent and his development of the Intercollegiate Strength Test are characteristic of this early era. It was soon realized, however, that strength testing alone could not measure the functional capacity of individuals. This realization led to cardiorespiratory testing. Schneider expressed this concept when he said:

Physical exertion overtaxes the circulatory mechanism long before it exhausts skeletal musculature; and while it is not easy to overwork the muscles, the heart can quite readily be overworked. The convalescent from infectious disease is limited in his exercise not by what his muscles can do but by the strength of his heart. Hence today the general opinion is that strength tests do not permit us to draw satisfactory conclusions regarding the efficiency of the entire body.†

As a result of this emphasis on functional capacity, many tests were developed, most of which involved changes in frequency of heart rate and blood pressure as a result of exercise. Examples of these are Tuttle's Pulse Ratio Test, McCurdy-Larson's Organic Efficiency Test, Carlson's

---

*President's Council on Physical Fitness: Youth physical fitness—suggested elements of a school-centered program, parts 1 and 2, Washington, D. C., July, 1961, The Council.
†Schneider, E. C.: Physical efficiency and the limitations of efficiency tests, American Physical Education Review 28:405, 1923.

Fatigue Test Curve, and Brouha's Step Test.

In 1925 strength testing was revived by Frederick Rand Rogers with his emphasis on physical capacity tests in the administration of physical education. More recent developments in strength testing have been accomplished by Harrison Clarke, who developed the tensiometer for use with orthopedic disabilities and by Hans Kraus and Ruth P. Hirschland, who devised a six-item test of "minimum muscular fitness" that appraises flexibility as well as strength.

During World War II, when physical fitness was a major objective, several performance type tests were developed. Some of these were the Army Air Force Test, the Army Physical Efficiency Test, the Navy Standard Physical Fitness Test, and the Victory Corps Tests.

Several tests with which to measure physical fitness are available today. Some of these have been scientifically validated, whereas others have been presented without objective evidence of validity. Validity and reliability are important criteria of a test, but administrative efficiency may place one test ahead of another. Validity, however, is the weak point in most physical fitness tests today.

Not all physical fitness tests measure the same kind of physical fitness. The evidence is that tests of physical fitness do not correlate very highly. Therefore, when selecting a fitness test it is necessary to select one that measures the kind of fitness the program is aiming to achieve.

It is difficult to identify the items we want to measure in physical fitness. Many experts feel we are a long way from having an all-purpose test and that it would be better to test component parts of physical fitness (posture, strength, balance, endurance), by means of several tests of each component. Then, through a partial correlation process it would be possible to determine the most valid test of each component. In turn, these most valid tests could be combined into a battery. Most physical fitness tests measure component factors that are not truly comprehensive.

GIRLS' PHYSICAL FITNESS TEST RECORD

Name _____ Grade _____ Period _____

School _____ Age ___ Ht. ___ Wt. ___ Test 1 Classification _____

Age ___ Ht. ___ Wt. ___ Test 2 Classification _____

Test No.	1		2	
Date				
Event	Score	Percentile	Score	Percentile
Modified Pull-Ups				
Sit-Ups (Max 50)				
Broad Jump				
50-yd. Dash				
Shuttle Run				
Modified Push-Ups				
600-yd. Run-Walk				
Softball Throw				
P.F.I.—Average percentile of 5 events				

They stress primarily arm strength, leg strength, and endurance. However, there are other considerations. For example, a husky body requires more strength for one pull-up than does a slight one. In addition to body build, physiologic age (when dealing with children) should also be considered. These and similar factors may account for the difficulty in validating tests.

The possibility of a universal battery of tests is remote because of disagreement among experts as to the nature of physical fitness. How much of it is esthetic and how much is a matter of health or expediency? Many physical education leaders feel it is important that the profession consider the adoption of a single tool of measurement. They feel this is of utmost importance if we are to propose a program that will become widely adopted and provide an answer to the present demand for an emphasis on physical fitness.

Tables 11-1 and 11-2 list the physical fitness components and tests that measure these components, as well as the selected tests of physical fitness.

The American Association for Health, Physical Education, and Recreation* has developed its own physical fitness test for national use. It consists of seven basic items plus a swimming test:

1. Pull-ups (modified for girls to flexed arm hang); to test arm and shoulder girdle strength
2. Sit-ups: to test strength of abdominal muscles and hip flexors
3. Shuttle run: to test speed and change of direction
4. Standing broad jump: to test explosive power of leg extensors
5. 50-yard dash: to test speed
6. Softball throw for distance: to test skill and coordination
7. 600-yard walk or run: to test cardiovascular system
8. Swimming test (jump into water, rest, and swim 15 yards): to test protective powers in the water

Norms have been established for girls and boys in grades five through twelve

*AAHPER youth fitness test manual, American Association for Health, Physical Education, and Recreation, 1201 16th St. N. W., Washington, D. C. 20036.

PHYSICAL FITNESS TEST RECORD

Name | Grade | Age | Wt. | Ht.

School | Period | Squad

Test No.	1		2		3	
Date						
Event	Score	Points	Score	Points	Score	Points
Pull Ups						
Sit Ups						
Push Ups						
Burpee 60						
Broad Jump						
	Total Points		Total Points		Total Points	
	Quartile		Quartile		Quartile	
Superior	277-Up		329-Up		400-Up	
Excellent	243-276		289-328		336-399	
Average	208-242		248-288		290-335	
Fair	174-207		208-247		245-289	
Unsatisfactory	Below 174		Below 208		Below 245	

Table 11-1. Physical fitness components and tests*

Component	Selected tests
Arm and shoulder strength	Pull-ups, push-ups, parallel bar, dips, rope climb
Speed	50-yard dash, 100-yard dash
Agility	Shuttle run, agility run
Abdominal and hip strength	Sit-ups, sit-ups with knees flexed, 2-minute sit-ups
Flexibility	Trunk flexion standing, trunk flexion sitting, trunk extension (prone position)
Cardiorespiratory endurance	600-yard run, half-mile run, mile run, 5-minute step test
Explosive power	Standing broad jump, vertical jump
Static strength	Grip strength, back lift, leg lift
Balance	Bass test, Brace test, tests on balance beam
Muscular endurance	Push-ups, chest raisings (prone position, hands behind neck, legs held down), V-sit (against time)

*From Hunsicker, P.: Physical fitness—what research says to the teacher, Washington, D. C., 1963, National Education Association, p. 17.

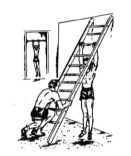

Improvised equipment for pull-up.

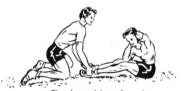

Final position for sit-up.

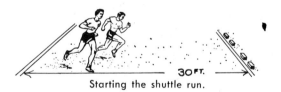

Starting the shuttle run.

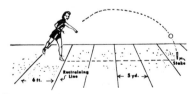

Measuring the softball throw for distance.

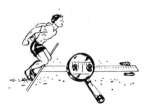

Measuring the standing broad jump.

Test items from AAHPER Youth Fitness Test Manual. (From NEA Journal **51**:33, 1962.)

Table 11-2. Selected tests of physical fitness*

Test	Source
AAHPER Youth Fitness Test	American Association for Health, Physical Education, and Recreation, 1201 16th St. N.W. Washington, D. C. 20036.
AAHPER-U. S. Office of Education Committee on Physical Fitness for Girls	Journal of HPER, pp. 308-311, 354-355, June, 1945.
All-round Muscular Endurance	Anderson, John E.: Endurance of young men, Society for Research in Child Development, vol. X, serial No. 40, No. 1, Washington, D. C., 1958, American Association for Health, Physical Education, and Recreation.
Army/Air Forces Physical Fitness Test	AAHPER Research Quarterly 15:12-15, March, 1944.
Army Physical Fitness Test	War Department, FM 21-20, 1945.
California Physical Fitness Test	California State Department of Education, Feb., 1948.
Harvard Step Test	AAHPER Research Quarterly 14:31-36, March, 1943.
Illinois Physical Fitness Test for High School Boys	Illinois State Department of Public Instruction, Bulletin No. 6, 1944.
Indiana High School Physical Condition Test	Indiana State Office of Public Instruction, Bulletin No. 136, Sept., 1944.
The JCR Test	AAHPER Research Quarterly 18:12-29, March, 1947.
Kraus-Weber Test of Minimum Muscular Fitness	AAHPER Research Quarterly 25:178-188, May, 1954.
Larson Muscular Strength Test	AAHPER Research Quarterly 11:82-96, Dec., 1940.
McCloy Strength Test	McCloy, H. C., and Young, N. E.: Tests and measurements in health and physical education, ed. 3, New York, 1954, Appleton-Century-Crofts, pp. 128-152.
Navy Standard Physical Fitness	Bureau of Naval Personnel, Training Division, Physical Fitness Section, 1943.
New York State Physical Fitness Test	New York State Education Department, 1948.
Youth Physical Fitness	President's Council on Youth Fitness: Youth physical fitness, Washington, D. C., 1961, United States Government Printing Office.
Rogers Strength Test	Clarke, H. Harrison: Application of measurement to health and physical education, ed. 3, New York, 1959, Prentice-Hall, Inc. pp. 182-213.

*From Hunsicker, P.: Physical fitness—what research says to the teacher, Washington, D. C., 1963, National Education Association, p. 17.

and for college students and may be obtained from the Association. A manual gives, in addition, complete directions for testing each item.

The State Department of Education of New York State* is an example of many state groups that have developed their own physical fitness tests for local use. The New York test consists of seven components that

---

*New York State physical fitness test, The University of the State of New York, The State Education Department, Albany, New York.

are measured to obtain a total physical fitness score:

1. Posture—evaluated by means of a posture rating chart
2. Accuracy—measured by means of a target throw, utilizing a softball and a circular target
3. Strength—evaluated by pull-ups for boys and modified pull-ups for girls
4. Agility—evaluated by means of the sidestep
5. Speed—evaluated by means of the 50-yard dash

6. Balance—evaluated by means of the squat-stand

7. Endurance—evaluated by means of the treadmill

Norms have been established and are listed in a manual, together with a description of the test.

Resources and materials for physical fitness*

At the present time the quantity of materials for teaching physical fitness continues to increase. Nationwide interest in this problem, fostered by the President's Council on Physical Fitness and Sports, as well as increased emphasis on health status, drugs, and medical care, has all brought this about. Physical educators have found greater interest in the reception for their programs among parents and lay people and have found it an ideal time to expand and extend their programs and facilities.

There is a wealth of material presently available to teachers for use in physical education classes. Following are some of the more well-known physical fitness test batteries and exercise programs which have been developed recently as part of this campaign for fitness:

1. *Youth Physical Fitness*—suggested elements of a school-centered program, President's Council on Youth Fitness, July, 1961, Superintendent of Documents, Washington, D. C., 40¢.

Part One—A discussion of the current concept and foundations of physical fitness programs, including suggested standards for instruction and complementary programs.

Part Two—Suggested tests and activities and developmental exercises for boys and girls, grades 4 to 12. Standards for different age levels are included with suggested test items, all of which have been adapted from the AAHPER test.

2. *Youth Fitness Test Manual*, American Association for Health, Physical Education, and Recreation, Washington, 1965, $1.00.

This booklet contains explanations for the administration of seven suggested test items, together with percentile scores for boys and girls at different age levels.

The association has also developed record forms for this testing program, and special awards and emblems which may be presented to students participating in this program.

3. *Vim*—A complete exercise plan for girls 12 to 18 years of age, and

4. *Vigor*—A complete exercise plan for boys 12 to 18 years of age, President's Council on Physical Fitness, May, 1964, Superintendent of Documents, Washington, D. C., 25¢ each.

These booklets contain helpful hints and facts about fitness for youngsters and include a daily exercise plan suitable for them to follow.

5. *Adult Physical Fitness*—A program for men and women, President's Council on Physical Fitness, Superintendent of Documents, Washington, D. C., 35¢.

This is an adult program for home exercising with which the teacher should be familiar.

6. *Royal Canadian Air Force Exercise Plans for Physical Fitness*—5BX, for men; 10BX, for women, Queen's Printer and Controller of Stationery, Ottawa, Canada, Revised, 1962, $1.00.

This, too, is an adult home exercise plan with which the teacher should be familiar.

7. *Physical Fitness for Girls*, William Hillcourt, and

8. *Physical Fitness for Boys*, William Hillcourt, A Golden Magazine Special, Golden Press, Inc., New York, 1967, $1.00.

There are many other materials available in this area of physical fitness. Many state departments of education have developed their own testing instruments (California, Oregon, Washington, Iowa, Virginia, New York) as have some cities (Tucson, Denver, Omaha, Louisville, Kansas City). A movie entitled *Why Physical Education?** which has been produced for use in junior and senior high schools discusses physical fitness and total fitness as the goal of physical education programs.

Some films and materials related to physical fitness are listed below:

Films

1. Girls are better than ever (13½ min.)   Free
   Modern Talking Picture Service
   1212 Avenue of the Americas
   New York, N.Y. 10036

2. Time of our lives (27 min.)   Free
   Associated Films, Inc.
   600 Madison Avenue
   New York, N.Y. 10022

---

*From Bucher, C. A., Koenig, C., and Barnhard, M.: Methods and materials for secondary school physical education, ed. 2, St. Louis, 1965, The C. V. Mosby Co.

*Why Physical Education? 16 mm., sound and color, 14 minutes, $150.00, produced by Wexler Film Productions, available from Henk Newenhouse, Inc., 1017 Longaker Road, Northbrook, Ill.

3. Badhe chalo (11 min.)

> Express postage collect

Information Service of India
Film Section
3 East 64th St.
New York, N.Y. 10021

4. Rhythmic ball exercises (1966) (13 min.)

> Free

Embassy of Finland
Press Section
1900 Twenty-Fourth St. N. W.
Washington, D. C. 20008

5. Physically fit (Don Schollander) (4½ min.)

> Free

Modern Talking Picture Service
1212 Avenue of the Americas
New York, N.Y. 10036

6. Focus of fitness (19 min.)   Free
Eastman Kodak Co.
Audio-Visual Service
343 State St.
Rochester, N.Y. 14650

Materials

	Single price	Per 100
Adolescent years		
As others see us	$.15	$.08
How teens set the stage for smoking	.10	.02
Why girls menstruate	.10	.02
Fitness		
Physical fitness	$.05	.02
Exercise and fitness	.05	.02
Safeguarding the health of the athlete	.05	.02
Seven paths to fitness	.10	.02
Tips of athletic training (vols. I-VI)	.05	.02

American Medical Association,
535 N. Dearborn St.
Chicago, Illinois 60610

Booklets, pamphlets, and articles on physical fitness.

AMA and AAHPER Joint Committee on Exercise and Fitness: Health problems revealed during physical activity, Journal of Health, Physical Education, and Recreation 37:7, 1967.

Bender, J. A., Kaplan, H. M., and Pierson, J. K.: Injury control through isometrics and isotonics, Journal of Health, Physical Education, and Recreation 38:2, 1967.

Brooks, B. W.: Views of physical fitness from four educational philosophies, The Physical Educator 24:1, 1967.

Collins, G. J.: Physical achievements and the schools, Bulletin 1965, no. 13, U. S. Department of Health, Education and Welfare, Office of Education, 1965, U. S. Government Printing Office.

Cooper, K. H., M.D.: How to feel fit at any age, Reader's Digest, March, 1968.

Doherty, J. K.: The nature of endurance in running, Journal of Health, Physical Education, and Recreation 35:44, 1964.

Flint, M. M.: Selecting exercises, Journal of Health, Physical Education, and Recreation 35:2, 1964.

Gerenstein, S.: Procedures and equipment for weight training in the high school program, Journal of Health, Physical Education, and Recreation 38:1, 1967.

Hillcourt, W.: Physical fitness for girls, New York, 1967, Golden Press, Inc.

Hillcourt, W.: Physical fitness for boys, New York, 1967, Golden Press, Inc.

Hunsicker, P. A., and Reiff, G. G.: A survey and comparison of youth fitness 1958-1965, Journal of Health, Physical Education, and Recreation 37:1, 1966.

Larson, L. A.: Research turns the spotlight on health and fitness, Journal of Health, Physical Education, and Recreation 36:4, 1965.

Marshall, J. W., and McAdam, R. E.: A buddy plan of active resistance exercise, Journal of Health, Physical Education, and Recreation 35:3, 1964.

McCarthy, J.: Fitness for activity, The Physical Educator 22:4, 1965.

Pennington, G.: Fitness honor roll, The Physical Educator 21:4, 1964.

Ponthieux, N. A., and Barker, D. G.: Relationship between socioeconomic status and physical fitness measures, The Research Quarterly 36:4, 1965.

Ponthieux, N. A., and Barker, B. G.: Relationship between race and physical fitness, The Research Quarterly 36:4, 1965.

Rosenstein, I., and Frost, R. B.: Physical fitness of senior high school boys and girls participating in selected physical education programs in New York State, The Research Quarterly 35:3, 1964.

Steinhaus, A. H.: Fitness beyond muscle, The Physical Educator 23:3, 1966.

Weiss, R. A.: Is physical fitness our most important objective? Journal of Health, Physical Education, and Recreation 35:2, 1964.

Yarnall, C. D.: Relationship of physical fitness to selected measures of popularity, The Research Quarterly 37:2, 1966.

Questions and exercises

1. Outline what you consider to be an effective physical fitness program for a high school.
2. Write an essay on the Kraus-Weber tests and their role in a school physical fitness program.
3. What were some of the high points of President Eisenhower's Conference on Fitness of American Youth?
4. Develop your own definitions of fitness and physical fitness.
5. What are the components of physical fitness?
6. Evaluate the statement of fitness made by the American Association for Health, Physical Education, and Recreation.
7. What are some of the tests for physical fitness? Evaluate each in the light of criteria in the chapter on Measurement and Evaluation.

Reading assignment in *Administrative Dimensions of Health and Physical Education Programs, Including Athletics:* Chapter 5, Selection 27.

Selected references

AMA and AAHPER Joint Committee: Exercise and fitness, Journal of Health, Physical Education, and Recreation 35:5, 1964.

American Association for Health, Physical Education, and Recreation: Youth fitness test manual, Washington, D. C., 1961, The Association.

Bookwalter, K. W., and Bookwalter, C. W.: Fitness of secondary youth, Washington, D. C., 1956, American Association for Health, Physical Education, and Recreation.

Bucher, C. A.: Highlights of President's Conference on Fitness of American Youth, unpublished paper, 1956.

Bucher, C. A.: Foundations of physical education, ed. 5, St. Louis, 1968, The C. V. Mosby Co.

Clarke, H. H.: Objective strength tests of affected muscle groups involved in orthopedic disabilities, Research Quarterly 19:11, 1948.

Collins, G. J., and Hunter, J. S.: Physical achievement and the schools, Bureau of Educational Research and Development, Office of Education Bulletin, 1965, No. 13.

Cureton, T. K.: Physical fitness appraisal and guidance, St. Louis, 1947, The C. V. Mosby Co.

Espenschade, A.: Restudy of relationships between physical performances of school children and age, height, and weight, Research Quarterly 34:144, 1963.

Gallagher, J. R., and Brouha, L.: Physical fitness, Journal of the American Medical Association 125:834, 1944.

Hunsicker, P.: Physical fitness—what research tells the teacher, Washington, D. C., 1963, National Education Association.

Johnson, W. R., editor: Science and medicine of exercise and sports, New York, 1960, Harper & Row, Publishers.

Journal of the American Association for Health, Physical Education, and Recreation, Sept., 1957, entire issue.

Kraus, H., and Hirschland, R. P.: Minimum muscular fitness tests in school children, Research Quarterly 25:178, 1954.

President's Conference on Fitness of American Youth: Fitness of American youth, Journal of Health, and Physical Education, and Recreation 28:3, 1957.

President's Council on Youth Fitness: Youth physical fitness—suggested elements of a school-centered program, parts 1 and 2, Washington, D. C., July, 1961, The Council.

Report of the National Conference on Fitness of Secondary School Youth: Youth and fitness: a program for secondary schools, Washington, D. C., 1958, American Association for Health, Physical Education, and Recreation.

Steinhaus, A. A.: Fitness—a definition and guide to its attainment, Journal of Health, Physical Education, and Recreation 16:175, 1945.

Weiss, R. A.: Is physical fitness our most important objective? Journal of Health, Physical Education, and Recreation 35:2, 1964.

PART

three

HEALTH PROGRAMS FOR STUDENTS

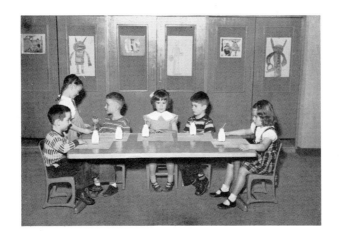

CHAPTER 12 THE HEALTH SCIENCE INSTRUCTION PROGRAM — WITH IMPLICATIONS FOR PHYSICAL EDUCATION*

The *health science instruction* phase of the total school and college program refers to the provision of learning experiences for the purpose of influencing knowledge, attitudes, and conduct relating to individual and group health.

Health science instruction is important in the educational program for many reasons, not the least of which are that healthy students learn more rapidly, are better adjusted, and get along better with their classmates. For these and other reasons schools and colleges should attempt to help each student to achieve and maintain a state of optimum health.

Throughout the history of education the schools and colleges have indicated an interest in health. In 1918 the report of a commission on education of the National Education Association listed health as its first objective. The Educational Policies Commission, an important policy-making group in education, pointed out that an educated person understands basic facts concerning health and disease, protects his own health and that of his dependents, and

strives to improve the health of the community. The American Council on Education, another policy-making group, has encouraged schools and colleges to help pupils improve and maintain their health. White House Conferences on Education have stressed physical and mental health as important educational objectives.

There are well-supported reasons for these statements emphasizing the importance of health in education. Research has shown that the healthy person has a better chance to be a success in school and college, to be more effective scholastically and academically, and to be more productive. In addition to these factors, it should be noted that the school acts in loco parentis and, as such, has a legal as well as a moral responsibility to concern itself with the health of the student.

If schools and colleges accept their responsibility for, and do an effective job in, health science instruction, the program should result in the following:

1. Students will become more intelligent citizens on matters concerning health; for example, they will understand the value in fluoridating water supplies.
2. Students will better understand the values of health and the contribution health can make to human productivity, happiness, and effectiveness.
3. Students will be better health consumers—they will not be taken in by quackery, frauds, and gimmicks that advertise shortcuts to health.

Many children and youth are attending

*The school and college attempt to promote health in children and youth through a specialized program that contributes to the understanding, maintenance, and improvement of the health of students and school personnel, including health services, health science instruction, and healthful school living. The healthful school and college living phase of the health program will be considered in Chapters 14 and 15. The health services phase of the total health program will be considered in Chapter 13.

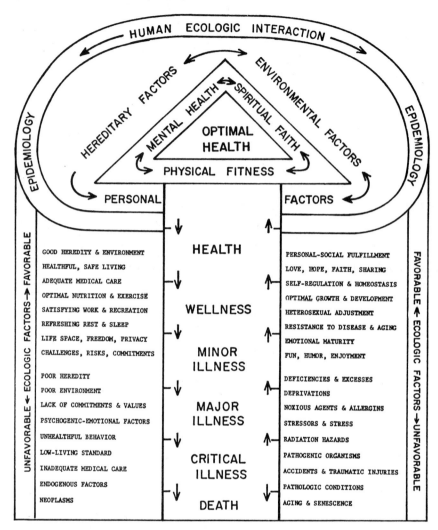

An ecologic model of health and disease. Examples of favorable and unfavorable dynamic, interacting, hereditary, environmental, and personal ecologic factors and conditions that are determinants of the levels of health and disease on a continuum extending from zero health (death) to optimal health. (From Hoyman, H. S.: Journal of School Health 35:113, 1965.)

schools and colleges with different kinds of health problems and disabilities, and few live at their optimum level of physical and emotional efficiency. Students are involved in accidents caused by carelessness. They suffer from remediable physical defects. They find it difficult to be realistic in respect to the demands of their environment. They contract needless diseases and infections.

A recognition of the need for health science instruction in the schools and colleges has developed through the years, as educators and the lay public have come to realize the importance of providing learning experiences that will result in healthful living for more people. Furthermore, they have come to see more clearly the relationship of knowledge, attitudes, and practices in respect to health.

The importance of health has been taught by educators since early times.

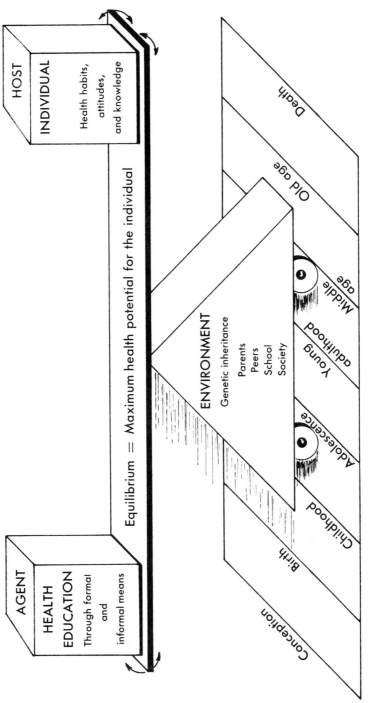

Epidemiology of health. From Mayshark, C.: Epidemiology of health, Journal of Health, Physical Education, and Recreation 39:49, 1968.

Older generations tell about how they received instruction in physiology, learned how to trace the flow of blood through the body, and memorized long definitions of various anatomic and physiologic aspects of the human body. This approach to health education has changed over the years. Toward the end of the nineteenth century some new ideas were introduced into school and college curricula. This resulted from a feeling on the part of certain individuals that the evil effects of alcoholic beverages should be taught. They also felt there should be a greater emphasis on the hygienic aspects of living. As a result, these concepts became an important part of health teaching, especially in colleges.

This emphasis continued until the early twentieth century. Then, the impact of World Wars I and II gave health education the impetus it needed to become firmly embedded as an important part of school and college programs. The public became aroused, for example, by the number of defects discovered in young men through Selective Service examinations. The results of such a disclosure included passing state laws, developing courses of study, publishing textbooks concerned with health education, and providing for the training of special teachers in this area. Today, there is increased recognition that health education can play a very important role in helping to make individuals aware of their responsibility for their own health and also that of others. Health is regarded as "everybody's business."

There is increased emphasis upon health teaching in our schools and colleges today and upon such topics as drugs, ecology, sex education, alcohol, tobacco, personality development, and accident prevention. Professional preparation institutions are placing greater emphasis on instructing teachers about their responsibilities in this area. There is closer cooperation between the school or college and community health officers. Medical doctors, dentists, and other representatives of professional services are taking more interest in health. School and college administrators and their teaching and professional staffs are voicing concern about students and their health. More research is providing new and better directions to help the schools and colleges in changing the health behavior of many boys and girls.

THE NATURE AND SCOPE OF HEALTH SCIENCE INSTRUCTION

One of the revealing studies in the area of health education and the schools is the School Health Education Study. This study has determined the nature and scope of health education in the public schools of the United States, the kind of instruction students receive, how much boys and girls know about health matters, who teaches these pupils, how the subject is organized and scheduled in the school program, the health content areas that are emphasized, and many other factors of importance to all educators and persons interested in health. The project involved such procedures as a survey of 135 public school systems regarding the health practices of approximately 16 million students in more than 1,000 elementary schools and 359 secondary schools. The following represents a sampling of some of the findings in this study:

Most health instruction in the elementary schools is taught by the classroom teacher, without supervisory assistance, and is included in the curriculum in combination with other subjects.

On the average, in those districts with secondary grades, a separate class in health education is offered in grades 7 and 8 by 61.2 percent of the large, 69.1 percent of the medium, and 48.0 percent of the small school districts. The average percentage of districts scheduling a separate class of health education in grades 9 through 12 is 52.2 percent of the large, 43.1 percent of the medium, and 31.8 percent of the small school districts.

On the average, health education is a required subject for all students in grades 7 and 8 in 55.6 percent of the large, 62.2 percent of the medium, and 48.0 percent of the small school districts of the sample group of districts that included secondary grades; in grades 8 through 12, 25.0 percent of the large, 37.5 percent of the medium, and 24.9 percent of the small districts require health education of all students.

In all districts, two-thirds or more of the health classes in grades 7, 8, and 9 and 90 percent or more in grades 10, 11, and 12 in all districts are taught by the teacher with a combined major in health and physical education, or with specialization in physical education only. The percentage reported varied by grades and within districts.

In the majority of secondary schools, boys and girls are separated for health instruction. In those instances where combined classes are scheduled, these tended to be the pattern more frequently in grades 7 and 8 than in the upper grades. Percentages of responses vary throughout the grades and among the districts. The majority of responses indicate that separate classes in health education for boys and girls are held because of staff, space, and scheduling problems. The nature of the subject matter as a reason for a separation was mentioned to a far lesser extent and then mainly by the medium and small districts only.

At the secondary level the large districts rely to a far greater extent than do the medium or small districts on local curriculum guides and local community influence in determining course content. The small districts depend heavily on the state course of study as a resource for deciding what to teach in health education.[*]

Some instructional problems involved with health science instruction, as cited by school administrators in the School Health Education Study, are ineffectiveness of instructional methods, parental and community resistance to certain health topics, insufficient time allocated for health instruction, lack of coordination, inadequate professional staff, lack of interest among teachers, and neglect of the health education course when combined with the physical education experience.

The School Health Education Study revealed that many health misconceptions exist among students. A brief sampling of these misconceptions includes the following:

1. Commercial medicines are safe to purchase if the label clearly indicates

---

[*]School Health Education Study: A summary report, Washington, D. C., 1964, National Education Association.

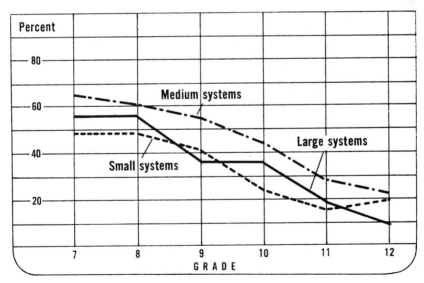

Percent of public school systems in sample group requiring a separate health class of all students. (From School Health Education Study: Summary report of a nationwide study of health instruction in the public schools, 1961 to 1963, Washington, D. C., 1964, School Health Education Study.)

the dose and contents, or if recommended by a pharmacist.

2. The use of "pep" pills and sleeping pills does not require medical supervision.

3. The purpose of fluoridating water supplies is to purify water and make it safe to drink.

4. Unrefrigerated chicken salad is not a potential source of food poisoning.

5. Chronic diseases can be transmitted from person to person.

6. Venereal disease can be inherited.

In respect to the basic health science course in colleges and universities, a survey conducted a few years ago showed that better than 80% of the institutions included in the survey offered a personal health course for their students. In some cases the course was offered on an elective basis, in other cases it was required. Teacher preparatory programs, in particular, provided the setting for most of the required courses.

The college survey also showed that in

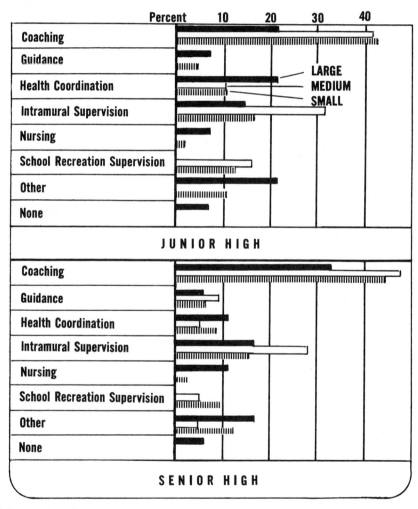

Responsibilities other than teaching for teachers assigned to health instruction on the secondary level in the sample group, 1961-1962. (From School Health Education Study: Summary report of a nationwide study of health instruction in the public schools, 1961 to 1963, Washington, D. C., 1964, School Health Education Study.)

most cases the basic health science course was offered by the Health and Physical Education Department. However, in other cases it was offered by Departments of Biology or Zoology, Science Department, De-

partment of General Education, Home Economics Department, College Health Service, College of Medicine, and College of Nursing.

The college survey further showed that

Table 12-1. Undergraduate majors of teachers of health*

Major	Teachers	Major	Teachers
Physical education	775	Psychology	4
Health education and physical education	289	Business	4
		Nursing	4
Science	173	Education	3
Biology	100	Special education	3
Home economics	99	Recreation	3
Social studies	32	Physiology	2
English	24	Physics	2
History	18	Guidance	2
Social science	16	Music	2
Health education	15	Industrial arts	1
Elementary education	13	French	1
Chemistry	8	Theology	1
Mathematics	6	Speech	1
Art	5	Political science	1
Physical science	4		

*From Michigan Department of Education: Patterns and features of school health education in Michigan public schools, East Lansing, 1969, Michigan State Department of Education, p. 7.

Table 12-2. Undergraduate minors of teachers of health*

Minor	Teachers	Minor	Teachers
Health education	258	Driver education	4
Physical education	128	Art	3
Science	68	Natural science	2
Biology	58	Spanish	2
Social studies	39	Physiology	2
English	34	Psychology	2
History	32	German	1
Social science	32	French	1
Mathematics	16	Journalism	1
Home economics	15	Conservation	1
Physical science	8	Economics	1
Elementary education	7	Political science	1
Business	7	Dance	1
Education	6	Language	1
Speech	6	Guidance	1
Geography	5	Commercial	1
Chemistry	5	Literature	1
Recreation	5	Nursing	1
Industrial arts	5	Zoology	1

*From Michigan Department of Education: Patterns and features of school health education in Michigan public schools, East Lansing, 1969, Michigan State Department of Education, p. 7.

the basic health science course was offered on the average for two or three semester or quarter hour credits and was taught by a variety of persons including health educators, physical educators, biologists, and physicians. Some of the topics covered in the courses included mental health, family health, nutrition, reproduction, tobacco, alcohol, narcotics, preparation for marriage, personal appearance, disease control, health appraisal, and care of the body.

The School Health Education Study and other research findings indicate more and more the need for health science instruction in schools and colleges. The growth and development characteristics of students, the social demands of dating, the preparation for marriage, and the pressures of the peer group are important considerations. Youth must be helped to make informed wise choices in meeting the pressing problems they face each day of their lives. These studies have shown that students are weak in health content concerning fatigue, sleep and rest, mental health, and habit-forming substances; that exposure to alcohol tends to occur first at 13 to 14 years of age; that dietary practices become increasingly worse throughout the teen-age years; that the greatest number of smokers begin smoking between 10 and 15 years of age; and that annually venereal diseases infect more than 250,000 young persons 15 to 19 years of age.

Tables 12-1 and 12-2 indicate the training that teachers of health in one state have had. As the tables show, physical educators play a major role in teaching health in today's schools.

ADMINISTRATION OF THE HEALTH SCIENCE INSTRUCTION PROGRAM

The manner in which health science instruction is administered will vary with the local situation. At the outset, however, it should be recognized that health education should be taught by individuals who are trained in the methodology of teaching. An individual who has studied educational psychology and other subjects that yield knowledges and techniques important to effective teaching is better prepared to do a good job of instruction in health than is the individual who does not have such training. This does not exclude using representatives of the health department and voluntary health agencies as consultants and resource persons. They can be invaluable in drawing up courses of study and in the presentation of various phases of the health education program.

Local administration will again determine where health science instruction should be located within the school or college structure. In some schools and colleges it is placed in such areas as physical education, science, and home economics. In other schools and colleges it is a separate area by itself. In most schools and colleges health is administratively located in the health and physical education department. In the larger schools especially, and in colleges and universities, there may be a separate health education department with full-time personnel who have been trained in the area of health education. Such an administrative arrangement is conducive to good interrelationships between the school and college and public health agencies, to the development of a health council, and to a well-coordinated and well-integrated health program. In smaller and medium-sized schools and colleges, there should also be full-time health educators charged with this important responsibility.

The physical education person many times is assigned such responsibilities as coaching, intramurals, and special events in addition to physical education classes. If the responsibility for health education is given to a teacher of physical education, in addition to these numerous other duties, some responsibility is going to suffer. In many cases, with pressure for winning teams, the class instruction program is neglected. School and college administrators should recognize that health education is a very important part of the school or college offering. It should be assigned only to qualified persons and should receive ample time and facilities to make it effective.

Every school and college, regardless of size, should have someone on its staff assigned to coordinate the various aspects of the health program. In larger schools and colleges this might be a full-time position. In smaller schools and colleges it could be the principal, chairman of the health department, or some qualified staff member who has interest and responsibility in this area.

The administration of the health education program should also include a health council or committee. The *health council* would be composed of representatives from the central administration, subject matter areas, students, parents, professional groups, custodial staff, and others whose duties have particular bearing on the health of the student. Such a group of individuals, regardless of type or size of school, can play an important part in planning and carrying out the health education program. They can be instrumental in providing the necessary funds, materials, staff, and experiences that make for an outstanding program. They would have as a major responsibility the identification and solution of health problems.

THE SCHOOL HEALTH TEAM

The following paragraphs discuss those persons who are participants in the school health team.

Teacher of health

The teacher of health is a key person if the health science program is to be effective. This person should possess an understanding of what constitutes a well-rounded health program and the teacher's part in it. Preparation should include a basic understanding of the various physical, biologic, and behavioral sciences that help to explain the importance of health

to the optimum functioning of the individual, including understanding of such areas as structure and growth of the human body, nutrition, and mental health. The teacher should be interested in the health needs and interests of pupils, possess personal characteristics that exemplify good health, and acquire knowledge and skill for presenting health knowledge in a meaningful and interesting manner to all students. The teacher should be competent to organize health teaching units in terms of the health needs and interests of students, motivate the child to be well and happy, and be aware of the individual differences of the pupils. The teacher should also be able and willing to interpret the school health program to the community and enlist its support in solving health problems.

Health coordinator

The health coordinator is a person on the staff who has special qualifications that enable him to serve as a coordinator, supervisor, teacher, or consultant for health education. He is concerned with developing effective working relationships with school, college, and community health programs and coordinating the total school or college health program with the general educational program. A health coordinator can render valuable service in seeing that a well-rounded health program exists. Health instruction can be more carefully planned. In addition to the direct health teaching, there can also be provision for the correlation and integration of health instruction with many subject matter areas. Resource materials can be provided for the classroom and other teachers involved in health teaching. School, college, and community relationships can be developed. The total health program can be guided to function as an integrated whole. Each administrator should recognize the importance of the position of health coordinator and designate a person qualified for such a responsibility. The Nebraska State

The school health coordinator should*:

Coordinate the health activities of all school personnel.

Provide leadership in the development of a health curriculum based upon the progression of health knowledge, concepts, and activities from kindergarten through high school.

Serve as a liaison person between school, public, and voluntary health agencies to establish desirable working relationships and coordination of school and community health efforts.

Be a resource person for teachers needing help with health education materials, references, teaching aids, and methods.

Establish good relationships with the community's professional medical and dental resources so that the school's program is properly understood.

Promote inservice training for the teaching of health through faculty meetings, small group meetings, workshop sessions with nurses and other school health personnel, and individual interviews with teachers.

With the assistance of the school health council, study needs and present activities of the school health program; from the findings make recommendations that will develop an improved program.

*From Health policies and procedures for Nebraska schools, Lincoln, Nebraska Department of Health and the Nebraska Department of Education, p. 8.

Departments of Health and Education outline the responsibilities for the health coordinator.

School or college administrator

The school or college administrator is a key figure in making important decisions in regard to health programs, such as the personnel appointed to teach health courses, the methods of instruction, the topics to be covered, and the budget essential to having the necessary equipment and supplies. Therefore, a school or college administrator, to be effective in the health science program, should be sympathetic and interested in meeting the health needs and interests of students, in seeing that the health courses include topics that meet these needs and interests, and in assuring that health is taught by competent faculty members in a way that will motivate behavior.

School or college physician

The school or college physician can be an effective member of the health team by discussing results of medical examinations with teachers, drawing implications from the medical examinations for health science instruction, stressing to administrators and the community in general the need for instruction in health, visiting classes, and periodically being a visiting lecturer in the health classes.

Nurse

The nurse works closely with medical personnel on one hand and with students, teachers, and parents on the other. As the person who engages in such duties as administering health tests, assisting in medical examinations, screening for hearing and vision, holding parent conferences, keeping health records, teaching health classes, helping to control communicable disease, and coordinating school, college, and community health efforts, she can play an effective and important role in giving support and direction to the health instruction program. The school nurse can help in the identification of the topics that need to be covered, emphasizing the health needs of the students, and interpreting to administrators the importance of health in the school or college program.

Physical educator

Although the physical educator may not be qualified or interested in teaching health courses, he can contribute much to the health program. His training in such areas as first aid and the foundational sciences and his direction of the physical education program places him in a position to impress upon students the importance of gaining desirable health knowledge, developing desirable health attitudes, and forming desirable health practices. Physical education can be a setting for correlated health teaching with the many opportunities that continually arise that are closely related to the health and fitness of students.

Dentist

The dentist employed to work with school children is frequently involved in such duties as conducting dental examinations of pupils, giving or supervising oral prophylaxis, and advising on curriculum material in dental hygiene. The health teacher can be helped by the dentist in the selection of curriculum material for classroom teaching, by discovering dental problems of students, and by participating himself in the classroom experiences of pupils as a resource person.

Dental hygienist

The dental hygienist usually assists the dentist and does oral prophylaxis. The teacher of health can therefore benefit from a close working relationship with this specialist in much the same way as she or he works with the dentist.

Custodian

All aspects of the school or college health program must be carefully coordinated— the health instruction program, health services, and healthful living. Therefore, the cleanliness of the building and a healthful physical environment are contributions to the health program. The custodian can be invited to help plan pertinent aspects of the health curriculum that specifically relate to his area of responsibility, to have the school or college be a model of cleanliness and of good health practices, and to adhere to proper health standards in respect to such items as lighting, ventilation, and heating.

Nutritionist

The nutritionist can contribute to health science instruction by contributing to the subject matter to be covered concerning nutrition, in speaking to classes about food and nutrition, and in discussing nutritional problems of students.

Guidance counselor

An individual on the school staff that is too frequently overlooked as an effective member of the school health team is the guidance counselor. Since many academic problems are health related and since the guidance counselor is interested in helping each student to have a successful school experience, his or her interest must at times concern itself with areas of health. As such, the guidance counselor can make suggestions for health topics to be discussed in classes, and he can be an effective guest speaker in health classes to discuss the relationship of health to scholastic and vocational success.

CONTENT AREAS FOR THE HEALTH SCIENCE INSTRUCTION PROGRAM

There is considerable knowledge and information that may be taught in health education. With all the literature that is available in such forms as textbooks, resource books, pamphlets, and promotional material, it is important that content be selected with care. At present there is little uniformity in the content of health education courses being taught in the schools and colleges throughout the country.

Some basic principles for selecting curriculum experiences in the health science instruction program are as follows:

1. The content of health science instruction should be based on the needs and interests of the students. Such considerations as developmental characteristics of children and youth and psychologic drives of students, such as security, approval, success in athletics, appearance, and peer-group approval, are considerations in relating teaching to the interests of students.

2. The problems and topics covered must be appropriate to the maturity level of the students.

3. The materials used should be current and scientifically accurate. The course should not be a textbook course. Many materials and experiences should be provided.

4. Pupils should be able to identify with the health problems discussed. As such, the problems should be geared to or related to the daily living experiences of the student body.

5. Health should be recognized as a multidisciplinary subject, and, as such, subject matter, projects, and methods of teaching should take cognizance of the new developments in the related sciences.

6. Health science instruction should be taught in light of a rapidly changing society, new knowledge, and ways of affecting the behavior of human beings.

7. Health teaching should take place in an environment that represents a healthful psychologic and physical environment.

8. The teacher of health science, in order to be most effective in her subject, must exemplify good health, be well informed, and be a happy and successful individual.

9. The basic concepts in health should be identified and taught.

10. The new technologic techniques and aids should be utilized in improving visual presentations of health material to students.

11. Considerations should be given to students' previous health experiences.

12. Planning for health science instruction should be a total school or college endeavor with teachers, specialists, and consultants participating. Furthermore, health instruction should permeate the entire school or college curriculum.

13. Objectives of the school or college health program, including knowledge, attitudes, practices, and skills, need to be reviewed and the program planned intelligently and meaningfully in light of these goals.

14. The community should be involved in health science instruction, including personnel from the health department, voluntary health associations, medical and dental professions, and other health associations and agencies.

15. School health science instruction should be closely integrated with home conditions.

16. New methods of organizing for teaching, including the nongraded school, team teaching, individualized instruction, and programmed instruction, should be considered.

17. Constant research and evaluation of the program should take place to provide the best instructional program for the students concerned.

18. Health instruction in general should share the same prestige and respect in the eyes of school or college administrators, teachers, and students as other respected school or college offerings, with time allotments and other considerations receiving equal attention.

19. Many interesting and meaningful experiences should be provided health classes to help in solving the health problems of students.

Student health needs and interests

It has been pointed out that content areas in health education should be selected on the basis of the needs and interests of the students being served. Therefore, the question arises as to how such interests and needs can be determined. Some ways in which this vital information may be obtained include an analysis of the health records that every school and college should keep in a cumulative manner and that contain such valuable information as the results of health appraisal and health counseling. Teacher observations offer some indication of student interests, desires, and health problems. Tests of knowledge, attitudes, and habits uncover superstitions and other health problems, together with the accuracy of the health knowledge possessed by the student. Conferences with parents, teachers, and students reveal many health interests and needs. A student interest survey will offer valuable information. A study of current literature concerned with scientific information in the field of health is essential. New knowledge and new health problems are revealed each day through experimentation and research on the part of the medical and other professions. Finally, a study of the community will show the health problems that are peculiar to the local setting.

The Joint Committee on Health Problems of the National Education Association and the American Medical Association suggests the following bases for determining needs and problems of students:

An analysis of biological needs of human beings.
An analysis of the characteristics of children of different age levels: their growth and developmental needs.
Health problems are revealed through a study of mortality records by age groups.
Health status by age groups as revealed on health records, accident and illness records, special studies, and surveys.
Analysis by age groups of activities related to health in which the majority of boys and girls engage.
Analysis of environmental health hazards at school and in the home and community.
Analysis of citizenship responsibilities relating to health.
Analysis of major social trends relating to health.
Analysis of vocational opportunities in health education.*

Although the specific health course of study will vary from community to community, it is still necessary to recognize that the basic health needs of students and the general content areas of health education are similar. To a great degree, what takes place is the specific adaptation of these general areas to local situations.

It seems important for the general information of the reader to point out some of the basic health needs of students and also the general health content areas, as listed by leaders in the field. Finally, it seems essential to discuss briefly some of the controversial content areas.

A Denver, Colorado, research project, concerned with a study of health needs, examined textbooks and programs of health in use throughout the United States and discussed health needs of students with teachers and physicians. The study resulted in the following list of eighteen broad areas that represented health needs of students†:

1. Keeping physically fit
2. Group health
3. Cause of disease
4. Protection from disease
5. Structure and function of the body
6. Dental health
7. Good eating habits
8. Selection and composition of food
9. Stimulants and narcotics
10. Rest and relaxation
11. Personal appearance
12. Personality development
13. Social health
14. Heredity and eugenics

---

*Joint Committee on Health Problems in Education of National Education Association and American Medical Association: Health education, Washington, D. C., 1961, National Education Association, pp. 127-129.
†Corliss, L. M.: A report of the Denver research project on health interests of children, The Journal of School Health 32:355, 1962.

15. First aid
16. Home nursing
17. Safety
18. Vocations in health

Health content areas based on needs and interests of students

The Joint Committee on Health Problems in Education of the National Education Association and the American Medical Association* suggests the following areas of health content at the junior high school educational level:

Physical growth and development
Living practices
Health maintenance and improvement
Food and nutrition
Mental health
Personality development
Family life
Sex adjustment
Safety and first aid
Community health

For the senior high school educational level the Joint Committee on Health Problems in Education of the National Education Association and the American Medical Association suggested the following areas of health content:

1. Structure and function of the human body; scientific concepts relative to normal and abnormal function; contributions of scientific research and medical practice to information relative to maintenance of normal function.
2. The balanced regimen of food, exercise, rest, sleep, relaxation, work, and study; evaluation of individual health needs.
3. Mental health, personal adjustment, development of emotional maturity, establishment of maturing sex roles, boy-girl relations.
4. Preparation for marriage, family life, child care; health implications of heredity and eugenics; good budgeting; health aspects of housing; budgeting for health insurance, medical and dental services; spending the health dollar wisely.

5. Communicable and noncommunicable diseases with emphasis on adolescent and adult disease problems; prevention and control of disease and illness including heart disease, cancer, diabetes, mental illness, alcoholism.
6. Consumer health education: choosing health products and services; scientific health care as contrasted with fads, quackery, and charlatanism; evaluating sources of information; awareness of nature of advertising appeals and "gimmicks" used to sell products.
7. Personal and community programs and practices in accident prevention and emergency care; driver education; recreational and occupational safety; fire prevention; civil defense and disasters.
8. Protection from hazards of poisons, drugs, narcotics; environmental hazards of radiation, air pollution, water contamination; chemical hazards in food production, processing, and distribution.
9. Community health: local, state, national, and international; tax-supported and voluntary health agency programs; contributions of individual citizens to community health.
10. Health careers in medicine, dentistry, nursing, public health, teaching, hospital administration, laboratory services, dietetics, physical therapy, occupational therapy, and allied professions.*

In Table 12-4 Hoyman presents a schematic health science spiral curriculum for kindergarten to grade twelve.

The health education content areas and the number of schools that include this area in their health science course, as reflected in a survey conducted in the fall of 1968 in which 810 schools returned the questionnaire, are shown in Table 12-3.

The content and basic aims of the New York State Health Education Programs are reflected in the diagram on p. 319.†

The health education program in Los Angeles includes the following topics and

---

*Joint Committee on Health Problems in Education of National Education Association and American Medical Association, op. cit., pp. 204-205.

*Joint Committee on Health Problems in Education of National Education Association and American Medical Association, op. cit., pp. 234-235.

†New York State Department of Education, New York State Program in the Health Sciences, Albany.

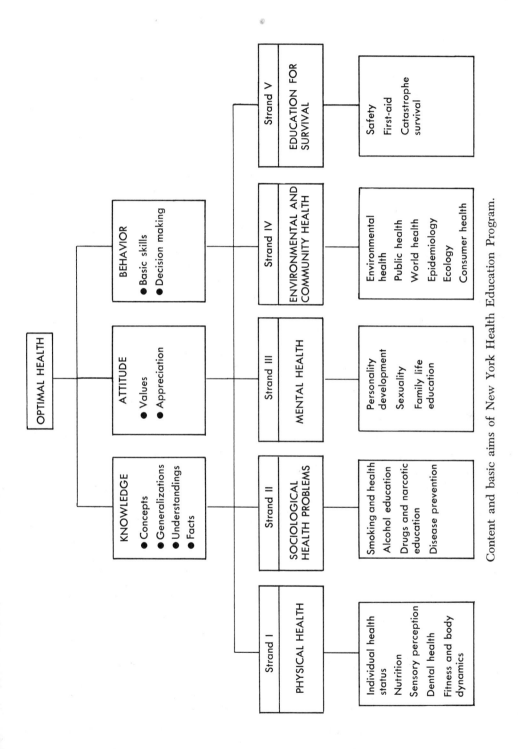

Content and basic aims of New York Health Education Program.

Table 12-3. Health education content areas*

Subject area	Schools	Subject area	Schools
Personal health	263	Hit and miss	5
Smoking, tobacco	155	Child care	4
Drugs	150	Menstruation	4
Sex education	150	Civil defense	3
Alcohol	148	Heart	3
Anatomy and physiology	113	Sanitation	3
First aid	112	Self-help	3
Communicable disease	109	Those required by	
Nutrition	81	state law	3
Mental health	52	Sight and hearing	3
Safety	41	Genetics	2
Growth and development	37	Major health problems	2
Physical fitness	30	School health	2
Marriage and family living	20	Immunization	1
Public and community health	19	Psychology	1
All areas	10	Recreation	1
Dental health	9	Young adult problems	1
Cancer	6	Regular physicial examination	1
Personality	6	Daily shower in physical	
Personal relations	5	education	1

*The Department of Education: Patterns and features of school health education in Michigan public schools, East Lansing, 1969, Michigan State Department of Education, p. 9.

units in their junior high and senior high school programs*:

Junior high school

    Unit 1—Introduction to health science
    Unit 2—Growing and maturing
    Unit 3—Achieving personal health
    Unit 4—Food for growth and health
    Unit 5—Addicting, habit-forming, and other
        dangerous substances
    Unit 6—Progress in community health
    Unit 7—First aid and safety

Senior high school

    Unit 1—Orientation to health needs
    Unit 2—Guidelines for improved nutrition
    Unit 3—Transitions to maturity
    Unit 4—Narcotics, alcohol, tobacco, and other
        harmful substances
    Unit 5—Progress in public health
    Unit 6—Consumer health protection
    Unit 7—Essentials of first aid

HEALTH CONCEPTS

The concept approach to teaching various subject matter fields of specialization has won much acclaim in educational cir-

*Langan, J. J.: Health education in Los Angeles schools, National Association of Secondary Schools Bulletin, March, 1968.

cles in recent years. It is felt that the decisions that people make and their behavior patterns are determined largely by their concepts. Concepts that evolve can have an impact on cognition (knowledge, intellectual abilities, and skills) and values, attitudes, and appreciations.

Recognizing the value of the concept approach, the school health study has developed an outline entitled *A Conceptual Approach to Health Education.*

The concept approach outlined by the school health education study recognizes the three dimensions of health—mental, physical, and social. These are closely interwoven. Furthermore, it stresses the triad of health education—the unity of man in respect to his physical, mental, and social aspects; the knowledges, attitudes, and practices as factors important to influencing health behavior; and the focus of health education upon the individual, family, and community. All these components of the triad are interdependent and constantly interacting.

The study identified three key concepts,

Table 12-4. A schematic health science spiral curriculum for kindergarten to grade twelve*†

Major health instruction areas	Primary grades				Intermediate grades			Junior high grades			Senior high grades		
	K	1	2	3	4	5	6	7	8	9	10	11	12
1. Human ecology and health, disease, longevity	X	X	X	X	X		X		X				X
2. Human growth, development, maturation, aging	X	X	X	X	X		X		X				X
3. Healthful living and physical fitness	X	X	X	X	X		X		X				X
4. Nutrition and personal fitness	X	X	X	X	X		X		X				X
5. Alcohol, tobacco, and narcotics	X	X	X	X	X		X		X				X
6. Prevention and control of disease	X	X	X	X		X			X			X	
7. Community and environmental health	X	X	X	X		X			X			X	
8. Consumer health education	X	X	X	X		X			X			X	
9. Rise of modern scientific medicine	X	X	X	X		X			X			X	
10. Safety education	X	X	X	X	X		X	X		X			X
11. First aid and home nursing	X	X	X	X		X			X		X		X
12. Personality development and mental health	X	X	X	X		X		X			X		X
13. Family-life and sex education	X	X	X	X		X		X			X		X
14. Current health events and problems	X	X	X	X	X	X	X	X	X	X	X	X	X

*From Hoyman, H. S.: An ecologic view of health and health education, The Journal of School Health 25:118, 1965.

†In kindergarten to grade three the X's denote topics, in grades four to twelve, units, or major parts of combined units.

Note: Separate health courses may be scheduled at the junior and senior high school levels as a part of the health science spiral curriculum where this method of scheduling is preferred.

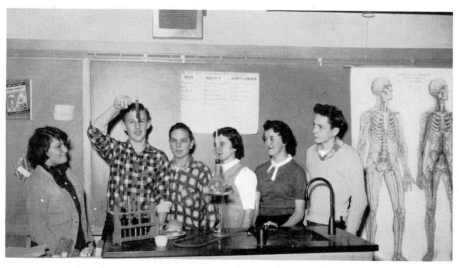

Nutrition instruction as part of the health education program.

ten conceptual statements, and thirty-one substantive elements that represent the conceptual framework for health. The ten concepts into which the key concepts are delineated are:

Growth and development influences and is influenced by the structure and functioning of the individual.

Growth and development follows a predictable sequence, yet is unique for each individual.

Protection and promotion of health is an individual, community, and international responsibility.

The potential for hazards and accidents exists, whatever the environment.

There are reciprocal relationships involving man, disease, and environment.

The family serves to perpetuate man and to fulfill certain health needs.

Personal health practices are affected by a complexity of forces, often conflicting.

Utilization of health information, products, and services is guided by values and perceptions.

Use of substances that modify mood and behavior arises from a variety of motivations.

Food selection and eating patterns are determined by physical, social, mental, economic, and cultural factors.*

SEX EDUCATION, DRUGS, AND OTHER CRITICAL CONTENT AREAS IN HEALTH SCIENCE INSTRUCTION

The question often arises as to whether such critical subjects as sex, narcotics, or alcohol education should be provided for in the health science instruction program. The fact that some of these problems are more pronounced in certain communities, and possibly restricted to some population groups, together with the fact that such education might tend to stimulate curiosity, are reasons put forth for not including them in courses of study.

On the other hand, instruction in regard to the ill effects of narcotics and alcohol is required by law in many states. Furthermore, it is felt that if children and youth

*From Sliepcevich, E. M., and Nolte, A. E.: The school health education study, The National Elementary Principal 47:43, 1968.

are provided with the facts, intelligent instruction in these subjects will act as a preventive measure. In the area of sex education, it is believed that the term *sex education* creates opposition among many parents and church groups and consequently should not be used. If it is introduced in the natural process of instruction without undue emphasis, much good can be done.

Some of the best thinking in the field emphasizes the fact that the nature of the instruction will depend upon the local situation. Where a narcotics or alcohol problem exists, there should be provision in the school curricula for the presentation of sociologic, physiologic, and psychologic facts, as well as the legal aspects of such a problem. Students should understand these facts and be guided intelligently in making the right decisions and establishing a sound standard of values.

Health education is not the only area in which discussions of sex, narcotics, and alcohol should take place. Social studies, biology, general science, physical education, and other classes also have a responsibility. Many phases of these subjects logically fit into certain aspects of these courses. Teachers must appreciate the importance of such instruction and the need for treating these subjects objectively on the basis of the facts. It is not necessary for the teacher to take a definite stand and act in the capacity of a minister preaching on the subject. Instead, if students obtain the necessary facts through research or some other method and then interpret them intelligently, the right answers will be clear. The students make their own decisions, not on the basis of the teacher's position but on the basis of the facts they have collected.

In regard to sex education, the emphasis should be on the psychologic and sociologic aspects rather than only on the biologic aspects. The end result should be to have students recognize what is desirable

RESOLUTIONS

DRUG ABUSE EDUCATION

Whereas, Drugs and medicines make a positive contribution to personal and community health, and
Whereas, A large segment of our population looks to drugs to alleviate a host of physiological, psychological and social discomforts, and
Whereas, The best deterrent to drug abuse is the individual's value system and his assessment of the consequences associated with drug involvement, and
Whereas, Those who develop school policies must be fully informed regarding the nature of drugs, psychosocial motivations, legal considerations, and the content and process of their communities' teacher inservice training and student instructional programs, and
Whereas, The nature of the problem is such that the school program must draw together the students, the total staff, and the community.
Be it Resolved:
1. That schools develop intensive inservice programs with assistance from specialists with experience and background in developing educational programs, including specialists in group process training and communications,
2. That planned programs be developed to involve and inform parents and community leaders regarding their roles in preparing young people to mature successfully in our culture,
3. That school programs for students be developed having these elements:
   a. a sequential plan beginning in the elementary years,
   b. emphasis on the decision-making process and why people use drugs,
   c. increasing understanding of the social conditions that promote drug use and abuse,
   d. a total institutional attitude which encourages acceptance of all children and an understanding that their individual needs, when frustrated, may lead to drug abuse,
4. That drug misuse education should be an important part of the total health education curriculum.

SEX EDUCATION

Whereas, Problems related to family life, sex education, and related interpersonal relationships are of concern to children and youth and have a bearing on their present and future welfare, and
Whereas, Children and youth need reliable information and interpretation from competent adults on issues bearing on their emotional and social well-being, and
Whereas, They learn best when there are cooperative relationships among families, schools, and communities, and
Whereas, There is concern that both critics and proponents have presented sex education issues in a sensational manner which inhibits the further development of a sound program,
Be it Resolved:
1. That a total institutional approach to human sexuality be initiated in the schools,
2. That schools develop sequential K-12 health education programs which encompass family life and sex education,
3. That schools assume leadership in involving parents and other responsible community leaders in the development and interpretation of school programs in family life and sex education,
4. That schools employ competent staff professionally prepared to assume leadership in the development and direction of comprehensive health education programs,
5. That inservice programs for better understanding of the schools responsibility be developed.

Adopted by the Representative Assembly of the American Association for Health, Physical Education, and Recreation, meeting at the 84th Anniversary Convention, Boston, Massachusetts, April 15, 1969.

Table 12-5. Suggested treatment of drugs in state health education curriculum guides (eleven states included)*

State	Grade level	Outline of content
A	7-12	Suggests collecting popular magazine articles on drugs and discussing reasons for A.M.A. acceptance or rejection (sic). Suggests pointing out the dangers to consumer health of over-gullibility to patent medicine advertising, and that the danger of patent medicines is delay in proper diagnosis and treatment. One of twelve content areas deals with stimulants and depressants.
B	1-12	Primary level—dangers in the incorrect use of medicines Junior high level—effects of alcohol, drugs, and tobacco on body and social functions Senior high level—analyzing effects of narcotics, drugs, tobacco and alcohol, and the use of patent medicines
C, D, E	7-12	Grades 7-9—suggests discussion of hazards of self-diagnosis and self-medication, review of medicine chest contents, evaluation of drug advertising Grades 10-12—suggests more comprehensive practice of the above and guest lectures on drugs by physicians and pharmacists
F	7-12	Discusses the importance of following prescription directions under the topic "Home Nursing." Mentions narcotics and stimulants with alcohol.
G	K-12	Defines the responsibility of informing students of dangers of drug abuse
H	K-12	Mentions narcotic drugs only in conjunction with alcohol and tobacco
I, J, K	1-12	Nothing on drugs

*From Smith, M. C., Mikeal, R. L., and Taylor, J. M.: Drugs in the health curriculum: a needed area, The Journal of School Health 39:334, 1969.

behavior and what constitutes a healthy sexuality rather than only to become acquainted with a body of factual knowledge such as that concerned with the reproductive organs. Students should be taught to live the finest type of lives possible. Sex education should not be a separate course but should be included and discussed in every course where its various aspects arise during regular discussions. Parents and representative community groups should be consulted and asked to participate in any discussions relative to the planning for instruction in this area. It is very important to have well-trained and qualified teachers handling such instruction. If the right type of leadership is provided, the result can be very beneficial to all concerned, but if poor leadership exists,

many harmful results can come from such discussion.

A resource unit in family life and sex education has been developed by the Committee on Health Guidance in Sex Education of the American School Health Association. The subunit titles for grades seven to twelve are listed here:

Grade 7
Unit 1. Understanding ourselves
Unit 2. The family
Unit 3. Review of male and female reproductive process

Grade 8
Unit 1. Emotions and behavior
Unit 2. Dating
Unit 3. The family
Unit 4. Review of the female reproductive process

Unit 5. Review of the male
reproductive process
Grade 9
Unit 1. Mental and emotional health
Unit 2. Family relationships
Unit 3. Boy-girl relationships
Grades 10 and 11
Unit 1. Psycho-social development
Unit 2. Boy-girl relationships in light of both
immediate and long-range goals
Unit 3. Family planning
Unit 4. Growth and reproduction
Grade 12
Unit 1. Preparation for marriage
Unit 2. Adjustments in marriage
Unit 3. Planning for parenthood
Unit 4. Family living
Unit 5. Attitudes toward sex and sexual behavior*

HEALTH SCIENCE INSTRUCTION AT THE PRESCHOOL AND ELEMENTARY SCHOOL LEVELS†

The committee on Health Education for Pre-School Children of the American School Health Association lists the following as a topical outline of content for preschool children:

Cleanliness and grooming
Dental health
Eyes, ears, nose
Rest and sleep
Nutrition
Growth and development
Family living

---

*As quoted from Mayshark, C., and Irwin, L. W.: Health education in secondary schools, ed. 2, St. Louis, 1968, The C. V. Mosby Co., pp. 136-137.

†The December, 1964, issue of *The Journal of School Health* has a detailed report of the study committee on health education in the elementary school of the American School Health Association. It presents in detail various health topics that may be covered at this grade level, together with basic understandings, and skills, motivational techniques and activities, materials, books, and visual aids pertinent to getting information across to students, together with suggestions for evaluation. There is also a section entitled "Workable ideas for the elementary school." The issue of *The Journal of School Health* should be of interest to those who want to know more about health science instruction at the elementary education level.

Understanding ourselves and getting along
Prevention and control of disease safety*

For each of these topics the committee has identified key concepts, suggested learning experiences, and means of evaluation.

Health education at the elementary level is aimed primarily at having the child develop good health habits and health attitudes, and at helping him live happily, healthfully, and safely. This is achieved in great measure by adapting good health practices to the regular routine of school and home living, rather than by dispensing technical, factual knowledge concerning health. The responsibility for the guidance, planning, and stimulation of good health practices and attitudes falls upon the classroom teacher. She is the guiding influence and her understanding of good health will determine to a great degree how effective such a program actually is.

The type of health program offered should be adapted to the child's level and planned in accordance with his or her interests and needs. It should also be remembered that health education is a continuous process and cannot be compartmentalized within a definite subject area or within a class period. It embraces all the activities and subjects that are a part of the child's life.

It is difficult to prescribe the amount of time that should be devoted to the teaching of health on the elementary level because the needs and interests of pupils vary. However, the amount of time devoted to health education should be equal to the other major areas of the curriculum.

At the primary grade level the emphasis should be more on the child and his daily routine as it is affected by certain health practices and attitudes. His various routines and associations at school and at home form the basis for the health emphasis. The importance of a healthful classroom

---

*Health instruction: suggestions for teachers, The Journal and School Health 39:11, 1969.

environment is stressed. Such items as cleanliness, eating, use of lavatories, safety, and good mental hygiene are brought out as the child plays, eats, and performs those many experiences that are common to all youngsters of his age.

The committee on Health Education for Elementary School Children of the American School Health Associations lists the following as a topical outline of content for this age group:

Grades 1, 2, and 3
   Cleanliness and grooming
   Rest and exercise
   Sleep and rest
   Growth
   Posture
   Role of physician and dentist
   Individual responsibility for one's health
   Responsibility for the health of others
   Dental health
   Vision and hearing
   Babies
   Nutrition
   Making new friends
   Being alone sometimes
   Family time
   Protection from infection
   Food protection
   Safety
Grades 4, 5, and 6
   Health care
   Cleanliness and grooming
   Vision and care of eyes
   Hearing and care of ears
   Heart
   Teeth
   Exercise, rest, and sleep
   Nutrition
   Growth and development
   Family living
   Understanding ourselves
   Getting along with others
   Making decisions
   Environmental health
   Prevention and control of diseases
   Safety and first aid*

For each of these topics the committee has identified key concepts, suggested learning experiences, and means of evaluation.

The Joint Committee on Health Prob-

lems in Education of the National Education Association and the American Medical Association* has suggested areas for health teaching in the kindergarten and primary grades. These areas pertain to school and home experiences relating to:
   Food and nutrition
   Exercise, rest, and sleep
   Eyes, ears, and teeth
   Clothing
   Cleanliness and grooming
   Mental and emotional health
   Communicable disease control
   Safety
   Home, schools, and neighborhoods

In the upper elementary years the values of certain health practices are brought out. A planned progression in instruction is developed. Although there is still stress on the actual practices and attitudes concerned with the daily routines and associations, more factual information is incorporated to form the basis for such habits. Furthermore, more and more responsibility is placed on the child for his own self-direction and self-control.

The utilization of trips and textbooks that point up the value of healthful living, interesting and inspiring stories, visual aids, class discussions, and projects can become a part of the experiences of each child so that the need for certain behavior is dramatically and effectively stamped upon his mind and total being.

Since health experiences should be based on the needs and interests of the child, the wise teacher will utilize various means of obtaining accurate information about these needs and interests. Such techniques as talks with parents and pupils, observations of children under various situations, a perusal of health records, a study of the home environment and community together with scientific measuring devices that have been developed to determine

---

*Health instruction: suggestions for teachers, The Journal of School Health **39:**22, 34, 1969.

*Joint Committee on Health Problems in Education of National Education Association and American Medical Association, op. cit., p. 149.

health knowledge and attitudes will be utilized. A health education program that is not based on accurate knowledge of needs and interests will fail to accomplish its objective of helping individuals to live a happier and healthier life.

HEALTH INSTRUCTION ACTIVITIES FOR THE ELEMENTARY SCHOOL

The Joint Committee on Health Problems in Education of the National Education Association and the American Medical Association has listed some of the health instruction activities in which pupils in intermediate and elementary grades can engage:

1. Conducting animal feeding experiments and experiments to test for food nutrients
2. Taking field trips to local dairies, markets, restaurants, bakeries, water supply and sewage treatment plants, and housing projects
3. Visiting museums
4. Preparing charts and graphs for visualizing class statistics, such as absence due to colds or school accidents
5. Making pin maps of sources of mosquitoes, rubbish depositories, and slum areas
6. Making health posters
7. Setting up room and corridor health exhibits
8. Preparing health bulletin boards and displays
9. Making murals and dioramas
10. Maintaining class temperature charts
11. Arranging a library corner of health materials on the subject being studied
12. Using sources of printed material—reference books, texts, bulletins, newspapers, and magazines—for the study of a particular topic
13. Giving reports in various ways—chalkboard talks, dramatizations, role-playing, panels
14. Serving on the safety patrol
15. Joining the bicycle safety club
16. Participating in a home or school cleanup campaign
17. Planning menus
18. Preparing meals for class mothers or other guests
19. Sharing health programs with primary grades
20. Securing a health examination
21. Having all dental corrections made
22. Taking inoculations
23. Keeping records of growth through charts or graphs
24. Keeping diaries of health practices
25. Studying text or references to find answers to problems
26. Thinking through solutions to problems
27. Applying in daily practices health principles learned*

Health suggestions for the classroom teacher

The classroom teacher is the key school person involved in the health of the elementary school child. The organization of the school with the self-contained classroom enables her to continually observe the pupils and to note deviations from normal. Continuous contact with the same children over a long period of time also makes it possible for her to know a great deal about their physical, social, emotional, and mental health. She can help them develop the right knowledge, attitudes, and practices. Some of the responsibilities that fall to the classroom teacher in regard to the health of her pupils require that she do the following:

1. Possess an understanding of what constitutes a well-rounded school health program and the teacher's part in it.

2. Meet with the school physician, nurse, and others in order to determine how she can best contribute to the total health program.

3. Become acquainted with parents and homes of her students and establish parent-school cooperation.

4. Discover the health needs and interests of her pupils.

5. Organize health teaching units that are meaningful and in terms of the health needs and interests of her students.

6. See that children needing special care are referred to proper places for help.

7. Be versed in first-aid procedures.

8. Participate in the work of the school health council. If none exists, interpret the need for one.

9. Provide an environment for children

---

*Joint Committee on Health Problems in Education of National Education Association and American Medical Association, op. cit., pp. 187-188.

while at school that is conducive to healthful living.

10. Continually be on the alert for children with deviations from normal behavior and signs of communicable diseases.

11. Provide experiences for living healthfully at school.

12. Help pupils assume an increasing responsibility for their own health as well as for the health of others.

13. Set an example for the child of what constitutes healthful living.

14. Motivate the child to be well and happy.

15. Be present at health examinations of pupils and contribute in any way helpful to the physician in charge.

16. Follow through in cooperation with the nurse to see that remediable health defects are corrected.

17. Interpret the school health program to the community and enlist its support in solving health problems.

18. Provide a well-rounded class physical education program.

19. Help supervise various activities that directly affect health—school lunch, rest periods, and so on.

20. Become familiar with teaching aids and school and community resources for enhancing the health program.

21. Be aware of the individual differences of pupils.

HEALTH SCIENCE INSTRUCTION AT THE SECONDARY LEVEL*

Since many aspects of health education at the secondary level are covered in this chapter under the topics of Content Areas

*The December, 1964, issue of *The Journal of School Health* has a detailed report of the study committee on health education in the junior high school and senior high school. It presents in detail various health topics pertinent to these educational levels, together with health problems, suggested learning experiences or activities, and evaluation techniques. Furthermore, there are many workable ideas presented.

for the Health Science Instruction Program, Concentrated, Correlated, Integrated, and Incidental Health Teaching, and Organization of Classes, this discussion will be limited to a brief summary of some of the points of emphasis in health education at the secondary level.

The changes taking place in American society and the research data available emphasize a need to stress certain areas of health instruction. These include alcohol education, community health problems, health careers, international health activities, sex education, venereal disease education, tobacco and narcotics, nutrition and weight control, environmental hazards, and consumer health education.

Health and the structural organization of the secondary school

The structural organization of the secondary level differs from the elementary level. At the elementary level, the classroom teacher frequently takes overall charge of a group of children. She teaches them in various subjects, stays with them throughout the entire day, and supervises their activities. At the secondary level, the student has many different teachers. These teachers specialize in subject matter to a greater degree than they specialize in pupils. There is departmentalization into such subject matter areas as mathematics, social studies, and English. This structural organization affects health education tremendously.

First, this structural organization points up the need for concentrated courses in health education, such as those found in the other subject matter areas. Health education as a subject should receive equal consideration with the other important subjects in the secondary school offering, in all aspects such as scheduling, facilities, and staff. The minimum time that should be allotted has been stated as a daily period for at least two semesters, at the seventh-, eighth-, or ninth-grade level, and a daily period for two semesters, preferably at the eleventh- or twelfth-grade level.

Second, this structural organization emphasizes the need for a specialist in the teaching of health education. Just as specialists are needed in English and the other subjects offered at the secondary level, so are they needed in the field of health education. The body of scientific knowledge, the training needed, and the importance of the subject make such a specialist a necessity.

Third, this structural organization stresses the need for coordination and cooperation. Health cuts across many subject matter areas, as well as the total school life of the child. In order that it may be properly treated in the various subject matter areas such as science, home economics, and social studies, in order that the physical environment and the emotional environment may be properly provided for, in order that health services may be most effectively administered, and in order that close cooperation and coordination between the school and the rest of the community may be obtained, there is an essential need for some type of coordinating machinery. There is a need for a school health council or committee where individuals representing various interests and groups can pool their thinking and bring about cooperative efforts. There is a need for some individual to act in the capacity of a health coordinator, to spearhead the movement for cooperation and coordination, and to develop good relationships among the various departments and interests represented in the total school situation, as well as with those in the broader community.

In order to have an effective, sound health education program at the secondary level, the central administration must provide the type of leadership that leaves no doubt as to the importance of health in the lives of the many children who attend the schools. Such administrative leadership will reflect itself from the very top to the very bottom of the school structure and be felt at the grass roots of all community enterprises.

The junior high school. The junior high school was created to meet the physical, mental, and socioemotional needs of the preadolescent and early adolescent boys and girls who make up grades seven, eight, and nine. These grades represent a period of transition when the characteristics of growth and development, although varying from individual to individual, form a relatively uniform pattern during the age period of 12 to 14 years.

Junior high school students are in need of knowledge and proper attitudes that will result in desirable health practices. The fact that students may not be interested in such information represents a challenge for the junior high school educational program. The consumption of many sweets as a substitute for essential foods, omission of breakfast, and other undesirable practices, an interest in personal grooming, a need to understand one's bodily makeup, the maturing sexual drive, and other factors make it imperative to get across health information at this time. Health education activities contribute feelings of satisfaction and understanding that may never be possible of accomplishment in the regular academic program.

Health content should be adapted to the needs and interests of the students in this age group. Stress should be on the personal health problems of the students themselves, and how hereditary factors affect their health, how good or poor health manifest themselves, and how health practices affect the attainment of life ambitions and goals. Such topics as food, rest, exercise, first aid, safety, alcohol and narcotics, mental health, communicable disease, growth and functions of the human body, personality development, family life, and community health would be covered.

The health teaching that takes place in

the junior high school should take into consideration the developmental tasks that characterize the early adolescent. These include the desire for independence of adults, self-respect, and peer identification, as well as accepting one's physical makeup, adjusting to the opposite sex, and establishing a standard of values.

The committee on Health Education for Junior High School of the American School Health Association lists the following as a topical outline of content for this age group:

Health status
Cleanliness and grooming
Rest, sleep, and relaxation
Exercise
Posture
Recreation and leisure-time activities
Sensory perception
Nutrition
Growth and development
Understanding ourselves
Personality
Getting along with others
Family living
Alcohol
Drugs
Smoking and tobacco
Environment
Air and water pollutions
Consumer health
Disease*

For each of these topics the committee has identified key concepts, suggested learning experiences, and means of evaluation.

The senior high school. During grades ten, eleven, and twelve, the stress continues to be on many subject-matter areas that were stressed for the health content in the junior high school years. However, the material and experiences presented would be more advanced and adapted to the age group found in the later high school years. Such topics as the structure and function of the human body could stress more scientific concepts as found

through research, evaluation of individual health needs in the light of proper balance in one's daily routine, and the means of attaining proper emotional maturity and mental health.

The committee on Health Education for Senior High School of the American School Health Association lists the following as a topical outline of content for this age group:

Health status
Fatigue and sleep
Exercise
Recreational activities
Sensory perception
Nutrition
Growth and development toward maturity
Family living
Alcohol
Drugs
Smoking and tobacco
Health protection
Noise pollution
Health agencies
Health careers
World health
Safety and accidents*

For each of these topics the committee has listed key concepts, suggested learning experiences, and means of evaluation.

Although personal health receives considerable attention during the high school years, a major part of the teaching is concerned with problems of adult and family living and community health. Such health areas as preparation for marriage and family life, communicable and noncommunicable disease control, evaluation of professional health services, environmental health, industrial health, Civil Defense, consumer health education, accident prevention, emergency care, protection from environmental hazards such as radiation, health agencies at the local, state, national, and international levels, and the various health careers open to high school students receive great stress.

---

*Health instruction: suggestions for teachers, The Journal of School Health 39:48, 1969.

*Health instruction: suggestions for teachers, The Journal of School Health 39:71, 1969.

Some students will not be going to college. This means that the senior high school years offer the last opportunity to impress boys and girls with their health responsibilities—to themselves, their loved ones, and the members of their community.

Health education at the secondary level can represent an experience that will have a lasting effect for the betterment of human lives. The leadership provided, the methods used, and the stress placed upon such an important aspect of living will determine in great measure the extent to which each school will fulfill its responsibility.

HEALTH SCIENCE INSTRUCTION AT THE COLLEGE AND UNIVERSITY LEVEL

The college and the university also have responsibilities for health science instruction. Health is important to everyone regardless of the type of work he may do.

Years ago the college and university health education offerings consisted mainly of lectures on various aspects of the anatomy and physiology of the human body. These were usually given by medical personnel and were often a collection of uninteresting facts unrelated to the student's interests and health problems. In more recent years this type of presentation has changed. The emphasis has shifted from the factual medical knowledge to health problems which students themselves encounter in day-to-day living and also to those subjects in which students are especially interested. Consequently, discussions are now held on subjects concerned with family living, personal and community health, mental health, drugs, environmental health, nutrition, the prevention of disease, and related subjects.

The Third National Conference on Health in Colleges recommended major health instruction courses appropriate to special groups of students. It also suggested "a minimum of 45 class hours or

three to four semester credits" for a basic or general health course in "personal and community health." Other recommended procedures for college health courses that have been set forth include (1) the 3- or 5-hour one-semester required or elective course, (2) the 2-hour per week course for two credits, (3) the 2-hour course shared with a physical education requirement, and (4) the 1-hour per week course for one credit. Such a course should meet frequently enough to maintain the student's interest and to cover the subject adequately. Furthermore, the lecture method of presentation should not be the only one used.

The President's Commission on Higher Education stressed the importance of health instruction for college students. It particularly stressed instruction based directly on the practical problems of personal and community health.

The American College Health Association has recommended that every college and university have a requirement in health education for all students who fall below acceptable standards on a college-level health knowledge test.

The junior college is in a particularly strategic position to offer health instruction. The 2-year college reaches a significant segment of the population that does not go on to the 4-year colleges and universities. Furthermore, research has shown that junior college students have demonstrated as much as 25% more interest in health problems than high school students. Junior college students are more mature and this may be an explanation of their increased interest in health problems. Topics such as sex instruction, marriage, mental health, emotional health, alcohol, tobacco, and narcotics are of particular interest to this segment of the college population.

It is generally felt that a health education department should be established to coordinate the instruction in health, that student needs should represent an important consideration for the determination of subject matter content, that only qualified faculty members be permitted to teach health education classes, and that classes be limited to a maximum of thirty-five students. Testing of new students is also recommended, after which those students who fall below desirable standards are required to take the required health education course.

Presently, health education courses offered in colleges and universities are listed in college catalogues under such names as Personal Hygiene, Health Education, Personal and Community Health, Health Science, Hygiene, Healthful Living, Health and Safety, Health Essentials, and Problems of Healthful Living. Courses are taught in such departments as health, physical education, and recreation; health education; biology; education; health and safety; basic studies; psychology; and biologic sciences. Students required to take such courses vary from only those students in schools of education or in departments of health, physical education, and recreation, or elementary education major students, to liberal arts students. In some institutions courses are required for women but not for men.

There is a need for a uniform requirement for all college students to demonstrate that they know basic facts in the field of health. Those students who fail to meet such standards should be required to take a course in this area. Such a requirement is basic to the general education, productivity, and health of each person.

HEALTH EDUCATON FOR ADULTS

Adults are the guiding force in any community. The prestige they have, the positions they occupy, and their interests determine the extent to which any project or enterprise will be a success. Therefore, if the schools are to have an adequate health education program, if the knowledge that is disseminated, attitudes that are developed, and practices that are encouraged are to become a permanent part of the child's being and routine, the adult must be taken into consideration. Unless this is done, the schools' efforts will be of no avail.

There is a great need for parental education and for education in regard to the many health problems that confront any community. Adults are interested not only in children's health problems but also in the causes of sickness and death in the population and ways in which they can live a healthier life. Adult education is rapidly spreading across the length and breadth of this country. It is important that health education become one of the areas considered in any such program.

Schools and colleges should play a key part in adult education programs through the facilities, staff, and other resources at their disposal. They should cooperate fully with the many official and voluntary health agencies and other interested community groups in the furtherance of health objectives. Adult education programs in the area of health should be designed to discover community health problems, understand the health needs of children, and understand school health programs. Such discovery and understanding should lead to active participation in meeting health needs and in solving health problems. Such a program would also lend itself to growth in respect to health knowledge, attitudes, and practices.

METHODS OF TEACHING HEALTH

Methods of teaching health, such as lecture, recitation, and assignments in the textbook, represent a limited array of approved techniques for the modern health class. Although good textbooks are important and the other methods have value under select conditions, there are many other methods that can motivate students and create interest in health topics.

The methods used should be adapted

to the group of students being taught, be in accordance with the objectives sought, be capable of use by the instructor, stimulate interest among the students, and be adaptable to the time, space, and equipment in the school program. Some of the more popular methods for teaching health are discussed in the following paragraphs.

Problem solving is one of the most effective and best methods for teaching health. Health topics can be stated in the form of problems and then a systematic approach can be utilized by the students to obtain an answer. For example, the problem can be stated: "What are the effects of narcotics on health?" A systematic approach to this problem might include (1) stating the nature and scope of the problem, (2) defining the various possible solutions to the problem, (3) collecting scientific information to support each of the various aspects of the problem, (4) analyzing the information gathered as to its source, authoritativeness, date of origin, and other pertinent factors, and (5) drawing conclusions for the solution of the problem.

Textbook assignments may be given, followed by class discussions based on the readings.

Field trips can include planned visits to an agency or place where health matters are of importance, such as a hospital, local health department, water purification plant, health clinic, or fire department.

Class discussions on health topics of interest can be encouraged among the members of the class.

Demonstrations are an excellent method to show how something functions or is constructed, such as good and poor forms of posture or first-aid procedures.

Experiments, such as observing the growth of animals when certain types of diet are administered, are informative.

Independent study in which the students are assigned health topics for investigation is helpful.

Resource people, such as doctors, dentists, firemen, or other specialists, can be brought in to speak to health classes.

Audiovisual aids, such as films, television, filmstrips, slides, radio, and recordings, are helpful in presenting certain types of health material to the students in an interesting and clear manner.

Graphic materials such as posters, graphs, charts, bulletin boards, and exhibits are valuable for motivating students in regard to health matters, arousing interest, attracting attention, and visualizing ideas.

Interviews can be arranged in which students may be assigned to interview such persons as officers of the local health department, representatives of safety councils, members of voluntary health agencies, and heads of medical and dental societies for the purpose of getting the views of specialists and their recommendations on health matters.

Panels can be made up of students for an informal exchange of ideas or points of view regarding pertinent health matters.

Buzz sessions in which a class is organized into small groups of students for the purpose of discussing health topics, permitting each student more opportunity for discussion, is an excellent method.

Class committees can be formed by dividing a class and assigning topics for exploration.

Dramatizations, such as a play or a skit, can be put on by a class to bring to the pupils' attention a health matter such as the importance of safety on the playground.

Surveys in regard to health problems in the school, college, or community that need investigation and more information as to their solution can be suggested. Survey forms can be constructed by pupils themselves or else standard forms may be available under certain conditions.

Games and quizzes patterned after popular shows on radio or television can provide interesting methods and challenge the thinking of students.

Health aids can be provided in which

community health agencies may offer opportunities for students to obtain experience by keeping records or engaging in various types of activities where the jobs do not require experience and special training. Working on a Red Cross blood program is an example.

CONCENTRATED, CORRELATED, INTEGRATED, AND INCIDENTAL HEALTH TEACHING

Four ways of including health education in the school offering are through concentrated, correlated, integrated, and incidental teaching. Each of these will be discussed.

Concentrated health teaching

Concentrated health education refers to the provision in the school offering for regularly scheduled courses that are confined solely to a consideration of health, rather than a combination with some other subject matter area. It implies a scheduled time for class meetings and a planned course of study. It is recommended that such courses be given on the secondary school level. Furthermore, such courses should be held for a daily class period at least one semester during the ninth or tenth grade and also during the eleventh or twelfth grade.

It is the general consensus that concentrated health education is a necessity. If the objectives for which the school health program has been established are to be achieved, time must be made available in the curricular offering of the school. Health has been listed as one of the main objectives in the field of education. Therefore, it would seem logical to assume that in order to achieve such an objective proper provisions must be made.

Concentrated health education courses required of all students result in many educational benefits. There is a specialized body of knowledge to impart that can best be given to students in a concentrated

manner, rather than by depending upon some other subject to provide this information. It allows for better planning, teaching progression, and evaluation. It further allows for the giving of credit, such as is given for any other course that is offered separately. It is more likely to result in health instruction by teachers who have specialized in this particular area and who are qualified and interested in participating in such a course. When offered as a separate course it enables boys and girls to be in the same class, as in other subjects. This is not true if it is combined with physical education, where boys and girls are usually in separate groups. It offers greater opportunities for discussion of personal health problems, with guidance and counseling in regard to these problems, and for the utilization of teaching methods appropriate to such a course.

The importance of concentrated health education is clearly recognized in the upper 6 years of school by one superintendent of schools who says:

. . . In the upper six years some of the health instruction may be provided for in other subjects, science and home economics, for example, but there must be at least a one-unit health course taught by a specialist. Only through such a course can justice be done to the extensive content of the complete health education course, since specialists in other subjects have their own objectives to satisfy and can be expected to subordinate satisfaction of health objectives. Moreover, maturing students, particularly those in the senior high school, need the challenge of being exposed to the teaching of a health specialist. Much can be said for diffusing health content through the high school program of studies, so long as diffusion does not result in confusion, if not chaos, and so long as provision is made for an adequate degree of specialization through the one-unit course.*

Correlated health teaching

Correlated health education refers to the practice of including health concepts in the

---

*Miller, J. L.: An administrator looks at the school health program, The Journal of Educational Sociology **22**:27, 1948.

various subject matter areas. For example, in the area of history the relationship of the rise and fall of various groups of people could be related to their health and the prevalence of disease, as could the increased speed of transportation and the transfer of disease from one country to the other. In the area of English, a study of the works of literature could be selected with a view to pointing up the health problems of individuals during various periods of history. The relationship of music and of art to mental health could be brought out. Mathematics could be used as a tool to figure the costs of various health projects. Science could bring out the health aspects in relation to the structure and functions of the human body. Home economics provides an excellent setting for teaching such things as nutrition and personal cleanliness. There is hardly a subject matter area that cannot be correlated with health education.

Correlated health education should be a part of every school health program. This necessitates definite planning to ensure that such an important subject is emphasized at every opportunity. Schools with health coordinators have found that such a person can perform an outstanding job in this area by meeting with teachers in the various subject matter areas and discussing and planning the contributions they can make to health education. Although correlated health education is very important and should be included in every school, it should not be regarded as a substitute for concentrated health instruction. Even when there is a concentrated health program there should also be a correlated health program that permeates the entire school offering. When both correlated and concentrated health education are provided for, in adequate amounts and in the right manner, the best results are obtained. A survey of Michigan schools shows the various subjects with which health is correlated in that state.

Integrated health teaching

In integrated health teaching, health learnings are integrated into other aspects of the classroom program. Learning experiences are organized around a central objective. Whereas in correlated teaching health

Table 12-6. Health education correlation*

Subject	Schools	Subject	Schools
Science	244	Conservation	1
Physical education	217	Driver education	1
Home economics	183	Educational guidance	1
Biology	165	Elective living	1
General science	34	Home arts	1
Family living	29	Home living	1
Sociology	11	Household mechanics	1
Social studies	10	Life adjustment	1
Psychology	6	Modern problems	1
Orientation	4	Nursing	1
Civics	3	Personal biology	1
Guidance	3	Personal living	1
Reading	3	Physics	1
Art	2	Political science	1
Chemistry	2	Sex education	1
Life science	2	Social living	1
Natural science	2	Teen living	1
Physiology	2		

*From State Department of Education: Patterns and features of school health education in Michigan public schools, East Lansing, 1969, Michigan State Department of Education, p. 4.

is brought into various subject matter areas, such as physical education and mathematics, in integrated health teaching various parts of a unit of study are related to a central theme. Two such themes might be that of living in a city or planning a visit to a foreign country. Health is one consideration involved in the planning, discussion, and assignments concerning this central theme. Health factors, for example, can be a very important consideration in living in a large metropolitan city or in going to a foreign country. There are problems concerned with water supply, sewage supply, fire prevention, disease control, immunizations, and medical examinations. Integrated health teaching finds its best setting in the elementary school.

Incidental health teaching

Incidental health education refers to that education that takes place during normal teaching situations, other than in regular health classes, where attention is focused on problems concerned with health. Such occasions may arise as the result of a question asked by a student; a problem that is raised in class; a personal problem that confronts a member of the class, a family, or the community; or a sudden illness, accident, or special project. It represents an opportunity for the teacher, physician, dentist, or nurse to provide information that is educational in nature. When a child has his eyes examined or his chest x-rayed, for example, many questions arise and opportunities are afforded to give the child information that will have a lasting and beneficial value. In many cases this will benefit the health of the child more than information given in more formalized, planned class situations. Teachers and others should constantly keep in mind the necessity for continually being alert to these "teachable moments." When a child is curious and wants information, this establishes a time for dynamic health education. Incidental health education can be planned for in advance. Situations and incidents should

be anticipated and utilized to their fullest in the interests of good health.

ORGANIZATION OF CLASSES

Many problems arise in connection with the organization of health science classes. Some of the more prevalent of these are concerned with whether boys and girls should meet together or separately, time arrangement, and scheduling.

Class membership

Boys and girls should be scheduled for health classes in a way that is in the best interests of all concerned. This would mean that where health science instruction is a combined program with physical education, and where the boys and girls are in separate classes, it would probably be best to conduct the health classes in a similar manner. On the other hand, if health science and physical education are not combined, it would seem that they should be handled in the same manner as any other subject. This would mean there would be mixed groups. The fact that the subject matter is health science should not mean separation of sexes. It should be pointed out, however, that some leaders in the field maintain this concept is wrong and advocate keeping the sexes separate as a means of getting better organization.

It is generally agreed that if boys and girls meet as a mixed group for health science they should continue as a mixed group throughout the entire course. It does not seem wise to have them meet separately when certain topics are considered. To do so tends to overstress and play up as "hush hush" certain aspects of health science. This creates confusion and encourages undue curiosity. It is best to treat the subjects in a natural and educational manner.

Time arrangement

There are many time arrangement patterns being followed in respect to health science. This is true especially on the secondary level.

The *Suggested School Health Policies— A Charter for School Health* recommends that "specific courses in health should be provided for all pupils in both junior and senior high schools. The minimum time allotment for the junior high school health course should be a daily period for at least two semesters, during the seventh, eighth, or ninth grade. The minimum time allotment for the health course in the senior high school should be a daily period for at least two semesters, preferably during the eleventh or twelfth grade. Health courses should receive credit equal to that given for courses in other areas. Health courses should be given in regular classrooms, adequately equipped. The classes should be comparable in size to those in other subject matter areas."*

The Joint Committee on Health Problems in Education of the National Education Association and the American Medical Association reaffirmed this stand when they pointed out that the trend appears to be toward concentrated health courses, one early in the high school, the other late in the senior high school period.

RESOURCES

The teacher or other individuals interested in obtaining help in planning, organizing, and administering a health education program can consult numerous persons and organizations for guidance and help. There are also many materials available for their use. Within the school itself, resource help exists in the form of staff members who possess specialized knowledge, such as the school physician, nurse, and home economics and physical education teachers. The community also offers numerous resources that can enrich the health education program immensely. In addition to the school and community, the state and nation also have rich resources that in many cases are available merely for the asking.

The organizations at the local, state, and national levels that offer resources for the field of health education can be listed and discussed under the following headings: (1) professional agencies and associations, (2) official agencies, and (3) commercial organizations.

Professional agencies and associations

Under professional agencies and associations can be listed such organizations as voluntary health agencies, medical, dental, and nursing associations, council of social agencies, and other health education associations. Some of the more prominent are listed here:

Voluntary health organizations

American Cancer Society, 219 E. 42nd St., New York, N. Y. 10017

American Heart Association, 44 E. 23rd St., New York, N. Y. 10010

American National Red Cross, National Headquarters, Washington, D. C. 20006

American Social Health Association, 1740 Broadway, New York, N. Y. 10019

American Hearing Society, 919 18th St. N. W., Washington, D. C. 20006

Child Welfare League of America, 44 E. 23rd St., New York, N. Y. 10010

National Committee for Mental Hygiene, 1740 Broadway, New York, N. Y. 10019

National Foundation, 800 2nd Ave., New York, N. Y. 10017

National Safety Council, 425 N. Michigan Ave., Chicago, Ill. 60611

National Society for the Prevention of Blindness, 16 E. 40th St., New York, N. Y. 10016

National Society for Crippled Children and Adults, 2023 W. Ogden Ave., Chicago, Ill. 60612

National Tuberculosis Association, 1740 Broadway, New York, N. Y. 10019

Professional associations

American Academy of Pediatrics, 1801 Hinman Ave., P. O. Box 1034, Evanston, Ill. 60201

American Association for Health, Physical Education, and Recreation, 1201 16th St. N. W., Washington, D. C. 20036

American Dental Association, 211 E. Chicago Ave., Chicago, Ill. 60611

---

*National Committee on School Health Policies: Suggested school health policies, ed. 3, Chicago, 1962, American Medical Association.

American Hospital Association, 840 N. Lakeshore Dr., Chicago, Ill. 60610

American Medical Association, 535 N. Dearborn St., Chicago, Ill. 60610

American Nurses Association, 10 Columbus Circle, New York, N. Y. 10010

American Public Health Association, 1740 Broadway, New York, N. Y. 10019

American School Health Association, 515 E. Main St., Kent, Ohio 44240

Child Study Association of America, 9 E. 89th St., New York, N. Y. 10019

National Education Association, 1201 16th St. N. W., Washington, D. C. 20036

National League of Nursing, 10 Columbus Circle, New York, N. Y. 10019

Official agencies

Official agencies, such as state departments of health, state departments of education, and public health departments, offer a rich source of help. They offer guidance and consultant services, disseminate information and materials in various forms for use in health classes, and make available films and other visual aids.

Government agencies on the national level provide resources in various forms, including consultant services, health reports, and grants-in-aid, and publish various materials of interest and use to all those teaching health education.

State colleges and universities, as well as private institutions, should be kept in mind when seeking resources for health. In many such institutions the staffs, with their various specialists, are available for use in the schools. Many times they will conduct workshops and institutes to provide inservice training to local schoolteachers. Many have libraries of films and other materials that may be rented at a very nominal fee.

Thought and planning are required in order to use these various resources effectively. The right persons to contact should be known, materials that are borrowed should be returned on time, and consultant services should be handled in a considerate manner.

The names of some official agencies follow:

Atomic Energy Commission, Washington, D. C.

Department of Agriculture, Washington, D. C. (Bureau of Animal Industry and Bureau of Home Economics and Human Nutrition)

Department of Commerce, Bureau of the Census, Washington, D. C.

Department of Health, Education, and Welfare, Washington, D. C. (Office of Education, Office of Special Services, Public Health Service, and Social Security Administration)

Department of the Interior, Bureau of Mines, Washington, D. C.

Department of State, Washington, D. C.

Executive Office of the President, National Security Resources Board, Civilian Defense Office (Federal Civil Defense Administration), Washington, D. C.

Government Printing Office, Superintendent of Documents, Washington, D. C.

State boards of health, located in the state capitals

State departments of education, located in the state capitals

State universities and colleges

Tennessee Valley Authority, Health and Safety Division, Knoxville, Tenn.

World Health Organization, Palais des Nations, Geneva, Switzerland

Commercial organizations

There are many commercial companies that dispense health materials. Although this material should be evaluated with care, much of it will prove helpful in the field of health education. Some of the commercial companies are listed:

The American Institute of Baking, 400 E. Ontario, Chicago, Ill. 60611

The Cereal Institute, 135 S. LaSalle St., Chicago, Ill. 60603

General Mills, Inc., 9200 Wayzata Blvd., Minneapolis, Minn. 55426

The Evaporated Milk Association, 228 N. LaSalle St., Chicago, Ill. 60601

The Florida Citrus Fruit Commission, Lakeland, Fla. 33802

The National Livestock and Meat Board, 36 S. Wabash Ave., Chicago, Ill. 60603

Sunkist Growers, Box 2706, Terminal Annex, Los Angeles, Calif. 90054

The United Fresh Fruit and Vegetable Association, 777 14th St. N. W., Washington, D. C. 20005

The Wheat Flour Institute, 309 W. Jackson Blvd., Chicago, Ill. 60606

RATING SCALE TO EVALUATE HEALTH EDUCATION MATERIALS*

Suitable material meets all of these criteria

	Yes	No
1. Is appropriate to the course of study.	___	___
2. Is a reinforcement of other materials.	___	___
3. Is significantly different.	___	___
4. Is impartial, factual, and accurate.	___	___
5. Is up-to-date.	___	___
6. Is nonsectarian, nonpartisan, and unbiased.	___	___
7. Is free from undesirable propaganda.	___	___
8. Is free from excessive or objectionable advertising.	___	___
9. Is free or inexpensive and readily available.	___	___

Pamphlets

	Excellent	Good	Fair	Poor
1. Readability of type.	___	___	___	___
2. Appropriateness of illustrations.	___	___	___	___
3. Organization of content.	___	___	___	___
4. Logical sequence of concepts.	___	___	___	___
5. Important aspects of topic stand out.	___	___	___	___
6. Material directed to one specific group such as teachers, pupils, or parents.	___	___	___	___
7. Reading level appropriate for intended group.	___	___	___	___
8. Based on interest and needs of intended group.	___	___	___	___
9. Positively directed in words, description, and actions.	___	___	___	___
10. Directed toward desirable health practices.	___	___	___	___
11. Minimal resort to fear techniques and morbid concepts.	___	___	___	___
12. In good taste; avoids vulgarity, stereotypes, and ridicule.	___	___	___	___
Total rating	___	___	___	___

Posters

	Excellent	Good	Fair	Poor
1. Realistic and within experience level.	___	___	___	___
2. Appeals to interest.	___	___	___	___
3. Emphasizes positive behavior and attitudes.	___	___	___	___
4. Message clear at a glance.	___	___	___	___
5. Little or no conflicting detail.	___	___	___	___
6. In good taste.	___	___	___	___
7. Attractive and in pleasing colors.	___	___	___	___
Total rating	___	___	___	___

Recommended for use

1. For use by:
   a. pupils ___ b. teachers ___ c. parents ___ d. adults ___
2. Appropriate grade level:
   a. primary ___ b. elementary ___ c. junior high school ___ d. secondary ___
   e. college ___ f. adult ___

Not recommended for use and why

Date _____ Evaluated by _____

*From Osborn, B. M., and Sutton, W.: Evaluation of health education materials, The Journal of School Health 34:72, 1964. (Rating scale prepared by members of the school activities subcommittee.)

EVALUATION

Chapters 17 and 18 discuss in detail the evaluation process concerning school and college health programs. These chapters should be reviewed by the reader for the evaluation of the health science instruction program.

Periodic evaluations of school and college health science instruction programs should provide information on the knowledge achieved by the students, the degree to which student needs are being met, the extent to which objectives are achieved, the value of certain methods of teaching, the effectiveness of the teaching, and the strengths and weaknesses of the program.

Instruments that have been found to be effective in evaluating the health science instruction program include the following:

1. Observation of students in respect to their behavior and skills
2. Checklists
3. Questionnaires
4. Rating scales
5. Interviews with students and parents
6. Tests—standardized and teacher-made
7. Examples of students' work
8. Diaries and other records kept by students
9. Case studies of individual students

CHECKLIST FOR EVALUATING THE HEALTH SCIENCE INSTRUCTION PROGRAM*

General

	Yes	No
1. The school has a clear statement of the philosophy and principles upon which an effective school health instruction program is based.	___	___
2. Teachers on the staff appreciate the importance of health instruction and understand the contributions it makes to the total education program.	___	___
3. The school administration has assigned a qualified person from the staff to coordinate the entire school health program and provides him time to carry out his duties and responsibilities.	___	___
4. The school has an active health committee that helps in planning and coordinating the school health program.	___	___
5. The school provides a physical environment and an emotional atmosphere that helps to make possible the achievement of the goals of the health instruction program.	___	___
6. Teachers and other school staff members set a good example, in terms of good physical and mental health habits and attitudes, as part of the health instruction program.	___	___
7. The health instruction program is based upon the health needs, problems, interests, and abilities of the pupils.	___	___
8. The school has developed a teaching guide outlining a progressive plan of health instruction from grades 1 through 12.	___	___
9. The school has established definite goals of achievement in relation to habits, understanding, attitudes, and skills for each.	___	___
10. The school administration promotes the integration of health and safety instruction with all curricular areas and extracurricular activities of the school.	___	___
11. The school includes in its in-service education program opportunities for its staff to become better qualified for conducting the health instruction program.	___	___

*From State of Ohio Department of Education: A guide for improving school health instruction programs, Columbus, Ohio, 1963, State of Ohio Department of Education, Division of Elementary and Secondary Education.

CHECKLIST FOR EVALUATING THE HEALTH SCIENCE INSTRUCTION PROGRAM—cont'd

General—cont'd

12. The school administration provides adequate materials, such as books, charts, filmstrips, and pamphlets needed for the program.   —— ——
13. Textbooks used in health classes are authoritative, up-to-date, written in an interesting manner, and suitable for the grade level in which they are used.   —— ——
14. The school evaluates its health instruction periodically to determine its effectiveness in achieving established goals.   —— ——

Elementary program

Yes No

15. In grades 1 to 3 sufficient time is provided during the school day for incidental and integrated teaching of health.   —— ——
16. In grades 4 to 6 a minimum of three periods a week is allotted for direct health instruction.   —— ——
17. The planned health instruction is supplemented in the upper grade by incidental teaching, correlation, and integration.   —— ——
18. Classroom teachers meet the state's minimum standards relative to college preparation in health education.   —— ——
19. The health instruction program centers around the daily living of the child instead of rote learning of health facts and rules.   —— ——
20. The program provides many interesting and worthwhile activities that are helpful to the child in solving his health problems related to growth, development, and adjustment.   —— ——
21. If the school attempts to integrate health instruction with large teaching units, the services of a health educator are utilized in planning those phases of unit dealing with health.   —— ——
22. The health instruction program includes the major health areas and problems.   —— ——

Junior and senior high schools

Yes No

23. The time required for direct health instruction at the junior high school level is equivalent to one full semester of daily classes.   —— ——
24. The time provided for direct health instruction in the senior high school is equivalent to one full semester of daily classes.   —— ——
25. In addition to specific health courses, health instruction is correlated with other subject areas and programs.   —— ——
26. Teachers of health classes in the school have at least a minor in health education or a major in health and physical education.   —— ——
27. The health teacher is keenly interested in the health instruction program and attempts to achieve the potentialities inherent in the program.   —— ——
28. The number of pupils assigned to health classes is no greater than those assigned to other classes in the school.   —— ——
29. The school provides suitable classrooms and adequate facilities for health classes.   —— ——
30. The teacher utilizes the films, materials, and other resources available to him from local and state health agencies.   —— ——
31. The content of the program is interesting and meaningful to the pupils and helps them meet their health problems.   —— ——
32. The school has established definite policies relative to the teaching of controversial areas in health education.   —— ——
33. The health instruction program in the junior high school includes the health areas recommended by leaders in the field.   —— ——
34. The health instruction program in the senior high school includes the health areas recommended by leaders in the field.   —— ——

Questions and exercises

1. What is the relationship of health education to the total school health program?
2. Write an essay of 250 words citing evidence to show the need for health education.
3. What part do the superintendent and principal play in the development of a desirable health education program for the schools?
4. If a physical education person is teaching health education, what should be his or her qualifications in order to do an acceptable job?
5. Identify: (a) health coordinator, (b) school health council, (c) health services, (d) concentrated health teaching, (e) incidental health teaching, (f) Joint Committee on Health Problems, (g) official agencies, and (h) problem-solving activities.
6. How should health education classes be organized?
7. What are eight content areas in health education? Which do you feel are most important in your school? What are the controversial content areas?
8. How does health education vary at the elementary, junior high school, senior high school, and college levels?
9. What are the resources available to individuals in the area of health education?

Reading assignment in *Administrative Dimensions of Health and Physical Education Programs, Including Athletics:* Chapter 9, Selections 48 to 54.

Selected references

A Report of the National Conference on Coordination of the School Health Program: Teamwork in school health, Washington, D. C., 1962, American Association for Health, Physical Education, and Recreation.

A Statement From the Society of State Directors of Health, Physical Education, and Recreation: Guidelines for effective health planning by schools and voluntary health agencies, Journal of Health, Physical Education, and Recreation 34:26, 1963.

American Academy of Pediatrics, Committee on School Health: School health policies, Chicago, 1954, The Academy.

American Association for Health, Physical Education, and Recreation: Children in focus, their health and activity, 1954 Yearbook, Washington, D. C., 1954, The Association.

Anderson, C. L.: Health principles and practices, ed. 6, St. Louis, 1970, The C. V. Mosby Co.

Anderson, C. L.: School health practice, ed. 4, St. Louis, 1968, The C. V. Mosby Co.

Bucher, C. A., Olsen, E., and Willgoose, C.: The foundations of health, New York, 1967, Appleton-Century-Crofts.

Byrd, O. E.: School health administration, Philadelphia, 1964, W. B. Saunders Co.

Cauffman, J. G.: Evaluating a health education curriculum guide, Journal of Health, Physical Education, and Recreation 34:20, 1963.

Grout, R. E.: Health teaching in schools, ed. 5, Philadelphia, 1968, W. B. Saunders Co.

Hanlon, J. J., and McHose, E.: Design for health, Philadelphia, 1963, Lea & Febiger.

Harris, W. H.: Suggested criteria for evaluating health and safety teaching materials, Journal of Health, Physical Education, and Recreation 35:26, 1964.

Hein, F. V.: Critical issues in health and safety education, The Journal of School Health 35:70, 1965.

Hoyman, H. S.: An ecologic view of health and health education, The Journal of School Health 35:110, 1965.

Joint Committee on Health Problems in Education of National Education Association and American Medical Association: Health education, Washington, D. C., 1961, National Education Association.

Joint Committee on Health Problems in Education of National Education Association and American Medical Association: The physical educator asks about health, Washington, D. C., 1951, National Education Association.

Kirkendall, L. A.: Sex education as human relations, New York, 1950, Inor Publishing Co.

Mayshark, C., and Irwin, L.: Health education in secondary schools, ed. 2, St. Louis, 1968, The C. V. Mosby Co.

National Committee on School Health Policies: Suggested school health policies, ed. 2, Washington, D. C., 1962, National Education Association.

National Tuberculosis Association: A health program for colleges, A report of the Third National Conference on Health in Colleges, New York, 1948, The Association.

Oberteuffer, D.: Vital ties between health and education, NEA Journal 53:57, 1964.

Oberteuffer, D., and Beyer, M. K.: School health education, ed. 4, New York, 1966, Harper & Row, Publishers.

Pollock, M. B.: The significance of health education for junior college students, The Journal of School Health 34:333, 1964.

Report of the Study Committee on Health Education in the Elementary and Secondary School of the American School Health Association: Health instruction—suggestions for teachers, The

Journal of School Health, vol. 34, 1964. (Entire issue.)

Richardson, C. E.: Community resources and the school health program, The Journal of School Health 33:314, 1963.

School Health Education Study: A summary report, Washington, D. C., 1964, School Health Education Study, 1201 16th St. N. W.

School Health Education Study: Health education: a conceptual approach, Washington, D. C., 1965, School Health Education Study, 1201 16th St. N. W.

Sheets, N. L.: Health can be interesting, The Journal of School Health 33:132, 1963.

Smith, S. L.: Implication of the report of the NEA project of instruction for health education, The Journal of School Health 34:432, 1964.

Smolensky, J., and Bonevchio, L. R.: Principles of school health, Boston, 1966, D. C. Heath & Co.

Willgoose, C. E.: Health education in the elementary school, ed. 3, Philadelphia, 1969, W. B. Saunders Co.

The health of school children and college students is a most important consideration for educators, parents, physicians, coaches, and others who desire to develop a fit populace. Effective school and college health service programs are essential in the achievement of this goal. Without satisfactory health services, the health of school children and college students cannot be adequately developed, maintained, and protected.

The history of health services shows that years ago schools and colleges stressed primarily provision for sanitary facilities and a clean environment. This was accomplished through a system of inspections and procedures. As more thinking has been given to this subject, however, there has been increased attention focused on those measures essential to the maintenance and improvement of the student's health. As a result, physicians, dentists, and other specialists have become more closely related to the schools and colleges. In turn, this has meant better detection of health defects, a more complete followthrough to ensure the correction of such defects, closer medical supervision of athletic programs, more adequate means for preventing and controlling communicable disease, an increased realization of the potentialities of the medical examination as an educational tool, and more attention to the eyes, throat, ears, nose, and teeth. As the need for better health services was recognized by the public at large, state laws were passed to provide these services. These laws required such procedures as periodic medical examinations and regular checking of vision and

hearing. They also stressed the need for nurses, who were trained not only in their particular area but also in the field of education. Today, there is a feeling that in order to adequately educate the student, health services must be an essential part of the program.

Health services cover a broad area. They include the procedures established to:

1. Appraise the health status of students and educational personnel
2. Counsel students, parents, and other persons concerning appraisal findings
3. Encourage the correction of remediable defects
4. Help plan for the health care and education of handicapped (exceptional) children
5. Help prevent and control disease
6. Provide emergency care for the sick and injured
7. Promote environmental sanitation
8. Promote the health of school and college personnel

THE HEALTH OF THE ATHLETE

The health of the athlete is of such importance to the students who read this text that this special section is being included. Although the entire chapter has implications for all who participate in physical education classes, this particular section emphasizes some of the essential health services for athletes. The growth of sports and athletic programs at both school and college education levels supports this emphasis.

Health services for athletes involves continuous medical attention, sound policies

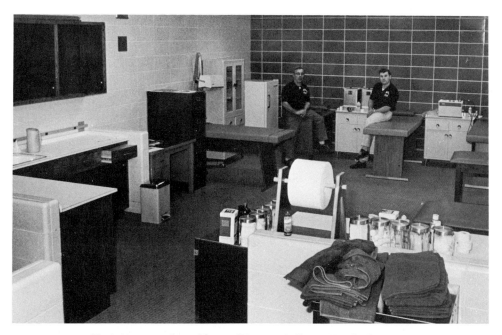

Training room for athletes. (Trinity College, Hartford, Conn.)

and procedures, and the availability of qualified personnel. A close working relationship should exist between coaches, trainers, athletic directors, and school and college administrators and medical society representatives if the athlete is to be adequately protected from injury and harm.

The American Medical Association, through its Committee on the Medical Aspects of Sports, the National Trainers' Association, and such athletic organizations as the National Federation of State High School Athletic Associations, has done an outstanding job in preparing materials, making recommendations to safeguard the health of the athlete, and outlining such procedures as first aid for athletic injuries. A few of the selected materials relating to health services for the athlete are included here. They include a checklist to help evaluate five major factors in the health supervision of athletes, disqualifying conditions for sports participation, and first aid procedures for athletic injuries. Furthermore, a suggested sports candidate's ques-

tionnaire, health examination form, and a student participation and parental approval form are also shown.*

THE PLACE OF HEALTH SERVICES IN SCHOOLS AND COLLEGES

The health services program must be well publicized so that educators, coaches, and the public in general will understand why such services are essential. Only as this need is understood will there be adequate planning and provision for such services.

*A Joint Statement of The Committee on the Medical Aspects of Sports of the American Medical Association and the National Federation of State High School Athletic Associations: Safeguarding the health of the athlete, Chicago, 1965, The American Medical Association.

The Committee on the Medical Aspects of Sports, American Medical Association: A guide for medical evaluation of candidates for school sports, Chicago, 1966, The American Medical Association.

The Committee on the Medical Aspects of Sports, American Medical Association: First aid chart for athletic injuries, Chicago, 1965, The American Medical Association.

SAFEGUARDING THE HEALTH OF THE ATHLETE*

A joint statement of the Committee on the Medical Aspects of Sports of the American Medical Association and the National Federation of State High School Athletic Associations

A checklist to help you evaluate five major factors in health supervision of athletics.

Participation in athletics is a privilege involving both responsibilities and rights. The athlete's responsibilities are to play fair, to keep in training, and to conduct himself with credit to his sport and his school. In turn he has the right to optimal protection against injury as this may be assured through good conditioning and technical instruction, proper regulations and conditions of play, and adequate health supervision.

Periodic evaluation of each of these factors will help to assure a safe and healthful experience for players. The checklist below contains the kinds of questions to be answered in such an appraisal.

PROPER CONDITIONING helps to prevent injuries by hardening the body and increasing resistance to fatigue.

1. Are prospective players given directions and activities for preseason conditioning?
2. Is there a minimum of three weeks of practice before the first game or contest?
3. Are precautions taken to prevent heat exhaustion and heat stroke?
4. Is each player required to warm up thoroughly prior to participation?
5. Are substitutions made without hesitation when players evidence disability?

CAREFUL COACHING leads to skillful performance, which lowers the incidence of injuries.

1. Is emphasis given to safety in teaching techniques and elements of play?
2. Are injuries analyzed to determine causes and to suggest preventive programs?
3. Are tactics discouraged that may increase the hazards and thus the incidence of injuries?
4. Are practice periods carefully planned and of reasonable duration?

GOOD OFFICIATING promotes enjoyment of the game and the protection of players.

1. Are players as well as coaches thoroughly schooled in the rules of the game?
2. Are rules and regulations strictly enforced in practice periods as well as in games?
3. Are officials qualified both emotionally and technically for their responsibilites?
4. Do players and coaches respect the decisions of officials?

RIGHT EQUIPMENT AND FACILITIES serve a unique purpose in protection of players.

1. Is the best protective equipment provided for contact sports?
2. Is careful attention given to proper fitting and adjustment of equipment?
3. Is equipment properly maintained, and are worn and outmoded items discarded?
4. Are proper areas for play provided and carefully maintained?

ADEQUATE MEDICAL CARE is a necessity in the prevention and control of injuries.

1. Is there a thorough preseason health history and medical examination?
2. Is a physician present at contests and readily available during practice sessions?
3. Does the physician make the decision as to whether an athlete should return to play following injury during games?
4. Is authority from a physician required before an athlete can return to practice after being out of play because of disabling injury?
5. Is the care given athletes by coach or trainer limited to first aid and medically prescribed services?

*From Committee on the Medical Aspects of Sports of the American Medical Association and the National Federation of State High School Athletic Associations: Tips on athletic training, XI, Chicago, Illinois, 1969, The American Medical Association.

SUGGESTED
SPORTS CANDIDATES' QUESTIONNAIRE

(To be completed by parents or family physician)

Name_____ Birth date_____

Home address_____

Parents' Name_____ Tel. No._____

1. Has had injuries requiring medical attention	Yes	No
2. Has had illness lasting more than a week	Yes	No
3. Is under a physician's care now	Yes	No
4. Takes medication now	Yes	No
5. Wears glasses	Yes	No
contact lenses	Yes	No
6. Has had a surgical operation	Yes	No
7. Has been in hospital (except for tonsillectomy)	Yes	No
8. Do you know of any reason why this individual should not participate in all sports?	Yes	No

Please explain any "Yes" answers to above questions:

_____

_____

9. Has had complete poliomyelitis immunization by inoculations (Salk) or oral vaccine (Sabin)	Yes	No
10. Has had tetanus toxoid and booster inoculation within past 3 years	Yes	No
11. Has seen a dentist within the past 6 months	Yes	No

Parent or Physician

Suggested sports candidates' questionnaire. (From Committee on the Medical Aspects of Sports, American Medical Association: A guide for medical evaluation of candidates for school sports, 1966, The Association, p. 2. Reprinted with permission of the American Medical Association.

The Joint Committee of the American Medical Association and the National Education Association[*] has listed the following as reasons why health services should exist:

1. They contribute to the learning experience and the realization of other educational aims.
2. They facilitate adaptation of school and college programs to individual needs.
3. They help in maintaining a healthful environment.
4. They help children secure the medical or dental care they need.
5. They possess inherent values for increasing students' understanding of health and health problems.

Health services contribute to the realization of educational aims. Educational committees, conferences, and other important groups have continually listed health as one of the objectives of education. Health services are necessary to attain this objective.

Health services minimize the hazards of school and college attendance. They make it possible for the student to attend school and college under safe conditions. Through emergency care, it is possible to greatly re-

---

[*]Joint Committee of American Medical Association and National Education Association: School health services, ed. 2, Washington, D. C., 1964, National Education Association, pp. 7-8.

SUGGESTED HEALTH EXAMINATION FORM

(Cooperatively prepared by the National Federation of State High School Athletic Associations and the Committee on Medical Aspects of Sports of the American Medical Association.) Health examination for athletes should be rendered after August 1 preceding school year concerned.

(Please Print)   Name of Student   City and School

Grade_____Age_____Height_____Weight_____Blood Pressure_____

Significant Past Illness or Injury_____

Eyes_____ R 20/ ; L20 /; Ears_____ Hearing R /15; L /15

Respiratory_____

Cardiovascular_____

Liver_____Spleen_____Hernia_____

Musculoskeletal_____Skin_____

Neurological_____Genitalia_____

Laboratory: Urinalysis_____Other:_____

Comments_____

Completed Immunizations: Polio_____Tetanus_____
                                          Date   Date

| Instructions for use of card | Other_____

I certify that I have on this date examined this pupil and find him (her) physically able to compete in supervised activities NOT CROSSED OUT BELOW.

BASEBALL	FOOTBALL	ROWING	SOFTBALL	TRACK
BASKETBALL	HOCKEY	SKATING	SPEEDBALL	VOLLEYBALL
CROSS COUNTRY	GOLF	SKIING	SWIMMING	*WRESTLING
FIELD HOCKEY	GYMNASTICS	SOCCER	TENNIS	OTHERS_____

*Weight loss permitted to make lower weight class: Yes_____ No_____; if "Yes" may lose _____pounds.

Date of Examination:_____Signed:_____
                                                      Examining Physician

Physician's Address_____Telephone_____

- -

STUDENT PARTICIPATION AND PARENTAL APPROVAL FORM

Name of student:_____Name of School:_____
                   First   Last   Middle Initial

Date:_____Date of Birth:_____Place of Birth:_____

This application to compete in interscholastic athletics for the above high school is entirely voluntary on my part and is made with the understanding that I have not violated any of the eligibility rules and regulations of the State Association.

| Instructions for use of card | Signature of Student:_____

PARENT'S OR GUARDIAN'S PERMISSION

I hereby give my consent for the above high school student to engage in State Association approved athletic activities as a representative of his high school, except those crossed out on reverse side of this form by the examining physician, and I also give my consent for the above student to accompany the team as a member on its out-of-town trips.

Signature of Parent or Guardian:_____

Date:_____Address:_____
                                          (Street)   (City or Town)

NOTE: This form is to be filled out completely and filed in the office of the high school principal or superintendent of schools before student is allowed to practice and/or compete.

Suggested health examination form. (From Committee on the Medical Aspects of Sports, American Medical Association: A guide for medical evaluation of candidates for school sports, 1966, The Association, p. 3. Reprinted with permission of the American Medical Association.)

duce the harmful effects of injuries in the event of accidents. Adequate precautions are taken against the spread of communicable disease. Medical examinations identify health defects, making for safer participation in athletics and other school activities. These are only a few of the many hazards that can be removed or minimized through effective health services.

Health services help youth to adapt better to school and college programs. Through careful and regular checking of vision and hearing and general physical condition and correction of defects, students will better assume their responsibilities. Deficiencies, defects, and weaknesses that are prevalent will be noted and provided for.

Health services have potentialities for educating the parents as well as the students. They have potentialities for developing proper attitudes toward health, developing proper habits, and imparting scientific information. Through the medical examination, for example, the teacher, nurse, physician, coach, and others have an opportunity to educate students and parents about various aspects of health.

The forty-first annual report of the Health Service Department of the Denver schools* includes a report on the basic functions that this department performs in the education of children and youth in that city. Since this school system has won national recognition for its school health services program, this information is given to provide a better understanding of what all schools should be trying to accomplish in this area:

Health services to assure a safe and wholesome school environment
1. Selection of healthy adult employees
2. Implementation of city health and building regulations
3. Application of control measures to stop the spread of illnesses.
   a. Implementation of official health rules
   b. Prompt attention to ill children and exclusion from school
   c. Immunizations for those who request it
4. Health consultations and periodic evaluations for adult personnel

Health services to detect conditions among pupils that would diminish their most effective participation in educational activities
1. Routine screening tests for vision, hearing, physical growth, and dental health
2. Periodic medical appraisals to evaluate general development and significant physical conditions and defects
3. Screening tests on preschool children for hearing and vision

*Corliss, L. M.: Forty-first annual report, 1965-1966, Health Service Department, Denver Public Schools, Denver, Colo.

Health services to assist in health instruction for all pupils
1. Cooperative efforts with instruction department on materials and inservice training
2. Educational emphasis on all health procedures
3. Work with faculties for classroom health units
4. Tuberculosis testing

Health services to promote followup care and correction of pupils' health problems and deficiencies
1. Nurse counseling with pupils, parents, teachers, social workers, and other school personnel
2. Intercommunications between school health personnel and private physicians and/or clinics
3. Cooperation with other community health agencies

Health services to assist with other needs of some pupils
1. Medical appraisal of those with physical, mental, and emotional problems that seem to interfere with learning
   a. Placement in special educational classes
   b. Assistance from consultant psychiatrists
2. Dental clinic services
3. Help in first-aid care of injuries
4. Medical reports on "battered" children

Additional health service department responsibilities
1. Continual evaluation of department activities
2. Close rapport and administrative planning with medical and dental profession and with official and nonofficial health agencies
3. Continued cooperative programs with other departments within the schools and with community and civic groups
4. Assistance with health, disability, and retirement leaves for adult personnel.

Table 13-1, taken from the Denver Report, indicates the recommended timing and frequency of routine school health services in respect to grades.

THE RESPONSIBILITY FOR SCHOOL HEALTH SERVICES

The question is frequently raised as to whether school health services should fall within the province of school personnel or public health department personnel. Both the school and the public health department are vitally interested in seeing that such services are provided. Both have specialized personnel who can render important contributions to the successful administration of health services. The school is especially interested in the educational aspects of such services and the vast potentialities they have for educating the children and the public. It has personnel who are specially trained in educational methods and techniques. In many communities it also has physicians on the staff who perform medical examinations and other health services. On the other hand, the public health department has specialists in sanitation, epidemiology, and other areas pertinent to the health services program.

Since both the school and the public health department have interests in health services, each local community should decide how such a program can best be carried out. In some communities the public health department is better staffed and qualified to perform many of the health services. In other communities the school has the better staff and other requisites. In many cases, health services should be a cooperative endeavor, where the health department and the school work together, sharing their resources and planning a program in the light of these conditions.

EDUCATION VERSUS TREATMENT

With the school becoming an increasingly important social organization of the community, the question often arises as to whether it should provide treatment as part of its health services program. The philosophy on which the school program is based establishes it mainly as an agency concerned with education. The educational aspects of the health services program represent the major contribution of the schools. By identifying health defects, making referrals to medical, dental, and other experts, counseling, providing for emergency care, making special provisions for the handicapped, and establishing and encouraging measures to prevent and control communicable diseases, the school is carrying out its responsibilities in health services. However, in some communities, as a result of agreement and consultation among public health, medical and dental professions, educators, and others, provisions have been made to provide dental treatment, occupational therapy, and other services. Such programs are exceptions to the rule, however, and usually are initiated as a result of a need for expediency and because it is felt that such a practice is the best way to handle certain health problems. Treatment is not usually a part of the school health program.

HEALTH SERVICES

The rest of the chapter will be concerned with a discussion of the various health services: (1) health appraisal, (2) health counseling, (3) correction of remediable defects, (4) care and education of exceptional children, (5) communicable disease control, (6) emergency care, (7) environmental sanitation, and (8) health of school and college personnel. Each of these health services will be considered in respect to how it fits into the total health program. Some of the various techniques that are used and administrative problems that arise, together with acceptable procedures to be followed, will be discussed.

Health appraisal

Health appraisal is that phase of health service that is concerned with evaluating the health of the student in as objective a way as possible, through examinations, observations, and records.

The cooperation of many individuals is needed to do an acceptable job in health service. Teachers, administrators, physicians, dentists, psychologists, public health officials, social workers, parents, and lay leaders must all work together. Through

Table 13-1. Recommended timing and frequency of routine health services*

Type of service	K	1	2	3	4	5	6	7	8	9	10	11	12
Medical appraisals													
All pupils with possible health problems at any grade level	X	X	X	X	X	X	X	X	X	X	X	X	X
When private physicians have not reported on pupils in grades 1, 6, and 9, or on new pupils at any other grade level		X					X			X			
All pupils who participate in varsity sports											X	X	X
All pupils who participate in school swimming classes								X	X	X	X	X	X
ROTC and NDCC members, if private physician reports are not obtained											X	X	X
All pupils being considered for placement in special education at any grade level	X	X	X	X	X	X	X	X	X	X	X	X	X
Weight and growth measurements													
In first semester (routinely) and on all new pupils and referred pupils; often done cooperatively with physical education teachers as part of fitness program	X	X	X	X	X	X	X	X	X	X			
Hearing screening tests													
At certain grades as shown on all new pupils, on referred pupils, and those with known defects	X	X		X				X					
Vision screening tests													
At certain grades as shown; on new pupils, referred pupils, and those with known defects	X	X		X		X		X			X		
Dental inspections													
At grades shown and at about 5-year intervals—high school pupils inspected and DMF rates ascertained	X	X	X	X	X	X	X		X				
Immunizations													
Once each year in each school for those in need of certain protections and at parents' request	X	X	X	X	X	X	X	X	X	X	X	X	X
Special services													
Tine test for tuberculosis								X					
Scalp ringworm inspections						All grades as needed							
Other nuisance diseases						All grades as needed							
Color vision rechecks								X					

*From Corliss, L. M.: Forty-first annual report, 1965-1966, Health Service Department, Denver Public Schools, Denver, Colo.

DISQUALIFYING CONDITIONS FOR SPORTS PARTICIPATION*

Conditions	Contact†	Noncontact endurance‡	Others§
General			
Acute infections:			
Respiratory, genitourinary, infectious mononucleosis, hepatitis, active rheumatic fever, active tuberculosis, boils, furuncles, impetigo	X	X	X
Obvious physical immaturity in comparison with other competitors	X	X	
Obvious growth retardation	X		
Hemorrhagic disease:			
Hemophilia, purpura, and other bleeding tendencies	X		
Diabetes, inadequately controlled	X	X	X
Jaundice, whatever cause	X	X	X
Eyes			
Absence or loss of function of one eye	X		
Severe myopia, even if correctable	X		
Ears			
Significant impairment	X		
Respiratory			
Tuberculosis (active or under treatment)	X	X	X
Severe pulmonary insufficiency	X	X	X
Cardiovascular			
Mitral stenosis, aortic stenosis, aortic insufficiency, coarctation of aorta, cyanotic heart disease, recent carditis of any etiology	X	X	X
Hypertension on organic basis	X	X	X
Previous heart surgery for congenital or acquired heart disease	X	X	
Liver			
Enlarged liver	X		
Spleen			
Enlarged spleen	X		
Hernia			
Inguinal or femoral hernia	X	X	
Musculoskeletal			
Symptomatic abnormalities or inflammations	X	X	X
Functional inadequacy of the musculoskeletal system, congenital or acquired, incompatible with the contact or skill demands of the sport	X	X	
Neurological			
History or symptoms of previous serious head trauma or repeated concussions	X		
Convulsive disorder not completely controlled by medication	X	X	
Previous surgery on head or spine	X	X	
Renal			
Absence of one kidney	X		
Renal disease	X	X	X
Genitalia			
Absence of one testicle	X		
Undescended testicle	X		

*Committee on the Medical Aspects of Sports, American Medical Association: A guide for medical evaluation of candidates for school sports, Chicago, Illinois, 1966, The Association, pp. 4-5.
†Lacrosse, baseball, soccer, basketball, football, wrestling, hockey, rugby, etc.
‡Cross country, track, tennis, crew, swimming, etc.
§Bowling, golf, archery, field events, etc.

the active cooperation of all, the necessary plans will be made for continuous evaluation and appraisal. If a health council exists, this body can play a major role in coordinating the various aspects of the program.

Planning should provide for desirable facilities and procedures for health appraisal. There should be provision for privacy and quiet so that the best type of examinations and other techniques can be used in an acceptable manner.

The aims of health appraisal include identifying students in need of medical or

---

NOTICE TO PARENTS ABOUT HEALTH APPRAISALS FOR SCHOOL PUPILS

Pupil's Name_____ Grade_____ Room or Section_____

It is important for the school to have some health information about every pupil. Health appraisals are strongly recommended for all pupils whenever they enroll in school and thereafter as your physician recommends.

If possible, please have your family or clinic physician send a report of a recent examination to the schools. Will you ask him to send it on special forms supplied by the schools?

Health clearance is required periodically for participation in swimming classes, ROTC, and certain other school activities. In addition, annual school medical appraisals are required for varsity sports.

In order to have health information of value to the school, we would appreciate your responses on the following:

1. Allergies_____
2. Convulsions or seizures_____
3. Diabetes_____
4. Frequent colds or sore throats_____
5. Frequent stomach-aches_____
6. Headaches_____
7. Heart trouble_____

8. Serious operations or accidents_____
_____
9. Known exposure to tuberculosis Yes_____ No_____
10. Vision_____ Hearing_____
11. Contagious diseases_____
_____
12. Other health problems, such as kidney trouble, ulcers, etc._____

HEALTH PRACTICES

1. *Eating:* Breakfast Yes_____ No_____ Between-meal snacks_____
2. *Rest and sleep:* Average hours_____
3. *Exercise and/or recreation outside of school:* Sports, clubs, music lessons, etc._____
_____
4. *Work activities outside of school*_____
5. *Emotional health:* Assuming responsibilities_____
   Getting along with others_____ Liking school_____

IMMUNIZATION RECORD AND TUBERCULIN TESTING (Please state year last given)

Smallpox vaccination_____   Rubeola (*measles*)_____ Mumps_____
Diphtheria-Tetanus_____   Rubella (*3-day measles*)_____
Polio: Type of Sabin (oral) doses I_____ II_____ III_____ Trivalent_____
Tuberculin test: Date_____ Negative_____ Positive_____

If a recent health examination has not been performed by a private or clinic physician, please indicate your choice below.

I will have our family or clinic physician give this
examination and send a report to school. . . _____
                                               (Sign here)

I wish the school medical appraisal. . . . . . _____
                                               (Sign here)

Date_____

(Please Return This Sheet Promptly to the School Nurse)

Notice to parents about health appraisals for school pupils. (Denver Public Schools, Denver, Colo.)

dental treatment, those who have problems relating to nutrition, and those who are in need of treatment by a psychiatrist or guidance clinic. In addition, the objectives of health services are to measure the growth of pupils; identify students with non-remediable defects so that modified programs may be provided, such as for crippled or mentally retarded pupils; identify students who need additional examinations, such as x-ray studies; and identify students who need programs apart from the school setting, such as the blind and deaf.

The techniques used in health appraisal that will be discussed here include medical, psychologic, and dental examinations, screening for vision and hearing, teacher observations, and health records.

Examinations. Examinations are effective means of health appraisal.

Medical examinations. There are many important considerations for the administrator to keep in mind if medical examinations are to fulfill their objective. The following are some administrative guides.

TYPES. Both periodic and referral examinations should be given to students. *Periodic* medical examinations are given at stated intervals. *Referral* examinations are those that are given to students who have health problems needing special attention and who have been referred to the proper professional source. Such students may be referred to the physician as a result of teacher's observations, screening examinations, health records, or other indications that special attention is needed. The *examination of athletes* is also a type of medical examination that needs to be considered.

PLANNING. Medical examinations require planning. Young children should be informed as to their nature and purposes. The teacher can play an important role in explaining some of these purposes and procedures. Desirable attitudes can be developed so that children and parents look forward to such an event with interest and anticipation. The various instruments that are used, such as the stethoscope, can be shown and discussed. Planning should also

---

I hereby give permission and request that

_____

be given the medical examination required for swimmers. I understand there is a small additional cost for this swimming program.

　　To my knowledge, my child does not have diabetes, epilepsy, chronic sinus or ear infection, or any other physical condition that would make it unsafe for him to swim.

| _____ | _____ |
| (Date) | (Signature of Parent) |

PARENT PERMIT FOR PUPIL TO PARTICIPATE IN SWIMMING CLASS

Department of Health Service
Department of Health Education
DENVER PUBLIC SCHOOLS

STOCK NO. 10753
FORM 853   DSP   4-59-15M   V-239-45140

take into consideration the provision of adequate facilities, having parents present, and making available the necessary health records.

FREQUENCY. At least four periodic medical examinations should be given during the time a child is in the elementary and secondary schools. There should be a minimum of one examination at the time of entrance to school, one at the intermediate grade level, one at the junior or early high school level when the student is entering the adolescent period, and one toward the termination of the high school period. The desirable procedure, however, would be to have a medical examination each year. Referral examinations should be given at any time that health problems are detected. There is also a need for more medical examinations for students who are engaging in the athletic phase of the physical education program and for those whose health conditions are such that the physician recommends examinations at more frequent intervals.

EXAMINER. There is a trend toward having the family physician conduct the medical examination. It is felt that through a more complete knowledge of the family history and a closer personal relationship, a better job can be done. However, since some families do not have their own physicians, since it means an additional outlay of funds, and for other reasons, many schools must rely on a school physician to administer the examination. The procedure that is utilized in each community should be a local prerogative and based upon the type of examination that will produce the best results.

PERSONNEL IN ATTENDANCE. The personnel that should be in attendance at the medical examination for young children would include the physician, nurse, child, teacher, and parents. At the secondary school level, the child should have progressed to the point where he or she assumes the responsibility for his own health, and so the need

for parents at the examination is not as great. Special attention should be given to sending a written invitation to parents, listing the date and time of the examination. The presence of parents at these medical examinations provides an excellent opportunity for educating them in regard to their child's health, as well as their own.

SETTING. The place where the examination is held should be conducive to good results. The physical and the emotional atmosphere should receive attention. There should be privacy for disrobing, so that interruptions will not occur, and quiet so that distractions will be reduced to a minimum. The examination room should also provide ample space for personnel, equipment, and supplies and should be attractive. Tension, hurry, and excitement should be reduced to a minimum. The entire setting should be friendly and informal.

RECORDS AVAILABLE. Essential health records should be brought up to date and be available at the time of the examination. These would include students' health cards, vision and hearing records, height-weight statistics, accident reports, and any other information that will help the physician to better interpret the results of the examination.

SCOPE. The periodic medical examination will include inspection or examination of such items as the following:

Eyes and lids	Nose
Throat and mouth	Teeth and gums
Heart: before and	Lymph node and
after exercise	thyroid gland
Nutrition	Lungs
Posture	Scalp and skin
Feet	Bones and joints
Speech	Nervous system
Behavior attitudes	Inguinal and um-
Ears: canal and	bilical region for
drums	hernia in males

TIME. The examination that is administered by the school physician should be of sufficient length to detect any health defects and also make the experience educational in nature. The minimum average

HEALTH RECORD

Parents or Guardians—Mr. and Mrs.

Occupation of Father   Session Teacher

Occupation of Mother   Family Doctor   Family Dentist

Last Name   *First Name*   *Address*   *Telephone*

MEDICAL EXAMINATION		1	2	3	4
1.	Date of Examination				
2.	Age				
3.	Weight				
4.	Height				
5.	Hearing	Rt.				
		Lt.				
6.	Eyes	Rt.				
		Lt.				
7.	Test with glasses		Yes No	Yes No	Yes No	Yes No
8.	Ring Worm					
9.	Plantar Warts					
10.	Hair					
11.	Personal Hygiene					
12.	Pulse before exercise					
13.	Pulse after exercise					
14.	Heart					
15.	Lungs					
16.	Tremor					
17.	Abdomen					
18.	Hernia					
19.	Ears					
20.	Nose					
21.	Tonsils					
22.	Adenoids					
23.	Teeth					
24.	Thyroid					
25.	Glands					
26.	Nutrition					
27.	Skin					
28.	P. E. Classification					
	Unrestricted (A or B)					
	Partially Restricted (C)					
	Rest Only (D)					
	Permanent Excuse					
	Temporary Excuse					
29.	Swimming					
	Permanent Excuse					
	Temporary Excuse					
Doctor's Initials						

HISTORY OF DISEASE

Chicken Pox	St. Vitus Dance	Diphtheria	Measles	Mumps	Pneumonia	Scarlet Fever	Rheumatic Fever	Whooping Cough	Tonsillitis	Hay Fever	Asthma	Date of Vaccination for Small Pox	T. B. in Family?	Date of Skin Test

Headaches:		Menstruation	
Never		Regular	
Occasionally		Irregular	
Frequently		Dysmenorrhea	

Operations:		Injuries	
Tonsils			
Others:			

Postural Findings Scoliosis	L	R	L	R	L	R	L	R
Shoulder High								
Hip High								
Feet: Pronation								
Long. Arch								
Transverse Arch								
Head Forward								
Round Shoulders								
Hollow Back								
Abdomen								
Body Balance								
Posture Grade								
Corrective Gym								

COMMENTS:

Explanation of Terms: "O"—Normal; "X"—Slight Defect; "XX"—Moderate; "XXX"—Marked.

Girl's health record. (Highland Park High School, Highland Park, Ill.)

time per student should be 15 minutes or four per hour.

Examination of athletes. Administrative guides for athletic examinations are as follows:

1. Medical examinations should be administered to all engaged in athletics previous to actual participation and as they are needed during the time the sport is in progress. This refers to all forms of strenuous athletics, whether it be interscholastic, intramural, or part of the class program.

2. There should be adequate provision for medical service at all athletic contests.

3. A physician's recommendation should accompany any athlete returning to competition after a period of illness.

4. Examinations for participation in athletics should preferably be conducted by the family physician. In instances where this is not feasible, the school physician should perform this service.

Psychologic examinations. With the increased emphasis on mental health, various psychologic examinations are being used more extensively. These examinations, however, represent only a very small part of the mental health services that should be available. Mental health programs are concerned with helping students to adjust satisfactorily to the school or college environment, detecting individual behavior problems, aiding the teacher, parent, and others to better understand human behavior, and helping in every way possible to appraise personality and to discover mental handicaps, emotional difficulties, and maladjustments.

Psychologic examinations and tests that appraise such factors as students' abilities, attitudes, personalities, intelligence, and social adjustment offer techniques for obtaining much information. The administration and interpretation of the findings of such techniques should be handled by qualified individuals.

Dental examinations and inspections. Following are administrative guides governing school dental services.

EMPHASIS. The emphasis in school den-

H-6 3M 9-36

LONG BEACH CITY SCHOOLS
HEALTH SERVICE DEPARTMENT
ATHLETIC PHYSICAL EXAMINATION REPORT

Name_____ School_____ Class_____

Age_____

Type of Athletic Activity—F. B., Basket Ball, Track, B. B., Class A. B. C.

Height_____Weight_____Standard_____Chest Circum.

In_____   Ex_____

Standing, Posture_____ Musculature_____ Nutrition_____

Skin_____ Superficial Glands_____

Hands_____ Arms_____ Abdomen_____

Hernia_____Genitalia_____ Leg_____

Feet_____

Sitting: Hair_____Teeth_____ Eyes, Reflexes_____

      R._____   R._____

Vision—   Corrected—

      L._____   L._____

      R._____

Hearing—   Nose_____Gums_____

      L._____

Tongue_____Tonsils_____ Pharynx_____

Ears_____Chest_____ Heart_____

Pulse, sitting_____ After exercise_____

2 min. later_____ Temp._____Lungs_____

Blood Pressure Systolic_____ Diastolic_____

Knee Reflexes_____

Urine Analysis: Sp. Grav._____ Alb._____ Sugar_____

Summary

Advice   Date_____

Athletic physical examination report. (Long Beach, Calif., Public Schools.)

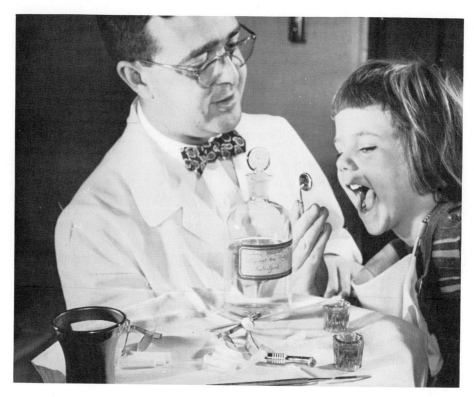

Dental inspection. (Indiana State Department of Health.)

FORM 79 3M 8-48 ◆

New Trier Township
High School

DENTAL CERTIFICATE

Winnetka
Illinois

This is to certify that I have examined the teeth of

STUDENT'S NAME _____ ADVISER _____
(Last)   (First)

RECORD OF EXAMINATIONS

Date	Clean	Under Repair	Under Treatment	Remarks	Dentist's Signature

tal services should be on health education. Children and parents should develop proper attitudes toward dental caries and oral hygiene. Periodically, they should consult their family dentist for the necessary examination, care, and advice.

PERSONNEL. The personnel in the school particularly concerned with dental health include the teacher, nurse, physician, and dental hygienist. The staff will depend upon the community philosophy concerning dental care. If the emphasis is upon education, it will be different than if it is on treatment. When a dental hygienist is a member of the school staff, she often has a variety of duties, including acting as a resource person for classroom teachers regarding dental health, making topical applications of sodium fluoride, cleaning children's teeth, and administering limited dental inspections.

NATURE. A difference of opinion exists as to whether or not schools should provide dental examinations for pupils. Those in favor of such a practice point to its value as a motivating device to encourage parents and children to visit the dentist. Furthermore, they say it helps children in the low-income classes and focuses attention on the dental needs of children. Those not in favor of such a practice argue that as a result of school examinations children and parents visit their dentist less often and in some cases even substitute this examination for regular dental care. They further point out that it is the responsibility of everyone to make provisions for his own dental care and that the school is not the agency responsible for providing such a service. The question of the school's responsibility should be decided in each local community through conferences with dentists, educators, parents, and others interested in the problem. It can then be resolved in a manner that will best meet the needs of the children.

DENVER PUBLIC SCHOOLS

APPOINTMENT FOR CARE AT SCHOOL DENTAL CLINIC

1350 Clarkson

Telephone 222-1055

PLEASE TAKE THIS APPOINTMENT WITH YOU TO THE CLINIC

Pupil's name_____ Room Number_____

Address_____

The above-named pupil has been approved for treatment at the school dental clinic and the "Parent Request" slip is on the Health Record. He/she is to begin such treatment on the date and at the hour stated below.

Date_____, 19_____   Hour_____

_____Nurse

_____School

IF FOR ANY REASON YOUR CHILD CANNOT KEEP HIS APPOINTMENT, NOTIFY THE DENTAL CLINIC IMMEDIATELY BY CALLING 222-1055.

Appointment for care at school dental clinic. (Denver Public Schools, Denver, Colo.)

SCOPE. The scope of the school dental program usually concerns itself with the dental inspections and prophylaxis or cleaning. There are a few schools, however, that treat emergency cases and provide other dental care for children of parents who cannot afford such services. Dental inspection may be used to determine dental needs, to help communities meet the needs, and for purposes of evaluating the dental health program.

DENTAL PROBLEMS. The problems concerned with dental health are dental caries, or decayed teeth; malocclusion, a condition in which the teeth do not uniformly fit together when the jaws are closed; and periodontal diseases in which the tissues surrounding the teeth become infected, such as gingivitis (inflammation of the gums) or Vincent's infection (trench mouth). Although dental caries is the most common problem, the others should receive due consideration.

Dental caries can best be prevented and controlled through good dental hygiene that includes frequent brushing, especially after eating; reducing sugar intake; topical fluoride applications; and fluoridation of water supplies, which experiments have shown reduces dental caries from 40% to 65%.

EDUCATIONAL IMPLICATIONS. The educational implications of dental health services are far reaching. Pupils and parents can be motivated to practice good oral hygiene and to visit their dentist regularly. The proper attitudes can be developed, resulting in good dental habits.

Screening for vision and hearing defects

Vision. Screening for vision requires a consideration of many factors.

VISION HEALTH SERVICES. The vision health services program in the school is concerned with the examinations given by physicians and appraisal of visual acuity. The appraisal of visual acuity is accomplished through continuous observations by the teacher and screening examinations. Both are necessary for the continual and satisfactory appraisal of the vision of school children.

FREQUENCY OF SCREENING TESTS. Tests of visual acuity should be given annually. The optimum time for such screening is immediately after the opening of school in the fall. They can be given to children in the early grades, as soon as they are old enough to cooperate satisfactorily. If possible, there should be a complete eye examination before the child enters school. A screening test for color acuity should be given during the early school years so that guidance can be given in regard to vocational opportunities.

ADMINISTRATION OF SCREENING TESTS. The teacher, after proper instruction and training, is qualified to administer various screening devices for vision. These devices, however, are only for purposes of detecting those individuals who need special care in respect to their vision. Their use is not a diagnostic technique.

SELECTION OF SCREENING DEVICES. The particular device that is utilized for checking visual acuity, together with the plans for appraisal, should be selected and arranged through conferences of school administrators, teachers, nurses, physicians, ophthalmologists, and optometrists.

It has been found that with young children, the Snellen E chart seems effective. For older children, the Snellen and Massachusetts Vision Tests have received wide recommendation. These devices should be administered according to prescribed instructions and pupils should be properly prepared for the examinations.

If needed, there are techniques for determining color acuity, such as the Holmgren test, and for determining muscle balance, such as the "cover test."

REFERRALS. The results of the screening examinations should be recorded and studied. In the light of these results and the teacher's observations, children with difficulties should be referred to the proper

DENVER PUBLIC SCHOOLS
Health Service Department

HOME REPORT ON VISION SCREENING

Date_____ School_____

Recently, _____
was given a vision screening test at school and seemed to have some visual
difficulty. Although glasses may not be needed, we urge you to have an
examination to recheck this condition. Would you please take this report
to an eye specialist to be completed so that it may be returned promptly to
the school nurse.

Thank you,

_____   _____
        (Principal)   (School Nurse)

Report From Eye Specialist

I have examined the above pupil on _____ and found the

following eye condition:_____

_____

_____

My recommendations are:_____

_____

_____

_____   _____
         (Date)   (Signature of Examiner)

Home report on vision screening. (Denver Public Schools, Denver, Colo.)

place for an eye examination. According
to the Joint Committee of the National
Education Association and the American
Medical Association, "parents should be
urged to secure eye examinations for children who are in the following categories:
(1) those who consistently exhibit symptoms of visual disturbance, regardless of
the results of the Snellen test, (2) older
children (eight years and older) who have
a visual acuity of 20/30 or less in either
eye, with or without symptoms, and (3)
younger children (seven years of age or
less) who have a visual acuity of 20/40
or less in either eye, with or without
symptoms."[*]

---

[*]Joint Committee of American Medical Association and National Education Association, op. cit.,
pp. 81-82.

DENVER PUBLIC SCHOOLS

Department of Health Service

PARENTS' NOTIFICATION OF VISION TEST

The school vision test of..
indicates that some difficulty with the vision exists. A more thorough examination should be made to determine the nature of the trouble and to make any correction, if such is necessary. If your child has not recently had his eyes tested by a doctor it would be advisable to consult your family physician.

School Nurse

Principal

FORM 973 DSP 6-51-50M P-312-36564

TEACHER'S OBSERVATIONS. The teacher as well as the parent should be alert to visual difficulties and problems among children. By being aware of certain actions and manifestations of the child from day to day under varying situations, it is possible to detect many eye difficulties that should be referred for examination. Many of these eye difficulties might go unnoticed unless the alert teacher or parent is aware of certain characteristics that indicate vision problems.

The Joint Committee has listed certain manifestations of visual difficulty in children before they begin to read and after reading activities have begun:

Before the child begins to read:
  Attempts to brush away blur
  Blinking more than usual
  Frequent rubbing of the eyes
  Squinting when looking at distant objects
  Frequent or continuous frowning
  Stumbling over small objects
  Undue sensitivity to light
  Red, encrusted, or swollen eyelids
  Recurring styes
  Inflamed or watery eyes

Crossed eyes, "wall" eye, or "wandering" eye (regardless of degree)
After reading activities have begun:
  Holding a book too far away from or too close to the face when reading
  Inattention during reading periods, chalkboard, chart or map work
  Difficulty in reading or in other work requiring close use of the eyes
  Inability, or lack of desire, to participate in games requiring distance vision
  Poor alignment in written work
  Tilting head to one side or thrusting head forward when looking at near or distant objects
  Irritability when doing close work
  Shutting or covering one eye when reading*

Hearing. Following are administrative guides for conduct of health services in regard to hearing.

SCOPE. The main responsibility of the schools in respect to auditory health services is to detect those pupils with hearing difficulties as early as possible. This can

---

*Joint Committee of American Medical Association and National Education Association, op. cit., p. 76.

be accomplished through such means as teacher observations and screening tests. A counseling and followthrough program that aims at remedying the defect should also be a part of the total plan.

FREQUENCY. Continuous observations should be a part of the school routine. Annual screening tests during the elementary years and one every 2 years at the secondary level are recommended. There should be a minimum of three tests during the first 8 years of school. It is also recommended that a preschool test of auditory acuity should be given wherever possible.

TECHNIQUE. The pure-tone audiometer is recommended as one of the most effective techniques for pupils of all school ages. This is a reliable instrument and allows for checking of either or both ears.

REFERRALS. Students with a hearing loss in one or both ears should be rechecked to determine the accuracy of screening. If results are consistent, parents should be informed and encouraged to follow through with more complete examination.

Teachers who observe mouth breathing, ear discharge, or other abnormalities or characteristics that might arouse suspicion of hearing loss should refer the case to the proper authorities.

TEACHER'S OBSERVATIONS. The teacher can play an important part in continually observing the child for indications of hearing loss. She is also a key person in administering screening techniques. She should be watchful for such mannerisms as speech difficulties, requests for repetition of questions, turning of head to better hear what is said, and inattention, together with such noticeable characteristics as discharging ears, earaches, and other departures from the normal makeup of the child. Through such observations the teacher will detect individuals who need to be referred for more careful study and examination. All teachers should be alert for such manifestations.

PERSONNEL. Teachers, nurses, or technicians may be utilized in administering the various screening devices. All should be well trained in the use and purpose of such instruments. They should recognize that these are screening instruments and not diagnostic devices. There should be a careful check to determine that the instruments are in good working order and yield accurate results.

Teachers' observations. Teachers' observations are of great importance in detecting the health needs of school children. Furthermore, they increase in importance in the absence of nurses and doctors. Although this subject has been discussed previously, it is of such great importance that it is considered again here in more detail. Teachers, through observations of the appearance and behavior of pupils from day to day, become very well acquainted with each individual child. Any deviations from normal in appearance and in action will be detected very quickly by the alert teacher. For many of the health needs this provides the only means of discovering problems. Very often they would not be detected through medical examinations and other health services. Therefore, the teacher's role in health services, through her continual association and observation of children, is a major one.

Such observations, after careful examination by nurses and physicians, may disclose various deficiencies. They may show that some children are maladjusted socially and emotionally, are undernourished, are in the early stages of a communicable or other disease, have some neurologic difficulties or other physical defects, or have developed poor health habits. Along with referral to nurses and physicians, the parents should also be informed of such discoveries. It should be reemphasized that in no case does the teacher diagnose. Instead, she refers the matter to the nurse, physician, and parent for further action.

The oft-quoted report from the health manual of the Massachusetts Department of Education and Department of Public Health* lists the various physical and behavior conditions for which the teacher should be alert in regard to the children with whom she associates each day:

1. *Eyes*
   a. Styes or crusted lids
   b. Inflamed eyes
   c. Crossed eyes
   d. Repeated headaches
   e. Squinting, frowning, or scowling
   f. Protruding eyes
   g. Watery eyes
   h. Rubbing of eyes
   i. Excessive blinking
   j. Twitching of the lids
   k. Holding head to one side

2. *Ears*
   a. Discharge from ears
   b. Earache
   c. Failure to hear questions
   d. Picking at the ears
   e. Turning the head to hear
   f. Talking in a monotone
   g. Inattention
   h. Anxious expression
   i. Excessive noisiness of child

3. *Nose and throat*
   a. Persistent mouth breathing
   b. Frequent sore throat
   c. Recurrent colds
   d. Chronic nasal discharge
   e. Frequent nose bleeding
   f. Nasal speech
   g. Frequent tonsillitis

4. *Skin and scalp*
   a. Nits on the hair
   b. Unusual pallor of face
   c. Eruptions or rashes
   d. Habitual scratching of scalp or skin
   e. State of cleanliness
   f. Excessive redness of skin

5. *Teeth and mouth*
   a. State of cleanliness
   b. Gross visible caries
   c. Irregular teeth
   d. Stained teeth

   e. Offensive breath
   f. Mouth habits such as thumb-sucking

6. *General condition and appearance*
   a. Underweight—very thin
   b. Overweight—very obese
   c. Does not appear well
   d. Tires easily
   e. Chronic fatigue
   f. Nausea or vomiting
   g. Faintness or dizziness

7. *Growth*
   a. Failure to gain regularly over 3-months' period
   b. Unexplained loss in weight
   c. Unexplained rapid gain in weight

8. *Glands*
   a. Enlarged glands at one side of neck
   b. Enlarged thyroid

9. *Heart*
   a. Excessive breathlessness
   b. Tires easily
   c. Any history of "growing pains"
   d. Bluish lips
   e. Excessive pallor

10. *Posture and musculature*
    a. Asymmetry of shoulders and hips
    b. Peculiarity of gait
    c. Obvious deformities of any type
    d. Anomalies of muscular development

11. *Behavior*
    a. Overstudious, docile, and withdrawing
    b. Bullying, overaggressive, and domineering
    c. Unhappy and depressed
    d. Overexcitable, uncontrollable emotions
    e. Stuttering or other forms of speech difficulty
    f. Lack of confidence, self-denial, and self-censure
    g. Poor accomplishment in comparison with ability
    h. Lying (imaginative or defensive)
    i. Lack of appreciation of property rights (stealing)
    j. Abnormal sex behavior
    k. Antagonistic, negativistic, continually quarreling

Health records. Following are some administrative guides in connection with health records:

1. As part of the overall school or college record, there should be a health record

---

*Commonwealth of Massachusetts: Health in the schools—a manual of the school health program, Boston, 1951, Massachusetts Department of Education with the collaboration of Massachusetts Department of Public Health, pp. 23-24.

that contains a complete appraisal of the student's health. This should include such items as health history, vision and hearing data, teacher's observations, results of various medical, psychologic, dental, and other examinations given, reports of all conferences held with student, health defects that have been corrected, and any other information that has a bearing on the health of the student.

2. The health record should follow the student wherever he goes—when he moves

---

HS-29
4-60-20M

COLUMBUS PUBLIC SCHOOLS

Elementary Immunization Record Card (K-6)

Name.. School.. Teacher..

Room..

This section pertains to pupils in **ALL GRADES.**	This section pertains to pupils in **ALL GRADES.**
SMALLPOX VACCINATION	**POLIOMYELITIS — 3 injections**
☐ Requirement met by a written statement of parent or physician, or by a scar	☐ School records show immunization completed
	☐ Completed by written statement of parent or physician
	☐ Received 1st injection................................ Date
	☐ Received 2nd injection (1-month interval)............... Date
	☐ Received 3rd injection (7-month interval)............... Date

This section pertains to all pupils in **GRADES K-2.**	This section pertains only to pupils in **GRADES 3-6** who did not receive injections for diphtheria and tetanus in grades K-2.
DIPHTHERIA, WHOOPING COUGH, TETANUS — **3 injections + 1 Booster**	
☐ School records show immunization completed	**DIPHTHERIA, TETANUS — 2 injections** **+ 1 Booster**
☐ Completed by written statement of parent or physician	
☐ Received 1st injection................ Date	☐ Completed by written statement of parent or physician
☐ Received 2nd injection (1-month interval)........ Date	☐ Received 1st injection................ Date
☐ Received 3rd injection (1-month interval)........ Date	☐ Received 2nd injection (1-month interval)........ Date
☐ Received booster injection (1-year interval)........ Date	☐ Received booster injection (1-year interval)........ Date

☐ Parental objection (written)

COLUMBUS PUBLIC SCHOOLS

Secondary Immunization Record Card (7-12)

Name.. School.. Teacher..

Room..

All **THREE** sections of this card pertain to **ALL PUPILS.**

(1) SMALLPOX VACCINATION

☐ Requirement met by a written statement of parent or physician, or by a scar

(2) POLIOMYELITIS — 3 injections	**(3) TETANUS — 2 injections plus 1 Booster**
☐ School records show immunization completed	☐ School records show immunization completed
☐ Completed by written statement of parent or physician	☐ Completed by written statement of parent or physician
☐ Received 1st injection................ Date	☐ Received 1st injection................ Date
☐ Received 2nd injection (1-month interval)........ Date	☐ Received 2nd injection (1-month interval)........ Date
☐ Received 3rd injection (7-month interval)........ Date	☐ Received booster injection (1-year interval)........ Date

☐ Parental objection (written)

from one community to another or when he is transferred from one school to another.

3. The records should be cumulative in nature, pointing out the complete health history of the student, together with a continuous appraisal of his health.

4. The health record should be made available to school or college medical and other personnel who are concerned with and who work toward the maintenance and improvement of a student's health. Professional ethics should govern the handling of such information.

5. The health record, if kept up to date and accurate, will prove a very useful and effective device in furthering the health of all students.

Health histories

1. The history of the student's health should be in recorded form as an aid to teachers, nurses, physicians, and others in order to understand better the total picture of the student's health.

2. This record should be kept on a prepared form and should contain a complete history of communicable diseases, operations, accidents, immunizations, dental history, emotional maladjustments, physical abnormalities, nutritional problems, athletic injuries, menstruation, and any other factors that would be of help in better interpreting the total health picture.

3. The health history should be brought up to date before the medical examination is given so that the examining physician may use it as an aid.

Height-weight records. Following are administrative guides in connection with height-weight records:

1. The teacher, or students under supervision, should measure and record the height and weight of pupils at least three times a year. It is recommended that this be done at the beginning, middle, and toward the end of the year.

2. Height-weight records should not be utilized as a device to diagnose such elements as nutritional status. Instead, they should be used as indications that some health problems may exist if, for example, a child's weight does not increase during

---

Form 750H 4M U—8-50

Name_____ Adviser_____

Street_____ Age_____ Date of Birth_____

Village_____ Tel. No._____ School Year_____

New Trier Township High School
Winnetka, Illinois

TUBERCULIN TEST RECORD

Skin test given_____, Read_____, Result_____ _____M. D.
          (date)   (date)   (reading)   (signed)

X-Ray_____Film_____X-Ray by_____M. D.
    (date)   (number)

Report on X-RAY FILM | X-Ray Diagnosis

No._____ | Signed_____M. D.

To — New Trier Township High School:
    I hereby authorize the tuberculin test (and if advised by physicians) an X-Ray for my (son) (daughter)

_____to be done with the rest of the student body at New Trier High School as
    (child's name)   explained in your letter.

I prefer that the above described test NOT be given } _____ _____ Signed_____
      (parent's signature)   (date)   (parent)

any 3-month period. They are best utilized not when compared against the height and weight of other children but when used as a comparison and history of a child's own growth from time to time.

3. Height-weight records provide an interesting and worthwhile phase of health education since students are interested in observing their growth and become curious as to some of the reasons that encourage or deter growth.

Accident records.* Accident records, as a means of health appraisal, provide information as to reasons for physical abnormalities and emotional maladjustment that may occur in children. They also provide a medium of promoting safety. They should be carefully kept and contain complete information.

Health counseling

In the light of the findings gathered through appraisal techniques, health matters are discussed with students and parents. Such problems as the need for medical and dental treatment, better health practices, diagnostic examinations, special services, and analysis of behavior problems are discussed. Through such counseling procedures a better understanding of the health of children and youth is achieved.

Health counseling is an important phase of the total health services program. As health needs and problems are revealed through medical examinations and other techniques, it is essential that defects be corrected, advice given, and a planned procedure established to provide for these needs and eliminate the problems. Health counseling by qualified persons can help in achieving these goals.

Purposes. One general objective of health counseling is to provide students and parents with a better understanding of their health needs and the procedures that should be followed in order to satisfy these needs. Also, health counseling serves as a device for health education. Through conferences and discussion regarding health problems it is possible to develop sound health attitudes. Facts are presented that indicate the need for following acceptable health practices. The parent and student are motivated to alter their behavior in accordance with acceptable health standards. In addition, health counseling can help to develop a feeling of responsibility in pupils and parents for the correction of health defects and for promoting school and community health programs.

The objectives of health counseling have been well stated by the Joint Committee on Health Problems in Education of the National Education Association and the American Medical Association:

1. To give students as much information about their health status, as revealed by appraisal, as they can use to good advantage.
2. To interpret to parents the significance of health conditions and to encourage them to obtain needed care for their children.
3. To motivate students and their parents so that they will want and accept needed treatment and to accept desirable modifications of their school programs.
4. To promote each student's acceptance of responsibility for his own health, in keeping with his stage of maturity.
5. To encourage students and their parents to utilize available resources for medical and dental care to best possible advantage.
6. To encourage, if necessary, the establishment or enlargement of treatment facilities for students from needy families.
7. To contribute to the health education of students and parents.
8. To obtain for exceptional students educational programs adapted to their individual needs and abilities.*

---

*For further discussion of accident records see Chapter 18 on Legal Liability and Insurance Management.

*Reprinted with permission of the Joint Committee on Health Problems in Education of National Education Association and American Medical Association, School health services, Chicago, 1964, National Education Association and American Medical Association, pp. 111-112.

In utilizing counseling as part of the health services program, it should be clearly recognized that it has limitations. Counselors cannot always change individuals. This has been true, for example, of some handicapped individuals who are subject to pity, ridicule, or scorn by their fellow beings. Counselors can only help individuals to understand themselves, realize their potentialities, and live out their natural lives in a happy and productive manner. In some individuals, however, the social and physical environments have left their stamp so indelibly that counseling can do only a limited amount of good.

The counselor. The classroom teacher, school principal, physician, nurse, psychologist, physical education teacher, social worker, recreation leader, guidance person, and others have potentialities as counselors in the field of health. All have relationships with students that place them in a position to offer helpful advice and guidance. Whether or not they carry out such responsibilities effectively will depend on certain basic requirements.

Basic requirements for the counselors are concerned with their interest in people, personality, and competency in counseling skills.

To be effective, a counselor must be interested in people from the standpoint of service. The desire to help others live a happy and successful life and to help eliminate those problems that handicap the achievement of such goals must predominate in the counselor's mind.

A second basic requirement is the counselor's personality. Counseling procedure involves divulging personal problems and other matters that are brought out only when there is good rapport between the counselor and student or parent. Personality is a key to the establishment of a warm and cooperative counselor-client rapport. The counselor's personality must reflect such essentials as friendliness, interest in others' problems, and the desire to help.

He must be a good listener and respecter of the views of others. A good counselor does not talk down to the pupil but confers with the student in an atmosphere of mutual understanding and respect.

A third requirement is competency in counseling skills. As in all specialized services, there are certain competencies that are essential to doing a good job. Studies have shown that the person who has developed competency in counseling gets more effective results and does a better job than the unskilled individual. Skills are necessary in establishing rapport with clients, understanding the implications of behavior patterns, communicating with students, analyzing pupil problems, conducting group discussions, administering conference procedures, and preparing records.

Conference method. The conference method of counseling that brings about a face-to-face relationship between the counselor, the pupil, and the parent is the best method for achieving desirable results. The use of written notices and standard forms is not recommended because of the possibility of misinterpretation and the lack of a clear understanding of the problems involved.

The success of the conference method will depend on the skill and the degree to which the counselor has planned for the conference. It is essential that the counselor have all the necessary records at hand, together with a complete understanding of the community, home, and problems surrounding the pupil in question.

The counselor must establish the proper relationship among the individuals who are present. A friendly and understanding atmosphere is necessary for the achievement of the desired results. The discussion of health matters must be carried on effectively and in a sound manner so that the pupil and parent will recognize the problems that exist and endorse the action that must be taken. No school person engaged in health counseling should attempt to di-

REQUEST FOR HEALTH INFORMATION

DENVER PUBLIC SCHOOLS

CONFIDENTIAL: for Professional Use Only.

IDENTIFICATION OF PUPIL

TO:_____

Physician or Clinic

_____

Address

_____

Clinic Number

We would appreciate your answering the items checked below to help us plan the best school program for this pupil for these reasons:

_____

(Name)

_____

(Address)

(School)   (Birth Date)

_____

(Father's Name)

_____

(Mother's Name)

Thank you,

_____M.D.

Date of request_____

Director, School Health Services
414 Fourteenth Street, Denver, Colorado

_____ Diagnosis?_____

_____ Is treatment completed?_____

_____ May pupil have full school activities?_____

_____ If pupil should have limited physical activities, how limited and for how long?_____

_____ Any other suggestions for this child's program at school?_____

Date of This Report   Signature of Physician

Request for health information. (Denver Public Schools, Denver, Colo.)

agnose diseases or select a physician or dentist for a pupil.

When the conference comes to an end there should be a common understanding among the counselor, pupil, and parent as to the next steps to be taken in the elimination of the health problems.

Correction of remediable defects

Two phases of school health services have been discussed. The student's health must first be appraised. Second, there must be a counseling procedure whereby the student and his parents are informed of health needs and problems so that the necessary action can be taken. After health appraisal and health counseling have been accomplished, the job is not completed. Next there must be a followthrough to see that remediable defects are corrected.

Students have many health defects that can be corrected. Dental caries is an example. It has been estimated that about 50% of 2-year-old children have one or more teeth that are carious. When they start school the number has risen to three and the number increases as the child progresses in school. In regard to vision defects it has been pointed out that eye problems increase from about 15% at 6 years of age to about 32% at 14 years of age.* Laxity in the correction of remediable defects seems to be especially prevalent in respect to teeth and eyes. There are also many other defects that can be corrected in the areas of malnutrition, hearing, speech, postural defects, diseased tonsils and adenoids, and emotional disorders.

The school has the responsibility for not only detecting such defects, whenever possible, but also putting forth every effort to see that they are corrected. The school's responsibility is to help every child attain optimum health; to encourage the removal of physical handicaps, defects, or anomalies that might constitute an obstacle to growth through correction or other helpful adjustment; and to guide parents, school staff, children, and others involved to a greater understanding of the factors related to better total health.

Community philosophy. The philosophy in respect to the methods that will be used to correct remediable defects will depend upon the community and the public at large. Although it is generally believed that the school should be concerned with educating parents and the public as to the importance of correcting such defects, rather than with becoming a treatment agency, this belief and practice do not exist in all communities. Basically, the schools should not treat. They are not equipped with the personnel, facilities, and other necessities for such a purpose. However, it is a community prerogative to decide such an issue. As a result, in some communities the school provides for the correction of dental, nutritional, postural, and other defects. In other communities this is considered a parental responsibility, and the school takes over only when indigent parents cannot afford such services. In many communities the school does not treat in any way. The community must decide which method is most effective for the correction of defects.

Getting results. To obtain the best results in the correction of remediable defects, there must be planning, conferences, and accurate record keeping.

The teacher, nurse, health counselor, principal, and school physician should play active roles in planning such a program. A written plan should be developed and distributed so that all will be acquainted with the procedure that is to be followed. The responsibility for record keeping, home visitation, periodic checkups to see if defects have been corrected, and all other essential phases of the plan should be clearly designated. Good results will not be obtained if planning is a "hit-and-miss" affair. It will be effective only if it is done in advance of the detection of defects. If necessary, it should also be reviewed and amended periodically.

A second requisite for getting results is home and school conferences. As has been previously pointed out, written notices are cold and formal and do not achieve the desired results, as do personal conferences. If possible, the parents should come to the school for such purposes, since it helps to give the school prestige. However, where parents are reluctant to come to school, there should be visits to the home, preferably by the nurse. This also affords an op-

---

*Joint Committee of American Medical Association and National Education Association, op. cit., p. 72.

portunity to observe home conditions that affect the health of the child. At these conferences or visitations every attempt should be made to interest the pupil and the parent in the correction of the defects.

Two of the main reasons why health defects are not corrected are lack of money to provide the necessary service and indifference on the part of both pupil and parent. Conferences should aim at eliminating the indifference and attempting to provide the ways and means when the money problem exists. In most communities there are charitable organizations, civic groups, or others who will be happy to defray such expenses.

A third requirement for getting good results is accurate record keeping. As a part of health appraisal the defects should be properly recorded. It is essential to keep a record of all conferences and home visitations. Progress that has been made should be noted. Accurate and complete records will make it possible to know the current status of each pupil.

Community resources. Community resources should be tapped for aid in the correction of remediable defects. Public clinics, welfare agencies, and voluntary organizations should be utilized to give aid to indigent families where financial status prevents such treatment. A list of the hospitals, specialists, and clinics for various types of treatment could be provided when parents want additional information. In most cases it is better to suggest the names of several specialists rather than just one.

The school should work cooperatively with the various community agencies interested in this work. In some cases, time during the school day might be provided for students who must have treatment. Literature and other information prepared by various community agencies might be distributed. Meetings between leaders in the school and community agencies might be held to plan a program. A community health council is an ideal place for discuss-

ing and formulating plans for the correction of remediable defects. By mobilizing and utilizing community resources, remediable defects will be corrected.

Care and education of exceptional students[*]

The term *exceptional* refers to those students who are handicapped mentally, physically, socially, or emotionally and also to those who are gifted intellectually or in other ways.

A democratic society rests on the premise that all individuals should have equal opportunities to develop the various talents that they possess. This means that all children and youth in our schools should be granted the right to have an education adapted to their particular physical, mental, social, and emotional endowments. Therefore, whether an individual is gifted, normal, or handicapped, he should have the right to pursue the educational program that is best adapted to his particular needs and that enables him to achieve his potentialities as a human being. This is an important consideration in a democratic society that recognizes the worth of each individual and his right to "life, liberty, and the pursuit of happiness."

In any discussion of the care and education of the exceptional child, it is important to consider (1) identifying the exceptional student, (2) discovering the exceptional child, (3) adapting the educational program, and (4) discussing the personnel that should be concerned with the care and education of the exceptional student.

Who are the exceptional students? Exceptional children include those students with superior intellectual capacity, the mentally retarded, those with handicaps derived from physical defects or disease, and those who are emotionally disturbed or socially maladjusted.

---

[*]See also Chapter 8 on The Adapted Program.

According to one source,* out of every 1,000 students about 59 will have some physical handicap that requires special attention. These 59 can be broken down as follows: partially seeing and blind, 2; hard of hearing and deaf, 15; speech defective, 15; crippled, 10; lowered vitality, 15; and epileptic, 2. In the same group of 1,000 students, about 40 will deviate markedly in respect to mental ability.

The prevalence of exceptional school children is evident in every community. These children should be identified and referred for special services, and the educational program should be adapted to their needs and abilities.

Discovering the exceptional student. It is very important that each school develop a planned procedure for determining those pupils who are exceptional. It is very simple to identify some cases, such as those that are crippled, defective in their speech, or socially maladjusted. However, in others, where cardiac defects or tuberculosis causes the handicap, it is not as easy.

The exceptional child may be identified through the various phases of health appraisal that are conducted as part of the health services program. Through a thorough medical examination, the cardiac-handicapped student, for example, will be identified; through a psychologic examination the mentally or emotionally maladjusted pupil will be singled out; and through screening procedures, those with vision and hearing handicaps will be known.

The health history that should be a part of every student's health record is another source for information leading to the identification of exceptional characteristics. A health history that lists all the significant diseases, accidents, and other aspects of the health history of a child should also list any exceptional characteristics that exist.

*Joint Committee of American Medical Association and National Education Association, op. cit., p. 129.

Teachers' observations also play a very important part. Through continuous observations on the part of a teacher, deviations from normal behavior will be identified. The individual who is listless might require further examination, a child who displays exceptional talent might be a genius in the class, or a child who finds it difficult to keep up with other boys his age in physical education activities should have further attention. Many of the children who fall into the exceptional group will have to be identified by teachers who work with them every day if they are to be singled out for special help.

Conferences with parents, teacher conferences with the school nurse, certain classroom tests, and reports from family physicians will help to identify exceptional individuals.

All of these methods should be carefully considered as potential media for identifying the many exceptional children who are regularly attending the public schools.

Adapting the educational program to the exceptional student. Some administrative guides for adapting the educational program and caring for the exceptional child are suggested here:

1. The school, as a general rule, should not undertake the treatment of handicapped students. However, it should do everything within its power to see that the necessary medical care is provided those who need such service. Through its referral service the school can carry out this responsibility.

2. Exceptional pupils should be treated as individuals rather than dealt with as groups of children with similar characteristics. Consideration should be given to each student.

3. Whether or not the exceptional individual is part of the regular group in the school situation, a part of a separate group, or in a separate school will depend upon the individual. The decision should be based on the question of which situa-

tion will allow the greatest possibility for improvement of the child's condition and for his total growth and development.

4. Special classes will aid certain individuals such as students who are hard of hearing, have speech and visual defects, and are severely crippled, homebound, or mentally retarded.

5. There is a need for an adequate supervisory program in connection with special classes for exceptional children. Good supervision will ensure periodic examinations to determine the status of the individual in respect to his exception, make sure that the program is as much like a regular school program as possible, and see that the child is returned to the regular class with normal children as soon as possible.

6. There are many different courses of action for the education and care of exceptional students. A few methods for making provisions for the various classifications are listed. This listing, however, is in no way complete, and special resources should be consulted for a more complete description of the school's responsibility.

The *deaf,* when so classified by a com-

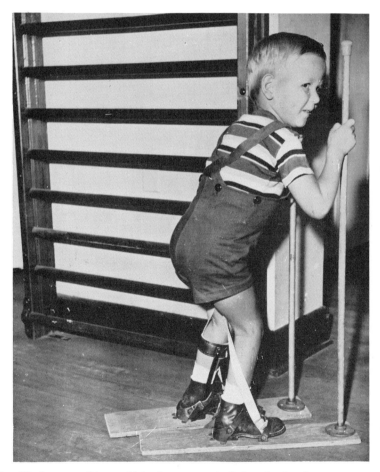

The school should do everything within its power to help obtain the necessary medical care for the handicapped child. (United States Office of Education, Department of Health, Education, and Welfare.)

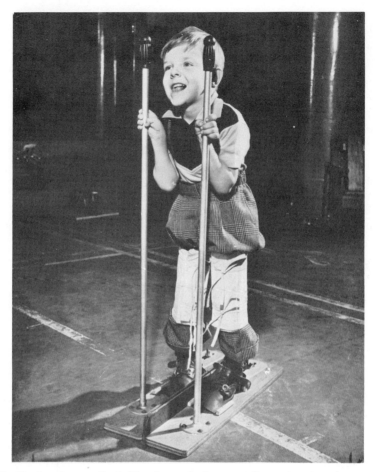

The orthopedically handicapped child. (United States Office of Education, Department of Health, Education, and Welfare.)

petent specialist, are those that have a hearing loss of 70 decibels or more. Generally, they should be placed in special schools.

The education and care of the *hard of hearing* will vary with hearing loss (slight—loss of 20 to 30 decibels; mild to moderate—loss of 30 to 40 decibels; moderate to severe—loss of 40 to 70 decibels; and severe—loss of more than 70 decibels). Provisions can be made, such as special arrangements for seating and instruction, hearing aids, speech and lipreading, special classes, and special schools.

The *blind* (20/200 in better eye with glasses) may be provided for either by a special school or by special classes where braille is used.

The *partially sighted* (between 20/70 and 20/200 with glasses) can be provided for by proper fitting of correct glasses, sight-saving classes, provision within regular classroom, proper seating, advantageous scheduling of classes, and special materials, such as typewriters.

The *orthopedically handicapped* child should be cared for in regular classes whenever it is possible. Special provisions for children handicapped in this group include: "(1) transportation in school buses with an attendant, (2) physical and occupational therapy, (3) speech therapy, if needed, and (4) general health supervision by the teacher under the general direction of the school medical adviser and nurse, if such are available."*

The *speech defective* student's first need is a complete examination with medical and surgical care, if necessary, to remove the cause of the speech defect. Speech defects such as stuttering, stammering, and phonetic difficulties can be aided through work with a speech correctionist, especially in the case of young children. Special classes are usually not needed; the student can attend regular classes and get the necessary treatment at a speech clinic or other place.

Malnourished and *undervitalized* children will usually be cared for on both an individual and a community basis. Health education aimed at raising the nutritional status of the home, a careful perusal of health histories to identify the causes, adjustment of the school program, and in some cases provision for special rest rooms will contribute to the solution of the defects.

The *mentally retarded* child (50 to 70 intelligence quotient, or I.Q.) should have a program that stresses, according to his individual abilities, proper health, safety, and social habits; information and skills essential to constructive community living, such as care of children, proper maintenance of the home, and the community health resources that are available; and skills for creative and leisure-time activities that will lead to cultural development.†

The *mentally gifted* child (I.Q. of approximately 140 or over) has been helped in at least four ways: (1) an accelerated program adapted according to his ability to achieve higher standards, (2) enrichment of his curriculum so that it is adapted more

to his abilities, (3) attendance in special classes, and (4) addition of elective courses.*

Cardiac-handicapped children should be provided for after complete examination by competent medical personnel. A few will require special classes, others will require modified programs, and some will need instruction to help them understand and live within certain restrictions.

The *tubercular-handicapped* child, if he has a case of active tuberculosis, should not be in school. The school programs for children who have had the disease should be adapted to their needs. This should be done in consultation with the appropriate medical person. This may mean only part-time attendance at school, provision for rest periods, limited physical activity, and special transportation.

Emotionally atypical students should be provided for in relation to their maladjustments. Some will need the help of a qualified psychologist or psychiatrist. Others will be helped by the guidance counselor or teacher. In most cases the teacher can play a key role in providing an emotional atmosphere where the child reacts favorably to the group.

The *socially exceptional* should also be provided for in relation to the extent of their maladjustments. Children with the most severe cases will need confinement to institutions; the rest will need rehabilitation, care, or developmental opportunities to restore them to normalcy.

The National Committee on School Health Policies points out other ways that the school can make special provisions for handicapped pupils:

Specially constructed chairs and desks—for the orthopedically disabled children.
Appropriate seating arrangements—"down front" for children with vision or hearing defects.
Provision of hearing aids.
Scheduling of classes all on one floor.

---

*Joint Committee of American Medical Association and National Education Association, op. cit., p. 136.
†Ibid., p. 143.

*Ibid., p. 145.

Rest periods and facilities (cots) for resting—for children with cardiac and other impairments.

Permission to attend school for only part of the day.

Adaptation of physical education requirements.

Transportation to and from school.*

Such provisions enable many handicapped pupils to attend regular classes.

Personnel. The teachers who work with exceptional children should be well trained for their duties. Whether or not the child is able to adjust satisfactorily to the group, improve, and be educated and cared for in a desirable manner will depend to a great degree upon the teacher.

Teachers should be well prepared for the particular grade or subject to which they are assigned. In addition, they should be trained to work with exceptional children with specific disabilities. The nature or type of disability will determine the training needed. The teacher should be emotionally stable and have the type of temperament that is suitable for working with abnormal children. The size of classes for exceptional children should be smaller than for regular classes. If progress is to be achieved, the individual approach must be applied as much as possible.

In addition to the teacher, there are other individuals in the school and community who can render contributions to this phase of the health service program. Where they are part of the school staff, the nurse, guidance director, school physician, psychologist, social worker, and director of special education should work closely with the teacher and school administrator in planning the program. Other individuals, such as ophthalmologists, psychiatrists, orthopedists, speech correctionists, otologists, directors of agencies dealing with the handicapped, and members of state departments of health and education, should be utilized for advice, planning, referrals, inservice education, and other contributions to this phase of the health service program.

Communicable disease control

Whenever students congregate there is the possibility of spreading disease. The school, as a place for children and youth to congregate, is unique in that the law requires attendance. Therefore, if it is compulsory to go to school, there should also be certain protective measures and precautions taken to ensure that everything is done to guard the health of the child. This includes the necessary procedures for controlling communicable disease. Although students are not required to go to college, higher educational institutions also have the responsibility for communicable disease control.

The problem of communicable disease control can be discussed under two main headings, first, responsibility, and second, the various measures that should be applied in the school situation.

Responsibility. The legal responsibility for communicable disease control rests with state and local departments of health. This means that public health officials have control over school and college personnel in this matter. In most cases, however, this is a case of cooperation rather than compulsion. School and college officials should work closely with public health officials so that cases of communicable disease are reported and proper measures taken to prevent other children from contracting the disease.

The responsibility for communicable disease control falls upon many individuals. These include public health personnel, school and college administrative personnel, nurse, school physician, teacher, custodian, and the parent. The teacher, parent, and nurse must be continually vigilant to notice symptoms of various communicable

---

*National Committee on School Health Policies: Suggested school health policies, ed. 3, Chicago, 1962, American Medical Association, p. 31.

diseases, isolate such individuals immediately, and refer these cases to the school, college, or family physician. There must be close cooperation among these three since all three play key roles in the control of communicable diseases. If the parent plays his or her role effectively and the child is isolated immediately, he will lessen considerably the exposure of other individuals to disease. If the child is in school, the alert teacher and nurse will take the necessary precautions.

The superintendent, principal, university physician, and other administrative officers have the responsibility for establishing policy, working cooperatively with public health officials, providing encouragement and inservice training for teachers, and developing among parents and the public in general an understanding that will be most conducive to communicable disease control.

The custodian, through his or her control over the sanitation of the equipment and facilities, can perform his responsibilities so effectively that a healthful environment is always in evidence and thus the spread of disease is decreased.

The school or college physician should

DENVER PUBLIC SCHOOLS
Department of Health Service

HOME CONTROL OF COMMUNICABLE DISEASES

TO PARENTS:

The control of communicable ("catching") diseases during the school year is a difficult problem and a grave responsibility for both parents and school. The first responsibility must fall upon the home. In addition to knowing your children are immunized against those communicable diseases which are preventable, the following information is given to help control acute illnesses. Because parents know the normal appearance of their children they should be the first to detect signs of illness.

1. Observe your child every morning and **do not send him to school if he shows any signs of illness.** Keep an ill child at home for his own safety as well as the safety of other children.

2. **Do not send a sick child to school** for the nurse or teacher to decide whether he should be in school. If in doubt, keep him at home, and when necessary call the family doctor.

3. Keep your child away from sick persons.

4. If your child is sick, keep other children away from him.

Some of the signs and symptoms of acute illness are:

1. Restlessness at night. (This is often the first sign of an acute illness.)
2. Running nose.
3. Sneezing and coughing.
4. Sore throat.
5. Rash.
6. Vomiting.
7. Red, watery eyes.
8. Flushed face.
9. Headache.
10. Unusually tired.

The cooperation of all parents is sincerely requested.

L. M. CORLISS, M.D.
Director of Health Service

STOCK NO. 10871
FORM 971 DSP

Enlisting parental support in communicable disease control.

advise the teacher, nurse, administrative officers, and others who are closely related to the whole problem of communicable disease control as to the necessary measures that should be provided. Through his specialized knowledge, he can contribute much toward the establishment of an effective and workable plan.

Control measures. There are many control measures that every school or college should follow to prevent the spread of disease. Some of the more important of these measures are discussed here.

*Healthful environment.** Some of the provisions for a healthful environment that are necessary for the control of communicable disease include sufficient space to avoid undue crowding, adequate toilet and washroom facilities, proper ventilation and heating, safe running water, properly installed drinking fountains, use of pasteurized milk, a system of exclusions and control of admissions for students who may have communicable disease, and policies toward student and teacher absences that do not require teachers to be in school when they may be ill and capable of spreading communicable disease germs.

Isolation of students. The student who is a "suspect" in regard to some communicable disease should immediately be isolated from the group. Isolating a student does not constitute diagnosis. The details and procedures followed in each school or college regarding isolation should be in writing and clearly understood by all concerned. The adopted plan should have the approval of the health service staff.

The teacher should be continually on the lookout for "suspects." Some indications of communicable disease that should be recognized by the teacher are the following:

Unusual pallor or flushed face
Unusual listlessness or quietness
Red or watery eyes
Eyes sensitive to light

Skin rash
Cough
Need for frequent use of toilet
Nausea or vomiting
Running nose or sniffles
Excessive irritability
Jaundice*

After the teacher isolates the "suspect" from the group, the student should not be left alone. Furthermore, the nurse or school or college physician should be notified. In the event neither of these individuals is available, the teacher and school administrator must decide on exclusion. The best solution is to arrange for the student to return to his home or to be sent to the infirmary, where the services of a physician should be procured as soon as possible. Furthermore, the case should be reported to the local health authorities.

Readmitting students to school or college. After having a communicable disease a student should not be readmitted to school or college until it is certain that his return is in the best interests of the health of both the student concerned and also the other students with whom he will come in contact. There should be strict conformance to the law that governs communicable diseases. In addition, there should be approval for such readmission indicated in writing by a qualified physician or the local health department. In minor cases a note from the parent or the decision of the nurse or other staff member may suffice.

Immunization. Every student should receive immunization against preventable diseases. Most of this should be done in the preschool years when danger from such diseases is prevalent. Every child should be immunized against tetanus, poliomyelitis, diphtheria, smallpox, and whooping cough. The school can play an important part in the health education of parents to see that children are immunized

---

*See also Chapter 14.

*Joint Committee of American Medical Association and National Education Association, op. cit., p. 210.

against these diseases before starting school. The children who come to school and have not received the benefit of such services need special attention. It is a public health and medical problem and should be dealt with through members of these professions. If the community decides that the school is the best place for immunization, the school should cooperate fully and keep complete records on initial immunizations and booster doses. Written permission should be secured from parents concerned.

Attendance. There should not be an overemphasis on perfect attendance for school children. This often results in children coming to school regardless of the condition of their health and the danger to others. Furthermore, state aid should be based on some method other than attendance.

Epidemics. The viewpoint on closing schools and colleges during epidemics has changed somewhat in recent years. Formerly, it was generally believed that schools should be closed. Today, it is felt that under many circumstances they should remain open. The deciding factor is whether or not the school provides regular inspections, observations, adequate staff, and facilities to screen out those who indicate signs of having the disease. If this service can be performed and if the closing of schools will result in many contacts on playgrounds and other places where children congregate, then, according to the latest thinking, the schools should remain open. This is particularly true in urban areas. Many times in rural areas, where children will not come in contact with each other if schools are closed, it may be advisable to have schools closed.

If an epidemic occurs during a vacation period it is often wise to postpone the opening of school, since such opening might result in increased contact with the disease.

Emergency care

Elementary and secondary schools are responsible for providing each student with the necessary protection and care. The school acts in loco parentis (in place of the parent) and it is assumed that the child will receive the same care and protection

---

SAN FRANCISCO DEPARTMENT OF PUBLIC HEALTH
IMMUNIZATION AND TEST CONSENT

Date_____

Name_____ Address_____ Phone No._____

School_____ Grade_____ Room_____ Phy. Ed. Period_____ P. E. Teacher_____ Birth-date_____

In looking over your child's health record, it is recommended that the following immunizations and/or tests be given. Please sign your name opposite the recommended procedure if you wish your child to have the benefit of the test or immunization.

If your child has had a positive Tuberculin Test in the past, it will probably remain positive and should not be repeated. If your child's test was ever positive, please indicate when or approximately when

Negative Tuberculin Tests may be repeated yearly.

F 1515 1-56

Immunizations and Tests	Recommended	Parent's Signature
Smallpox Vaccination		
Diphtheria Pertussis Tetanus } D.P.T.		
Polio Vaccination		
Tuberculin Test		

PLEASE RETURN TO PUBLIC HEALTH NURSE

Table 13-2. First-aid supplies and how to use them*

Suggested supplies	What they are for
Tincture of green soap	Washing injured parts
Hospital cotton, roll	Large soft pads or dressings
Absorbent cotton, sterilized, roll, box or "picking" package	Swabs or pledgets for applying medication or wiping wounds
Dressings, large or small pads, sterilized, in individual transparent envelopes	For protecting injuries
Dressings, finger, in envelopes	For protecting very small injuries
Adhesive tape, roll, one inch	Fastening dressings, or splints
Scissors, bandage or blunt	Cutting dressings
Toothpicks	For making swabs
Alcohol 70% (water 30%) or rubbing alcohol	Disinfecting skin and minor wounds
Mercurochrome, 2% aqueous	Minor injuries especially in young children
Other disinfectant, if ordered by physician	As ordered by physician
Mineral oil, bottle, or petroleum jelly, tube or jar, white or yellow, but not medicated	For removing ointments; in eye to relieve irritation from foreign body; for burns if no other ointment is at hand
Boric acid ointment U.S.P.	For very small minor first-degree burns only
Epsom salts	In hot water, a handful to a basin, for soaking sprains, bruises, or infection when ordered by a physician
Baking soda, powder	Teaspoonful to a pint of warm water for mouthwash, or gargle if ordered
Salt, crystal or tablets	Same as baking soda, or with baking soda as directed
Hot-water bottle with cover	Local relief of pain
Ice bag	Local relief of pain
Two warm blankets	For prevention of chilling
Tourniquet (three feet of soft rubber tubing and a stick or pencil)	USE ABOVE place from where red blood spurts. Call doctor at once. Release every 15 minutes to allow circulation to reach parts, then reapply if necessary
Eye droppers	Dropping liquid medicines. Cleanse after using and boil before using
Ear syringe, soft rubber	For ears only when ordered by physician
Graduated medicine glass†	For measuring liquid medicines
Drugs for internal use	Only when ordered by physician and as directed by him

*From American Association of School Administrators: Health in schools, Twentieth Yearbook, Washington, D. C., 1951, National Education Association, pp. 394-395. (Prepared by American Medical Association.)

†Graduated medicine glass is most accurate and should be used whenever possible. In emergency, this table may be used:

20 drops (water solution)	1 c.c. (metric)
1 teaspoon (measuring spoon, not table silver)	5 c.c.
1 tablespoon (measuring spoon, not table silver)	15 c.c.
1 wineglass	50 c.c.
1 tumbler	250 c.c.

during the hours of school that he normally would receive at home. Children often become sick or injured during school hours. Therefore, the school must provide the necessary attention until this can be undertaken by the parents.

According to the Joint Committee on Health Problems, the school has four responsibilities in respect to emergency care procedures. These are "(1) giving immediate care, (2) notifying the pupil's parents, (3) arranging for the pupil to get home, and, (4) guiding parents, when necessary, to sources of treatment."*

Some administrative guides for emergency care are as follows:

1. Every school and college should have a written plan for emergency care. It should be carefully prepared by the school administration with the help of the school or college physician, parents, medical and dental professions, hospitals, nurse, teachers, and others interested and responsible in this area. The time to plan and decide on procedure is before an accident occurs. This should be one of the first administrative responsibilities that is accomplished.

The written plan should contain such essentials as first-aid instructions; procedures for getting medical help, transportation, and notifying parents; staff responsibilities, supplies, equipment, and facilities available; and any other information that will help clarify exactly what is to be done in time of emergency.

The plan should be reviewed periodically and revised so that it is continually up to date. It should be posted in conspicuous places and discussed periodically with school staff and community groups, whenever necessary.

2. As many staff members as possible should be trained in first-aid procedures. There is a need for special knowledge and training in respect to emergency care that might entail first aid for broken bones, use of artificial respiration, control of hemorrhage, and proper care of patients suffering from shock. The more staff members that are trained in these specific first-aid procedures, the better coverage there is for accidents that may occur at any time when school activities are in progress.

Some schools have the American Red Cross give inservice courses in first-aid procedures. Such inservice training will help to ensure that the staff is competent along this line.

When a nurse is on duty it would usually be expected that her responsibility includes seeing that proper first-aid procedures are carried out.

Professional preparation institutions should give due consideration to instruction in first-aid and emergency care procedures as part of the training of all teachers and school and college personnel.

3. A health room for first aid and emergency care should be available.* It should possess the necessary equipment and supplies; have good lighting; be clean, of adequate size, and always available for emergency cases.

A basic list of first-aid supplies, together with a statement as to what they are for, has been developed by the American Medical Association. See p. 380.

In addition to furniture and routine equipment, the health room should also have available as a minimum the following:

Stethoscope	Tuning fork for
Thermometer, clinical	hearing tests
Sphygmomanometer	Mouth mirror
Electric ophthalmoscope	Probes, dental
Electric otoscope	Forceps
Reflex hammer	Syringes
Tape measure	Needles
Platform scale	Eye droppers
(not a spring model)	Graduated medicine
Illuminated eye	glasses
test charts	

*Joint Committee of American Medical Association and National Education Association, op. cit., pp. 222-223.

*See description in Chapter 15.

first aid chart for athletic injuries

FIRST AID, the immediate and temporary care offered to the stricken athlete until the services of a physician can be obtained, minimizes the aggravation of injury and enhances the earliest possible return of the athlete to peak performance. To this end, it is strongly recommended that:

ALL ATHLETIC PROGRAMS include prearranged procedures for obtaining emergency first aid, transportation, and medical care.

ALL COACHES AND TRAINERS be competent in first aid techniques and procedures.

ALL ATHLETES be properly immunized as medically recommended, especially against tetanus and polio.

Committee on the
Medical Aspects of Sports
AMERICAN MEDICAL ASSOCIATION

to protect the athlete at time of injury, FOLLOW THESE FIRST STEPS FOR FIRST AID

STOP play immediately at first indication of possible injury or illness.

LOOK for obvious deformity or other deviation from the athlete's normal structure or motion.

LISTEN to the athlete's description of his complaint and how the injury occurred.

ACT, but move the athlete *only* after serious injury is ruled out.

BONES AND JOINTS

fracture Never move athlete if fracture of back, neck, or skull is suspected. If athlete *can* be moved, carefully splint any possible fracture. Obtain medical care at once.

dislocation Support joint. Apply ice bag or cold cloths to reduce swelling, and refer to physician at once.

bone bruise Apply ice bag or cold cloths and protect from further injury. If severe, refer to physician.

broken nose Apply cold cloths and refer to physician.

HEAT ILLNESSES

heat stroke Collapse—with dry warm skin—indicates sweating mechanism failure and rising body temperature. THIS IS AN EMERGENCY; DELAY COULD BE FATAL. Immediately cool athlete by the most expedient means (immersion in cool water is best method). Obtain medical care at once.

heat exhaustion Weakness—with profuse sweating—indicates state of shock due to depletion of salt and water. Place in shade with head level or lower than body. Give sips of dilute salt water. Obtain medical care at once.

sunburn If severe, apply sterile gauze dressing and refer to physician.

IMPACT BLOWS

head If any period of dizziness, headache, incoordination or unconsciousness occurs, disallow any further activity and obtain medical care at once. Keep athlete lying down; if unconscious, give nothing by mouth.

teeth Save teeth, if completely removed from socket. If loosened, do not disturb; cover with sterile gauze and refer to dentist at once.

solar plexus Rest athlete on back and moisten face with cool water. Loosen clothing around waist and chest. Do nothing else except obtain medical care if needed.

testicle Rest athlete on back and apply ice bag or cold cloths. Obtain medical care if pain persists.

eye If vision is impaired, refer to physician at once. With soft tissue injury, apply ice bag or cold cloths to reduce swelling.

MUSCLES AND LIGAMENTS

bruise Apply ice bag or cold cloths and rest injured muscle. Protect from further aggravation. If severe, refer to physician.

cramp Have opposite muscles contracted forcefully, using firm hand pressure on cramped muscle. If during hot day, give sips of dilute salt water. If recurring, refer to physician.

strain and sprain Elevate injured part and apply ice bag or cold cloths. Apply pressure bandage to reduce swelling. Avoid weight bearing and obtain medical care.

OPEN WOUNDS

heavy bleeding Apply sterile pressure bandage using hand pressure if necessary. Refer to physician at once.

cut and abrasion Hold briefly under cold water. Then cleanse with mild soap and water. Apply sterile pad firmly until bleeding stops, then protect with more loosely applied sterile bandage. If extensive, refer to physician.

puncture wound Handle same as cuts; refer to physician.

nosebleed Keep athlete sitting or standing; cover nose with cold cloths. If bleeding is heavy, pinch nose and place *small* cotton pack in nostrils. If bleeding continues, refer to physician.

OTHER CONCERNS

blisters Keep clean with mild soap and water and protect from aggravation. If already broken, trim ragged edges with sterilized equipment. If extensive or infected, refer to physician.

foreign body in eye Do not rub. Gently touch particle with point of clean, moist cloth and wash with cold water. If unsuccessful or if pain persists, refer to physician.

lime burns Wash thoroughly with water. Apply sterile gauze dressing and refer to physician.

EMERGENCY PHONE NUMBERS		
Physician	Phone:	
Physician	Phone:	
Hospital	Ambulance	
Police	Fire	Other

The staff responsible for the health room should be fixed and such responsibility should include training and competency in first-aid procedures.

4. Proper emergency equipment and supplies, in addition to being located in the health room, should also be available in strategic school or college locations that are accident-prone because of activity courses and in places remote from the health room. Such locations might include gymnasium, laboratories, shops, school buses, annexes, and buildings housing school activities apart from the central unit.

5. School and college records should contain complete information on each student. This might include such information as his address; parent's name, address, and phone number; business address of parent and phone number; family physician, address, and phone number; family dentist, address, and phone number; parent instruction in case of emergency; choice of hospital; and any other pertinent information.

6. There should be a complete record of every accident, including first aid given and emergency care administered in the event of illness. Such information preserves for future reference the procedures followed in each case. This record is very important in the event questions arise in the future. Time results in forgetfulness, misinterpretation, misunderstanding, and inaccurate conclusions being drawn. Records can also be used to disclose hazards that should be eliminated and weak spots in procedures for emergency care that should be improved. Finally, such records aid in impressing upon students, staff, parents, and other individuals who are concerned the importance of good procedures for safe and healthful living.

7. The legal aspects of problems involved in regard to emergency care should be discussed and understood by the entire school or college staff. Such discussion will make for a better understanding of the laws of a particular state or locality and show the importance of avoiding negligence in duty.

8. Insurance plans for staff, athletes, and students should be made clear. They should be in writing and well publicized so that each individual will know the extent to which expenses, claims, and other items will be paid in event of accident, or the extent to which he can or should procure additional coverage.

9. Disasters in the form of fires, floods, tornadoes, and air raids can occur at any time. In order to provide proper emergency care under such circumstances, there must be advance planning. Schools and colleges should recognize their responsibility along this line. Adequate insurance coverage should be maintained. Supplies for emergency care should be on hand. Responsibilities should be fixed in key positions. Plans should be laid for taking children to safest place possible. Drills should be conducted. Close cooperation should exist between the schools and such organizations as Civil Defense or the Red Cross.

Environmental sanitation

Another health service responsibility of schools and colleges is that of ensuring a sanitary environment. Since many aspects of this topic are covered in Chapter 14, as well as earlier in this chapter, it will be discussed only briefly here. Some aspects of environmental sanitation that need particular attention are the school's or college's responsibility for ensuring a safe water supply; sanitary sewage disposal; and cafeterias, kitchens, locker rooms, showers, and swimming pools.

If desirable environmental sanitation standards are adhered to, it will not only help to reduce the incidence of the spread of disease but also will be conducive to a more comfortable, pleasant environment that will contribute to optimum learning.

Health of school and college personnel

Educational organizations need to give attention to the health of school and college personnel in order to ensure the most efficient carrying out of duties by teachers, administrators, and other members of the staff; to provide examples for children and young people that are worth emulating; and to promote the most healthful and pleasant environment possible. Boards of education, boards of trustees, and other persons who are involved in making pertinent decisions, therefore, need to concern themselves with such matters as sick leave, health insurance, sabbatical leaves, retirement provisions, maternity leaves, medical examinations, exclusion from school or college of teachers with health conditions that have implications for students' health and well-being, and other matters that concern the health of all employees of the school district or college. The health of school and college personnel is as important a consideration as health of school and college students.

Questions and exercises

1. What are the component parts of a school or college health service program? What is the importance to the student of each part?
2. What is the relationship between health services and the other phases of the school or college health program?
3. Prepare a speech to be given in class that could be used to point out to the parent-teacher association the importance of the development of a desirable health services program.
4. What should be the relationship between the public health department and the school or college health department in relation to school health services?
5. Discuss the advantages and disadvantages of the theory: "The school is a place for both education and treatment."
6. Outline what you consider to be a sound health appraisal program for an elementary school.
7. Describe the nature and scope of the school medical examination. Relate how it can be an educational experience for boys and girls.
8. Prepare a list of arguments to be presented to the board of education to justify the addition of a psychologist to the school staff.
9. What part do the teacher's observations play in a health services program? What are his or her responsibilities in the matter?
10. Identify pure-tone audiometer, whisper test, Massachusetts Vision Test, caries, Snellen E Chart, followthrough, and exceptional child.
11. What are the essential health records that should be maintained to conduct a desirable health services program?
12. Prepare a mock health counseling conference with a child and his mother after a medical examination that has revealed several defects that need correction.
13. What recommendations could you make in order to ensure the greatest possible correction of remediable health defects?
14. Take one type of exceptional child, do considerable research on the type of educational program that is best suited to this particular individual, and make recommendations to the class.
15. After careful study of all factors involved, outline a program for a particular community as to how the public health department and school health education division can most effectively work together for communicable disease control.
16. Prepare a written plan for emergency care of injuries for your school or college, which will then be submitted to the class for approval and then presented to the school health services division of your institution for comment.

Reading assignment in *Administrative Dimensions of Health and Physical Education Programs, Including Athletics:* Chapter 10, Selections 55 to 58.

Selected references

Committee on the Medical Aspects of Sports of the American Medical Association: The team physician, The Journal of School Health 37:497, 1967.

Corliss, L. M.: Multiple handicapped children—their placement in the school education program, The Journal of School Health 37:113, 1967.

Day, H. P.: University administration views the health service, American College Health Association Journal 15:140, 1966.

DeBoer, L.: Application of screening method for the detection of heart disease in children, Journal of School Health 33:81, 1962.

Eiserer, P. E.: The school psychologist, New York, 1963, The Center for Applied Research in Education, Inc. (The Library of Education).

Ferguson, D. G.: Pupil personnel services, New

York, 1963, The Center for Applied Research in Education, Inc. (The Library of Education).

Forbes, O.: The role and functions of the school nurse as perceived by 115 public school teachers from three selected counties, The Journal of School Health 37:101, 1967.

Gibbons, H.: Recognizing the educational implications of visual problems, Journal of School Health 32:280, 1962.

Goolishian, H. A.: School health services, The Journal of School Health 44:313, 1968.

Hein, F. V.: Health classification vs. medical excuses from physical education, Journal of School Health 32:14, 1962.

Joint Committee on Health Problems in Education of National Education Association and American Medical Association: Health appraisal of school children, ed. 2, Washington, D. C., 1961, National Education Association.

Joint Committee on Health Problems in Education of National Education Association and American Medical Association: Health education, Washington, D. C., 1961, National Education Association.

Joint Committee on Health Problems in Education of National Education Association and American Medical Association: School health services, ed. 2, Washington, D. C., 1964, National Education Association.

Kleinschmidt, E. E.: Current problems in school health service, Journal of School Health 32:222, 1962.

Lampe, J.: For the medical director, Journal of School Health 32:269, 1962.

Lowman, L.: A message to school health services, Journal of School Health 32:17, 1962.

National Committee on School Health Policies: Suggested school health policies, ed. 3, Chicago, 1962, American Medical Association.

Neilson, E. A.: Health education and the school physician, The Journal of School Health 39:377, 1969.

Ryan, A. J.: Providing medical services for athletes, School Activities, November, 1967.

Schneeweiss, S. M., and Locke, A.: New horizons in school health services: the computer, The Journal of School Health 37:349, 1967.

Shaffer, T. E.: What health services do school-age children need? Journal of the American Association for Health, Physical Education, and Recreation 23:16, 1962.

Tower, B., and Fay, P.: Can contracted school health services work? The Journal of School Health 38:339, 1968.

Wetzel, N. C.: New dimensions in the simultaneous screening and assessment of school children, Journal of Health, Physical Education, and Recreation, vol. 37, January, 1966.

Yankauer, A., Jr., and others: Study of case-finding methods in elementary schools; methodology and initial results, American Journal of Public Health 53:656, 1962.

CHAPTER 14 PROVIDING A HEALTHFUL ENVIRONMENT FOR STUDENTS

A healthful school or college environment means not only having safe physical facilities, proper equipment, water, and other essentials, but it also means having a healthful psychologic environment where students benefit from practices and conditions conducive to their mental and emotional health. Therefore, this chapter concerns itself with both the physical and psychologic environment.

THE PHYSICAL ENVIRONMENT

The general health features of the physical environment will be discussed here under the following headings: site, building, lighting, heating and ventilation, furniture, plant sanitation, and acoustics.

Site

There are many aspects to consider in the selection of a suitable site. These considerations will differ, depending on the community. Whether it is a rural or an urban community will have a bearing on the location of the site. In an urban community it is desirable to have the school situated near transportation facilities, but at the same time located away from industrial concerns, railroads, noise, heavy traffic, fumes, and smoke. Consideration should be given to the trends in population movements and future development of the area in which the buildings are planned. Adequate space for play and recreation should be provided. Some standards recommend 5 acres of land for elementary schools, 10 to 12 acres for junior high schools, and 20 acres for senior high schools. The play area should consist of a minimum of 100 square feet for every child. The National Council on Schoolhouse Construction* has suggested that, although larger sites may be used, standards that provide a minimum of 5 acres plus an additional acre for each 100 pupils of projected enrollment for elementary schools and a minimum of 10 acres plus an additional acre for each 100 pupils of projected enrollment for junior and senior high schools should be followed. Thus an elementary school of 200 pupils would have a site of 7 acres, for example, and a high school of 500 pupils a site of 15 acres.

Attention should be given to the esthetic features of a site because of its effect on the physical and emotional well-being of students and staff. The surroundings should be well landscaped, attractive, and free from disturbing noises or odors.

The American Association of School Administrators and the National Council on Schoolhouse Construction can supply detailed information on the selection of a site.

Building

Some trends in modern building construction have already been discussed and consideration of some of the special areas is still to come. Suffice it to say here that the trend is toward one-story construction at the precollege educational level, where that is possible, with stress on planning from a functional rather than an ornamen-

---

*National Council of Schoolhouse Construction, East Lansing, Michigan.

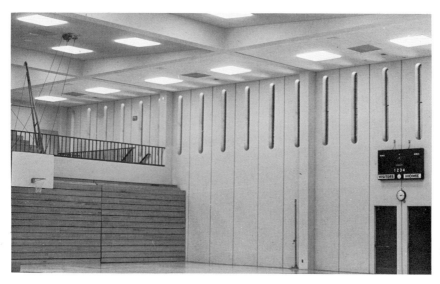

Lighting for gymnasium at University of California at Irvine.

tal point of view. The building should be constructed from the standpoint of use. As much natural lighting as possible should be utilized. The materials used should make the building attractive and safe. According to the National Safety Council a high percentage of children's accidents occur in school buildings. Every precaution should be taken to protect against accidents from fire, slippery floors, and other dangers. The walls should be painted with light colors and treated acoustically. Doors should open outward. Space for clothing should be provided.

These are only a few of the considerations in planning a school building. It is important that an architect plan such facilities with special regard to the educational needs of those who utilize it. Educators should formulate a plan and use it in discussions with the architect.

Lighting*

Proper lighting is important to conserve vision, to prevent fatigue, and to improve morale. There should be proper lighting as to both quality and quantity. In the past it has been recommended that natural light should come into the room from the left and that artificial light should be provided as needed. There is a trend now toward allowing natural light from more than one direction. Artificial light, moreover, should come from many sources rather than one, so as to prevent too much concentration of light in one place. Switches for artificial light should be located in many parts of the room.

Light intensity in most classrooms, according to expert opinion, usually varies from 15 to 100 footcandles.* Most authorities suggest between 30 and 70 footcandles for reading and close work. In gymnasia and swimming pools it is recommended that intensity range from 10 to 50 footcandles. Glare is undesirable and should be eliminated. Fluorescent lights should be properly installed and adjusted for best results. Strong contrasts of color such as light walls and dark floors should be avoided.

Windows, according to most experts,

---

*A good source of information for acceptable standards on lighting is the Illuminating Engineering Society, New York, N. Y.

*A footcandle is the unit by which light is measured in intensity at a given point.

should extend as far up toward the ceiling as possible and should consume space equal to about one-fourth to one-fifth of the floor area.

Window shades aid in controlling light. They should be durable, of light color, and located in the middle of the window so that they may be adjusted either up or down.

Heating and ventilation*

Efficiency in the classroom, gymnasium, special activities rooms, and other places is determined to some extent by thermal comfort. Thermal comfort is determined in the main by heating and ventilation.

The purposes of heating and ventilation are many. Some of the more common are to remove excess heat, unpleasant odors, and, in some cases, gases, vapors, fumes, and dust from the room; to prevent rapid temperature fluctuations; to diffuse the heat within a room; and to supply heat to counteract loss from the human body through radiation and otherwise.

Heating standards vary according to the activities engaged in, the clothing worn by the participants, and section of the country. The following represents an approximate average of various suggested standards for temperatures:

1. Classrooms, offices, and cafeterias— 68° to 76° F. (30 inches above floor)
2. Kitchens, closed corridors, shops, and laboratories—65° to 68° F. (60 inches above floor)
3. Gymnasia and activity rooms—55° to 65° F. (60 inches above floor)
4. Locker and shower rooms—70° to 78° F. (60 inches above floor)
5. Swimming pools—80° to 85° F. (60 inches above the deck)

In respect to ventilation, the range of recommendations is from 8 to 21 cubic feet of fresh air per minute per occupant.

---

*A good source for ventilating and heating information is the American Society of Heating, Refrigerating, and Air-Conditioning Engineers, New York, N. Y.

Adequate ventilating systems are especially needed in dressing, shower, and locker rooms, toilet rooms, gymnasia, and swimming pools. The recommended humidity ranges from 35% to 60%. The type and amount of ventilation will vary with the specific needs of the particular area to be served.

Furniture

The furniture that students use most is desks and chairs. Seats and desks that are adjustable and movable are recommended by most educators. There are many different kinds of seats and desks that are available in both wood and metal. The desk should be of proper height and fit the pupil comfortably and properly. Desks should be arranged to provide the best light for the students.

Plant sanitation

Various items concerned with plant sanitation should not be overlooked. Sanitation facilities should be well provided and well maintained. The water supply should be safe and adequate. If any question exists, the local or state health department should be consulted. In regard to water supply, one authority suggests that at least 20 gallons per pupil per day is needed, for all purposes.

Drinking fountains of various heights should be recessed in corridor walls and should be of material that is easily cleaned. Approximately one drinking fountain should be provided for every 75 students. A stream of water should flow from the fountain in such a manner that it is not necessary for the mouth of the drinker to get too near the drain bowl.

Water closets, urinals, lavatories, and washroom equipment such as soap dispensers, toilet paper holders, waste containers, mirrors, bookshelves, and hand-drying facilities should be provided as needed.

Waste disposal should be adequately cared for. There should be provision for cleanup and removal of stray paper and other materials that make the grounds and buildings a health and safety hazard as well as unsightly. Proper sewage disposal and prompt garbage disposal should also be provided.

Acoustics

Concentration is necessary in many kinds of school, college, and recreational work. Noise distracts attention, causes nervous strain, and results in the loss of many of the activity's benefits. Therefore, noise should be eliminated as effectively as possible. This can be achieved by acoustical treatment of such important places as corridors, gymnasia, swimming pools, shops, music rooms, and libraries.

Acoustical materials include plasters, fibers, boards, tiles, and various types of fabrics. Some areas should be given special attention. Floor covering that reduces noise can be used in corridors, and acoustical material can be used in walls. In classrooms, special attention should be given to materials that absorb sound in the upper walls and to tight floor coverings. In cafeterias there should be sound-absorption materials on floors, tables, counter tops, ceilings, and walls. Furthermore, the kitchen with its noises should be separated from the dining room. The music room and shop areas should be isolated as much as possible in addition to having acoustically treated walls. Swimming pools and gymnasia need special treatment to control the various noises associated with joyous and enthusiastic play participation. Ceiling and wall acoustical treatment will help control noises in the gymnasium, while the use of mineral acoustical material, which will not be affected by high humidity, will be found helpful in the swimming pool.

Special considerations for a healthful environment for physical education

Physical educators including teachers, coaches, and others should contribute to a healthful environment by providing safe and sanitary conditions for their program and the construction and maintenance of safe facilities.

Outdoor physical education facilities. Playing fields and playgrounds should have good turf and be clear of rocks, holes, and uneven surfaces. A dirty, dusty surface, for example, can aggravate such conditions as emphysema, chronic bronchitis, and allergies. Artificial turf is now coming into use and has been proved to be very satisfactory. Safety precautions should be provided in terms of well-lined areas, regularly inspected equipment, and fenced-in playfields and playgrounds, particularly where there is heavy traffic adjoining these facilities. Rubber asphalt, synthetic materials, and other substances that require little maintenance and help to free an area from cinders, gravel, stones, and dust are being used more and more on outdoor surfaces. In some sections of the country limited shelters are also being used to provide protection from the rain, wind, and sun. All outdoor areas should provide for sanitary drinking fountains and toilet facilities as needed.

Indoor physical education facilities. Just as safe and properly constructed equipment should be a part of outdoor facilities, so should they be a part of indoor physical education facilities. There should be adequate space provided for all the activity phases of the program whether they be in the gymnasium, swimming pool, or auxiliary areas. Mats should be used as a protective measure on walls and other areas where participants may be injured. Drinking fountains should be recessed and doors should open away from the playing floor. Proper flooring should be used—tile-cement floors are sometimes undesirable where activity takes place. Space should be provided for the adapted physical education program where students in wheelchairs and on crutches can be accommodated.

Clothing and equipment. Clothing and equipment used in physical education activities should meet health standards. If not, odors and germs will thrive, causing an unpleasant environment that may help to spread disease. Gymnasium mats, for example, should be kept clean. Regular physical education clothing, not street clothes, should be worn in most classes. Social dancing or similar activities, of course, would be exceptions. Clean clothing, including all types of athletic costumes, should be required. Footwear should be fitted properly. Socks should be clean. Many schools provide facilities for laundering physical education clothing.

Shower and locker facilities. Special attention should be paid to shower facilities. The shower room should be kept clean and plenty of soap and warm water should be available. Proper heating and ventilation should be provided; a nonslip floor surface should be installed; and ceilings should be constructed so as to prevent condensation. The drying area should be washed daily so as to prevent athlete's foot and other contaminations. A towel service should be initiated if it doesn't already exist. Adequate time should be allowed in the program to take a good shower.

Locker rooms should provide dressing as well as storage lockers for all students starting with the upper-grade elementary

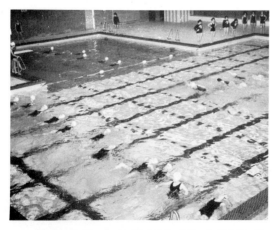

Richwoods Community High School, Peoria Heights, Ill.

school. Adequate space should be provided so that dressing is not done in cramped quarters. Occasional locker inspections are considered to be necessary.

Swimming pools. Swimming pools need special attention whether they are of the indoor or outdoor variety. First, the pool should be properly constructed to provide for adequate filtration, circulation, and chlorination. There should be a daily diary kept of such things as temperature of water, hydrogen ion concentration, residual chlorine, and other important matters. Regulations should be established and students acquainted with them in regard to pool use. A list of pool regulations advocated by the National Education Association and the American Medical Association include:

1. Everyone using the pool should have an overall bath, in the nude, with soap and water, washing carefully the armpits, the genital and rectal areas, and the feet.
2. Before taking a shower, the bladder should be emptied. Pupils needing to urinate during the swimming period should be excused to go to the toilet.
3. Anyone leaving the pool to go to the toilet must take another cleansing bath with soap and water before returning.
4. Pupils should expectorate only in the overflow trough.
5. Boys and men should swim in the nude or wear sanitized trunks. Girls and women should wear sanitized tank suits.
6. Girls and boys with long hair should wear rubber bathing caps. Caps keep hair, dandruff, and hair oil from contaminating the water. They also keep hair out of the eyes.
7. Each pupil should be inspected by the instructor or the pool guard before he enters the pool. Pupils with evidence of skin infection, eye infection, respiratory disease, open cuts or sores, or bandages should be excluded.
8. There must be no rough or boisterous play and no running or playing tag in or around the pool area.
9. Pupils should wear ear plugs or nose clips if these have been recommended by their physicians. Some pupils, on medical recommendation, may need to be excused, at least temporarily, from participation in the aquatic program.

10. A qualified person, either the instructor or other person qualified as a lifeguard, should be on duty whenever the pool is in use. No pupil should enter the pool unless a guard is present. All doors leading to the pool should be locked when the pool is not in use and a guard on duty.
11. Since dirt from shoes may be tracked into the pool and contaminate the water, spectators should be prohibited from entering the pool deck.*

Athletics. All the suggestions previously stated for a healthful environment refer to athletics as a phase of the total physical education program. In addition, athletes need some special considerations. All athletes should have medical examinations and medical supervision. The coach should be concerned about the health of the athlete at all times. This responsibility ranges from not putting undue pressure on an athlete to win to providing proper competition with teams of comparable ability. The coach also has great influence on the health habits of the athlete and as such should use it in a way that will reduce the amount of cigarette smoking, use of drugs, undue weight reduction brought about by crash diets, and improper nutrition.

The Joint Committee on Health Problems of the National Education Association and the American Medical Association has set forth a set of guidelines for safeguarding the health of the athlete. These can be found in Chapter 13, p. 346.

THE PSYCHOLOGIC ENVIRONMENT

The World Health Organization defines health as follows: "Health is a state of complete physical, mental, and social well-being, and not merely the absence of disease or infirmity." In order to have a mentally healthful and educational en-

vironment, therefore, one should not be concerned merely with providing the proper physical facilities. It is necessary also to take into consideration the administrative practices that play such an important part in providing for the total health of the child. It has been estimated that one of every ten school children is emotionally disturbed. This fact shows the necessity for coming to grips with this problem in every way possible. Health and physical educators should be especially concerned with mental and emotional health because of their close relationship with physical health and illness. During the last few years the psychosomatic aspects of education have increasingly been given more attention.

Mental health implies a state of mind that allows the individual to adjust in a satisfactory manner to whatever life has to offer. Good mental health cannot be thought of as a subject included in the school curriculum. Instead, it must permeate the total life of the educational institution. It means that programs are flexible and geared to individual needs, a permissive climate prevails, children are allowed considerable freedom, and students become self-reliant and responsible for their own actions. It means that the child is recognized and has a satisfying educational experience. The National Association for Mental Health points out that the well-adjusted person is the one who has the right attitudes and feelings toward himself, other people, and the demands that life places upon him. George Preston* has listed the qualities of mental health and says it consists of being able to live (1) within the limits imposed by bodily equipment, (2) with other human beings, (3) happily, (4) productively, and (5) without being a nuisance.

School and college programs offer an

*Joint Committee on Health Problems in Education of the National Education Association and the American Medical Association: Healthful school environment, Washington, D. C., 1969, The Association, pp. 234-235.

*Preston, G. H.: The substance of mental health, New York, 1943, Holt, Rinehart & Winston, Inc., p. 112.

excellent laboratory for developing good human relations, democratic methods, responsibility, self-reliance, and other essentials to happy and purposeful living. The degree to which this laboratory is utilized for such purposes depends upon administrative officers, teachers, custodians, and other staff members. Such important considerations as the administrative policies established, teachers' personalities, program, human relations, and professional help that is given will determine to what extent educational programs justify their existence in human betterment. Some of the important implications for a healthful and educational environment are discussed in more detail.

Administrative practices

A few of the administrative practices that have a bearing upon the mental and emotional health of the students and participants deal with organization of the school day, student achievement, play and recreation, homework, attendance, personnel policies, administrative emphasis, and discipline.

Organization of the school day. The organization of the school day will have a bearing upon whether a healthful environment is provided for the child. The length of the school day must be in conformance with the age of the child. Classes should be scheduled in a manner that does not result in excessive fatigue. Subjects that require considerable concentration should be scheduled when the individual is more mentally efficient. Usually this is during the early part of the day. Boredom and tension will arise from scheduling similar classes close together, without any breaks. The program should be flexible to allow for variety, new developments, and satisfying children's interests. Adequate periods of rest and play should be provided, not only as a change from the more arduous routine of close concentration but also as a necessity for utilizing the big muscles of the body. "Big-muscle" activity is essential during the growing years. The length of classes should be adequate for instructional purposes but not so excessively long that the law of diminishing returns sets in.

Student achievement. Success is an experience essential to the development of self-confidence and an integrated person. One who experiences success will be better stimulated to do good work than one who consistently fails. The child or youth who consistently fails is likely to have behavior disorders. In view of this, it is important that educational programs recognize their responsibility for developing each individual. Experiences should be provided that are adapted to the individual and are planned so that each person will have a series of successful experiences.

Individual differences. It is important to recognize that individuals differ. They differ in respect to intellect, physique, skill, personality, and many other qualities. In a fifth-grade class, for example, although the average chronologic age may be 11 years, the mental age could range from 6 to 16 years. Similar differences abound in other characteristics.

It is very important for administrators, teachers, and leaders to recognize that these differences do exist and that programs must be planned accordingly. The same goals cannot be established for all. If goals are standardized, some individuals will become frustrated because it is impossible for them to achieve the standards, and others will become very bored because there is no challenge. Goals that are within reach for everyone should be established. Administrators and teachers sometimes become so engrossed in the idea of setting high standards that they forget to consider the individual.

Grades. Excessive emphasis should not be placed on marks. Too often the individual is interested more in the mark received than in the knowledge, attitudes, and self-improvement inherent in the activity. It seems that, if marks must be given, as broad a category as possible should be used. These could be stated in terms such as "passed" and "did not pass" or "satisfactory" and "unsatisfactory." Whenever possible, descriptive statements of the student's progress should be given without any marks whatsoever. Parent-teacher conferences are probably the best way to evaluate a student's progress in the most effective manner. These procedures are being followed in some elementary schools with excellent results.

Marks, although supposedly an index of the quality of work done, are poor guides for such purposes. Many tests that are given as a basis for marks do not measure what they are supposed to measure and have been found to be unreliable when rated by various persons. Furthermore, the human element always enters the picture.

Marks stimulate competition that is unhealthy in many of its aspects. Too often the underlying reason for such competition is to prove superiority over someone rather than to prove a mastery in a particular subject matter field or skill. Under such circumstances harm frequently results to the mental health and personalities of students.

Tests and examinations. It is generally agreed that some method is needed to check on the progress that has been made in the acquisition of knowledge, skills, or attitudes. Harmful effects of such tests and examinations result when they are used by teachers and leaders to instill fear in the individual. Frequently, individuals harm themselves physically, mentally, and emotionally when they become worked up over an approaching examination. They stay up all night cramming, cannot sleep, are tense, and generally find it a very trying experience. This is especially true at the college educational level. Students should understand that examinations are a means by which greater help can be given to them. Such help is not possible unless information

is gained as to what the person knows at certain points along the way.

Intelligence ratings. Intelligence ratings can be of some value in the hands of a trained person. It is important to recognize, however, that such measuring devices are not definite, exact, and accurate in indicating the mental capacity of an individual. Furthermore, intelligence is only one factor that makes for success of an individual. In fact, it has been shown through Terman's study of gifted children, where all received high intelligence ratings, that intelligence does not necessarily ensure the achievement of prominent position in life.

Furthermore, intelligence ratings are often in error. One test should never be used as the criterion. Instead, several tests should be given before definite conclusions are drawn. Even then, as the work of Allison Davis and others at the University of Chicago has shown, intelligence tests measure a person's environment and the cultural experiences open to him to a greater extent than they do his native intelligence.

Play and recreation. The impression that achievement in so-called academic subjects is the only criterion necessary to ensure successful living is erroneous. In addition, there should be achievement in the areas of human relations, personality development, physical development, acquisition of skills for leisure hours, and other areas even more vital to the success of the individual than so-called scholastic achievement.

Dr. William Menninger and other experts in the field of psychiatry point to the contributions of play and recreation to mental health. Furthermore, to achieve success in the competitive society of today, a person needs a sound body that possesses stamina and endurance and that will support long hours of work. Also, the skills in physical activities, music, industrial arts, and allied areas that are learned during the early years of an individual's life will determine to a great degree his hobbies or leisure-time pursuits during adult years.

For these and other reasons, it is important that physical education and other subjects falling into this category be recognized for the contribution they can make to the total growth of the individual. There are many persons in mental institutions today who were capable of working out the most difficult problems in calculus and were expert in their knowledge of geography and other subjects. Many of these individuals might have been spared their illness if they had recognized the importance of developing other skills that would have afforded a more balanced life.

Homework. Educators are increasingly recognizing that homework should be assigned in a manner that is in the best interest of the whole child. If it is given for the purpose of busywork, to keep someone occupied during hours after dinner at night, or solely for enabling a person to surpass his classmates, it cannot be justified. Children as well as adults need time for play and recreation. They are entitled to time after school for such purposes. For young children in elementary school, homework assignments should take into consideration that young bodies need great amounts of physical activity. Ample exercise is necessary for body organs and muscles that are developing and gaining strength for future years. In junior high school, the homework assigned should be reasonable in nature. In high school it should not be given in such large amounts that it requires late hours of work. Instead, it should promote achievement and allow the student opportunity for independent work and help to promote the development of the whole individual.

Attendance. In many states financial aid is based upon school attendance. In some cases this has resulted in harmful effects to the health of children. Administrators have been known to stress attendance to the point at which students come to school with colds and other illnesses when they should be home in bed. This not only endangers their own health, but at the same time it exposes many innocent children to harmful germs.

It is important to have regular attendance at school. However, if the student is ill and in need of rest or parental and medical care, it is much better that he stay home. In order not to abuse this privilege, administrators, teachers, and others should try to educate the parents as to what constitutes good reasons for absences from school.

Furthermore, if the student is well enough to attend school, then it would seem that he should attend all classes. Too often a student is dismissed from a physical education class because of some minor disorder. If the program is adapted to the needs of the individual, special consideration can be given to such cases. It is just as important that regular attendance prevail in physical education as in social studies, mathematics, or any other subject.

Personnel policies. The administration's personnel policies in regard to teachers and other staff members will determine in some measure whether or not a healthful environment is created. A teacher who is required to punch a clock when she comes to work in the morning and leaves at night, is never greeted with a smile, never experiences an enjoyable conversation with the principal, is held responsible for many unnecessary details, is required to be at work regardless of how she feels, receives no administrative support when subject to community prejudices, and finds that the administrative policies that are established do not give her happiness, security, and confidence in doing her job cannot help but reflect such policies in her dealings with students and colleagues.

Administrators should try to establish the best possible working conditions for all members of a staff. Only if they feel

Table 14-1. Analysis of 193 student discipline provisions in negotiation agreements*

Clause	Agreements with clause	
	Number	Percent
Joint committee established to study disciplinary policy	11	5.7%
Board disciplinary policy or public law tied into agreement by contract language	22	11.4
General statement of teacher board disciplinary philosophy	156	80.8
Reasons for disciplinary action		
Disruptive behavior	52	26.9
Persistent misbehavior	40	20.7
Gross offenses	39	20.2
Physical violence (assault, fighting)	18	9.3
Gambling, drugs, alcohol, tobacco, pornography, weapons	14	7.3
Disrespect or insubordination	10	5.2
Vandalism, arson, theft, extortion	9	4.7
False bomb reports, inciting violence	6	3.1
Abusive language	5	2.6
Threatening or belligerent manner	4	2.1
Truancy/skipping	3	1.6
Health/physical appearance	3	1.6
Procedures for initial identification and handling of disciplinary problems		
Reasonable force for protection and restraint	19	9.8
Child sent to office or principal notified	6	3.1
Teacher reports punishable offenses and points out emotional or disciplinary problem students to principal	47	24.4
Parents called to conference	28	14.5
Punishment for offenses		
Temporary exclusions from class		
By teacher	56	29.0
By principal	1	9.5
Detention	6	3.1
Corporal punishment	14	7.3
Transfer to another class (before suspension)	13	6.7
Suspension	32	16.6
Expulsion	4	2.1
Limitation on punishment	6	3.1
Special consideration given to teachers with one or more children who have emotional or behavior problems		
Reduced class size only	1	0.5
More or longer relief periods and/or reduced class size	2	1.0
Equal distribution of problem children among teachers	1	0.5
General statement	1	0.5
Need for help from specialists recognized		
Psychiatrists, psychologists, physicians, counselors	103	53.4
Law enforcement personnel	80	41.5
Special classes or services for emotional and behavior problem children		
Special classes exist	6	3.1
Expansion of special education	2	1.0
Board to prepare program	1	0.5
Removal from classroom of those who cannot adjust	6	3.1
Record of disciplinary cases kept	4	2.1
Miscellaneous clauses	7	3.6

*From NEA Research Bulletin 47:59, 1969.

happy and well adjusted in their jobs will a healthful environment exist.

Administrative emphasis. The administrative emphasis should be on the children and on those experiences that will help them to grow and develop into healthy and educated human beings. It should not be on subject matter material, with rigid and inflexible programs designed to pump as much factual knowledge as possible into the heads of students. Administrative policies should be established that reflect human beings as the center of the program, allow for flexibility, encourage initiative on the part of the teacher, are adapted to the needs and interests of the participants, and provide in every way for a healthful physical and nonphysical environment.

Discipline. The school and college should be a place where individuals receive joy and satisfaction from their experiences. A spirit of cooperation should exist among the administration, staff, and members of the organization. The emphasis in student discipline should be on self-government. As much freedom as possible should be given. The individual who is surrounded on all sides by restrictions and who is not trusted will rebel. As many educators have discovered, abrupt use of authority invites resistance. There should be a permissive attitude toward individual variations from acceptable behavior, coupled with a firm but kind insistence upon higher standards of conduct. Responsibility should go along with freedom. A climate of opinion should be established that allows as much freedom as possible without encroaching on the rights of others. A strong student government can be one of the best educational devices for self-discipline.

Regulations should not be accepted just because they are regulations. Rather, they should be accepted because they are essen-

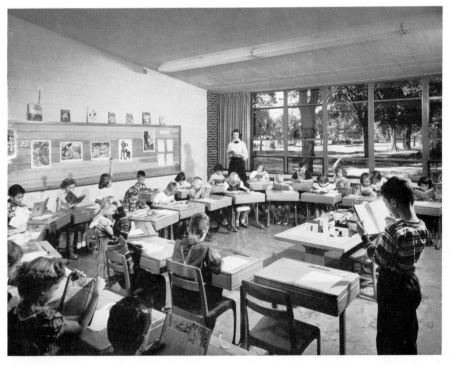

Burnett and Logan, Chicago.

The school should be a place where individuals receive joy and satisfaction from their experiences. (Washington Irving Elementary School, Waverly, Iowa.)

tial to securing the rights of everyone so that all can enjoy and benefit from the programs that are offered.

If antisocial behavior develops, it is important to look into the reasons for such behavior and work to eliminate the causes, rather than to abruptly and harshly discipline some person. Unless this is done, such antisocial behavior will continue to show itself. Furthermore, in time it may become so obstreperous as to require isolation of the individual from society. If a constructive approach is taken, such measures may be avoided.

The teacher

Good mental health in a school program is tied up very closely with the teacher. The manner in which the teacher and student interact with one another is very important. It is important for the teacher to think of youngsters as living, feeling, and developing human beings who pursue different and varied courses on their ways to maturity. They are not inanimate objects or receptacles into which the instructor pours knowledge.

One of the main responsibilities of any teacher in health or physical education should be student counseling. Quite frequently specialists in these areas are the ones to whom the child goes in search of information. Anyone who is to perform such an important job as counseling should be well adjusted, understand himself, and get along well with others.

The teacher must be in good physical condition in order to do a good job. A teacher may come to a job in excellent physical condition, but if large classes are assigned, the salary is insufficient, and outside work is necessary, physical harm may result. Furthermore, if there is no provision for sick leave and as a result the teacher must be on the job even when sick or ill, her physical condition will suffer. When this happens, the students also suffer.

The teacher's personality has important implications for the mental and emotional health of those with whom he or she comes in contact. The teacher who is happy, wears a smile, is kind, considerate, and likes people in general will impart these qualities to the students. It is bound to "rub off" in the daily interaction that takes place. Conversely, the teacher or leader who is sarcastic, depressed, prejudiced, and intolerant will also impart these qualities to the children with whom he or she associates. The leader's personality is also reflected in the appearance of the classroom and the teaching methods employed.

Administrators should be cognizant of the factors that result in maladjusted personalities for members of their staffs. A few years ago the National Educational Association found that many faculty members were plagued by personal and working conditions that influenced their mental outlooks. Some of these were as follows: financial difficulties, economic problems, serious illness of relatives or friends, unsatisfactory progress of pupils, matters of personal health, being unmarried and without normal family relationships, disciplinary problems, an official rating by a superior, possible loss of position, work on a college course, being unhappily married, and religious problems. Many of these frustrating factors could have been eliminated.

All teachers should have satisfactory working conditions. They should receive an adequate salary to eliminate financial worries, be encouraged to develop out-of-school interests in the community, have hobbies in which they can engage after school hours and during vacation periods, and have adequate provisions for sick and sabbatical leaves and leaves of absence so that proper rest and adequate educational standards may be assured. Furthermore, there should be ample opportunities provided for affiliation with professional groups and the development of cultural and other interests conducive to better leadership qualifications. By providing such essentials teachers and leaders will be made happier and have better mental and emotional health. In turn, this will be reflected in the total health of the children with whom they come in contact.

Human relationships

Human relationships are a most important consideration if one is to grow into a happy, successful, and well-adjusted individual. Of all the traits that should be developed in health and physical education, human relationships rank toward the top of the list. Through counseling, participation in group games and activities under good leadership, and other phases of the programs, the potentialities are great for developing good human relationships.

Each individual should be made to feel that he belongs to the group and has something to contribute in its behalf. There

must never be an attempt to make a member of the group feel insignificant and unimportant. More praise should be dispensed than criticism. Every attempt should be made to help each person maintain his self-respect. The atmosphere that pervades the classroom, gymnasium, or recreation center should be relaxed and friendly. The emotional needs of every individual should be taken into consideration in the class or group activities that are held.

The teacher should have good relationships with his or her colleagues. Any faculty or staff that is infested with cliques, jealousies, and strife communicates these attitudes to the students. This is just as true here as in the case of quarreling parents who communicate their feelings to their children. If one is to help others develop good human relationships, one must set an example worthy of emulation.

There must be good human relationships among the children themselves. They are

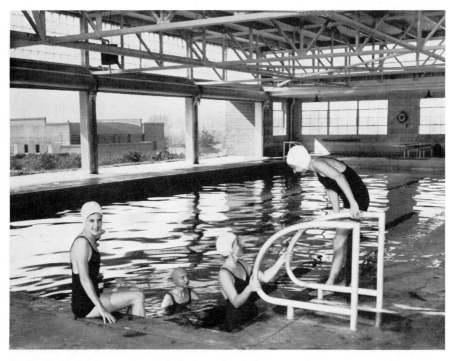

Each individual should be made to feel that she belongs to the group and has something to contribute in its behalf. (Alabama College, Montevallo, Ala.)

dependent upon the feeling of the group toward them and whether or not they are accepted. It is important to have status among one's associates. The teacher can play an important part in helping to see that everyone gains recognition. This is especially important with such individuals as the dull child in the classroom, the awkward, uncoordinated youngster on the playfield, and the intellectually gifted student in a recreation setting.

The teacher should be careful not to accentuate any characteristic that makes a child markedly different from the rest of the group. This applies to the whole realm of deviations, including scholastic, physical, mental, social, and economic.

Professional services

The factors discussed thus far in respect to the nonphysical environment have been largely preventive in nature. They have attempted to show the importance of providing an environment where the individual has freedom, self-respect, and security and experiences satisfaction in his activities. However, despite emphasis upon preventive measures, there will always be some individuals who become behavior problems and will need professional help.

The teacher can play an important part by identifying those individuals who need help. He can also render guidance and such other aid as is possible in the school or college situation. The teacher can often do a great deal of good by studying the student thoroughly in respect to his school, home, and community environment. Through such study and by working closely with parents, many minor maladjustments can be eliminated. If further help is needed, he should refer the child to the proper professional persons.

In some schools there are counselors who have had preparation that goes beyond that of the ordinary teacher or leader. Their special knowledge of guidance and mental hygiene should be utilized in dealing with problem cases.

With the increasing emphasis being placed upon mental hygiene, many schools and colleges are utilizing the services of social workers, psychologists, and psychiatrists. The more serious cases should be referred to such professional people. They are trained in dealing with such problems and can render a great deal of personal help as well as promote a more healthful environment.

Recently, there has been a marked growth of child guidance clinics across the country. These are sponsored by various organizations interested in securing professional guidance for individuals with behavior problems. These clinics guide parents and community groups in good mental hygiene practices and needs, aid children who have various mental maladjustments, and seek support and understanding within the community to help promote better mental hygiene. They have trained people on their staffs who are competent to assist in preventing and solving problems that involve psychology.

CHECKLIST FOR ADMINISTRATIVE PRACTICES FOR A HEALTHFUL ENVIRONMENT

Organization of the school day

Length of the school day   *Yes*   *No*

1. The length of the school day should be adapted to the age of the child, starting with one-half day in kindergarten. ____ ____
2. Play and rest periods are provided in accordance with pupil needs. ____ ____

Continued.

CHECKLIST FOR ADMINISTRATIVE PRACTICES FOR A HEALTHFUL ENVIRONMENT—cont'd

Scheduling   Yes   No

1. Subjects demanding diligent application are scheduled early in the day.   ___   ___
2. Subjects requiring more mental concentration and academic effort are interspersed with those requiring less mental effort.   ___   ___
3. The amount of time devoted to a specific task is assigned with regard to the age, readiness, and needs of the child.   ___   ___
4. There is ample time between classes to ensure student promptness without excessive haste.   ___   ___
5. A leisurely lunch break is provided for each pupil.   ___   ___
6. The educational program is a flexible one, so that it is possible to schedule special programs or activities without hindering the regular program.   ___   ___

Student achievement

Individual differences

1. There is provision in the school program for individual differences among children in respect to physical handicaps, readiness to learn, academic ability, and environmental background.   ___   ___
2. Consideration is given to the physical and mental growth of each child.   ___   ___
3. The abilities of each child are recognized and instruction is adjusted to individual ability.   ___   ___

Grades

1. Provision is made for clerical and special assistance in helping the teacher to spend more time with teaching responsibilities.   ___   ___
2. The program is planned so that each child experiences a series of educational successes.   ___   ___
3. Goals are adjusted to fit each pupil, and marks are used to indicate progress toward stated goals.   ___   ___
4. Provision is made for a descriptive evaluation along with the grade.   ___   ___

Reporting pupil progress

1. The means used to report pupil progress include personal conferences, checklists, graphs, letters, progress reports, and report cards.   ___   ___
2. Problems, weaknesses, and potential of child are items for teacher-parent conferences.   ___   ___

Tests and examinations

1. Examinations are used as a means of helping pupil and teacher discover the progress that has been made in the acquistion of knowledge.   ___   ___
2. Tests help the learner attain satisfaction and a sense of achievement when he is doing as well as he should.   ___   ___
3. Tests help the teacher judge how effective his teaching methods are.   ___   ___
4. Tests assist in making administrative judgments in respect to grouping and other procedures.   ___   ___
5. Tests provide emphasis on diagnosis rather than on rating of overall merit, upon individual improvement rather than comparison with others, and are used more as guides than as final measures.   ___   ___

Intelligence ratings

1. Intelligence tests are selected and administered by a trained person.   ___   ___
2. Tests are used with a view to how the children can profit with suitable instruction.   ___   ___

CHECKLIST FOR ADMINISTRATIVE PRACTICES FOR A HEALTHFUL ENVIRONMENT—cont'd

Physical education and recreation   *Yes   No*

1. Physical education class size ranges from thirty to forty pupils.   —— ——
2. Physical education is offered daily and stresses basic skills and movement experiences.   —— ——
3. The physical education program is concerned with the social, mental, and emotional aspects of the child, as well as the physical.   —— ——
4. Recreational activities are based on pupil interests.   —— ——

Homework

1. Homework is assigned in accordance with the age, interest, ability, and needs of the child.   —— ——

Pupil attendance

1. The school nurse determines whether the child should attend school and when he should be sent home.   —— ——
2. The child does not return to school after sickness until he is able to attend all classes.   —— ——
3. The nurse and attendance officer play a major role in communication with the parent regarding proper health practices.   —— ——

Discipline

1. Behavior is evaluated with the knowledge that misconduct is a sign of maladjustment and an attempt is made to find the cause.   —— ——
2. The staff upholds the same general standards of behavior.   —— ——
3. All pupil abilities are recognized and an effort is made to maintain the self-respect of the child through the use of praise.   —— ——
4. Fear is not used as a technique of control.   —— ——
5. Children are encouraged to assist in developing standards of behavior and to assist in their enforcement.   —— ——

Student grouping

1. Grouping is flexible so that administration and organization exist only to expedite the process of learning.   —— ——
2. Differences in learners and subject matter are considered in grouping.   —— ——
3. Promotion practices are flexible.   —— ——
4. Grouping is such that children do not bear labels, for example, "fast group" or "slow learner."   —— ——

Teacher-pupil relationships

1. There is cooperative thinking and effort between teachers and pupils rather than emphasis upon the sole direction and authority of the teacher.   —— ——
2. The teacher sets a good example for the pupil.   —— ——
3. A primary teacher responsibility is that of pupil counseling.   —— ——
4. The pupil is made to feel that he is part of the group and contributes to it.   —— ——
5. The atmosphere of the classroom is relaxed and friendly.   —— ——
6. The teacher shows interest in each pupil.   —— ——
7. The teacher recognizes the various environmental factors that compose pupil personality and behavior.   —— ——
8. The teacher has good relationships with his colleagues.   —— ——
9. The teacher has an enthusiastic and confident attitude.   —— ——
10. The teacher enjoys his work and takes pride in it.   —— ——
11. The teacher is secure in his job.   —— ——

Continued.

CHECKLIST FOR ADMINISTRATIVE PRACTICES FOR A HEALTHFUL ENVIRONMENT—cont'd

Professional services

1. The administration provides for guidance, psychologist, psychiatrist, and social worker services. ___ ___
2. Specialists in "1" work closely with the home in providing necessary help for the child. ___ ___

Personnel policies

1. Relationships between administrators and teachers are harmonious. ___ ___
2. The administration promotes good social and professional relations among members of the staff. ___ ___
3. Administrators help educate the public to its true responsibilities to the schools and seek the support and assistance of the public in the promotion of educational goals. ___ ___

The teacher

Qualities

1. The teacher likes children. ___ ___
2. The teacher is well adjusted and mentally healthy. ___ ___
3. The teacher understands the growth and development of children. ___ ___
4. The teacher is able to identify children with serious problems and knows how and when to refer them for help. ___ ___
5. The teacher helps pupils meet their basic emotional needs. ___ ___
6. The teacher has a pleasing appearance and manner and is physically healthy, patient, and impartial. ___ ___
7. The teacher respects the child's personality, understands his limitations, and creates an overall atmosphere of security. ___ ___

Working conditions

1. The physical conditions of the job are good (salary, sick leave, class load). ___ ___
2. Administration is aware of factors that might affect the mental health of the teacher and help to eliminate such problems. ___ ___

Improving instruction

1. Administration utilizes opportunities to commend teacher achievement and effort. ___ ___
2. The beginning teacher is helped over the rough spots and is also assisted in obtaining a broad professional orientation. ___ ___

Questions and exercises

1. Define what is meant by the "physical" and "nonphysical" environments. What are the implications of each for total health?
2. Prepare a research report on administrative practices for a healthful and educational environment as they relate to a school with which you are very familiar.
3. Prepare a list of administrative practices in health, physical education, or recreation that are nationally in evidence and should be eliminated in order to provide greater total health.
4. What part does each of the following play in mental health of school children: (a) organization of the school day, (b) achievement, (c) marks, (d) play and recreation, (e) homework, (f) attendance, and (g) discipline?
5. How does the mental and emotional health of a teacher affect the mental and emotional health of school children?
6. Consult case studies in some social agency and report on the teacher's role in these cases.
7. To what degree are the physical features of

a school related to mental and emotional health?

8. Why is it so important to have good human relationships within the school?

9. How can the school and community coordinate their efforts to further better physical, mental, emotional, and social health for all residents?

10. What is the role of professional services in the school program?

Reading assignment in *Administrative Dimensions of Health and Physical Education Programs, Including Athletics:* Chapter 11, Selections 59 to 62.

Selected references

Ahmann, J. S., and Glock, M. D.: Evaluating pupil growth, Boston, 1958, Allyn & Bacon, Inc., pp. 6, 449, 501-504.

Ahmann, J. S., Glock, M. D., and Wardeberg, H. L.: Evaluating elementary school pupils, Boston, 1960, Allyn & Bacon, Inc., pp. 8-9.

American Association for Health, Physical Education, and Recreation: Administrative problems in health education, physical education, and recreation, Washington, D. C., 1953, The Association, chaps. 2, 4-7.

American Association for Health, Physical Education, and Recreation: School safety policies with emphasis on physical education, athletics, and recreation, Washington, D. C., 1964, The Association.

American Association of School Administrators: Health in schools, Twentieth Yearbook, Washington, D. C., 1951, National Education Association, chap. 6.

American Medical Association, Committee on Medical Aspects of Sports: Proceedings of the National Conference on the Medical Aspects of Sports—I through IX, Chicago, 1960-1967, The Association.

American Medical Association, Committee on Medical Aspects of Sports: Tips on athletic training—I through IX, Chicago, 1960-1967, The Association.

American Public Health Association: Suggested ordinance and regulations covering public swimming pools, New York, 1964, The Association.

Association for Supervision and Curriculum Development: Fostering mental health in our schools, 1950 Yearbook, Washington, D. C., 1950, The Association, a department of the National Education Association.

Carroll, H. A.: Mental hygiene, New York, 1951, Prentice-Hall, Inc.

Daniels, A. S., and Davies, E. A.: Adapted physical education, ed. 2, New York, 1965, Harper & Row, Publishers.

Educational Policies Commission: Educational objectives—education for all-American youths: a further look, Washington, D. C., 1952, The Commission, p. 15.

Florida State Department of Education: A checklist, as evaluation in physical education, Tallahassee, Fla., 1961, The Department.

Grout, R. E.: Health teaching in schools, Philadelphia, 1968, W. B. Saunders Co.

Illinois Office of Public Instruction: Guidelines for evaluating programs in physical education, Springfield, Ill., Office of Public Instruction.

Indiana State Board of Health: Indiana physical education score card, Indianapolis, 1960, The Board.

Jacobs, L.: Mental health in the school health program, The Journal of School Health **22**:288, 1952.

Joint Committee on Health Problems in Education of National Education Association and American Medical Association: Mental hygiene in the classroom, Washington, D. C., 1949, National Education Association.

Joint Committee on Health Problems in Education of National Education Association and American Medical Association: School health services, Washington, D. C., 1964, National Education Association.

Joint Committee on Health Problems in Education of National Education Association and American Medical Association: Healthful school living, Washington, D. C., 1957, National Education Association.

Joint Committee on Health Problems in Education of National Education Association and American Medical Association: Health education, Washington, D. C., 1961, National Education Association.

Michigan Department of Education: A suggested checklist for evaluating the physical education program, Lansing, Mich., 1962, The Department.

Miller, F., chairman: Evaluative criteria, Washington, D. C., 1960, National Study of Secondary School Evaluation.

New York Department of Education: A guide for the review of secondary school physical education, Albany, N. Y., 1964, The Department.

Oberteuffer, D., and Beyrer, M. K.: School health education, ed. 4, New York, 1966, Harper & Row, Publishers.

Ohio Association of Health Physical Education and Recreation: Evaluative criteria for physical education, Columbus, Ohio, 1963, Ohio Department of Education.

Texas Education Agency: Suggestions for planning the secondary school physical education program, Austin, Texas, 1961, The Agency.

PART

four

ADMINISTRATIVE FUNCTIONS

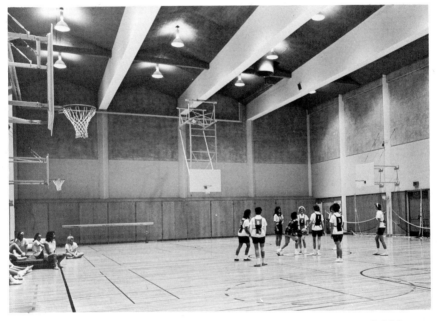

Women's gymnasium. (College of San Mateo, San Mateo, Calif.)

Estimates of that portion of the total school or college plant devoted to health and physical education programs range as high as 50% to 75%. This large investment of money, time, and personnel requires considerable thought and planning. Physical education facilities should reflect the program in action. Furthermore, administrators, teachers, and other personnel in these special areas should participate in this planning, and, as such, they need to be knowledgeable about facilities and the various procedures for developing a healthful and efficient school plant. They need to know the needs of the programs involved, the latest trends in facilities, the common errors that are made, how they can work most effectively with the architect, and health features that should be considered.

BASIC CONSIDERATIONS IN PLANNING

At the outset, two principles should be very much in the minds of health and physical educators in relation to facility management: (1) facilities emanate as a result of program needs and (2) cooperative planning is essential to avoid common mistakes. The objectives, activities, teaching methods and materials, administrative policies, and equipment and supplies represent program considerations regarding facilities. The educational and recreational needs of both the school and community, the thinking of both school administrators and health and physical educators, and the advice of both architects and lay persons are other considerations if facilities are to be planned wisely.

Another set of principles basic to facility planning relate particularly to the optimum promotion of a healthful environment for the students. Included in this set of principles is the provision for facilities that take into account physiologic needs of the student, including proper temperature control, lighting, water supply, and noise level. A second principle would be the provision of facilities that take into account protection against accidents. The facilities would be planned so that the danger of fire, the possibility of mechanical accidents, and the hazards involved in student traffic would be eliminated or kept to a minimum. A third principle would concern itself with protection against disease. This would mean attention to such items as proper sewage disposal, sanitation procedures, and water supply. Finally, a fourth principle is the need to provide a healthful psychologic environment. This would have implications for space, location of activities, color schemes, and elimination of distractions through such means as soundproof construction.

A third set of principles has been developed by Bookwalter.* These may be used as guides for the planning, construction, and utilization of facilities for school health and physical education programs:

1. *Validity.* Standards for space, structure, and fixtures must be compatible with

---

*Bookwalter, K. W.: Physical education in the secondary schools, Washington, D. C., 1964, The Center for Applied Research in Education, Inc. (The Library of Education), pp. 84-86.

407

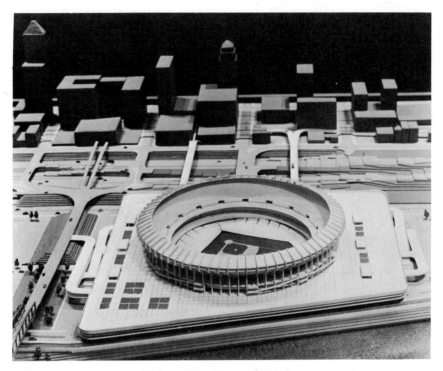

Home of the Cincinnati Reds.

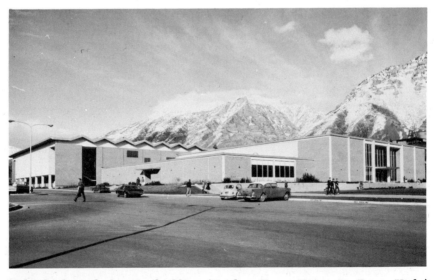

Richards physical education building. (Brigham Young University, Provo, Utah.)

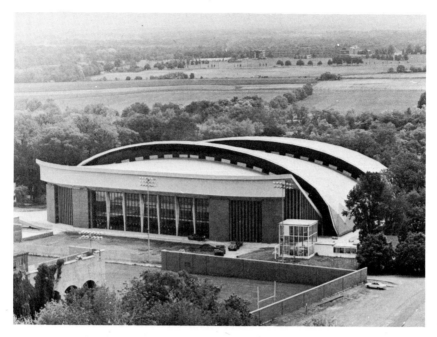

Gymnasium. (Princeton University, Princeton, N. J.)

the rules essential for the effective conduct of the program. According to the New York State Department of Education, the number of teaching stations needed for a school will depend upon school enrollment, physical education class size, periods of physical education scheduled each week for a teaching station, the number of periods of physical education each week for which a pupil is scheduled, activities offered, and pupils in out-of-class programs.

2. *Utility.* Facilities should be adaptable for different activities and programs without affecting such items as safety and effective instruction.

3. *Accessibility.* Facilities should be readily and directly accessible for the individuals who will be using them.

4. *Isolation.* Facilities should be planned so as to reduce to a minimum distractions, offensive odors, noise, and undesirable activities and groups.

5. *Departmentalization.* Functionally related services and activity areas should be continuous or adjacent for greatest economy and efficiency.

6. *Safety, hygiene, and sanitation.* The maintenance of proper health standards should be a major consideration in all facility planning.

7. *Supervision.* Facilities should take into consideration the need for proper teacher supervision of activities under his jurisdiction. Therefore, visibility and accessibility are essential considerations.

8. *Durability and maintenance.* Facilities should be easy and economical to maintain and should be durable.

9. *Beauty.* Facilities should be attractive and esthetically pleasing with the utilization of good color dynamics and design.

10. *Flexibility and expansibility.* Changes in enrollments, program, and other considerations for future expansion should be considered. Modern thinking has stressed the principle of flexibility in regard to physical education facilities. Flexibility should provide for immediate change through folding partitions, such as doors that separate gymnasia, for overnight change with very little effort in cases in which partitions cannot be removed

immediately, and for greater change that can be made within a period of 1 or 2 months, such as during the summer vacation.

11. *Economy.* The best use of money, space, time, energy, and other essential factors should be considered as they relate to facility planning.

A summary of some of the important guidelines and principles for facility planning for school and college health and physical education programs include the following:

1. All planning should be based on goals that recognize that the total physical and nonphysical environments must be safe, attractive, comfortable, clean, practical, and adapted to the needs of the individual.

2. The planning should include a consideration of the total school or college health and physical education facilities and the recreational facilities of the community. The programs and facilities of these areas are essential to any community. Since they are closely allied, they should be planned coordinately and based on the needs of the community. Each should be part of the overall community pattern.

3. Facilities should be geared to health standards. They play an important part in protecting the health of individuals and in determining the educational outcomes.

4. Facilities play a part in disease control. The extent to which schools and colleges provide for play areas, ample space, sanitary considerations, proper ventilation, heating, and cleanliness will to some extent determine how effectively disease is controlled.

5. Administrators must make plans for facilities long before an architect is consulted. Technical information can be procured in the forms of standards and guides from various sources, such as state departments of education, professional literature, building score cards, and various manuals. Information may also be secured from such important groups as the American Association of School Administrators, National Council on Schoolhouse Construction, and American Institute of Architects.

6. Standards should be utilized as guides and as a starting point. They will prove to be very helpful. However, it is important to keep in mind that standards cannot always be used entirely as developed. They usually have to be modified in the light of local needs, conditions, and resources.

7. Building and sanitary codes administered by the local and state departments of public health and the technical advice and consultation services available through these sources should be known and utilized by administrators in the planning and construction of facilities. Information concerned with acceptable building materials, specifications, minimum standards of sanitation, and other details may be procured from these informed sources.

8. Health, physical education, and recreation personnel should play important roles in the planning and operation of facilities. The specialized knowledge that such individuals have is very important. Provisions should be made so that their expert opinion will be utilized in the promotion of a healthful and proper environment.

9. Facilities should be planned with an eye to the future. Too often, facilities are constructed and outgrown within a very short time. Units should be sufficiently large to accommodate peak-load participation in the various activities. The peak-load estimates should be made with future growth in mind.

10. Planning should provide for adequate allotment of space to the activity and program areas. They should receive priority in space allotment. The administrative offices and service units, although important, should not be planned and developed in a spacious and luxurious manner that goes beyond efficiency and necessity.

Text continued on p. 415.

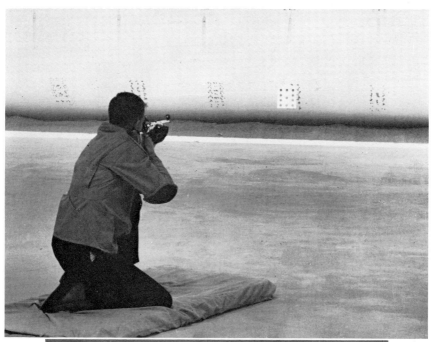

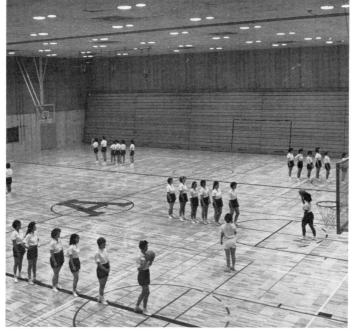

Rifle range and gymnasium of physical education building. See also next two illustrations.
(University of Alaska, College, Alaska.)

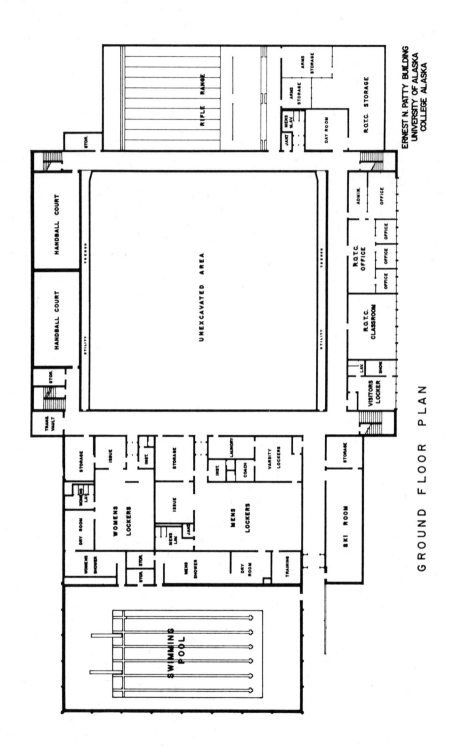

GROUND FLOOR PLAN

ERNEST N. PATTY BUILDING
UNIVERSITY OF ALASKA
COLLEGE ALASKA

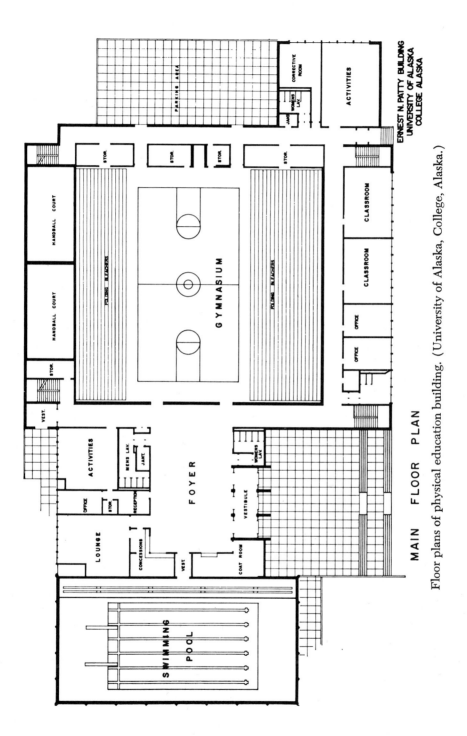

MAIN   FLOOR   PLAN

Floor plans of physical education building. (University of Alaska, College, Alaska.)

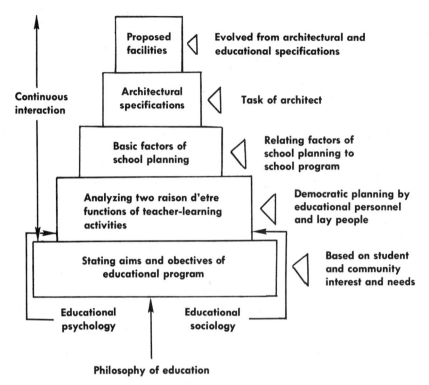

A procedure for planning facilities for schools. (From MacConnell, J. D.: Planning for school buildings, Englewood Cliffs, N. J., 1957, Prentice-Hall, Inc. Reprinted by permission.)

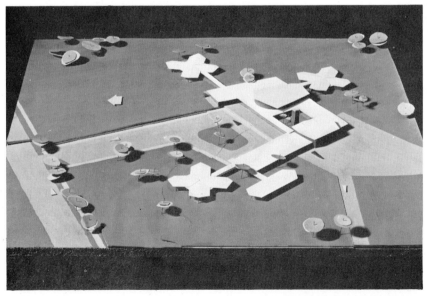

Suter, Hedrich-Blessing, Chicago.

Planning should include consideration of the total school health and physical education facilities as well as the recreational facilities of the community. (Model of Heathcote School, Scarsdale, N. Y.)

11. Geographic and climatic conditions should be taken into consideration in planning facilities. By doing this, the full potentialities for conducting activities outdoors as well as indoors can be realized.

12. Architects do not always pay as much attention as they should to the educational and health features when planning buildings and facilities. Therefore, it is important that they be briefed on certain requirements that educators feel are essential in order that the health and welfare of children, youth, and adults may be provided for. Such a procedure is usually welcomed by the architect and will aid him in rendering a greater service to the community.

13. Facilities should take into consideration all the necessary safety features so essential in programs of health, physical education, and recreation. Health service substations near the gymnasium and other play areas, proper surfacing of activity areas, adequate space, and proper lighting are a few of these considerations.

14. It should be kept in mind that the construction of school or college health, physical education, and recreational facilities often tends to set a pattern that will influence parents, civic leaders, and others. This in turn will promote a healthful and safe environment for the entire community.

COMMON ERRORS OF HEALTH AND PHYSICAL EDUCATION PERSONNEL IN FACILITY MANAGEMENT

Some common mistakes made by health and physical educators in facility management include the following:
1. Failure to adequately project enrollments and program needs into the future (Facilities are difficult to expand or change, so this is a significant error.)
2. Failure to provide for multiple use of facilities
3. Failure to provide for adequate accessibility for students in health and

physical education classes and also for community groups for recreation purposes
4. Failure to observe basic health factors in planning facilities in regard to lighting, safety, and ventilation
5. Failure to provide adequate space for the conduct of a comprehensive program of physical education activities
6. Failure to provide appropriate accommodations for spectators
7. Failure to soundproof areas of the building where noise will interfere with educational functions
8. Failure to meet with the architect to present views on program needs
9. Failure to provide adequate staff offices
10. Failure to provide adequate storage space
11. Failure to provide adequate space and privacy for medical examinations
12. Failure to provide large enough entrances to transport equipment
13. Failure to observe desirable current professional standards
14. Failure to provide for adequate study of cost in terms of durability, time, money, and effective instruction
15. Failure to properly locate teaching stations with service facilities

THE PLANNING TEAM

Planning for meaningful facilities is a team effort. It includes such persons as members of the board of education or board of trustees, representatives of the administration, students, custodians, curriculum specialists, educational consultants, members of the community, and selected teachers and department heads.

WORKING WITH THE ARCHITECT

The architect is the specialist in facility planning and the leader in the designing of school and college buildings. As such, he is an important consideration for all persons engaged in health and physical education work. The architect, through his training and experience, is a specialist who is competent to give advisory service in all aspects of facility management.

The qualifications of the architect include:

1. The architect should be legally qualified to practice in the state and should be in good standing in his profession. He must be a man of unquestioned professional character and integrity and must possess high ethical standards.
2. The architect should have had previous successful experience in designing buildings that demonstrate his competence in architectural work. The buildings previously designed by the architect should also reflect a careful study of the peculiar needs of each client.
3. The architect should possess the vision and imagination to translate the educational aims and program specified by the educator into functional buildings. There should be an avoidance of stereotypes. The architect should not possess set, preconceived ideas which are hard to change. He must be able and willing to mold design to fit needs.
4. The architect must have a record of working cooperatively and harmoniously with his clients, educational advisors, and contractors.
5. The architect must have an adequate staff of trained personnel to carry out the building program without undue delay. The architect should either have qualified engineering services available in his own organization or should specify qualified engineering specialists who will work with him.
6. The architect should keep abreast of recent research and study concerning materials and mechanical equipment used in school buildings.
7. The architect should show such economy in the use of space and materials as is consistent with educational needs.
8. The architect should be competent in the field of site planning and the utilization of space for educational and recreational purposes.
9. The architect must give adequate supervision to his buildings. This is a very important part of the architect's services.
10. The architect should be informed concern-

ing state and municipal building regulations and codes and must show care in complying with them.
11. The architect must demonstrate sound business judgment, proper business procedures, and good record keeping on the job.[*]

Physical educators should carefully think through their own ideas and plans for their special facilities and submit them in writing to the architect during the early stages of school and college planning. There should also be several conferences in which the architect and physical education specialist exchange views in regard to the educational and architectural possibilities to be considered.

Many architects know little about programs of health and physical education and therefore welcome the advice of specialists in these fields. The architect might be furnished with such information as the names of school or college plants where excellent facilities exist, kinds of activities that will constitute the program, space requirements for various activities, storage and equipment areas needed, temperature requirements, relation of dressing, showering, and toilet facilities to program, teaching stations needed, best construction materials for activities, and lighting requirements. The physical educator may not have all this information readily available, including some of the latest trends and standards recommended for his field and endeavor. However, such information can be obtained through professional organizations, other schools where excellent facilities have been developed, and facility books developed by experts in the area.

Mr. William Haroldson, Director of Health and Physical Education for the Seattle, Washington, Public Schools, has developed a procedural outline in cooperation with three architectural firms, in

[*]From Leu, D. J.: Planning education facilities, New York, 1965, The Center for Applied Research in Education, Inc. (The Library of Education), p. 50.

which are listed some essential considerations for health and physical educators in their relationships and cooperative planning with architects. Some of the main points stressed in this outline are discussed.

Educational specifications

Adequate educational specifications provide the basis for good planning by the architect:

1. General description of the program, such as the number of teaching stations necessary to service the health and physical education programs for a total student body of approximately _____ boys and _____ girls.

2. Basic criteria as pertain to the gymnasium: the number of teaching periods per day, capacities, number and size of courts, lockers, and projected total uses contemplated for the facility.

   a. Availability to the community

   b. Proximity to parks

   c. Parking

   d. Size of groups that will use gymnasium after school hours

   e. Whether locker rooms will or will not be made available to public use

3. Specific description of aspects of the health and physical education programs that are of concern to the architects.

   a. Class size and scheduling, both present and possible future; number of instructors, present and future

   b. Preferred method of handling students, for example, flow of traffic in classrooms, locker rooms, shower rooms, and going to outside play area (This item has a direct bearing on the design of this area.)

   c. Storage requirements and preferred method of handling all permanent equipment and supplies (Here, unless a standard has been established, requirements should be specific—for example, request should state number and size of each item rather than "ample storage.")

   d. Team and other extracurricular use of facilities (It is of assistance to the architect if the educational specifications can describe a typical week's use of the proposed facility, which would include a broad daily program, afterschool use, and potential community use.)

Meeting with the architect

At this point, it is advisable to meet with the architect to discuss specifications in order to ensure complete understanding and to allow the architect to point out certain restrictions or limitations that may be anticipated even before the first preliminary plan is made.

Design

The factors to be considered in the design of the facility and discussed with the architect should include the following:

1. *Budget.* An adequate budget should be allowed. Gymnasia are subject to extremely hard usage, and durability should not be sacrificed for economy.

2. *Acoustics.* Utilize the service of acoustical consultants.

3. *Public address system.* How is it to be used—for instruction, athletic events, general communication?

4. *Color and design.* Harmonize with surrounding neighborhood if it is a new school or match other areas if it is an addition to an old school.

5. *Fenestration* (window treatment). Consider light control, potential window breakage, vision panel; gymnasium areas should have safety glass (preferred) or wire protectors.

6. *Ventilation.* The area should be zoned for flexibility of usage. This means greater ventilation when a larger number of spectators are present, or a reduction for single class groups, or isolated areas, such as locker rooms. Special attention must be given to proper ventilation of uni-

form drying rooms, gymnasium storage areas, locker and shower areas. (Current and off-season uniform storage areas require constant ventilation when plant is shut down.) Ventilation equipment should have a low noise level.

7. *Supplementary equipment in the gymnasium.* Such equipment should be held to a minimum. Supplementary equipment, such as fire boxes, should be recessed.

8. *Compactness and integration.* Keep volume compact—large, barnlike spaces are unpleasant, costly to heat and maintain. Integrate as far as budget permits.

9. *Mechanical or electrical features.* Special attention should be given to location of panel boards, chalk boards, fire alarm, folding doors, and so on.

Further critique with the architect

1. The architect begins the development of his plans from his understanding of the initial requirements that he has considered in relation to the design factors listed.

2. When it becomes evident that the basic plan is set, the architect usually will call in consulting engineers to discuss the structural and mechanical systems prior to approval of the plan by the school district. These systems will have been given previous attention by the architect but cannot be discussed with the consultants other than in generalities before the plan is in approximate final form.

3. A further series of meetings are then held with school personnel regarding approval of preliminary plans and proposed structural and mechanical systems and the use of materials after the incorporation in the preliminary plans.

4. If supplementary financing by governmental agencies other than the school district is involved, the drawing or set of drawings will have been submitted to those agencies with a project outline or specifications as soon as the plan has been sufficiently developed to establish the area. If the other agency approves the application as submitted by the architect, the final preliminary working drawings are started.

Final processing

It is advisable that all matters that can be settled are decided during preliminary planning in order to save time. If this method is used, greater clarity is assured and less changing or misunderstanding results. Preliminary plans are drawn with the intent of illustrating the plan for the school district; working drawings are technical in nature and are often difficult to interpret. However, should school personnel wish to check the working drawings before their completion, they should be welcome to do so.

GENERAL TRENDS IN FACILITY CONSTRUCTION

In respect to educational buildings in general, there has been considerable change. Traditionally rectangular in shape, buildings of all shapes and sizes have appeared in recent years, including round, semicircular, quadrangular, hexangular, oval, and pentangular buildings. New types of rooms have also been introduced, including large rooms for team teaching and large lecture groups; classrooms of various shapes and sizes; special rooms including those for dramatics, science, band, choral groups, business machines, and television broadcasting; and more office and conference rooms for such people as counselors and health program and administrative assistants. Furthermore, with the greater use of overhead lighting, there has been a trend to more windowless rooms. In fact, some buildings have no windows whatsoever.

School sites are getting larger and are being located away from busy industrial centers. More space is also being provided for parking.

The designs of school buildings and other facilities concerned with health and physical education programs and recreation today stress two factors: the educational needs of the children and others who pursue programs in such areas and the need for economy at a time when construction costs are so high.

The trend is to do away with many of the so-called frills in order to achieve economy but at the same time not to compromise educational standards. Educational leaders advocate taking greater advantage of labor-, material-, and space-saving devices. For example, they suggest that the ceilings in regular classrooms be cut down from the traditional 12 feet to 8 feet. They maintain that good lighting can be gained under most conditions with only 8-foot ceilings. Also, multipurpose halls can be constructed to double as exhibit and social areas, and gymnasia can be used for physical education and community purposes rather than merely for spectator entertainment.

It has further been pointed out that several practices are not economical in some of the construction going on today. An example of this is the application of Gothic and Colonial architecture merely to enhance appearance. Buildings should be planned with emphasis on the functional, inside aspects, rather than on the outside ornamentation. Also, it is not economical to have a large auditorium constructed that will be only half filled except on commencement day.

These features have received the support of the American Association of School Administrators. Bright plastic floor covering, improved lighting, and colorful painted walls are important. Classrooms should be large, with movable furniture, work alcoves, and conference rooms. Large, well-planned play areas are important features in the selection of a school site, with 10 to 20 acres of land frequently being used for such sites. Both on the elementary and secondary levels, one-story buildings are becoming increasingly common. Single-story construction is safer more economical and decreases noise. Walls are being constructed with special attention to acoustical treatment to reduce noise. Ceilings

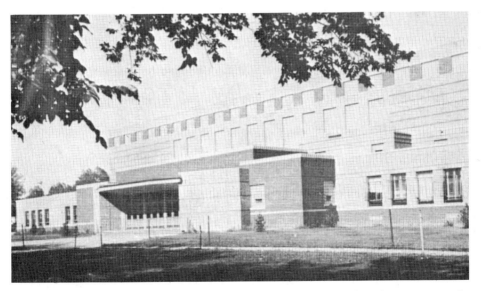

Main entrance to Storey gymnasium. (Cheyenne Public Schools, Cheyenne, Wyo.)

that slope are being increasingly utilized in order to improve light distribution and to reduce the space to be heated. Many rooms and facilities are being located to facilitate community use. Finally, there is evidence of the practicability of single-loaded corridors, which run along the outer walls of the building. In this way classrooms open onto the hall from only one side.

Flexibility of design is an important trend in facility management today, with the inclusion of folding partitions and multiple use of facilities for different types of activities.

Some new materials that are being used are as follows:

1. *Structural steel.* One of the most versatile of building materials, used in various shapes, sizes, and strengths, providing for greater stability, flexibility, and adaptability.

2. *Structural pine.* Used for such purposes as laminated beams to form roof structures and uprights of buildings and other purposes, providing economy of design, beauty, safety, and ease of maintenance.

3. *Concrete block.* Increasingly being used to enclose framework and as interior walls; economical and easily removed from non–load-bearing walls to develop flexibility.

4. *Stone.* Used to a great extent for attractive exteriors on schools and for permanence.

5. *Corrugated steel.* Provides an economical method of long-span roofing.

6. *Carpeting of classrooms.* Helps eliminate noise and is easy to clean and maintain with less man hours required.

NEW FEATURES IN THE CONSTRUCTION OF PHYSICAL EDUCATION FACILITIES

There are many new trends in facilities and materials for physical education programs. New paving materials, new types of equipment, improved landscapes, new construction materials, new shapes for swimming pools, partial shelters, and synthetic grass are just a few of the many new developments. Combination indoor-outdoor pools, physical fitness equipment for outdoor use, all-weather tennis courts, and lines that now come in multicolors for various games and activities are other new developments.

In gymnasium construction some of the new features include the utilization of modern engineering techniques and materials. This has resulted in welded steel and laminated wood modular frames; arched and gabled roofs; domes that provide areas completely free from internal supports; exterior surfaces of aluminum, steel, fiber glass, and plastics; different window patterns and styles; several kinds of floor surfaces of nonslip material; prefabricated wall surfaces; better lighting systems with improved quality and quantity and less glare. Facilities are moving from use of regular glass to either plastic and fiber glass panel or to overhead skydome. Lightweight fiber glass, sandwich panels, or fabricated sheets of translucent fiber glass laminated over an aluminum framework are proving popular. They require no painting, the cost of labor and materials is lower, there is no need for shades or blinds to eliminate glare, and the breakage problem is reduced or eliminated.

Locker rooms and service areas are including built-in locks that involve combination locks with built-in combination changers that permit the staff to change combinations when needed. There is more extensive use of ceramic tile because of its durability and low-cost maintenance. Wall-hung toilet compartment features permit easier maintenance and sanitation with no chance for rust to start from the floor. Odor control is being effectively handled by new dispensers. New thin-profile heating, ventilating, and air-conditioning fan coil units are now being used.

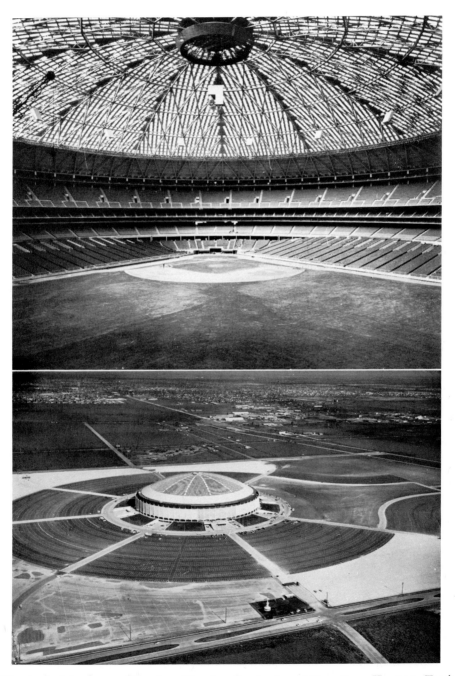

Houston's Astrodome. (Courtesy Houston Sports Association, Inc., Houston, Tex.)

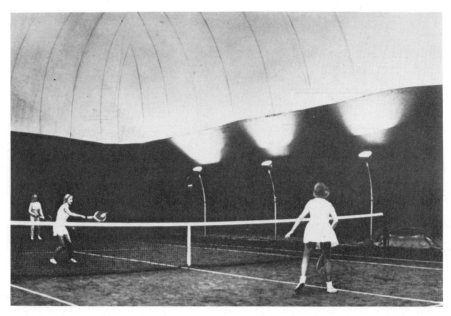

Air-supported tennis court enclosure. (Airshelters, Division of Birdair Structures, Inc., Buffalo, N. Y.)

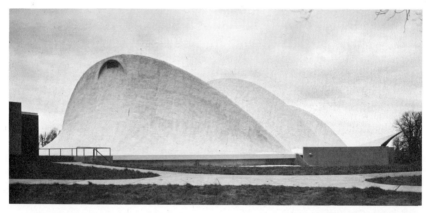

Shaver & Company, Salina, Kan.

Graceland Fieldhouse, Lamoni, Iowa.

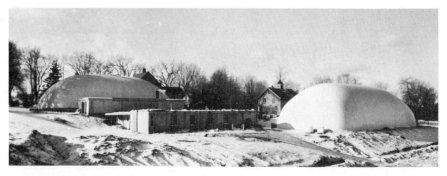

Forman School, Litchfield, Conn. (Courtesy Educational Facilities Laboratories, New York, N. Y.)

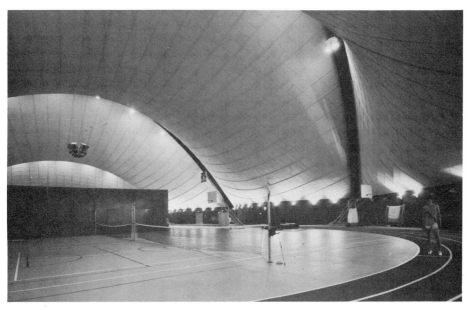

Graceland Fieldhouse, Lamoni, Iowa.

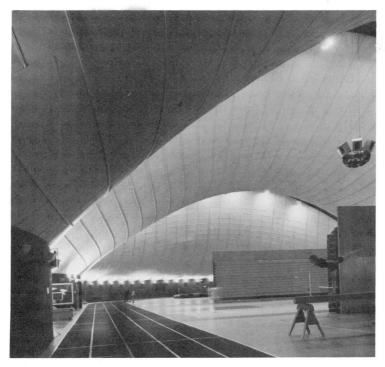

Graceland Fieldhouse, Lamoni, Iowa.

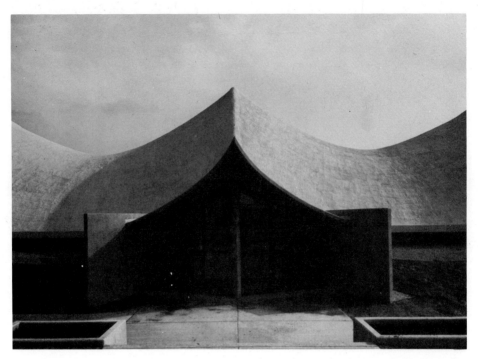

Shaver & Company, Salina, Kan.

Graceland Fieldhouse, Lamoni, Iowa.

The health suite is being modernized by making it more attractive and serviceable. There is also a trend toward better ventilation, heating, and lighting and more easily cleaned materials on walls and floors to guarantee improved sanitation.

New developments in regard to indoor swimming pools include automatic control boards, where one person can have direct control over all filters, chlorinators, chemical pumps, and level controllers; much larger deck space area constructed of non-slip ceramic tile; greater use of diatomaceous earth rather than sand filters to filter out small particles of matter including some bacteria; underwater lighting; water-level deck pools (where the overflow gutters are placed in the deck surrounding the pool instead of in the pool's side walls and provision is made for grating that is designed so that the water that overflows is drained to a trench under the deck without the possibility of debris returning to the pool); air-supported roofs that can serve as re-movable tops in a combination indoor-outdoor pool; and movable bulkheads.

New developments in regard to outdoor swimming pools involve new shapes—including oval, wedge, kidney, figure eight, cloverleaf, and bean shaped—as well as modern accessories, including gas heaters, automatic water levelers, and retractable roofs and sides. More supplemental recreational facilities, such as shuffleboard courts, volleyball, and horseshoes, and more deck equipment, including guard rails, slides, and pool covers, are being included around larger pools.

A brief listing of some new features that are being used in many school buildings in the area of health and physical education have been developed by the Educational Facilities Laboratories.* This is a nonprofit organization financed by the Ford Foundation. It enters into joint research projects

---

*Educational Facilities Laboratories, 477 Madison Ave., New York, N. Y. 10022.

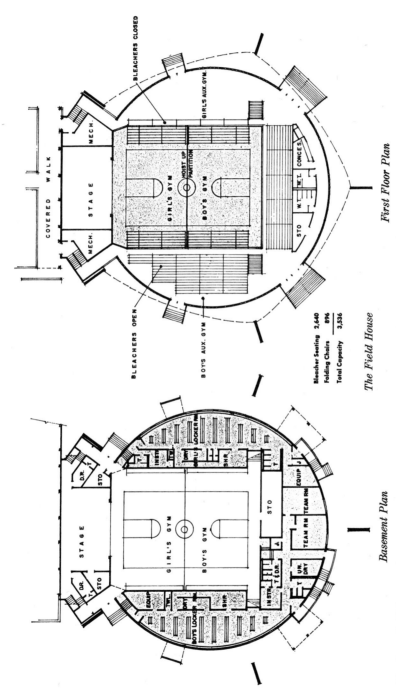

Basement Plan

The Field House

First Floor Plan

Bleacher Seating	2,640
Folding Chairs	896
Total Capacity	3,536

Geodesic field house. (From *Conventional gymnasium vs. geodesic field house: case studies of educational facilities No. 1*, New York, Educational Facilities Laboratories, Inc.)

with schools interested in testing the practicality of some new kind of facility, design, or material.

The geodesic field house has been compared, in cost of construction, with a conventional gymnasium (see accompanying illustration) and found to be slightly less expensive. This type of structure has applicability primarily to programs in which strong emphasis is placed on athletics and spectator appeal or to communities that need a very large auditorium. For these reasons it seems that the geodesic field house has limited value for the general physical education program.

Bubble tops for swimming pools and tennis courts make it possible to use them as outdoor facilities in summer and as indoor facilities in the winter. The roof made of vinyl-coated fabric costs less per square foot in contrast to a wooden dome or a geodesic dome.

Partial shelters for physical education activities have been studied and are in use in many Texas public schools. They are considered practical for elementary school physical education in which change from school clothes many times is not required. These partial shelters protect children from extremes of climate and, at the same time,

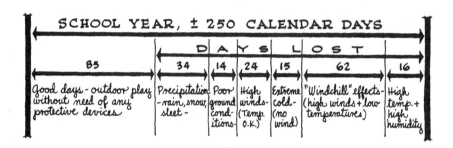

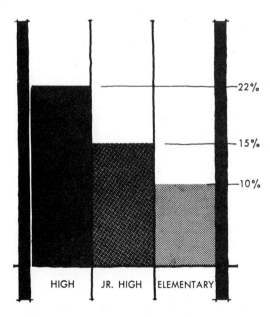

BUILDING SPACE DEVOTED TO PHYSICAL ACTIVITIES

Charts showing amount of space devoted to physical activities in schools, the implications of weather conditions for the physical education program, and some ideas for partial shelters for physical education programs. (From Shelter for physical education: a study of the feasibility of the use of limited shelters for physical education, College Station, Texas, Texas Engineering Experiment Station, Texas A & M University.)

allow for exercise in the open air. They are of course more economical than traditional facilities.

New artificial turf has been developed and successfully tried. The initial reaction of students and teachers is that the turf provides excellent traction and helps the acoustics. It is easily cleaned with a vacuum.

Rubber-cushioned tennis courts are being used in some places. They consist of tough durable material about 4 inches thick, with the individual advantages of clay, turf, and composition courts being combined into one type of surfacing.

Other new developments in health and physical education facilities that have come into use in schools across the country are

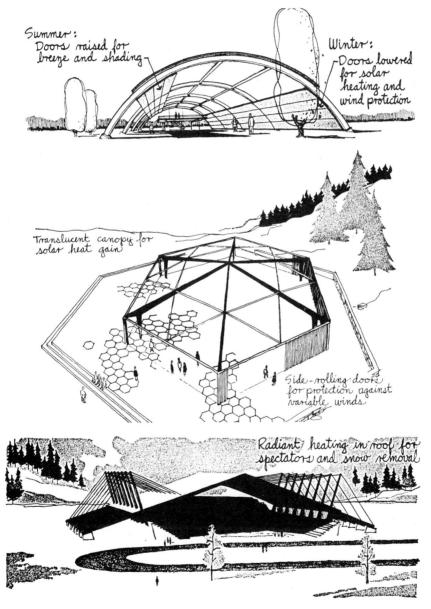

For legend see opposite page.

numerous. Sculptured play apparatus has been produced by a number of firms. It is designed to be more conducive to imaginative movements and creativity than conventional equipment. Hard-surfaced, rubberized, all-weather running tracks, radiant heating of decks on swimming pools, floating roofs with the elimination of non–load-bearing walls, interior climate control, better indoor and outdoor lighting, rubber padding for use under apparatus, park-school concept with land being used for school and recreational purposes, outdoor skating rinks, translucent plastic materials for swimming pool canopies and other uses, electrically operated machinery to move equipment and partitions and bleachers, and auxiliary gymnasia used for both activity and classroom use are a few more of the new developments in facilities for health and physical education programs.

Park-school facilities

The park-school complex is another innovation that should be mentioned. In this type of setup the school is erected near a park, and the park facilities are used by both the school and the community. This has implications particularly for physical education and recreation programs, since the school usually uses the park facilities during school hours and the recreation department uses them after school hours, on weekends, and during vacation periods.

TEACHING STATIONS

The teaching station concept should be taken into consideration when scheduling physical education classes. A teaching station is the space or setting where one teacher or staff member can carry on physical education activities for one group of students. The number and size of teaching stations available together with the number of teachers on the staff, the size of the group, the number of times the group meets, the number of periods in the school or college day, and the program of activities are important items to consider in planning.

According to the participants in the National Facilities Conference,* the following formulas are listed for determining the number of teaching stations needed.

---

*Participants in National Facilities Conference: Planning areas and facilities for health, physical education, and recreation, Washington, D. C., 1965, American Association for Health, Physical Education, and Recreation, p. 83.

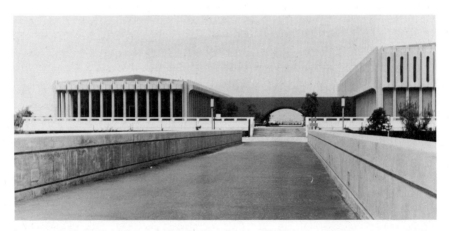

Overpass to athletic facilities. A unique feature of overall campus planning permits access to facilities from parking lots and academic buildings without the necessity of crossing a main thoroughfare. (University of California at Irvine.)

Secondary schools and colleges

The formula for computing the number of teaching stations needed for physical education in colleges and secondary schools would be as follows:

$$\text{Minimum number of teaching stations} = \frac{\dfrac{\text{Number of students}}{\text{Average number of students per instructor}} \times \text{Number of periods class meets each week}}{\text{Total number of class periods in school work}}$$

For example, if a school system projects its enrollment to 700 students and plans six class periods a day with an average class size of thirty students, and physical education is required daily, the formula would read as follows:

$$\text{Minimum number of teaching stations} = \frac{\dfrac{700 \text{ students}}{30 \text{ per class}} \times 5 \text{ periods per week}}{30 \text{ periods per week}} = \frac{3,500}{900} = 3.9$$

Colleges could substitute pertinent facts into the same formula to determine the number of teaching stations they would need.

Elementary schools

The formula for computing the number of teaching stations needed for physical education in the elementary schools would be as follows:

$$\text{Minimum number of teaching stations} = \frac{\dfrac{\text{Number of class-rooms of students}}{} \times \text{Number of physical education periods per week per class}}{\text{Total periods in school week}}$$

For example, in an elementary school with six grades, with three classes at each level (approximately 450 to 540 students), ten 30-minute physical education periods per day, and physical education conducted on a daily basis, the teaching station needs would be calculated as follows:

$$\text{Minimum number of teaching stations} = 18 \text{ classroom units} \times \frac{5 \text{ periods per week}}{50 \text{ periods per week}} = \frac{90}{50} = 1.8$$

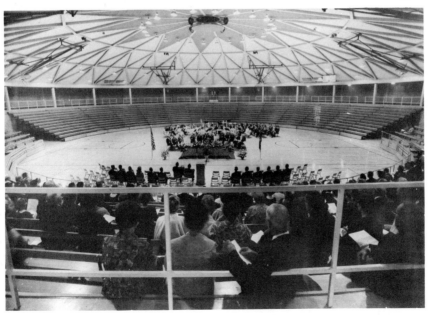

Shaver & Company, Salina, Kan.

Gymnasium. (McPherson High School, McPherson, Kan.)

ROOMS	FLOORS									LOWER WALLS					UPPER WALLS						CEILINGS		
	Asphalt, Rubber Linoleum Tile	Cement, Abrasive and Non-absorbent	Maple, hard	Terrazzo Abrasive	Tile, ceramic	Brick	Brick, glazed	Cinder Block	Concrete	Plaster	Tile, ceramic	Wood Panel	Moisture-proof	Brick	Brick, glazed	Cinder Block	Plaster	Acoustic	Moisture-resistant	Concrete or Structure Tile	Plaster	Tile, acoustic	Moisture-resistant
Apparatus Storage Room	1	2			1	2	2	1	C														
Classrooms	2	1				2	2	2	1		2				2	1				C	C	1	
Clubroom	2	1				2	2		1		2				2	1				C	C	1	
Corrective Room		1		2	1			2	1		2		2	2	1	2				C	C	1	
Custodial Supply Room				2																			
Dance Studio	1		2																	C	C	1	
Drying Room (equip.)	1	1	2	2	2	1	1	1		1			1		1								
Gymnasium		1	2	2	2	1	2		1	2	2		2	2	1	2	*			C	C	1	
Health-Service Unit	1	1					2			C					2	1	*				1	*	
Laundry Room	2			2	1	2	2	2	1			*	1		1	2		*			1	*	
Locker Rooms	3			2	1	2	2	3				*	1		1	2				C	1		
Natatorium	1			2	1	3	2		1	1		*	2	2	1		*	*		C	C	1	*
Offices	2	1				2	2	2	1	1	1				2	1				C	1		
Recreation Room	2	1		2		2	2	2	1	1	1	*	2		1	2		*		C	1		
Shower Rooms	2		1		2			2	1	1		*	1	2	1	2		*		1	1	*	
Special-activity Room	2	1		2			2	1	1	1		*	1	1	1	1				C	1		
Team Room	3	2	1	2	1	2	2	3	1	1		*	1	1	1	2				C	1		
Toilet Rooms	3	2	1	1	1	1	2	2	1	1		*	1	1	1	2				C	1		
Toweling-Drying Room (bath)	3	2	1	1	1	2	2	2	1	1		*	2	1	2	2		*		1	1	*	

Note: The numbers in the Table indicate first, second, and third choices. "C" indicates the material as being contrary to good practice. An * indicates desirable quality.

Suggested indoor surface materials. (From Participants in National Facilities Conference: Planning areas and facilities for health, physical education, and recreation, revised, Chicago, 1965, The Athletic Institute.)

INDOOR FACILITIES

Several special areas and facilities are needed by programs of health, physical education, and recreation. A few of the indoor areas that are important and prominent in the conduct of these specialized programs are briefly discussed in this section.

Administrative and staff offices*

It is important, as far as it is practical and possible, for professional persons working in health, physical education, and recreation to have a section of a building set aside for administrative and staff offices. As a minimum there should be a large central office with a waiting room. The central office will provide a place where the secretarial and clerical work can be performed, space for keeping records and files, and storage closets for office supplies. The waiting room can serve as a reception point where students and visitors can wait until staff members are ready to see them.

Separate offices for the staff members should be provided, if possible. This allows for a place where conferences can be held in private and without interruption. This is a very important consideration for health counseling and for discussing scholastic, family, recreational, and other problems. If separate officers are not practical, a desk should be provided for each staff member. In this event, there should be a private room available to staff members for conferences.

Other facilities that make for a more efficient and enjoyable administrative and staff setup are staff dressing rooms, departmental library, conference room, and toilet and lavatory facilities.

Locker, shower, and drying rooms

Health, physical education, and recreation activities require facilities for storage of clothes, showering, and drying. These

*See also Chapter 21 on Office Management.

are essential to good health and for a well-organized program. The reason such facilities are often not fully utilized is that poor planning makes them inadequate and uncomfortable.

Locker and shower rooms should be readily accessible to activity areas. Locker rooms should not be congested places that students want to get out of as soon as possible. Instead, they should provide ample room, both storage and dressing type lockers, stationary benches to sit upon, mirrors to aid in dressing, recessed lighting fixtures, and drinking fountains.

An average of 14 square feet per individual at peak load, exclusive of the space utilized by the lockers, is required to provide proper space.

Storage lockers should be provided for each individual in the school or recreational program. An additional 10% should be installed for purposes of expanded enrollments or membership. These are lockers for the permanent use of each individual and can be utilized to hold essential clothing and other supplies. They can be smaller than the dressing lockers and some recommended sizes are these: 7½ by 12 by 24

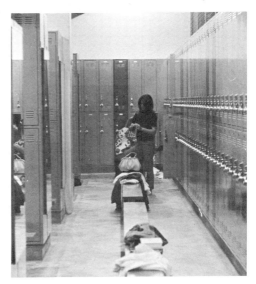

Women's locker room. (University of California at Irvine.)

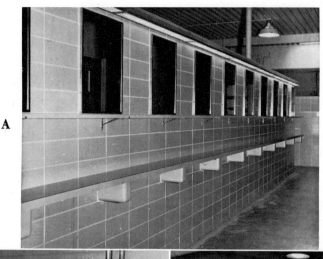

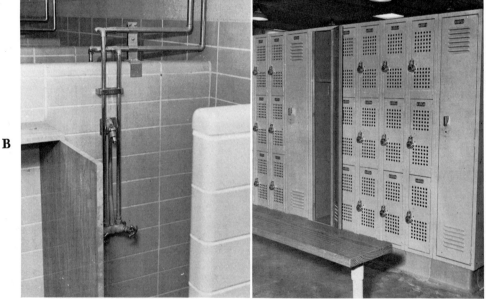

A, Dual-shelf system in the girls' dressing room. Books, purses, and other in-hand objects go on the lower shelf. Bobby pins, combs, compacts, and lipstick, of course, need to be at hand on the smaller upper shelf. **B,** A girl's shower stall. Picture taken from an upper angle. **C,** Locker arrangement utilized in both girls' and boys' locker rooms. The perforated storage lockers are 9 inches wide, 20 inches high, and 15 inches deep. Hook hangers provide a place to hang gymnasium wear. Each student has his own personal lock rented from the school. Shelves in the dressing lockers were lowered from 12 inches to 16 inches to make room for the large folios that many students carry. The dressing lockers are 8 inches high, 12 inches wide, and 15 inches deep. There is room for books, shoes, and clothes. (Courtesy Spring Branch Independent School District, Houston, Tex.)

inches, 6 by 12 by 36 inches, and 7½ by 12 by 18 inches. The basket type lockers are not looked upon with favor by many experts, because of the hygiene factor, the fact that an attendant is required for good administration of this system, and the necessity of carting the baskets from place to place.

Dressing lockers are utilized by participants only when actually engaging in activity. They are large in size, usually 12 by 12 by 54 inches or 12 by 12 by 48 inches in elementary schools and 12 by 12 by 72 inches for secondary schools and colleges and for community recreation programs.

Shower rooms should be provided that have the gang type shower for boys and a combination of the gang and cubicle type showers for girls. Some facility planners recommend that girls have a number of shower heads equal to 40% of the enrollment at peak load and the boys, 30% of the enrollment at peak load. Another recommendation is one shower head for four boys and one for three girls at peak load. These should be 4 feet apart. If showers are installed where a graded change of water temperature is provided and where the individual progresses through such a gradation, the number of shower heads can be reduced. The shower rooms should also be equipped with liquid soap dispensers, good ventilation and heating, floors constructed of nonslip material, and recessed plumbing. The ceiling should be dome-shaped so that it will more readily shed water.

The drying room adjacent to the shower room is an essential. This should be equipped with proper drainage, good ventilation, towel bar, and a ledge that can be used to place a foot upon while drying.

A report of a conference on the planning of facilities for health, physical education, and recreation lists the following common errors in service facilities:

Failure to provide adequate locker and dressing space

Failure to plan dressing and shower area so as to reduce foot traffic to a minimum and establish clean, dry aisles for bare feet
Failure to provide a nonskid surface on dressing, shower, and toweling room floors
Failure to properly relate teaching stations with service facilities
Inadequate provision for drinking fountains
Failure to provide acoustical treatment where needed
Failure to provide and properly locate toilet facilities to serve all participants and spectators
Failure to provide doorways, hallways, or ramps so that equipment may be moved easily
Failure to design equipment rooms for convenient and quick check-in and check-out
Failure to provide mirrors and shelving for boys' and girls' dressing facilities, and lipstick tissues for girls
Failure to plan locker and dressing rooms with correct traffic pattern to swimming pool
Failure to construct shower, toilet, and dressing rooms with sufficient floor slope and properly located drains
Failure to place shower heads low enough and in such a position that the spray is kept within the shower room.
Failure to provide shelves in the toilet room[*]

Gymnasia

The type and number of gymnasia that should be part of a school or recreational plant will depend upon the number of individuals who will be participating, the variety of activities that will be conducted in this area, and the school level concerned.

General construction features to which most individuals will agree include smooth walls, hardwood floors (maple preferred—laid lengthwise), recessed lights, recessed radiators, adequate and well-screened windows, and storage space for the apparatus and other equipment utilized. It is also generally agreed that in schools it is best to have the gymnasium located in a separate wing of the building to isolate the noise and also as a convenient location for

[*]Planning facilities for health, physical education, and recreation, revised edition, Chicago, 1956, The Athletic Institute, Inc., p. 70.

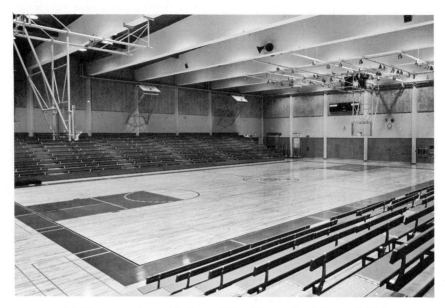

Men's gymnasium. (College of San Mateo, San Mateo, Calif.)

community groups that will be anxious to use such facilities.

The American Association for Health, Physical Education, and Recreation has listed several important factors to keep in mind when planning the gymnasium:

1. Hard maple flooring which is resilient and nonslippery.
2. Smooth interior walls to a height of 10 or 12 feet.
3. Upper walls need not be smooth.
4. The ceiling should reflect light and absorb sound, and there should be at least 22 to 24 feet from the floor to exposed beams.
5. Windows should be ten to twelve feet above floor and placed on long side of room.
6. Heating should be thermostatically controlled, radiators recessed with protecting grill or grate if placed at floor level.
7. Sub-flooring should be moisture- and termite-resistant and well ventilated.
8. Prior consideration must be given concerning the suspension of apparatus from the ceiling and the erection of wall-type apparatus.
9. Mechanical ventilation may be necessary.
10. Proper illumination meeting approved standards and selectively controlled for various activities must be designed.
11. Floor plates for standards and apparatus

must be planned, as well as such items as blackboards, electric clocks and scoreboards, public address system, and provisions for press and radio.
12. Floor markings for various games should be placed after prime coat of seal has been applied and prior to application of the finishing coats.*

The number of teaching stations desired will play an important part in deciding the size and number of the gymnasia. A teaching station is a place where a group meets with a teacher or leader for the conduct of certain activities. The degree to which a varied program is offered, the facilities available, and the number of staff members assigned will determine the number of teaching stations utilized in any program.†

In addition to an adequate number of teaching stations, it is also important to give attention to official size courts, ade-

---

*American Association for Health, Physical Education, and Recreation: Administrative problems in health education, physical education, and recreation, Washington, D. C., 1953, The Association, p. 83.

†See also pp. 428-429.

This unit provides:

Two teaching stations

One standard inter-school basketball court

Two court areas for instruction and intra-mural basketball

Two court areas for volleyball, newcomb, etc.

Four court areas for badminton, paddle tennis, etc.

Two circle areas for instruction, dodge ball, and circle games

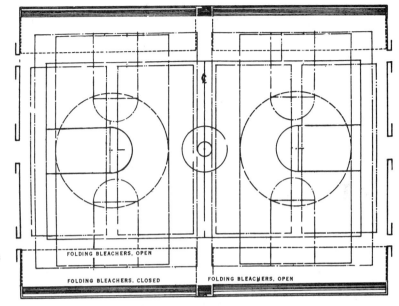

A

This unit provides:

Two teaching stations

One standard inter-school basketball court

Two court areas for instruction and intra-mural basketball

Three court areas for volleyball, new-comb, etc.

Six court areas for badminton, paddle tennis, etc.

Four circle areas for instruction, dodge ball, and circle games

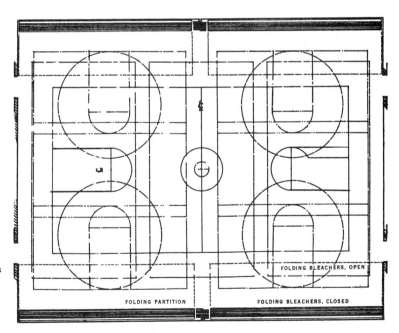

B

A, Illustrative plan of two teaching stations for junior high school gymnasium. **B,** Illustrative plan of two teaching stations for senior high school gymnasium. (From Participants in National Facilities Conference: Planning areas and facilities for health, physical education, and recreation, revised, Chicago, 1965, The Athletic Institute.)

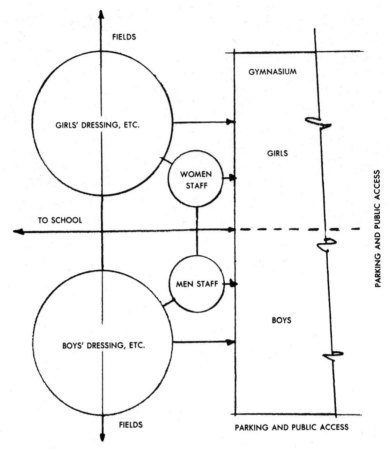

Orientation of gymnasium to related areas. (From Participants in National Facilities Conference: Planning areas and facilities for health, physical education, and recreation, revised, Chicago, 1965, The Athletic Institute.)

quate space for safe and enjoyable participation, and spectator space, if such is desired. When spectator space is provided, bleachers that can be telescoped and recessed in the walls are advisable, as they do not take space away from activity participation.

Many gymnasia have folding doors that divide them into halves, thirds, or fourths and allow for activities to be conducted simultaneously on each side. This has proved satisfactory where separate gymnasia could not be provided.

In elementary schools that desire only one teaching station a minimum floor space of 36 feet by 52 feet is required. Where two

teaching stations are desired, floor space of 52 feet by 72 feet may be divided by a folding partition. In junior and senior high schools where only one teaching station is desired, a minimum floor space of 48 feet by 66 feet is necessary. If two teaching stations are necessary, an area 66 feet by 96 feet of floor space, exclusive of bleachers, will provide these teaching stations of minimum size. The folding partition that provides the two teaching stations should be motor driven. Where seating capacity is desired, additional space will be needed. If more than two teaching stations are desired, the gymnasium area may be extended to provide an additional

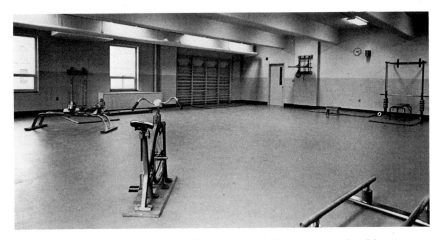

Special exercise room. (University of Maine at Portland.)

station or activity rooms may be added. Of course, the addition of a swimming pool will also provide an additional teaching station.

Other considerations for gymnasia should include provisions for basketball backboards, mountings for various apparatus that will be used, recessed drinking fountains, places for hanging mats, outlets for various electric appliances and cleaning devices, proper line markings for activities, bulletin boards, and other essentials to a well-rounded program.

Common errors in construction of gymnasia are as follows:

Provision for spectator space at the sacrifice of instructional space.
Failure to mark floor for possible court games such as badminton, basketball, and volleyball.
Construction of a combination auditorium-gymnasium when separate facilities could be provided.
Installation of permanent bleachers instead of folding bleachers, resulting in loss of maximum use of floor space.
Failure to provide ventilated space below a built-up gymnasium floor.
Natural lighting construction permitting leakage and glare problems.*

---

*Planning facilities for health, physical education, and recreation, revised edition, Chicago, 1956, The Athletic Institute, Inc., p. 63.

Special activity areas

Although gymnasia are large and take up considerable space, there should still be additional areas for activities essential to school programs of health, physical education, and recreation.

Wherever possible additional activity areas should be provided for remedial or adapted activities, apparatus, handball, squash, weight lifting, dancing, rhythms, fencing, and dramatics and for various recreational activities such as arts and crafts, lounging and resting, and bowling. The activities to be provided will depend on interests of participants and type of program. The recommended size of such auxiliary gymnasia is 30 by 50 by 24 feet, or preferably 40 by 60 by 24 feet.

Another special room especially desirable in the elementary school is the all-purpose room that could be used for all types of activities, including games, music, dramatics, and social events.

In reference to special activity areas, it should also be pointed out that regulation classrooms can be converted into these special rooms. This may be feasible where the actual construction of such costly facilities may not be practical.

The remedial or adapted activities room should be equipped with such items as horizontal ladders, mirrors, mats, climbing

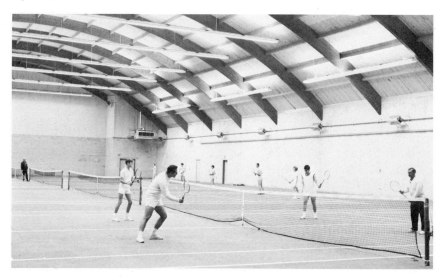

Special tennis structure. (Brigham Young University, Provo, Utah.)

ropes, stall bars and benches, pulley weights, dumbbells, Indian clubs, shoulder wheels, and such other equipment as is suited for the particular needs of the individuals participating.

Auxiliary rooms

The main types of auxiliary areas found in connection with school and college health and physical education and recreation facilities are supply, checkout, custodial, and laundry rooms.

Supply rooms should be easily accessible from the gymnasium and other activity areas. In these rooms will be stored balls, nets, standards, and other equipment needed for the programs that are offered. The size of these rooms will vary according to the number of activities offered and the number of participants.

Checkout rooms should be provided on a seasonal basis. They will house the equipment and supplies used in various seasonal activities.

Custodial rooms provide a place for storing equipment and supplies utilized in the maintenance of these specialized facilities.

Laundries should be adequate in size to accommodate the laundering of such essential items as towels, uniforms, and swimming suits.

SWIMMING POOLS

In the year 1900 there were very few indoor swimming pools in the public schools in the United States. Today, however, there are approximately 2,500 swimming pools in public schools.

According to Gabrielsen,[*] schools should have swimming pools for many reasons. Swimming is the number one recreation activity in America, and it is often listed by elementary and secondary school students as their favorite activity. Teaching all children how to swim could reduce the more than 8,000 deaths by drowning that occur in the United States each year. Knowing how to swim leads to many other excellent aquatic activities such as surfing, sailing, canoeing, fishing, scuba diving, and water skiing.

Gabrielsen in his report cited the major

[*]Professor M. A. Gabrielsen, New York University. From a speech given at the Conference on Planning, Constructing, Utilizing Physical Education, Recreation, and Athletic Facilities, sponsored by the Ohio Department of Education, Columbus, Ohio, December 10, 1969.

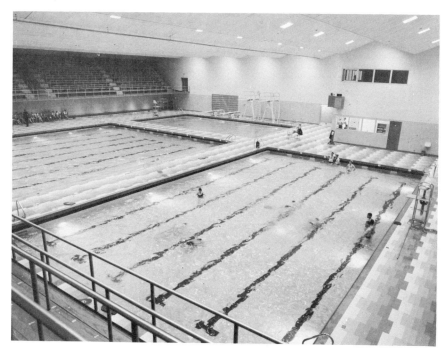

Swimming pool complex. (Brigham Young University, Provo, Utah.)

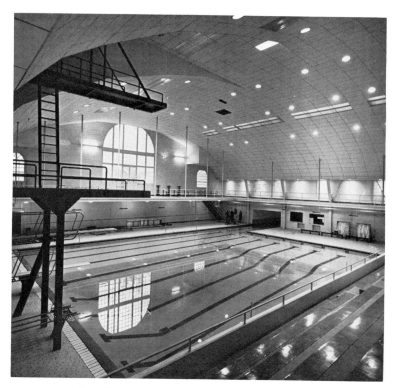

Dartmouth College swimming pool. See also pp. 440 and 441.

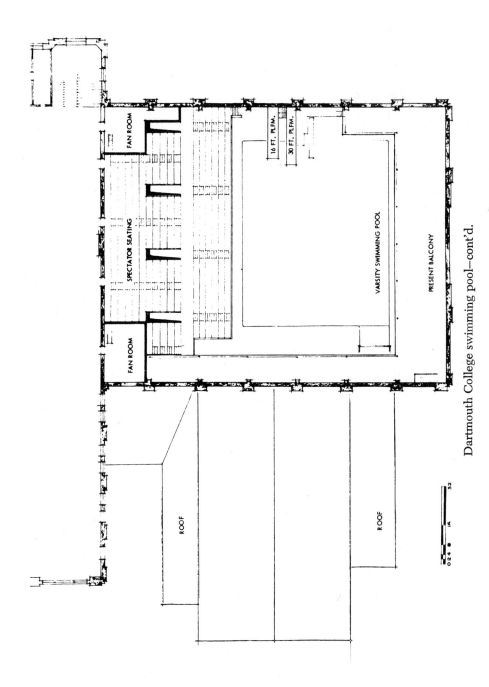

Dartmouth College swimming pool–cont'd.

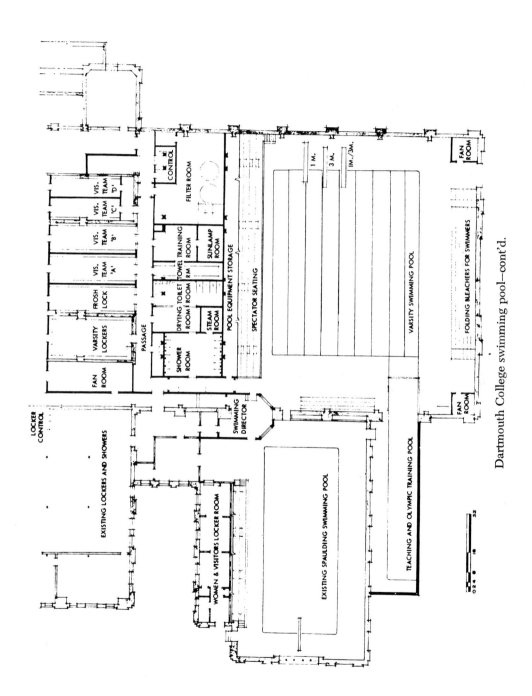

Dartmouth College swimming pool—cont'd.

design decisions that must be made if a school or college decides to construct a pool. These include such items as the nature of the program to be conducted in a pool, type of overflow system to be used, dimensions and shape of pool, depth of the water, type of finish, type of filters and water treatment system, construction material to be used, amount of deck area, climate control, illumination, and number of spectators to be accommodated. The range in cost of pools can vary from $2.65 per square foot to $17.00 per square foot depending upon the material used, the design, and the geographic location. Cost of pool enclosures vary from about $2.50 to $3.50 per square foot for air structures, to $7.00 to $9.00 per square foot for prefabricated, lightweight aluminum dome frames supporting reinforced plastic roof tents of acrylic panels, to $18.00 to $25.00 per square foot for steel frame with masonry or fireproof panel walls, steel roof trusses, beams, or joints, and fire-resistive metal or concrete plank roof deck.

Some mistakes that Gabrielsen says should be avoided in the construction of a pool include entrances to the pool from the locker rooms opening onto the deep rather than the shallow end of the pool, pool base finished with slippery material such as glazed tile, insufficient depth of water for diving, improper placement of ladders, insufficient rate of recirculation of water to accommodate peak bathing loads, inadequate storage space, failure to use acoustical material on ceiling and walls, insufficient illumination, slippery tile on decks, and an inadequate overflow system at the ends of the pool.

Finally, in this report are listed some trends and innovations in pool design and operation. These include: the Rim-Flow Overflow System, inflatable roof structure, the skydome design, pool tent cover, floating swimming pool complex, prefabrication of pool tanks, automation of pool recirculating and filter systems, regenerative cycle filter system, adjustable height diving platform, variable depth bottoms, fluorescent underwater lights, automatic cleaning systems, and wave making machines.

Present types of swimming pools have in the main two objectives, one to provide instructional and competitive programs and the other for recreation.

The swimming pool should be located on or above the ground level, have southern exposure, be isolated from other units in the building, and be easily accessible from the central dressing and locker rooms. Materials that have been found most adaptive to swimming pools are smooth, glazed, light-colored tile or brick.

The standard indoor pool is 75 feet in length. The width should be a multiple of 7 feet, with a minimum of 35 feet. Depths vary from 2 feet 6 inches at the shallow end to 4 feet 6 inches at the outer limits of the shallow area. The shallow or instructional area should comprise about two-thirds of the pool. The deeper areas taper to 9 to 12 feet in depth. An added but important factor is a movable bulkhead that can be used to divide the pool into various instructional areas.

The deck space around the pool should be constructed of a nonslip material and provide ample space for land drills and demonstrations. The area above the water should be unobstructed. The ceiling should be at least 25 feet above the water if a 3-meter diving board will be used. The walls and the ceiling of the pool should be acoustically treated.

The swimming pool should be constructed so as to receive as much natural light as possible, with the windows located on the sides rather than on the ends. Artificial lighting should be recessed in the ceilings. Good lighting is especially important in the areas where the diving boards are located. Underwater lighting is beautiful but not an essential.

There should be an efficient system for adequately heating and circulating the

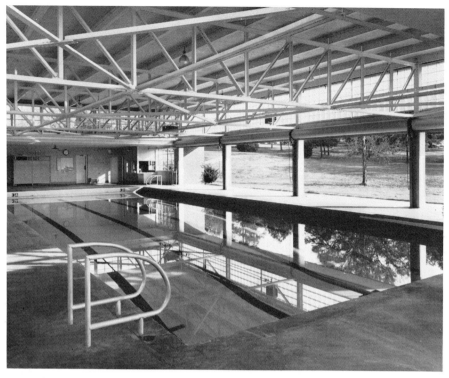

Swimming pool. (Alabama College, Montevallo, Ala.)

water. The temperature of the water should range from 75° to 80° F.

If spectators are to be provided for, it is recommended that a gallery that is separate from the pool room proper be erected along the length of the pool.

An office adjacent to the pool where records and first-aid supplies can be kept is advisable. Such an office should be equipped with windows that overlook the entire length of the pool. Also, there should be lavatory and toilet facilities available.

The swimming pool is a costly operation. Therefore, it is essential that it be planned with the help of the best advice obtainable. Specialists who are well acquainted with such facilities and who conduct swimming activities should be brought into conferences with the architect, a representative from the public health department, and experts in such essentials as lighting, heating, construction, and acoustics.

The checklist at the end of this chapter should be consulted for further standards regarding swimming pools.

HEALTH SCIENCE INSTRUCTION FACILITES

The health science instruction program should have facilities especially designed to meet the needs of educating students in respect to health matters. The National Facilities Conference stresses the following standards:

1. Space for 35 square feet per pupil, maximum of 30 pupils
2. Flexible teacher location
3. Provision for various teaching methods, including laboratory demonstration
4. Flexibility of seating
5. Hot and cold running water and gas outlet
6. Educational-exhibit space
7. Storage space
8. Provision for using audio-visual devices (electrical outlets, window shades, screens)
9. Access to health service unit
10. Exemplary environmental features

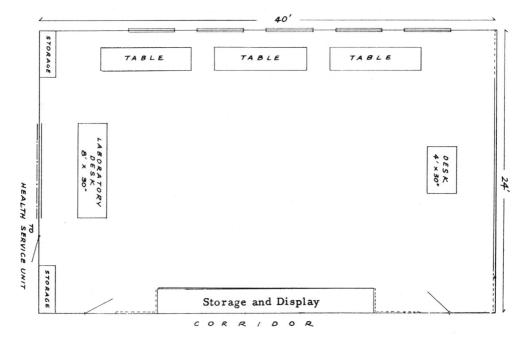

Health instruction laboratory. (From Participants in National Facilities Conference: Planning areas and facilities for health, physical education, and recreation, revised, Chicago, 1965, The Athletic Institute.)

11. Adequate handwashing facilities, drinking fountains, and toilets
12. Air-conditioning
13. Accessible to and usable by the disabled
14. Planned jointly for community use*

The recommended sizes in square feet for a floor plan for a health instruction laboratory are given in Table 15-1.

Classrooms

Classrooms utilized for health instruction should include the requirements discussed in relation to seating, lighting, color of walls and ceilings, heating and ventilation, acoustics, and sanitation. All classrooms should be healthful, comfortable, and adaptable, regardless of whether they are

*Participants in National Facilities Conference: Planning areas and facilities for health, physical education, and recreation, Washington, D. C., 1965, American Association for Health, Physical Education, and Recreation, p. 209.

being used for health instruction or some other subject.

There is one feature, however, that should receive consideration if there is not a special room set aside for such a purpose. This is the use of audiovisual equipment. There are ample resources for audiovisual material that can be utilized very effectively in any health instruction program. There should be available projection and sound equipment including an opaque projector, slide projector, filmstrip projector, motion picture projector, and turntables. There should also be outlets for electrical connections. Projection equipment should be installed in the rear of the room and audio equipment outlets in the front. There should be shades or other facilities for darkening the room. Finally, a screen should be available.

Another consideration in any health instruction room is a large display board that

Table 15-1. Recommended sizes in square feet of health service facilities for schools of various sizes*

	Enrollment					
	200 to 300	301 to 500	501 to 700	701 to 900	901 to 1,100	1,101 to 1,300
Waiting room	80	80	100	100	100	120
Examining room†	200	200	200	240	240	240
Rest room (total area for boys and girls)‡	100	180	220	260	300§	340§
Toilets (48 square feet total area—provide one for girls and one for boys)						

Optional areas
Dental clinic   100 square feet for all schools
Office space   80 square feet for each office provided
Eye examination   120 square feet minimum for all schools

*From Participants in National Facilities Conference: Planning areas and facilities for health, physical education, and recreation, Chicago, 1965, The Athletic Institute, p. 211. Based on data from State Department of Education: School planning manual, School Service Section, vol. 37, 1954, Richmond, Va.
†Examining room areas include 6 square feet for clothes closet and 24 square feet for storage closets.
‡For determining the number of cots, allow one cot per 100 pupils up to 400 pupils, and one cot per 200 pupils above 400. Round out fractions to nearest whole number. Allow 50 square feet of floor space for each of the first two cots and 40 square feet for each additional cot.
§In schools enrolling 901 to 1,100, a three-cot rest room is suggested for boys and a four-cot rest room for girls, and in 1,101-pupil to 1,300-pupil schools, a three-cot rest room is suggested for boys and a five-cot rest room for girls.
Note: For larger schools, add multiples of the above areas to obtain total needs.

can be used to illustrate the material that is presented.

Health service facilities

The health services are a very important part of the health program and require adequate facilities to carry out the responsibilities that are assigned to this health area. DeWeese and Moore* made an extensive study of the health service facilities and concluded that at least 720 square feet of floor surface should be provided and include the following:

1. Administrative office

*DeWeese, A. O., and Moore, V. M.: The organization of a school health service comprising from 500 to 1000 pupils from kindergarten through high school, Journal of School Health 34:415, 1964.

2. Library for health science instruction material
3. Rest rooms
4. Examination room
5. Conference facilities
6. Space for first-aid care and treatment
7. Space for scientific and educational displays
8. Storage and toilet facilities

Health service suite. To have a practical health service setup that can accommodate examination work, a suite is needed rather than just one room. Experts recommend at least four rooms, which include examining, waiting, and rest rooms for boys and for girls. In addition there should be toilet facilities for each sex. Several exits from the examining room are recommended as a means of expediting the conduct of health services and eliminating confusion.

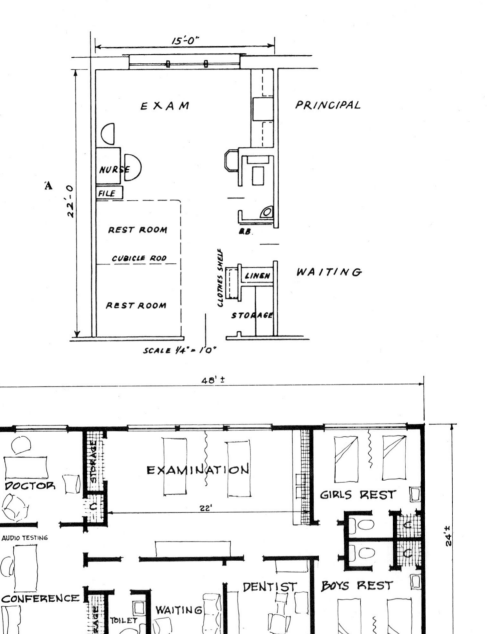

A, Health suite for elementary school—seven classrooms. **B,** Suggested health suite for over 1,100-pupil school. **C,** Suggested health suite for up to 700-pupil school. (From Participants in National Facilities Conference: Planning areas and facilities for health, physical education, and recreation, revised, Chicago, 1965, The Athletic Institute.)

The health service suite may also become the nurse's headquarters. In this case, there should be room for various items that are needed in her work, such as health records, desk, and files.

The color and furnishings of the waiting room should provide an attractive and cheerful atmosphere. A desk for clerical help can also be provided. There should be screens, if necessary, to give privacy to the examining and rest rooms that are part of the health suite and attached to the waiting room.

The examining room should be large enough to accommodate all the necessary equipment, supplies, and measuring devices. Provisions for eye testing, weighing, first aid, examining procedures, parent interviews, and other essentials should be kept in mind.

The rest rooms should be large enough to hold necessary cots, tables, and other items. They should also be equipped with subdued lighting, walls and ceilings that keep noise to a minimum, and other conveniences that contribute to rest.

A Committee on School Health Service Facilities of the American School Health Association conducted an extensive study of health service units throughout the country. This committee, recognizing that there could be no standard health unit that would meet the needs of schools everywhere, did, however, indicate what an average health unit might be, on the basis of statistical information gathered from their survey. According to this committee, the elementary school health service unit consisting of approximately 400 square feet would probably contain the following:

Examination room	Waiting room
Cot room	Dental ex-
Toilet room	amination room,
Storage spaces	in some cases
Testing and dressing room	

Health service units for secondary schools would require approximately 600 to 700 square feet of floor space and consist of the following:

Examination room	Storage spaces
Two cot rooms	Waiting room
Two toilet rooms	Testing room

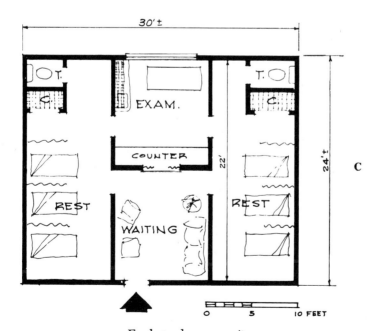

For legend see opposite page.

The following general statements help describe some essential considerations for a health service unit:

1. Future expansion should be considered.
2. The unit should be located near the administrative area, for ease of supervision, and away from noisy areas such as the shops, gymnasia, and music rooms.
3. Finishes should be of a type that can be easily maintained.
4. Attractive colors are important.
5. Service facilities such as sinks, lavatories, counters, and toilets should be of appropriate size for the pupils to be served.
6. Telephones are a necessity.

Cafeteria

The school lunch is a vital factor in the general health of any child and is an important part of his educational experiences. Furthermore, the cafeteria in any school or college recreational or other building is an important consideration and concern of individuals engaged in health, physical education, and recreation work.

The cafeteria should be easily accessible from anywhere within the building, as well as the service driveway. The size depends upon the number of individuals to be served. In general, from 10 to 12 square feet per person is required at peak load for the dining area.

The kitchen area will depend in size upon the number of meals to be prepared. The kitchen should contain all the equipment and supplies essential to the preparation and serving of good meals. Such equipment as ranges, ovens, sinks, dish-washing machines, refrigerators, tables, service trucks, counters, and kitchen machines such as mixers, peelers, and slicers should be provided.

The dining-room part of the cafeteria should be equipped with the necessary tables and chairs, serving counter, refrigerated counters, silver, napkins, plates, trays, drinking fountain, and other essentials.

The physical appearance of the cafeteria should be attractive, with adequate lighting, light colors, and floors that are easy to clean. The cafeteria should be quiet and conducive to enjoyable and satisfactory eating conditions.

OUTDOOR FACILITIES

The outdoor facilities that will be discussed in this section are (1) play areas, (2) game areas, (3) outdoor swimming pools, and (4) camps.

Play areas

Many things must be taken into consideration when planning outdoor facilities for schools and colleges. The location, topography, soil drainage, water supply, size, shape, and natural features are a few important considerations before a site is selected. The outdoor facilities should be as near the gymnasium and locker rooms as possible and yet far enough from the classrooms so that the noise will not be a disturbing factor.

The play areas should serve the needs and interests of the students for the entire school year and at the same time should provide a setting for activities during vacation periods. The needs and interests of the citizens of the community must also be taken into consideration, since the play areas can be used for part of the community recreation program. This is especially important in some communities where such facilities can be planned as education and recreation centers. Since the community uses the areas after the school day is over, the plan is feasible.

The size of the playground area should be determined on the basis of activities offered in the program and the number of individuals who will be using the facilities at peak load. Possibilities for expansion should also be kept in mind.

Playground and recreation areas will be discussed under the three headings of elementary, junior high, and senior high school.

Elementary school. The activities program in the elementary school suggests what facilities should be available. Children of the primary grades engage in big muscle activity involving adaptations of climbing, jumping, skipping, kicking, throwing, leaping, and catching. The children in the intermediate and upper elementary grades utilize not only these activities but also such other ones as games of low organization, team games, and fundamental skills used in playing these games.

The playground area for an elementary school should be located near the building and should be easily accessible from the elementary classrooms. The kindergarten children should have a section of the playground for their exclusive use. This should be at least 5,000 square feet in size and separated from the rest of the playground. It should consist of a surfaced area, a grass area, and a place for sand and digging. The sand area should be enclosed to prevent the sand from being scattered. It is also wise to have a shaded area where storytelling and similar activities may be conducted. Some essential equipment would include swings, slides, seesaws, climbing structures, tables, and seats.

The children older than kindergarten age in the elementary school should have play space that includes turf, apparatus, shaded, multiple-use paved, and recreation areas.

The turf area provides space for many field and team games. Provisions for speed ball, soccer, field hockey, softball, and field ball could be included.

The apparatus area should provide such equipment as climbing bars in the form of a Jungle Jim, horizontal bars, and Giant Strides. There should be ample space to provide for the safety of the participants.

The shaded area may provide space for

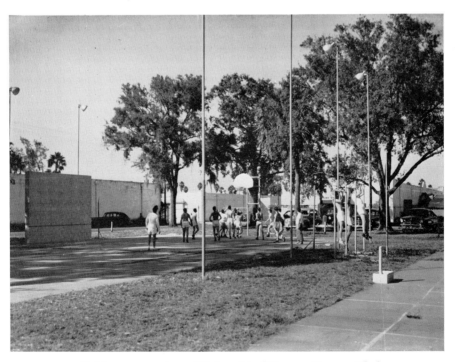

Outdoor gymnasium. (University of Tampa, Tampa, Fla.)

such activities as marbles, hopscotch, or ring toss and also storytelling.

The multiple-use paved area may serve for a variety of purposes and activities on a year-round basis by both school and community. It can house basketball, tennis, and handball courts, games of minimum organization, and other activities. This area should be paved with material that takes into consideration resiliency, safety, and durability. Rapid and efficient drainage is essential. Lines may be painted on the area for the various types of games. Schools should allow additional space adjacent to this area for possible future expansion.

Other recreation areas that have important implications for the community are a landscaped, parklike area, a place for quiet activities such as dramatics and informal gatherings, a wading pool, a place for older adults to congregate, and a place for children to have gardening opportunities.

Junior high school. The junior high school play and recreation area, planned and developed for the children who attend the school and also for the adults in the community, should be located on a larger site than that for the elementary school.

Some suggestions have been made that it consist of from 10 to 25 or more acres. Local conditions will play a part in deciding the amount of area available.

Many of the facilities of the elementary school will be a part of the junior high school. In many cases, however, the various areas should be increased in size. There should be a place for small children, apparatus, quiet games, and a wading pool, as in the elementary schools. The multiple-use paved area of turf area for games should be increased in size.

The program for junior high school girls will stress a broad base in fundamentals for participation in such activities as archery, volleyball, tennis, and hockey.

The boys' program will include soccer, touch football, baseball, speed ball, softball, and golf. A track should also be included. Therefore, the necessary facilities should provide for those activities that will be part of the regular physical education class as well as the intramural program.

A landscaped, parklike area should be provided for the various recreational activities in which people in the community will like to engage, such as walking, picnicking, skating, and fly casting.

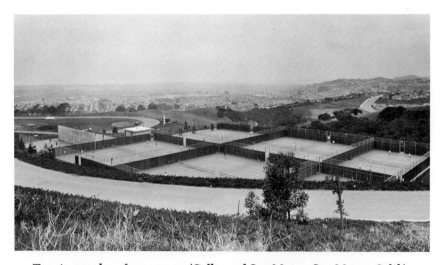

Tennis complex of ten courts. (College of San Mateo, San Mateo, Calif.)

Senior high school. The senior high school physical education program is characterized to a more pronounced degree by a team game program in various activities. This emphasis, together with the fact that facilities are needed for the recreational use of the community, requires an even larger area than those for the two previous educational levels. Estimates range from 10 to 40 acres for such a site.

Most of the areas that have been listed in discussing the elementary and junior high schools should again be included at the senior high school. This means there would be facilities for young children, such as apparatus, pool, and a place for quiet activities. Where there was an increase in size of many areas at the junior high over the elementary level, there should again be an increase in size at the high school level over the junior high.

There should be considerably more space for the various field games so that not only can physical education class instruction take place but also at the same time full-sized official fields will be available for such activities as softball, field hockey, soccer, speed ball, lacrosse, football, and baseball. This would be on an intramural as well as an interscholastic basis. Also, the community recreation program could make use of these facilities.

Football and track can be provided for in an area of approximately 4 acres, with the football field being placed within the track oval. A baseball field is questionable in such an area, because track and baseball are both spring sports. Baseball needs an

Table 15-2. Recommended dimensions for game areas*†

	Elementary	Upper grades	High school (adults)	Area size (sq. ft.)
Basketball	40′ × 60′	42′ × 74′	50′ × 84′	5,000
Volleyball	25′ × 50′	25′ × 50′	30′ × 60′	2,800
Badminton			20′ × 44′	1,800
Paddle tennis			20′ × 44′	1,800
Deck tennis			18′ × 40′	1,800
Tennis		36′ × 78′	36′ × 78′	7,200
Ice hockey			85′ × 200′	17,000
Field hockey			180′ × 300′	54,000
Horseshoes		10′ × 40′	10′ × 50′	1,000
Shuffleboard			6′ × 52′	648
Lawn bowling			14′ × 110′	7,800
Tetherball	10′ circle	12′ circle	12′ circle	
Croquet	38′ × 60′	38′ × 60′	38′ × 60′	2,275
Handball	18′ × 26′	18′ × 26′	20′ × 34′	1,280
Baseball			350′ × 350′	122,500
Archery		50′ × 150′	50′ × 300′	20,000
Softball (12″ ball)‡	150′ × 150′	200′ × 200′	250′ × 250′	62,500
Football—with 440-yard track—220-yard straightaway			300′ × 600′	180,000
Touch football		120′ × 300′	160′ × 360′	68,400
6-man football			120′ × 300′	49,500
Soccer			165′ × 300′	57,600

*From Planning facilities for health, physical education, and recreation, revised edition, Chicago, 1956, The Athletic Institute, Inc., p. 26.
†Table covers a single unit; many of above can be combined.
‡Dimensions vary with size of ball used.

area of about 350 feet by 350 feet. This allows for a minimum of 50 feet from home plate to the backstop and also allows for adequate space outside the first and third base lines.

Game areas

The recommended dimensions for game areas for school physical education programs have been outlined by a group of experts as shown in Table 15-2. An area of about 1 acre will accommodate four tennis courts, four handball courts, three badminton courts, and two volleyball courts.

There should be a separate area for high school girls with a minimum area of 320 feet by 280 feet, which is approximately 2 acres in size. Such an area will permit basic physical education instructional classes to be held and also provide fields for softball, field hockey, soccer, speedball, lacrosse, and other activities.

High school boys should also be adequately provided for in addition to the many courts areas that include basketball, softball, and other activities. There should be proper space for track if desired, an oval one-fourth mile in length or at least a straightaway of 380 feet and 15 to 20 feet in width. Of course, there is also the need for the interschool athletic area, which usually includes football, track, baseball, and soccer.

Not to be forgotten should be the winter activities. With such activities gaining increased popularity, provision should be made for skiing, sleds, skating, and other winter activities.

The New York State Department of Education* recommends that the outdoor facilities for the basic needs of a physical education and recreation program, from kindergarten to grade twelve, should consist of a minimum of 12 acres of land. This

area should be divided into an elementary area of 3 acres; courts area of 1 acre; high school girls' area of 2 acres, a high school boys' intramural area of 3 acres, and an interschool athletic area of 3 acres. The interschool athletic area would be used for baseball in the spring and summer and football or soccer in the fall. A quarter-mile track could also be added, but in this case the interschool athletic program should have 7 acres of land. The recommendation further points out that if archery, golf, natural theater, picnic area, skiing, and tobogganing area are desired, additional land will be necessary.

Outdoor swimming pools

The outdoor swimming pool is a popular and important facility in many communities. To a great degree climatic conditions will determine the advisability of such a facility.

Outdoor pools are built in various shapes, including oval, circular, T-shaped, and rectangular. Rectangular pools are most popular because of easier construction and because they lend themselves better to competitive swimming events.

The size of pools varies, depending upon the number of persons they are to serve. One recommendation has been made that 12 square feet of water space per swimmer be allotted for swimming purposes or, if the deck is taken into consideration, 20 square feet of space for swimming and walking area per swimmer.

The decks for outdoor pools should be larger than those for indoor pools. This larger space will serve to accommodate more people and also provide space for sunbathing.

Shower facilities should be provided to ensure that every swimmer takes a soapy shower in the nude before entering the water. A basket system for storing clothes has been found practical instead of the locker type of system that is used inside. In cases where the pool is located adjacent to

---

*New York State Department of Education: Planning the outdoor physical education facilities, Albany, 1964, The Department.

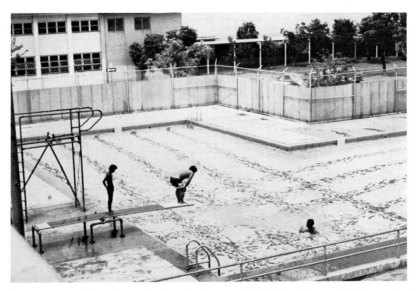

Swimming pool. (Wallace Rider Farrington High School, Honolulu, Hawaii.)

the school, it sometimes is practical to use the locker and shower facilities of the school. However, it is strongly advised that wherever possible separate shower and basket facilities be provided. Toilets should also be provided for the convenience of the swimmers.

Since swimming is popular at night as well as in the daytime, lights should be provided in order that a great percentage of the population may participate in this healthful and enjoyable activity.

Diving boards generally are of wood or metal, but in recent years glass and plastic ones have proved popular. The standard heights of boards are 1 and 3 meters. The 1-meter board should be over water 9 to 10 feet in depth and the 3-meter board over water 10 to 12 feet in depth. The board or any diving takeoff area should have a nonskid covering. The boards should be securely fastened to the ground or foundation.

The rules and regulations concerning diving equipment should be clearly posted near the diving areas. Roping off and patrolling the area is a good safety precaution.

The checklist at the end of the chapter provides further information on swimming pool standards.*

Camps†

Since camping is becoming an increasingly popular activity in both school and recreational programs, it should receive consideration.

Camps should be located within easy reach of the school and community. They should be in locations that are desirable from the standpoints of scenic beauty, safety, accessibility, water, and natural resources pertinent to the program offered. Activities usually offered include fishing, hiking, swimming, campcraft, boating, nature study, and appropriate winter sports. The natural terrain and other resources can contribute much toward such a program.

There should be adequate housing, eating, sanitary, waterfront, and other facilities essential to camp life. These do not have to be as elaborate as those in the home or school but instead can be very simple. Adequate facilities for protection

---

*For more information on swimming pools, see pp. 438-443.

†See Chapter 25.

against the elements are essential, however. Facilities should also meet acceptable standards of health and sanitation. In general, camp structures should be adapted to the climatic conditions of the particular area in which the camp is located. It is wise to consult public health authorities when selecting a camp site. Sometimes existing facilities can be converted to camp use. The camp site should be purchased outright or a long-term lease acquired.

CHECKLIST FOR FACILITY PLANNERS*

General

	Yes	No
1. A clear-cut statement has been prepared on the nature and scope of the program, and the special requirements for space, equipment, fixtures, and facilities dictated by the activities to be conducted.	___	___
2. The facility has been planned to meet the total requirements of the program as well as the special needs of those who are to be served.	___	___
3. The plans and specifications have been checked by all governmental agencies (city, county, and state) whose approval is required by law.	___	___
4. Plans for areas and facilities conform to state and local regulations and to accepted standards and practices.	___	___
5. The areas and facilities planned make possible the programs which serve the interests and needs of all the people.	___	___
6. Every available source of property or funds has been explored, evaluated, and utilized whenever appropriate.	___	___
7. All interested persons and organizations concerned with the facility have had an opportunity to share in its planning (professional educators, users, consultants, administrators, engineers, architects, program specialists, building managers, and builder—a team approach).	___	___
8. The facility and its appurtenances will fulfill the maximum demands of the program. The program has not been curtailed to fit the facility.	___	___
9. The facility has been functionally planned to meet the present and anticipated needs of specific programs, situations, and publics.	___	___
10. Future additions are included in present plans to permit economy of construction.	___	___
11. Lecture classrooms are isolated from distracting noises.	___	___
12. Storage areas for indoor and outdoor equipment are adequately sized. They are located adjacent to the gymnasia.	___	___
13. Shelves in storage rooms are slanted toward the wall.	___	___
14. All passageways are free of obstructions; fixtures are recessed.	___	___
15. Facilities for health services, health testing, health instruction, and the first-aid and emergency-isolation rooms are suitably interrelated.	___	___
16. Buildings, specific areas, and facilities are clearly identified.	___	___
17. Locker rooms are arranged for ease of supervision.	___	___
18. Offices, teaching stations, and service facilities are properly interrelated.	___	___
19. Special needs of the physically handicapped are met, including a ramp into the building at a major entrance.	___	___
20. All "dead space" is used.	___	___
21. The building is compatible in design and comparable in quality and accommodation to other campus structures.	___	___
22. Storage rooms are accessible to the play area.	___	___

*Adapted from Participants in National Facilities Conference: Planning areas and facilities for health, physical education, and recreation, Washington, D. C., 1965, American Association for Health, Physical Education, and Recreation, pp. 256-260.

CHECKLIST FOR FACILITY PLANNERS–cont'd

General–cont'd

	Yes	No

23. Workrooms, conference rooms, and staff and administrative offices are inter-related.

24. Shower and dressing facilities are provided for professional staff members and are conveniently located.

25. Thought and attention have been given to making facilities and equipment as durable and vandalproof as possible.

26. Low-cost maintenance features have been adequately considered.

27. This facility is a part of a well-integrated master plan.

28. All areas, courts, facilities, equipment, climate control, security, etc. conform rigidly to detailed standards and specifications.

29. Shelves are recessed and mirrors are supplied in appropriate places in rest rooms and dressing rooms. Mirrors are not placed above lavatories.

30. Dressing space between locker rows is adjusted to the size and age level of students.

31. Drinking fountains are conveniently placed in locker-room areas or immediately adjacent thereto.

32. Special attention is given to provision for the locking of service windows and counters, supply bins, carts, shelves, and racks.

33. Provision is made for the repair, maintenance, replacement, and off-season storage of equipment and uniforms.

34. A well-defined program for laundering and cleaning of towels, uniforms, and equipment is included in the plan.

35. Noncorrosive metal is used in dressing, drying, and shower areas except for enameled lockers.

36. Antipanic hardware is used where required by fire regulations.

37. Properly placed hose bibbs and drains are sufficient in size and quantity to permit flushing the entire area with a water hose.

38. A water-resistant, coved base is used under the locker base and floor mat, and where floor and wall join.

39. Chalkboards and/or tackboards with map tracks are located in appropriate places in dressing rooms, hallways, and classrooms.

40. Book shelves are provided in toilet areas.

41. Space and equipment are planned in accordance with the types and number of enrollees.

42. Basement rooms, being undesirable for dressing, drying, and showering, are not planned for those purposes.

43. Spectator seating (permanent) in areas which are basically instructional is kept at a minimum. Roll-away bleachers are used primarily. Balcony seating is considered as a possibility.

44. Well-lighted and effectively displayed trophy cases enhance the interest and beauty of the lobby.

45. The space under the stairs is used for storage.

46. Department heads' offices are located near the central administrative office, which includes a well-planned conference room.

47. Workrooms are located near the central office and serve as a repository for departmental materials and records.

48. The conference area includes a cloak room, lavatory, and toilet.

49. In addition to regular secretarial offices established in the central and department chairmen's offices, a special room to house a secretarial pool for staff members is provided.

50. Staff dressing facilities are provided. These facilities may also serve game officials.

Continued.

CHECKLIST FOR FACILITY PLANNERS–cont'd

General–cont'd

	Yes	No

51. The community and/or neighborhood has a "round table"—planning round table.

52. All those (persons and agencies) who should be a party to planning and development are invited and actively engaged in the planning process.

53. Space and area relationships are important. They have been carefully considered.

54. Both long-range plans and immediate plans have been made.

55. The body comfort of the child, a major factor in securing maximum learning, has been considered in the plans.

56. Plans for quiet areas have been made.

57. In the planning, consideration has been given to the need for adequate recreation areas and facilities, both near and distant from the homes of people.

58. Plans recognize the primary function of recreation as being enrichment of learning through creative self-expression, self-enhancement, and the achievement of self-potential.

59. Every effort has been exercised to eliminate hazards.

60. The installation of low-hanging door closers, light fixtures, signs, and other objects in traffic areas has been avoided.

61. Warning signals—both visible and audible—are included in the plans.

62. Ramps have a slope equal to or greater than a 1-foot rise in 12 feet.

63. Minimum landings for ramps are 5 feet × 5 feet, they extend at least 1 foot beyond the swinging arc of a door, have at least a 6-foot clearance at the bottom, and have level platforms at 30-foot intervals on every turn.

64. Adequate locker and dressing spaces are provided.

65. The design of dressing, drying, and shower areas reduces foot traffic to a minimum and establishes clean, dry aisles for bare feet.

66. Teaching stations are properly related to service facilities.

67. Toilet facilities are adequate in number. They are located to serve all groups for which provisions are made.

68. Mail services, outgoing and incoming, are included in the plans.

69. Hallways, ramps, doorways, and elevators are designed to permit equipment to be moved easily and quickly.

70. A keying design suited to administrative and instructional needs is planned.

71. Toilets used by large groups have circulating (in and out) entrances and exits.

Climate control

1. Provision is made throughout the building for climate control—heating, ventilating, and refrigerated cooling.

2. Special ventilation is provided for locker, dressing, shower, drying, and toilet rooms.

3. Heating plans permit both area and individual room control.

4. Research areas where small animals are kept and where chemicals are used have been provided with special ventilating equipment.

5. The heating and ventilating of the wrestling gymnasium have been given special attention.

Electrical

1. Shielded, vaporproof lights are used in moisture-prevalent areas.

2. Lights in strategic areas are key controlled.

3. Lighting intensity conforms to approved standards.

CHECKLIST FOR FACILITY PLANNERS–cont'd

Electrical–cont'd

	Yes	No

4. An adequate number of electrical outlets are strategically placed.
5. Gymnasium and auditorium lights are controlled by dimmer units.
6. Locker-room lights are mounted above the space between lockers.
7. Natural light is controlled properly for purposes of visual aids and other avoidance of glare.
8. Electrical outlet plates are installed 3 feet above the floor unless special use dictates other locations.
9. Controls for light switches and projection equipment are suitably located and interrelated.
10. All lights are shielded. Special protection is provided in gymnasia, court areas, and shower rooms.
11. Lights are placed to shine between rows of lockers.

Walls

1. Movable and folding partitions are power-operated and controlled by keyed switches.
2. Wall plates are located where needed and are firmly attached.
3. Hooks and rings for nets are placed (and recessed in walls) according to court locations and net heights.
4. Materials that clean easily and are impervious to moisture are used where moisture is prevalent.
5. Shower heads are placed at different heights—4 feet (elementary) to 7 feet (university)—for each school level.
6. Protective matting is placed permanently on the walls in the wrestling room, at the ends of basketball courts, and in other areas where such protection is needed.
7. An adequate number of drinking fountains is provided. They are properly placed (recessed in wall).
8. One wall (at least) of the dance studio has full-length mirrors.
9. All corners in locker rooms are rounded.

Ceilings

1. Overhead-supported apparatus is secured to beams engineered to withstand stress.
2. The ceiling height is adequate for the activities to be housed.
3. Acoustical materials impervious to moisture are used in moisture-prevalent areas.
4. Skylights, being impractical, are seldom used because of problems in waterproofing roofs and the controlling of sun rays (gyms).
5. All ceilings except those in storage areas are acoustically treated with sound-absorbent materials.

Floors

1. Floor plates are placed where needed and are flush-mounted.
2. Floor design and materials conform to recommended standards and specifications.
3. Lines and markings are painted on floors before sealing is completed (when synthetic tape is not used).
4. A coved base (around lockers and where wall and floor meet) of the same water-resistant material used on floors is found in all dressing and shower rooms.

Continued.

CHECKLIST FOR FACILITY PLANNERS–cont'd

Floors—cont'd

5. Abrasive, nonskid, slip-resistant flooring that is impervious to moisture is provided on all areas where water is used—laundry, swimming pool, shower, dressing, and drying rooms.   ____ ____
6. Floor drains are properly located and the slope of the floor is adequate for rapid drainage.   ____ ____

Gymnasia and special rooms

1. Gymnasia are planned so as to provide for safety zones (between courts, end lines, and walls) and for best utilization of space.   ____ ____
2. One gymnasium wall is free of obstructions and is finished with a smooth, hard surface for ball-rebounding activities.   ____ ____
3. The elementary school gymnasium has one wall free of obstructions; a minimum ceiling height of 18 feet; a minimum of 4,000 square feet of teaching area; and a recessed area for housing a piano.   ____ ____
4. Secondary school gymnasia have a minimum ceiling height of 22 feet; a scoreboard; electrical outlets placed to fit with bleacher installation; wall attachments for apparatus and nets; and a power-operated, sound-insulated, and movable partition with a small pass-through door at one end.   ____ ____
5. A small spectator alcove adjoins the wrestling room and contains a drinking fountain (recessed in the wall).   ____ ____
6. Cabinets, storage closets, supply windows, and service areas have locks.   ____ ____
7. Provisions have been made for the cleaning, storing, and issuing of physical education and athletic uniforms.   ____ ____
8. Shower heads are placed at varying heights in the shower rooms on each school level.   ____ ____
9. Equipment is provided for the use of the physically handicapped.   ____ ____
10. Special provision has been made for audio and visual aids, including intercommunication systems, radio, and television.   ____ ____
11. Team dressing rooms have provisions for:
    a. Hosing down room   ____ ____
    b. Floors pitched to drain easily   ____ ____
    c. Hot- and cold-water hose bibbs   ____ ____
    d. Windows located above locker heights.   ____ ____
    e. Chalk, tack, and bulletin boards, and movie projection   ____ ____
    f. Lockers for each team member   ____ ____
    g. Drying facility for uniforms   ____ ____
12. The indoor rifle range includes:
    a. Targets located 54 inches apart and 50 feet from the firing line   ____ ____
    b. 3 feet to 8 feet of space behind targets   ____ ____
    c. 12 feet of space behind firing line   ____ ____
    d. Ceilings 8 feet high   ____ ____
    e. Width adjusted to number of firing lines needed (1 line for each 3 students)   ____ ____
    f. A pulley device for target placement and return   ____ ____
    g. Storage and repair space   ____ ____
13. Dance facilities include:
    a. 100 square feet per student   ____ ____
    b. A minimum length of 60 linear feet for modern dance   ____ ____
    c. Full-height viewing mirrors on one wall (at least) of 30 feet; also a 20-foot mirror on an additional wall if possible   ____ ____
    d. Acoustical drapery to cover mirrors when not used and for protection if other activities are permitted   ____ ____

CHECKLIST FOR FACILITY PLANNERS–cont'd

Gymnasia and special rooms–cont'd

	Yes	No
e. Dispersed microphone jacks and speaker installation for music and instruction	—	—
f. Built-in cabinets for record players, microphones, and amplifiers, with space for equipment carts	—	—
g. Electrical outlets and microphone connections around perimeter of room	—	—
h. An exercise bar (34 inches to 42 inches above floor) on one wall	—	—
i. Drapes, surface colors, floors (maple preferred), and other room appointments to enhance the room's attractiveness	—	—
j. Location near dressing rooms and outside entrances	—	—
14. Training rooms include:		
a. Rooms large enough to administer adequately proper health services	—	—
b. Sanitary storage cabinets for medical supplies	—	—
c. Installation of drains for whirlpool, tubs, etc.	—	—
d. Installation of electrical outlets with proper capacities and voltage	—	—
e. High stools for use of equipment such as whirlpool, ice tubs, etc.	—	—
f. Water closet, hand lavatory, and shower	—	—
g. Extra hand lavatory in the trainer's room proper	—	.—
h. Adjoining dressing rooms	—	—
i. Installation and use of hydrotherapy and diathermy equipment in separate areas	—	—
j. Space for the trainer, the physician, and the various services of this function	—	—
k. Corrective-exercise laboratories located conveniently and adapted to the needs of the handicapped	—	—
15. Coaches' rooms should provide:		
a. A sufficient number of dressing lockers for coaching staff and officials	—	—
b. A security closet or cabinet for athletic equipment such as timing devices	—	—
c. A sufficient number of showers and toilet facilities	—	—
d. Drains and faucets for hosing down the rooms where this method of cleaning is desirable and possible	—	—
e. A small chalkboard and tackboard	—	—
f. A small movie screen and projection table for use of coaches to review films	—	—

Handicapped and disabled

Have you included those considerations that would make the facility accessible to, and usable by, the disabled? These considerations include:

	Yes	No
1. The knowledge that the disabled will be participants in almost all activities, not merely spectators, if the facility is properly planned.	—	—
2. Ground-level entrance(s) or stair-free entrance(s) using inclined walk(s) or inclined ramp(s).	—	—
3. Uninterrupted walk surface; no abrupt changes in levels leading to the facility.	—	—
4. Approach walks and connecting walks no less than 4 feet in width.	—	—
5. Walks with a gradient no greater than 5%.	—	—
6. A ramp, when used, with rise no greater than 1 foot in 12 feet.	—	—
7. Flat or level surface inside and outside of all exterior doors, extending 5 feet from the door in the direction that the door swings, and extending 1 foot to each side of the door.	—	—
8. Flush thresholds at all doors.	—	—
9. Appropriate door widths, heights, and mechanical features.	—	—
10. At least 6 feet between vestibule doors in series, i.e., inside and outside doors.	—	—
11. Access and proximity to parking areas.	—	—

Continued.

CHECKLIST FOR FACILITY PLANNERS–cont'd

Handicapped and disabled–cont'd

Yes   *No*

12. No obstructions by curbs at crosswalks, parking areas, etc.   ___   ___
13. Proper precautions (handrails, etc.) at basement-window areaways, open stairways, porches, ledges, and platforms.   ___   ___
14. Handrails on all steps and ramps.   ___   ___
15. Precautions against the placement of manholes in principal or major sidewalks.
16. Corridors that are at least 60 inches wide and without abrupt pillars or protrusions.   ___   ___
17. Floors which are nonskid and have no abrupt changes or interruptions in level.   ___   ___
18. Proper design of steps.   ___   ___
19. Access to rest rooms, water coolers, telephones, food-service areas, lounges, dressing rooms, play areas, and all auxiliary services and areas.   ___   ___
20. Elevators in multiple-story buildings.   ___   ___
21. Appropriate placement of controls to permit and to prohibit use as desired.   ___   ___
22. Sound signals for the blind, and visual signals for the deaf as counterparts to regular sound and sight signals.   ___   ___
23. Proper placement, concealment, or insulation of radiators, heat pipes, hot-water pipes, drain pipes, etc.   ___   ___

Swimming pools

1. Has a clear-cut statement been prepared on the nature and scope of the design program and the special requirements for space, equipment, and facilities dictated by the activities to be conducted?   ___   ___
2. Has the swimming pool been planned to meet the total requirements of the program to be conducted as well as any special needs of the clientele to be served?   ___   ___
3. Have all plans and specifications been checked and approved by the local board of health?   ___   ___
4. Is the pool the proper depth to accommodate the various age groups and types of activities it is intended to serve?   ___   ___
5. Does the design of the pool incorporate the most current knowledge and best experience available regarding swimming pools?   ___   ___
6. If a local architect or engineer who is inexperienced in pool construction is employed, has an experienced pool consultant, architect, or engineer been called in to advise on design and equipment?   ___   ___
7. Is there adequate deep water for diving (minimum of 9 feet for 1-meter boards, 12 feet for 3-meter boards, and 15 feet for 10-meter towers)?   ___   ___
8. Have the requirements for competitive swimming been met (7-foot lanes; 12-inch black or brown lines on the bottom; pool 1 inch longer than official measurement; depth and distance markings)?   ___   ___
9. Is there adequate deck space around the pool? Has more space been provided than that indicated by the minimum recommended deck/pool ratio?   ___   ___
10. Does the swimming instructor's office face the pool? And is there a window through which the instructor may view all the pool area? Is there a toilet-shower-dressing area next to the office for instructors?   ___   ___
11. Are recessed steps or removable ladders located on the walls so as not to interfere with competitive swimming turns?   ___   ___
12. Does a properly constructed overflow gutter extend around the pool perimeter?   ___   ___
13. Where skimmers are used, have they been properly located so that they are not on walls where competitive swimming is to be conducted?   ___   ___

CHECKLIST FOR FACILITY PLANNERS–cont'd

Swimming pools–cont'd

	Yes	*No*
14. Have separate storage spaces been allocated for maintenance and instructional equipment?	____	____
15. Has the area for spectators been properly separated from the pool area?	____	____
16. Have all diving standards and lifeguard chairs been properly anchored?	____	____
17. Does the pool layout provide the most efficient control of swimmers from showers and locker rooms to the pool? Are toilet facilities provided for wet swimmers separate from the dry area?	____	____
18. Is the recirculation pump located below the water level?	____	____
19. Is there easy vertical access to the filter room for both people and material (stairway if required)?	____	____
20. Has the proper pitch to drains been allowed in the pool, on the pool deck, in the overflow gutter, and on the floor of shower and dressing rooms?	____	____
21. Has adequate space been allowed between diving boards and between the diving boards and sidewalls?	____	____
22. Is there adequate provision for lifesaving equipment? Pool-cleaning equipment?	____	____
23. Are inlets and outlets adequate in number and located so as to ensure effective circulation of water in the pool?	____	____
24. Has consideration been given to underwater lights, underwater observation windows, and underwater speakers?	____	____
25. Is there a coping around the edge of the pool?	____	____
26. Has a pool heater been considered in northern climates in order to raise the temperature of the water?	____	____
27. Have underwater lights in end racing walls been located deep enough and directly below surface lane anchors, and are they on a separate circuit?	____	____
28. Has the plan been considered from the standpoint of handicapped persons (e.g., is there a gate adjacent to the turnstiles)?	____	____
29. Is seating for swimmers provided on the deck?	____	____
30. Has the recirculation-filtration system been designed to meet the anticipated future bathing load?	____	____
31. Has the gas chlorinator (if used) been placed in a separate room accessible from and vented to the outside?	____	____
32. Has the gutter waste water been valved to return to the filters, and also for direct waste?	____	____

Indoor pools

1. Is there proper mechanical ventilation?	____	____
2. Is there adequate acoustical treatment of walls and ceilings?	____	____
3. Is there adequate overhead clearance for diving (15 feet above low springboards, 15 feet for 3-meter boards, and 10 feet for 10-meter platforms)?	____	____
4. Is there adequate lighting (50 footcandles minimum)?	____	____
5. Has reflection of light from the outside been kept to the minimum by proper location of windows or skylights (windows on side walls are not desirable)?	____	____
6. Are all wall bases coved to facilitate cleaning?	____	____
7. Is there provision for proper temperature control in the pool room for both water and air?	____	____
8. Can the humidity of the pool room be controlled?	____	____
9. Is the wall and ceiling insulation adequate to prevent "sweating"?	____	____
10. Are all metal fittings of noncorrosive material?	____	____
11. Is there a tunnel around the outside of the pool, or a trench on the deck which permits ready access to pipes?	____	____

Continued.

CHECKLIST FOR FACILITY PLANNERS—cont'd

                                                                              Yes   No

Outdoor pools

1. Is the site for the pool in the best possible location (away from railroad tracks, heavy industry, trees, and open fields which are dusty)?   ——   ——
2. Have sand and grass been kept the proper distance away from the pool to prevent them from being transmitted to the pool?   ——   ——
3. Has a fence been placed around the pool to assure safety when not in use?   ——   ——
4. Has proper subsurface drainage been provided?   ——   ——
5. Is there adequate deck space for sunbathing?   ——   ——
6. Are the outdoor lights placed far enough from the pool to prevent insects from dropping into the pool?   ——   ——
7. Is the deck of nonslip material?   ——   ——
8. Is there an area set aside for eating, separated from the pool deck?   ——   ——
9. Is the bathhouse properly located, with the entrance to the pool leading to the shallow end?   ——   ——
10. If the pool shell contains a concrete finish, has the length of the pool been increased by 3 inches over the "official" size in order to permit eventual tiling of the basin without making the pool "too short"?   ——   ——
11. Are there other recreational facilities nearby for the convenience and enjoyment of swimmers?   ——   ——
12. Do diving boards or platforms face north or east?   ——   ——
13. Are lifeguard stands provided and properly located?   ——   ——
14. Has adequate parking space been provided and properly located?   ——   ——
15. Is the pool oriented correctly in relation to the sun?   ——   ——
16. Have windshields been provided in situations where heavy winds prevail?   ——   ——

Questions and exercises

1. Prepare a sketch of what you consider to be an ideal physical education plant. In your plans consider both outdoor and indoor facilities.
2. Plan a health suite that you consider to be ideal.
3. What are ten basic considerations in planning facilities?
4. Discuss the following statement: The trend in schoolhouse construction is away from the so-called frills.
5. Develop a list of standards for outdoor play areas and locker, shower, and drying room facilities in the following areas: (a) lighting, (b) heating and ventilation, (c) plant sanitation, (d) furniture.
6. What are some of the essential factors to keep in mind when planning the gymnasium?
7. What should be provided in the school in the way of special activity areas?
8. What are some of the essential factors to keep in mind when planning the swimming pool?
9. What considerations should be made in school facilities for recreation?

10. Draw up a list of references for obtaining authoritative information on various aspects of facility construction and maintenance.

Reading assignment in *Administrative Dimensions of Health and Physical Education Programs, Including Athletics:* Chapter 12, Selections 63 to 69.

Selected references

American Association for Health, Physical Education, and Recreation: Planning areas and facilities for health, physical education, and recreation, Washington, D. C., 1965, The Association.

Architectural Research Group: Shelter for physical education, College Station, Texas, 1961, Publications Department, Texas Engineering Experiment Station, A & M College of Texas.

Athletic Institute and American Association for Health, Physical Education, and Recreation: Equipment and supplies for athletics, physical education, and recreation, Chicago, 1960, The Institute.

California State Department of Education: Brief statement of principles involving the construction of school health unit, State Health Committee Bulletin, Sacramento, The Department.

California State Joint Committee on School Health: Guide and check list for healthful and safe school environment, Sacramento, The Committee.

DeWeese, A. O., and Moore, V. M.: The organization of a school health service comprising from 500 to 1000 pupils from kindergarten through high school, Journal of School Health **34**:415, 1964.

Dickey, D. D.: Athletic lockers for schools and colleges, Minneapolis, Minnesota, Post Office Box 6630, 1967.

Educational Facilities Laboratories, Inc.: Air structures for school sports, New York, 1964, The Laboratories.

Gabrielsen, M. A.: Swimming pool planning and utilization, a speech to the Conference on Planning, Constructing, Utilizing Physical Education, Recreation, and Athletic Facilities at Columbus, Ohio, December 10, 1969.

Gabrielsen, M. A., and Miles, C. M.: Sports and recreation facilities for school and community, Englewood Cliffs, N. J., 1958, Prentice-Hall, Inc.

Grieve, A.: Legal considerations of equipment and facilities, The Athletic Journal **47**:38, 1967.

Joint Committee on Health Problems in Education of National Education Association and American Medical Association: Healthful school environment, Washington, D. C., 1969, The Association.

Leu, D. J.: Planning educational facilities, New York, 1965, The Center for Applied Research, Inc. (The Library of Education).

New York State Department of Education: Planning the indoor physical education facilities, Albany, 1962, The State Department of Education.

Scott, H. A., and Westkaemper, R. B.: From program to facilities in physical education, New York, 1958, Harper & Row, Publishers.

The State Education Department, The University of the State of New York: Planning the outdoor physical education facilities for central schools, Albany, 1964, The Department.

Wetzel, C. H.: Planning gym seating for long-range needs, Scholastic Coach **30**:48, 1961.

Annuals and periodicals

Professional architectural and educational magazines devote considerable space to the planning, designing, constructing, equipping, and managing of school facilities. The school facilities articles appearing in the annuals and periodicals listed below are usually concerned with specific school plants of recent construction and are illustrated with drawings and photographs. Some of these periodicals issue special editions that are devoted entirely to school facilities.

Architectural

Architectural Forum, Time, Inc., 9 Rockefeller Plaza, New York, N. Y. 10020

Architectural Record, F. W. Dodge Corp., 119 W. 40th St., New York, N. Y. 10018

Progressive Architecture, Reinhold Publishing Corp, 430 Park Ave., New York, N. Y. 10022

Educational

American School and University, Buttenheim Publishing Corp., 470 Park Ave. South, New York, N. Y. 10016 (annual).

American School Board Journal, Bruce Publishing Co., Milwaukee, Wis.

Nation's Schools, Modern Hospital Publishing Co., Inc., 1050 Merchandise Mart, Chicago, Ill. 60654

Overview, Buttenheim Publishing Corp., 470 Park Ave. South, New York, N. Y. 10016

School Management, School Management, Inc., 22 W. Putnam Ave., Greenwich, Conn.

School Planning, School Planning, Inc., 75 E. Wacker Dr., Chicago, Ill. 60601

Budgeting and financial accounting provide the necessary administrative machinery and operations to request funds, make them available for special facilities, programs, projects, and individuals, and then exercise control to see that they are used in an efficient manner. Administration is responsible for this function. It is an important duty and one that requires special qualities of integrity, foresight, wisdom, and firmness.

Fiscal management reflects the administrative program. It shows where the emphasis is, what is considered important in long-term planning, and the activities that need developing. The administration must therefore closely coordinate program with budgeting and financial accounting. The two go hand in hand.

IMPORTANCE OF FISCAL MANAGEMENT

The services that a school system provides, whether personal help, facilities, instructional materials, or other items, usually involve the disbursement of money. This money must be secured from proper sources, be expended in the light of educational purposes, and be accounted for item by item. The budget, the master financial plan for the entire school or college system or any subdivision, is constructed with this purpose in mind.

There must be well-thought-through policies for the raising and spending of school or college money. Educators should know the procedures for handling such funds with integrity, the basic purposes for which the educational program exists, the school

laws, and the codes and regulations concerning fiscal management. Education is big business and is rapidly occupying a major role in the fiscal planning of national, state, and local units of government. Only as the funds are used wisely and in the best interests of the students and all people concerned can the large outlay of monies be justified.

PLACE OF FINANCIAL MANAGEMENT IN HEALTH AND PHYSICAL EDUCATION PROGRAMS

Of all the subject matter areas in elementary, secondary, or college and university educational systems, health and physical education require one of the largest outlays of funds in order that the educational programs may be conducted effectively. The cost of personnel, health services, facilities, and supplies and equipment are only a few of the items that amount to large sums of money. As much as 25% of many school and college plants are devoted to these programs. There are probably 200,000 physical educators and coaches getting paid at least $1 billion annually in salaries. More than 60 million children and young people are the focus of attention in health and physical education.

Gymnasia, swimming pools, health suites, playgrounds, and other facilities are being constructed at the cost of astronomical sums to taxpayers.

With such a great outlay of funds for health and physical education programs, there must be sound financial management to see that the monies are utilized in the best way possible. This is one of the most important responsibilities that educators, and particularly administrators, have.

Purposes of financial management

Some of the principal purposes for which financial management exists in health and physical education programs are as follows:

1. To prevent misuse and waste of funds that have been allocated to these special fields.
2. To help coordinate and relate the objectives of health and physical education programs with the money appropriated for achieving such outcomes.
3. To ensure that monies allocated to health and physical education will be based upon research, study, and a careful analysis of the pertinent conditions that influence such a process.
4. To involve the entire staff in formulating policies and procedures and in preparing budgetary items that will help ensure that the right program directions are taken.
5. To utilize funds in a manner that will develop the best programs of health and physical education possible.
6. To exercise control over the process of fiscal management in order to guarantee that the entire financial process has integrity and purpose.
7. To make the greatest use of personnel, facilities, supplies, equipment, and other factors involved in accomplishing educational objectives.

Responsibility

The responsibility for fiscal management, although falling largely upon the shoulders of the administration, involves every person who is a member of the school staff, as well as the pupils themselves.

Formulation and preparation of the budget, for example, is a cooperative enterprise in many respects. It is based on information and reports that have been forwarded by faculty and staff through the various departments and subdivisions of the organization. These reports must contain information on programs, projects, obligations that exist, funds that have been spent, and monies that have been received from various sources. Staff members help in this process. Administrators must have an overall picture of the entire enterprise at their fingertips. They must be cognizant of the work being done throughout the establishment, functions that should be carried out, needs of every facet of the organization, and other items that must be considered in the preparation of the budget. The larger the organization, the larger should be the budget organization under the administrator. The efficiency of the enterprise depends upon expert judgment in fiscal matters. Students themselves play a part in many school and college systems. For example, through general organizations, budgets are prepared and outlays of funds relating to many activities, such as plays and athletics, are either approved, amended, or rejected. Fiscal management involves many people, but the job of leadership and direction falls upon the administration.

COST ANALYSIS

Cost analysis of materials consumed or used in a program is a derivative of cost accounting. The need for cost analysis is to aid the administrator to evaluate present operations as well as to project future planning. Cost analysis is limited to the types of accounting systems being used as well as designating the unit to be compared. For example, some schools operate on grades one to eight, kindergarten to grade twelve, or some other educational pattern. Naturally, there would be a great difference in expenditures per pupil in the various patterns or organization.

Various units are used in cost analysis for the general education fund. The number of pupils in attendance, the census, average daily attendance, and average daily membership are some of those that are used. There are advantages and disadvantages to each of the various units.

Knezevich and Fowlkes* found in their study that the most common raw per capita unit used in cost analysis is per pupil in average daily attendance. In other words, educational costs are figured on a per pupil basis and the total number of pupils involved is computed by determining what the average daily pupil attendance is in a school or educational system. This figure is arrived at by adding the aggregated days of attendance of all pupils and then dividing by the number of days school was in session. The number of pupils in average daily attendance is then divided into the total of the educational costs in order to obtain the cost per pupil in average daily attendance. It should be recognized, however, there is no universally accepted definition of average daily attendance. Whereas some states would permit all pupils to be counted in attendance when teachers are attending a state teachers meeting, others would not.

Knezevich and Fowlkes also pointed out that as a raw measure of educational burden, the average daily membership is a better measure than the average daily attendance. Teachers' salaries must be paid whether pupils are in 90% or 100% attendance, and desks and school books must be available whether pupils are in attendance or not. As raw per capita units go, the average daily membership is a better unit to measure the educational burden than the more commonly used average daily attendance unit. Tradition, however, has favored the average daily attendance

unit over that of average daily membership.*

Cost analysis as it relates to equipment and supplies for health and physical education may be simply handled by allowing a certain number of dollars per pupil enrolled in the district or on the various levels in the school system. The New York State Education Department, for example, publishes an analysis of the monies spent on different budget categories on a pupil basis, depending on the type and size of the school.† This is very helpful and offers the business administrator a guide to the problem of budget allocation.

Good business administration should allow a space on the budget sheet for personnel in all departments to list any needs over the specified allocations and a place to state reasons for the listing. One of the drawbacks of using cost analysis sheets is that it is physically impossible for the data to be current.

Some experts in fiscal management feel that a per capita expenditure allocation for health and physical education represents a good foundation program. However, they recommend, in addition, (1) an extra percentage allocation for program enrichment, (2) an extra percentage allocation for variation in enrollment, and (3) a reference to a commodity index (current prices of equipment and supplies) that may indicate need for changes in the per capita expenditure because of current increase or decrease in the value of the items being purchased.

Cost analysis in practice in physical education programs

In order to provide the reader with an understanding of the amount of money

---

*Knezevich, S. J., and Fowlkes, J. G.: Business management of local school systems, New York, 1960, Harper & Row, Publishers, p. 157.

*Knezevich, S. J., and Fowlkes, J. G., op. cit., p. 15.

†Bureau of Statistical Services: Expenditures per pupil in average daily attendance, Division of Educational Management Services, State Education Department, The University of the State of New York, Albany, N. Y.

allocated to physical education programs throughout the United States and how it is determined, a survey of selected school systems was accomplished. The following paragraphs are cited examples of money allocation in several cities.

California. A large city system in California reports that physical education

supplies are included in each school's allocation for instructional supplies, with the amount being based upon the number of pupils enrolled—elementary schools, $3.25 per pupil; junior high schools, $2.44 per pupil; and senior high schools, $2.15 per pupil.

Physical education equipment was in-

AVERAGE P.E. BUDGETS
(NOT INCLUDING INTERSCHOLASTIC ATHLETIC PROGRAM)

Level	Cost/student	Avg'e cost/District
ELEMENTARY	$ .67	$ 6,000.00
JR. HIGH	2.34	6,670.00
HIGH SCHOOL (By District Enrollment) under 1000	13.70	6,610.00
1000-5000	10.20	11,120.00
over 5000	2.40	22,200.00

COST - HIGH SCHOOL INTERSCHOLASTIC ATHLETIC PROGRAM

District Enrollment	Cost/student	Avg'e cost/District
under 1000	No. of participants not known	$ 8,585.00
1000 - 5000		20,900.00
over 5000		95,625.00

DEFICIT SPENDING - HIGH SCHOOL INTERSCHOLASTIC ATHLETIC PROGRAM

District Enrollment	% of Districts reporting cost of program exceeds gate receipts	Am't of deficit reported by individual schools Min.	Max.
under 1000	62%	$ 21.00	$ 22,296.00
1000-5000	43%	1500.00	20,500.00
over 5000	37%	15,652.00	164,445.00

Cost analysis in physical education. Reports on sixty-eight school districts in forty states. (From A study of the feasibility of the use of limited shelters for physical education: partial shelter for physical education, College Station, Texas, 1961, Texas Engineering Experiment Station, Texas A & M University.)

cluded in the budget for the year at a figure of $32,000. The maintenance of physical education equipment was provided for, as needed, by the board of education. The board of education also provided the towels and laundry service. In regard to the athletic program, the board of education provided extra pay for coaches and intramural directors, all the necessary athletic uniforms, the cleaning and repair of these uniforms and equipment, officials, and accident insurance for all boys and girls participating in the extramural and interschool athletic programs.

In another large school district in California, there was an allocation of $1.35 per pupil (boys) in junior and senior high schools for physical education programs. Girls were allocated the amount of $1.05 per pupil at the same educational level for the same period. The amount varied from year to year based upon need and prior experience. If the total amount allocated was not used during the school year, an amount not to exceed 20% of the total year's allocation could be carried over. The school district provided the expenses of transportation and instruction for the athletic program. Supplies needed in connection with the athletic program were provided through student body funds derived from student fees, sales at student stores, and admissions to athletic activities.

Florida. As reported to the author, Florida as a general policy does not favor earmarked funds for any single program in the schools. The procedure recommended is that county school districts receive what is called a teacher-unit allocation from the state for each twenty-seven students in average daily attendance. Each unit carries with it a certain amount of money for expendable supplies. The local school district holds a percentage of this money for general district-wide use and reallocates the remaining amount to individual schools based on formulas such as pupil enrollment. Each individual school is encouraged to involve its faculty in determining the priority of needs for the coming year. Therefore, health and physical education could have a high priority one year and a low one another year. As a general rule, health and physical education appear to have the same consideration as other phases of the curriculum. In a few instances, physical education needs are met through such fund-raising activities as dances and PTA drives.

Illinois. A high school in Illinois reported that no set figure or set formula was used to arrive at the allocation for health or physical education programs. The board of education subsidized the program of physical education beyond the gate receipts. At the time of the survey there was an equipment budget of $1,000 and a supplies budget of $1,300. The board of education reviews the anticipated budget each year for approval. The Director of Health and Physical Education submits a list of anticipated expenditures for such items as equipment, supplies, transportation, and officials. Gate receipts are also estimated. The difference between the two figures is the amount the board must approve or adjust before approval.

Indiana. One medium-sized school system in Indiana reported that each school (elementary, junior high, senior high, and so on) is allocated so much money for each student enrolled, and then the principal assigns the amount for each phase of the school program.

A county school corporation in Indiana budgets 10 cents per pupil for elementary schools in two accounts—one for instructional supplies and one for repair and replacement. Junior high and senior high schools are budgeted 35 cents per pupil in both accounts. In addition to the above-mentioned accounts, each junior and senior high school principal is budgeted 35 cents per pupil per school as additional money that he can use where he feels the greatest need exists.

A large city school system in Indiana does not have a formula for determining the amount of money allocated for physical education. Budget requests are prepared by the high school department heads for grades nine to twelve and by the supervisor of health and physical education for grades one to eight. The amount requested is based on inventory, program needs of individual schools, and requirements for supplying new schools and additions to present plants.

Another Indiana school system finances the entire interscholastic athletic program from gate receipts. Extra pay for coaches and maintenance of athletic facilities is financed through the general fund. In respect to the physical education program, each department is given an allocation of funds based on the number of students served.

New Jersey. One large school system in New Jersey reported an allocation of 50 cents per student for physical education supplies, and a smaller school system reported an allocation of $3,000 to $6,000 for supplies and coaches' salaries for athletics. Most school districts in New Jersey, it was reported, do not seem to have difficulty in getting reasonable physical education supplies based on needs. For athletics, most schools in New Jersey are subsidized in whole or part by board of education funds.

New York. Twenty-five New York State schools were surveyed to determine the amount of money allocated to their physical education programs. The amounts allocated were then changed into a per pupil allotment so as to provide a means of comparison. The items for which said money was allocated included athletic and gymnasium supplies and equipment, various athletic fees, officials, transportation, police, reconditioning of equipment, supplies and equipment needed in physical education

classes, and intramurals and extramurals for both men and women. In those schools in which the administrative pattern grouped grades seven to twelve, the highest allocation per pupil was $33.86 and the lowest was $10.07. In those schools in which budgets were figured on a kindergarten to grade twelve school administrative pattern, the highest per capita allocation was $13.22 and the lowest was $5.30. In those schools in which the administrative pattern included grades nine to twelve, the highest per capita allocation was $35.24 and the lowest was $13.68.

Each school surveyed was asked how the amount that was allocated per student was determined. The general practice was that the Director of Health and Physical Education submitted and substantiated the following:

1. Needs—for the coming school year
2. Increased expenditures—a sound estimate of projected increases in regard to pupil program participation based on increased enrollments, pupil interest, program changes, and the anticipated cost of equipment and supplies to be used
3. Inventory—present equipment and supplies on hand and the condition of these items
4. Previous year's budget—amounts allocated in previous year or years

These four items represent the basis on which most allocations of funds to programs of health and physical education were determined.

Directors of health and physical education programs surveyed felt that where they were granted increases in per capita allocations it was the result of such factors as increase in the number of participants, a careful evaluation of the number of participants and the time they spent using the equipment and supplies, the cost per hour (for example, it was determined in one community that it cost less than 50 cents per hour per child to participate in football), and an excellent working rapport with the board of education.

The survey also disclosed that most schools have a contingency fund to meet emergency needs, that many schools used the money that was saved when the proposed budget allocation was in excess of the actual bid price on certain supplies and equipment, that some schools used part of the money received from gate receipts, and that some other schools used part of the money from the sale of general organization tickets.

Oklahoma. A city school system in Oklahoma reported that budget allocations for health and physical education programs for boys and girls vary according to pupil en-

rollment. The superintendent of schools and the board of education decide the amount that will be allocated to each of the special programs. Athletics are self-supporting and the board of education does not allocate money directly to them.

Texas. An independent school district in Texas pointed out that they do not have a formula for physical education or health education. The board of education and school administration decide the total budget.

BUDGETING

Budgeting is the formulation of a financial plan in terms of work to be accomplished and services to be performed. All

---

SCHOOL DISTRICT			TAX BUDGET.	
Assessed Valuation		......$59,681,265.00		
Rate per $1,000.00		32.34		
Amount of Budget to be Raised by Taxation		1,930,067.00		

GENERAL CONTROL:

2/2	Board of Education—Legal, Auditing	$	1,225.00	
2/3	Board of Education—Supplies, Travel, etc.		5,700.00	
2/7	Central Office—Salaries		66,680.00	
2/8	Central Office—Supplies, Travel, etc.		4,600.00	
2/10	Attendance & Census Service—Salaries		450.00	
2/11	Attendance & Census Service—Supplies		165.00	
	Total General Control	$		78,820.00

INSTRUCTIONAL SERVICE:

3/3	Salaries of Principals	$	87,225.00	
3/4	Salaries of Clerical & Other Help		36,405.00	
3/6	Other Expenses of Supervision— Supplies, Travel, etc.		8,850.00	
3/9	Salaries of Teachers		1,277,015.00	
3/10	Textbooks		18,800.00	
3/11	Supplies Used in Instruction		38,250.00	
3/13	Tuition to Other Districts		12,600.00	
3/14	Other Expenses of Instruction		10,100.00	
	Total, Instructional Service (Day Schools)		$ 1,489,245.00	

OPERATION OF SCHOOL PLANT:

4/1	Wages—Building Service Employees	$	110,575.00	
4/2	Fuel Oil		20,900.00	
4/3	Water		3,875.00	
4/4	Light & Power		21,800.00	
4/5	Custodial Supplies		5,600.00	
4/7	Services Other Than Personal (Telephone, Laundry, Piano Tuning)		7,100.00	
	Total, Operation of School Plant	$		169,850.00

MAINTENANCE OF SCHOOL PLANT:

5/1	Upkeep of Grounds	$	8,175.00	
5/2	Repair of Buildings		57,160.00	
5/3	Repair & Replacement of Heating, Lighting & Plumbing Equipment		20,400.00	
5/4	Repair & Replacement of Instructional Equipment		14,182.00	
5/5	Repair & Replacement of Furniture		9,920.00	
5/6	Repair & Replacement—Other Equipment		5,457.00	
5/11	Other Expenses of Maintenance		1,985.00	
	Total, Maintenance of School Plant	$		117,279

FIXED CHARGES:

6/1	Pensions—State Teachers' Ret. System	$	226,000.00	
6/2	Pensions—Other Employees		35,525.00	
6/3	Insurance		37,410.00	
6/4	Taxes		3,200.00	
6/5	Membership—State School Boards Assn.		400.00	
6/6	Employers Contrib. to F.I.C.A. (Soc. Sec.)		37,500.00	
	Total, Fixed Charges	$		340,035.00

DEBT SERVICE:

7/1	Payment of Bonds	$	175,000.00	
7/4	Payment of Interest on Bonds		56,555.00	
7/7	Refunds			
7/8	Other Expenses of Debt Service		225.00	
	Total, Debt Service	$		231,780.00

CAPITAL OUTLAY:

8/2	Improvement of Grounds	$	800.00	
8/3	Architect & Engineer Fees		2,500.00	
8/4	New Buildings & Bldg. Equipment			
8/9	Alteration of Bldgs. (Not Repairs)		1,920.00	
8/11	Instructional Equip. & Furniture		19,157.00	
8/12	Other Equipment		1,971.00	
8/15	New Library Books		5,700.00	
8/14	Gift Fund			
	Total, Capital Outlay	$		32,048.00

AUXILIARY AGENCIES AND OTHER SUNDRY ACTIVITIES:

9/1	Library Salaries	$	20,800.00	
9/2	Library—Repair & Repl. of Books		3,500.00	
9/3	Library—Other Expenses		1,350.00	
9/4	Health Service—Med. Inspection		5,100.00	
9/5	Health Service—Nurses' Salaries		32,800.00	
9/6	Health Service—Dental Hyg. Salary		500.00	
9/7	Health Service—Other Expenses		1,400.00	
9/8	Transportation Services		19,000.00	
			22,500.00	
9/10	Cafeteria		8,400.00	
9/12	Recreation & Sports		4,135.00	
9/13	Other Expenses		50.00	
9/14	Psychological Services		11,175.00	
	Total, Auxiliary Agencies	$		130,710.00
	Grand Total of Budget	$		2,596,067.00
	Amount of State Aid (Estimated)			550,000.00
	Miscellaneous Receipts (Estimated)			53,000.00
				$ 1,930,067.00
	Reduction of Contingent Fund			63,000.00
	Amount to be Raised by Taxes			$ 1,930,067.00
	Assessed Valuation			$59,681,265.00
	Tax Rate per $1,000.00 (Estimated)		$	32.34

Certified to be a true and correct copy

Sgd:
Sgd: District Clerk

Sample budget summary for a school system.

of the expenditures should be closely related to the objectives that the organization is trying to achieve. In this aspect the administration plays a very important part in the budgeting process.

Budgets should be planned and prepared with a thought to the future. They are an important part of the administration's 3-, 5-, or 7-year plan and the program of accomplishment that has been outlined for a fiscal period. Projects of any size should be integrated progressively over many years. Thus the outlay of monies to realize such aims requires long-term planning.

According to the strict interpretation of the word, a budget is merely a record of receipts and expenditures. As used here, however, it reflects the long-term planning of the organization, pointing up the needs with their estimated costs, and then ensuring that a realistic program is planned that will fit into the estimated income.

The budget forecasts revenues and expenses for a period of 1 year, known as the fiscal year, which is not always synonymous with the school or college year.

Purposes of budgets

The purposes of budgets are as follows:

1. They express the plan and program for the departments of health and physical education. They determine such things as (a) size of classes, (b) supplies, equipment, and facilities, (c) methods used, (d) results and educational values sought, and (e) personnel available.

2. They reflect the school's or college's educational philosophy and policies and those of the professional fields of health and physical education. They provide an overview of these specialized areas.

3. They determine what phases of the program are to be emphasized. They aid in an analysis of all aspects of health and physical education programs.

4. They interpret to the principal, superintendent of schools, board of educa-

tion (or trustees), dean, and the public in general the needs of health and physical education.

5. They assist, together with the budgets of other educational subdivisions, in determining the tax levy for the school district.

6. They make it possible, upon approval by the recognized officials, to authorize expenditures for the program of health and physical education.

7. They make it possible to administer the health and physical education program economically by improving accounting procedures.

Types of budgets

There are short-term and long-term budgets. The short-term is usually the annual budget that runs for a 12-month period. The long-term budget represents long-term fiscal planning, possibly for a 10-year period. Most health and physical education personnel will be concerned with short-term or annual budgets whereby they plan their financial needs for a period covering the school year.

Responsibility for budgets

The responsibility for the preparation of the overall school or college budget may vary from one locality to another. In most systems the superintendent of schools is responsible. In colleges it is the responsibility of the president and the dean. Where these situations exist, it is often possible for principals, department heads, teachers, and professors to participate in preparation of the budget by submitting various requests for budget items. In other situations the budget may be first prepared in nearly all its details and then submitted to the subdivisions for consideration.

In some large school systems the superintendent of schools frequently delegates much of the budget responsibility to a business manager, a clerk, or an assistant or associate superintendent.

The final official school authority in re-

THE ROLE OF THE ADMINISTRATOR IN BUDGETING*

A. Preliminary considerations in preparing the budget
    1. Program additions or deletions
    2. Staff changes
    3. Inventory of equipment on hand

B. Budget preparation: additional considerations
    1. Athletic gate receipts and expenditures — Athletic Association fund
    2. Board of education budget — allocations for physical education, including athletics
    3. Coaches requests and requests of teachers and department heads
    4. Comparison of requests with inventories
    5. Itemizing and coding requests
    6. Budget conferences with administration
    7. Justification of requests

C. Athletic association funds: considerations
    1. Estimated income
        a. Gate receipts
        b. Student activities tickets
        c. Tournament receipts
    2. Estimated expenditures
        a. Awards
        b. Tournament fees
        c. Films
        d. Miscellaneous
        e. Surplus

D. General budget: considerations
    1. Breakdown
        a. By sport or activity
        b. Transportation
        c. Salaries of personnel
        d. Insurance
        e. Reconditioning of equipment
        f. Supervision
        g. General and miscellaneous
        h. Equipment
        i. Officials
    2. Codes
        a. Advertising
        b. Travel
        c. Conferences
        d. Others

E. Postbudget procedures
    1. Selection of equipment and supplies
    2. Preparation of list of dealers to bid
    3. Request for price quotations
    4. Requisitions
    5. Care of equipment
    6. Notification of teachers and coaches of amounts approved

F. Ordering procedures
    1. Study the quality of various products
    2. Accept no substitutes for items ordered
    3. Submit request for price quotations
    4. Select low quotes or justify higher quotes
    5. Submit purchase orders
    6. Check and count all shipments
    7. Record items received on inventory cards
    8. Provide for equipment and supply accountability

*Adapted from recommendations of Director's Workshop, New York University, 1968.

THE ROLE OF THE ADMINISTRATOR IN BUDGETING—cont'd

G. Relationships with administration
 1. Consultation — program plans with building principal and/or superintendent
 2. Make budget recommendations to administration
 3. Advise business manager of procedures followed
 4. Discuss items approved and deleted with business manager
 5. Advise teachers and coaches of amounts available and adjust requests
H. Suggestions for prospective directors of physical education programs
 1. Develop a philosophy and approach to budgeting
 2. Consult with staff for their suggestions
 3. Select quality merchandise
 4. Provide proper care and maintenance of equipment and supplies
 5. Provide for all programs on an equitable basis
 6. Budget adequately but not elaborately
 7. Provide a sound well-rounded program of physical education
 8. Emphasize equality for girls and boys
 9. Provide for basic instructional, adapted, intramural and extramural, and interscholastic parts of the program
 10. Conduct a year-round public relations program
 11. Try to overcome these possible shortcomings:
  a. Board of education not oriented to needs of physical education
  b. Program not achieving established goals
  c. Staff not adequately informed and involved in administrative process

---

spect to school budgets is the board of education. This body can approve, reject, or amend. But even beyond the board of education rests the authority of the people, who in most communities have the right to approve or reject the budget.

In colleges the budget may be handled in the dean's office, or the director or chairman of the physical education department may have the responsibility. In some cases the director of athletics is responsible for the athletic budget.

Within school departments of health and physical education the chairman, supervisor, or director is the person responsible for the budget. However, he or she will usually consult with members of the department and receive their suggestions.

Criteria for a good budget

A budget for health and physical education should meet the following criteria:
1. The budget will clearly present the financial needs of the entire program in relation to the objectives sought.

2. Key persons in the organization have been consulted.

3. The budget will provide a realistic estimate of income to balance the expenditures that are anticipated.

4. The possibility of emergencies is recognized through flexibility in the financial plan.

5. The budget will be prepared well in advance of the fiscal year so as to leave ample time for analysis, thought, criticism, and review.

6. Budget requests are realistic, not padded.

7. The budget meets the essential requirements of students, faculty, and administrators.

Budget preparation and planning

Four general steps for procedure in budget planning that health and physical education personnel might consider are as follows:

1. Actual preparation of the budget by the chairman of the department with his or her staff, listing the various estimated receipts, expenditures, and any other information that needs to be included.

2. Presentation of the budget to the principal, superintendent, dean, board of education, or other person or group that represents the proper authority and has the responsibility for reviewing it.

3. After formal approval of the budget, its use as a guide for the financial management and administration of the department or organization.

4. Critical evaluation of the budget periodically to determine its effectiveness in meeting educational needs, with notations being made for the next year's budget.

The preparation of the budget, representing the first step, is a long-term endeavor that cannot be accomplished in a day or two. The budget is something that can be well prepared only after a careful review of program effectiveness and appraisal over an extended period of time. However, the actual finalization of the budget usually is accomplished in the early spring after a detailed inventory of program needs has been taken. The director of health and/or physical education, after close consultation with staff members and the principal, dean, superintendent of schools, or other responsible administrative officer, should formulate the budget.

In preparing the budget many records and reports will be of value. The inventory of equipment and supplies on hand will be useful, and copies of inventories and budgets from previous years will provide good references. Comparison of budgetary items with those in schools and colleges of similar size may be of help. Accounting records will be valuable.

The preparation of the budget should be accomplished in such a way that it is flexible and will allow for readjustments to be made, if necessary. It is difficult to accurately and specifically list each detail in the way that it will be needed and executed.

The budget should represent a schedule that can be justified. This means that each budgetary item must satisfy the most meaningful educational needs and interests of all concerned. Furthermore, each item that constitutes an expenditure should be reflected in budget specifications.

Richard G. Mitchell, writing on "administrative planning," lists these five important considerations in budget preparation:

1. What was planned last year? This constitutes the tying together of the proposed budget with the one approved last year to check on long-term planning goals.
2. What was accomplished last year? This step relates last year's accomplishments to the achievement of the department's long-term objectives.
3. What can realistically be accomplished this year? In light of past years, future trends, and the master plan, what can be accomplished this year?
4. What needs to be done? This constitutes the minimum essentials that must be accomplished this year. These items have priority.
5. How is it to be done? Such items as staff, equipment, supplies, and other requirements for accomplishment and meeting of needs would be outlined.*

Budget organization

Budgets can be organized in many ways. One pattern that consists of four sections or divisions and that might prove useful for a health or physical education administrator is described here:

1. An introductory message enables the administration to present the financial proposals in terms that a board of education or person outside the specialized fields might readily understand. This section offers to persons who have specialized in these areas an opportunity to discuss some

*Mitchell, R. G.: Administrative planning—its effective use, Recreation **44:**426, 1961.

aspects of the program in lay terms and some of the directions that need to be taken in order to provide for the health and physical fitness of the students.

2. The second section presents an overall view of the budget, with expenditures and anticipated revenues arranged in a clear and systematic fashion so that any person can compare the two.

3. A third section, with an estimate of receipts and expenditures in much more detail, should enable a principal, superintendent of schools and/or board of education, or other interested person or group to understand the budget specifically and to follow up any item of cost.

4. A fourth section might include supporting schedules to provide additional evidence for the requests outlined in the budget. Many times a budget will have a better chance of approval if there is sufficient documentation to support some items. For example, extra pay for coaching may be thought to be desirable. Salary schedules for coaches in other school systems could be included to support such a proposition.

Another type of budget organization might be one that consists of the following three parts: (1) an introductory statement of the objectives, policies, and program of the health and physical education department; (2) a résumé of the objectives, policies, and program interpreted in terms of proposed expenditures; and (3) a financial plan for meeting the educational needs during the fiscal period.

Not all budgets are broken down into these four or three divisions. All budgets do, however, give an itemized account of receipts and expenditures.

In a physical education budget common inclusions are items concerning instruction, such as extra compensation for coaches; matters of capital outlay, such as a new swimming pool or handball court; the replacement of expendable equipment, such as basketballs and baseball bats; and pro-

vision for maintenance and repair, such as refurbishing football uniforms or doing some grading on the playground. It is difficult to estimate many of these items without making a careful inventory and analysis of the condition of the facilities and equipment.

Sources of income

The sources of income for most school and college health and physical education programs include the general school or college fund, gate receipts, health, general organization, and activity fees, and some other revenues.

General school or college fund. At the elementary and secondary levels the health program would be supported, usually entirely, through general school funds, and the physical education program would be financed in the same way, to a large extent. At the college and university level the general fund of the institution would also represent a major source of income.

Gate receipts. Gate receipts play an important part in some schools in the financing of at least part of the physical education program. Although there is usually less stress on gate receipts at lower educational levels, colleges and universities sometimes finance their entire athletic, intramural, and physical education programs through such a medium. At a few high schools throughout the country, gate receipts have been abolished because of the feeling that if athletics represent an important part of the education program, they should be paid for in the same way that science and mathematics programs, for example, are financed.

Health, general organization, and activity fees. Some high schools either require or make available to students separate health, general organization, or activity fees and tickets or some other inducement that enables them to attend the athletic, dramatic, and musical events that are offered. In colleges and universities a similar plan is generally used, thus providing students

Table 16-1. General organization athletic account — financial report (September-December)

Expenses		
Football		
Officials (four home games)	$ 240.00	
Equipment and supplies	1,182.01	
Transportation	87.50	
Supervision (police, ticket sellers and takers)	476.00	
Reconditioning and cleaning equipment	656.60	
Medical supplies	62.70	
Scouting	30.00	
Film	15.68	
Guarantees	260.00	
Football dinner	115.50	
Miscellaneous (printing tickets, meetings)	86.00	
Total football expense		$3,211.99
Cross country		
State and county entry fees	$ 5.00	
Transportation	32.00	
Total cross country expense		$ 37.00
Basketball		
Supervision (three games)	$ 18.00	
Custodian (three games)	13.00	
Police (one game)	6.00	
Total basketball expense		$ 37.00
Cheerleaders		
Transportation	$ 26.10	
Sixteen sweaters	160.00	
Cleaning sweaters	48.00	
Total cheerleader expense		$ 234.10
Total expenses		$3,520.09
Receipts		
Football		
Newburgh game	$ 655.85	
Norwalk game	909.80	
Yonkers game	564.75	
Bridgeport game	550.00	
Guarantee (New Haven)	60.00	
Total receipts		$2,740.40

with reduced rates to the various out-of-class activities offered by the institution. A health fee also is quite common at higher education levels. Table 16-1 shows a general organization financial statement.

Other sources of income. Some other sources of income, not so common to all educational levels, are (1) *special foundation, governmental, or individual grants or gifts* intended to promote physical fitness, athletics, or some phase of health and physical education programs; (2) the sale of *radio and television rights* at the college level, especially for those institutions that have nationally ranking teams and where the athletic contests have great public appeal; (3) *concessions* at athletic contests and other activity events; and (4) *special fund-raising events* such as a faculty-varsity basketball game or a gymnastic circus.

Linn* has listed some steps that might profitably be followed for estimating receipts in the general school budget and that are also application to the preparation of budgets for health and physical education:

1. Gathering and analyzing historical data
2. Collecting current data
3. Preparing income estimates
4. Organizing and classifying receipts into proper categories
5. Preparing revenue estimates from accumulated data
6. Making comparisons with estimates for preceding years and preparing final draft of receipts

Expenditures

In health and physical education budgets, typical examples of expenditures are items of *capital outlay,* such as a dental chair or swimming pool; *expendable equipment,* such as tongue depressors or basketballs; and a *maintenance and repair provision,* such as towel and laundry service and the repair of pure-tone audiometers or refurbishing of football uniforms. See Table 16-2 for a sample list of expenditures for athletics.

Some expenditures are very easy to estimate but others are more difficult, requiring the keeping of accurate inventories, examination of past records, and careful

*Linn, H. H.: School business administration, New York, 1956, The Ronald Press Co.

Table 16-2. A sample list of expenditures for athletics

	Baseball	Basketball	Football	Cross country	Girls' sports	Golf	Hockey	Soccer	Swimming	Tennis	Track	Total
Equipment and supplies	$369.55	$116.70	$278.68	$ 45.80	$ 41.60	$36.10	$251.65	$ 70.40	$ 80.05	$27.20	$231.77	$1,549.50
Transportation	208.50	248.70	39.60	83.20	84.98	48.40	495.00	63.70	108.80	8.80	120.90	1,510.48
Officials	122.00	391.35	50.00					52.00				615.35
Cleaning	65.70	30.95	129.40				95.60	57.20			141.10	519.95
Supervision		66.00										66.00
Custodian		37.00										37.00
Additional coaching			350.00					100.00				450.00
Entry fees						7.00			17.21	4.00	22.50	50.75
Rental, boys' club pool									250.00			250.00
Totals	$765.75	$890.70	$847.68	$129.00	$126.58	$91.50	$842.25	$343.20	$456.10	$40.00	$516.27	$5,049.03

analysis of the condition of the equipment. Some items and services will need to be figured by averaging costs over a period of years, such as cleaning and mending athletic equipment. Other examples of items that require careful consideration in order to list expenditures accurately are awards, new equipment needed, guarantees to visiting teams, and medical services for emergencies.

Linn* suggests some sound procedures to follow in estimating expenditures:

1. Prepare a budgetary calendar that will include what is to be accomplished and when.
2. Gather and analyze historical data.
3. Collect current information and data pertinent to expenditures.
4. Prepare estimates from accumulated data.
5. Organize and classify various items of expenditure, stating the purposes for which money will be expended.
6. Clarify expenditure estimates to show how they represent meaningful educational needs.
7. Compare estimates with expenditures for previous years.
8. Reevaluate estimates and prepare final draft.

Budget presentation and adoption

Budgets in health and physical education, after being prepared, should usually be submitted to the superintendent through the principal's office. The principal represents the person in charge of his particular building and, therefore, subdivision budgets should be presented to him for his approval. Good administration would mean, furthermore, that the budgetary items would have been reviewed with him during their preparation so that approval is usually a routine matter.

In the case of college and university, the

*Linn, H. H., op. cit.

proper channels should be followed. This might mean clearance through a dean or other administrative officer. Each person, of course, who is responsible for budget preparation and presentation should be very familiar with the proper working channels.

For successful presentation and adoption, the budget should be prepared in final form only after careful consideration so that little change will be needed. Requests for funds should be justifiable, and ample preliminary discussion of the budget with persons and groups most directly concerned should be held so that needless difficulty will be avoided.

Budget administration

After the presentation and approval of the budget, the next step is to see that it is administered properly. This means that it should be followed as closely as possible with periodic checks on expenditures to see that they fall within the budget appropriations that have been provided. The budget should function as a good guide for economical and efficient administration.

Budget appraisal

Periodic appraisal calls for an audit of the accounts and an evaluation of the school program resulting from the administration of the current budget. Such appraisal should be done in all honesty and with a view to eliminating weaknesses in current budgets and strengthening future ones. It should also be remembered that the budget will be only as good as the administration makes it and that the budget will improve only as the administration improves.

FINANCIAL ACCOUNTING

The great amount of money involved in health and physical education programs means that strict accountability must be observed. This means the maintenance of accurate records, proper distribution of materials, and adequate appraisal and evaluation of procedures. Financial accounting should provide:

1. A record of receipts and expenditures for all departmental transactions
2. A permanent record of all financial transactions for future reference
3. A pattern for expenditures that is closely related to the approved budget
4. A tangible documentation of compliance with mandates and requests either imposed by law or by administrative action
5. Some procedure for evaluating, to see that funds are dealt with honestly, and proper management in respect to control, analysis of costs, and reporting

Most of the state departments of education publish manuals on school accounting. Each chairman of health and physical education should have a copy of his or her own state's school accounting procedure and should read and follow it carefully.

Reasons for financial accounting

Some reasons why financial accounting is needed in health and physical education include those listed below:

1. To provide a method of authorizing expenditures for items that have been included and approved in the budget. This means proper accounting records are being used.
2. To provide authorized procedures for making purchases of equipment, supplies, and other materials and to let contracts for various services.
3. To provide authorized procedures for paying the proper amounts (a) for purchases of equipment, supplies, and other materials, which have been checked upon receipt, (b) for labor that actually has taken place, and (c) for other services that have been rendered.
4. To provide a record of each payment

Table 16-3. Sample sports program, general organization, and board of education report of expenditures and receipts

Sports	Board of education	General organization	Total
Total expenditures			
Baseball	$ 765.75		$ 765.75
Basketball	890.70	$ 106.34	997.04
Football	847.68	3,943.09	4,340.77
Cross country	129.00	37.00	166.00
Girls' sports and cheerleaders	126.58	249.10	375.68
Golf	91.50		91.50
Hockey	842.25	48.95	891.20
Soccer	343.20		343.20
Swimming	456.10	41.10	497.20
Tennis	40.00	4.00	44.00
Track	516.27	15.03	531.30
Total	$5,049.03	$3,994.61	$9,043.64
Total general organization receipts			
Football		$2,740.40	
Basketball		381.30	
Total			$3,121.70

that has been made, including the date, to whom, for what purpose, and other pertinent material.

5. To provide authorized procedures for handling various receipts and sources of income.

6. To provide the detailed information that is essential for proper auditing of accounts, such as confirmation that money has been spent for accurately specified items.

7. To provide material and information for the preparation of future budgets.

8. To provide a tangible base for the development of future policies relating to financial planning.

Administrative principles and policies for financial accounting

The Athletic Institute* has prepared some excellent material on accountability, in which it brings out such important principles and policies as the following:

1. The administrative head has the final responsibility for accountability for all equipment and supplies in his or her organization.

2. Departments should establish and enforce policies covering loss, damage, theft, misappropriation, or destruction of equipment and supplies or other materials.

3. A system of accurate record keeping should be established and be uniform throughout the department.

4. Accountability should demonstrate the close relationship that exists between equipment and supplies and the program objectives.

5. A system of policies should be developed that will guarantee the proper use and protection of all equipment and supplies within the department.

6. The person to whom equipment and supplies are issued should be held accountable for these materials.

---

*The Athletic Institute: Equipment and supplies for athletics, physical education and recreation. Chicago, 1960, The Institute, chap. 5.

7. Accurate inventories are essential to proper financial accounting.

8. A system of marking equipment and supplies as proof of ownership should be instituted.

9. A meaningful procedure should be established for the proper distribution of all equipment and supplies.

10. The discarding of equipment and supplies should take place only in accordance with established procedures and by authorized persons.

Accounting for receipts and expenditures

A centralized accounting system is very advantageous, with all funds being deposited with the school treasurer or business manager. Purchase orders and other procedures are usually then countersigned or certified by the school treasurer, thus better guaranteeing integrity in the use of funds. A system of bookkeeping wherein books are housed in the central office by the finance officer helps to ensure better control of finances by the school and allows for all subdivisions or departments in an educational system to be financially controlled in the same manner. Such a procedure also provides for better and more centralized record keeping. The central accounting system fund accounts, in which are located the physical education and health funds, should be audited annually by qualified persons not associated with the school funds. Finally, an annual financial report should be made and publicized to indicate receipts, expenditures, and other pertinent data associated with the enterprise.

All receipts and expenditures should be recorded in the ledger in the proper manner, providing such important information as the fund in which it has been deposited, or from which it was withdrawn, and the money received from such sources as athletics and dues to school organizations should be shown with sufficient cross references and detailed information. Supporting vouchers should also be at hand. Tickets to athletic and other events should be numbered consecutively and checked to get an accurate record of ticket sales. Students should not be permitted to handle funds except under the supervision of some member of the administrative staff or faculty. All accounts should be properly audited at appropriate intervals.

Purchase orders on regular authorized forms issued by the school should be used, so that accurate records may be kept. To order verbally is a questionable policy. By preparing written purchase orders, on regular forms and according to good accountability procedure, legality of contract is better ensured, together with prompt delivery and payment. For more information see Chapter 17 on the purchase and care of supplies and equipment.

CHECKLIST FOR BUDGETING AND FINANCIAL ACCOUNTING

	Yes	No
1. Has a complete inventory been taken and itemized on proper forms as a guide in estimating equipment needs?	___	___
2. Does the equipment inventory include a detailed account of the number of items on hand, size and quantity, type, condition, etc.?	___	___
3. Is the inventory complete, current, and up-to-date?	___	___
4. Are budgetary estimates as accurate and realistic as possible without padding?	___	___
5. Are provisions made in the budget for increases expected in enrollments, increased pupil participation, and changes in the cost of equipment and supplies?	___	___
6. Have supply house and the school business administrator been consulted on the cost of new equipment?	___	___
7. Has the Director of Health and Physical Education consulted with his staff on various budget items?	___	___
8. Has the Director of Health and Physical Education consulted with the school business administrator in respect to the total budget for his department?	___	___
9. Are new equipment and supply needs for health and physical education determined and budgeted at least one year in advance?	___	___
10. Was the budget prepared according to the standards desired by the chief school administrator?	___	___
11. Are statistics and information for previous years indicated as a means of comparison?	___	___
12. Is there a summary of receipts and expenditures listed concisely on one page so that the total budget can be quickly seen?	___	___
13. If receipts from athletics or other funds are to be added to the budget, is this shown?	___	___
14. Are there alternate program plans with budgetary changes in the event the budget is not approved?	___	___
15. Has a statement of objectives of the program been included that reflects the overall educational philosophy and program of the total school and community?	___	___
16. Has the budget been prepared so that the major aspects may be viewed readily by those persons desiring a quick review and also in more detail for those persons desiring a further delineation of the budgetary items?	___	___
17. Is the period of time for which the budget has been prepared clearly indicated?	___	___
18. Is the health and physical education budget based on an educational plan developed to attain the goals and purposes agreed upon by the		

Continued.

CHECKLIST FOR BUDGETING AND FINANCIAL ACCOUNTING—cont'd

	Yes	No

director and his staff within the framework of the total school's philosophy? _____ _____

19. Is the health and physical education plan a comprehensive one reflecting health science instruction, health services, and a healthful environment, physical education class, adapted, intramural and extramural, and interscholastic program? _____ _____

20. Does the plan include a statement of the objectives of the health and physical education programs and are these reflected in the budget? _____ _____

21. Are both long-range and short-range plans for achieving the purposes of the program provided? _____ _____

22. Have provisions been made in the budget for emergencies? _____ _____

23. Are accurate records kept on such activities involving expenditures of money as transportation, insurance, officials, laundry and dry cleaning, awards, guarantees, repairs, new equipment, medical expenses, and publicity? _____ _____

24. Are accurate records kept on the receipt of monies from such sources as gate receipts and advertising revenue? _____ _____

25. Once the budget has been approved, is there a specific plan provided for authorizing expenditures? _____ _____

26. Are specific forms used for recording purchase transactions? _____ _____

27. Are purchases on all major items based on competitive bidding? _____ _____

28. Are requisitions used in obtaining supplies and equipment? _____ _____

29. Are requisitions numbered and do they include such information as the name of the person originating the requisition, when the item to be purchased will be needed, where to ship the item, the description and/or code number, quantity, unit price, and amount? _____ _____

30. With the exception of petty cash accounts, is a central purchasing system in effect? _____ _____

31. Is the policy of quantity purchasing followed wherever possible and desirable in the interests of economy? _____ _____

32. If quantity purchasing is used, is advanced thought and planning given to storage and maintenance facilities and procedures? _____ _____

33. Are performance tests made of items purchased? Are state, regional, or national testing bureaus or laboratories utilized where feasible? _____ _____

34. Are receipts of equipment and supplies checked carefully? _____ _____

35. Is an audit made of all expenditures? _____ _____

36. Are specific procedures in effect to safeguard money, property, and employees? _____ _____

37. Is there a check to determine that established standards, policies, and procedures have been followed? _____ _____

38. Are procedures in operation to check condition and use of equipment and supplies? _____ _____

39. Is a financial report made periodically? _____ _____

40. Are there proper procedures for the care and maintenance and accountability of all equipment and supplies? _____ _____

41. Are accurate records kept on all equipment and supplies including condition, site, and age? _____ _____

42. Have established procedures been developed and are they followed in regard to the issuance, use, and return of equipment? _____ _____

43. Have provisions been made for making regular notations of future needs? _____ _____

Questions and exercises

1. Prepare a budget for a high school or college department of physical education.
2. What are five reasons for fiscal management in health and physical education?
3. Collect budgets from five school systems or colleges and critically evaluate them.
4. Where does the responsibility fall for budget preparation?
5. Outline the procedure you would follow in the preparation of a budget if you were chairman of the department of health and physical education for a city educational system.
6. What are the criteria for a good budget?
7. What are the most common sources of receipts and expenditures in a health and/or physical education department?
8. What records would you keep in order to ensure good financial accounting?
9. Formulate ten policies to ensure good financial accounting.

   Reading assignment in *Administrative Dimensions of Health and Physical Education Programs, Including Athletics:* Chapter 13, Selections 70 to 76.

Selected references

Athletic Institute: Equipment and supplies for athletics, physical education, and recreation, Chicago, 1960, The Institute.

Casey, L. M.: School business administration, New York, 1964, The Center for Applied Research in Education, Inc. (The Library of Education).

Cosgrove, J. N., editor: Budgeting—experts say it's wise planning, not pinching pennies, The National Underwriter 50:42, 1967.

Gehric, E. A.: Budget procedure for extracurricular organizations, Business Education World 32: 17, 1951.

Knezevich, S. J., and Fowlkes, J. G.: Business management of local school systems, New York, 1960, Harper & Row, Publishers.

Linder, I. H., and Gunn, H. M.: Secondary school administration, Columbus, Ohio, 1963, Charles E. Merrill Books, Inc.

Ranney, D. C.: The determinants of fiscal support for large city educational systems, Administrators Notebook, vol. 15, December, 1966.

Roe, W. H.: School business management, New York, 1961, McGraw-Hill Book Co.

Thomas, J. A.: Education decision-making and the school budget, Administrators Notebook, vol. 12, December, 1963.

Wilsey, C. E.: Budget for equipment replacement, School Board Journal, p. 10, May, 1967.

CHAPTER 17 THE PURCHASE AND CARE OF SUPPLIES AND EQUIPMENT INCLUDING AUDIOVISUAL MATERIALS

Health and physical education programs utilize many supplies and equipment that cost thousands of dollars. *Supplies* are those materials that are expendable and that need to be replaced at frequent intervals, such as shuttlecocks and adhesive tape. *Equipment* is the term used for those items that are not considered expendable but are utilized over a period of years, such as parallel bars and audiometers.

Since so much money is expended upon supplies and equipment and since such materials are vital to school and college health and safety, to good playing conditions, and to values derived from the programs, it is important that this administrative phase of the specialized fields of health and physical education be considered carefully.

Many different sources for purchasing equipment exist, many grades and qualities of materials are available, and many methods of storing and maintaining such merchandise are prevalent. Some of these sources, grades, and methods are good and some are questionable. In order to obtain the greatest values for the amount of money spent, basic principles of selecting, purchasing, and maintaining need to be known and understood. This chapter includes a brief discussion of these matters and also a discussion of audiovisual materials. In Appendix A the reader will find a listing of organizations and companies where various health and physical education supplies and equipment may be purchased. Appendix B contains an extensive chart on the subject of the care, repair, and storage of physical education supplies and equipment. All types of health, physical education, and athletic equipment and supplies are included.

SUPPLY AND EQUIPMENT NEEDS VARY

Supplies and equipment needed in a school or college system will vary according to certain influencing factors. These include, first, the programs themselves and the activities that are to be offered. The geographic location of the school will help to determine the activities scheduled, as will such other elements as the interests of students and their physiologic, psychologic, and sociologic needs. A second factor would be the other facilities and the health rooms and playing space available. Some schools and a few colleges do not have a health suite and have only limited physical education facilities. Under such conditions the supplies and equipment needed will differ from those required in settings where spacious accommodations exist. Other factors that will need to be taken into consideration are the nature of the clientele (in regard to age, sex, and number of students), the money available, the length of playing seasons, and provisions for the health and safety of participants. Those persons responsible for purchasing supplies and equipment should carefully study their own particular situations and estimate their own needs in an objective and realistic manner.

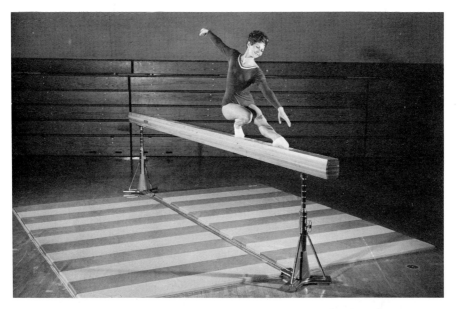

Gymnastic equipment courtesy Nissen Corporation, Cedar Rapids, Iowa.

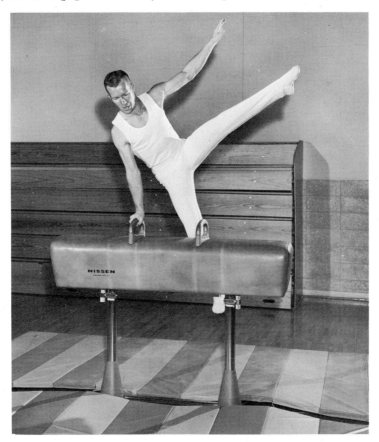

Gymnastic equipment courtesy Nissen Corporation, Cedar Rapids, Iowa.

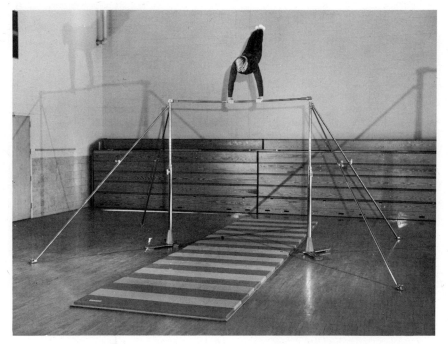

Gymnastic equipment courtesy Nissen Corporation, Cedar Rapids, Iowa.

As pointed out previously, the types of equipment and supplies will vary with the program. In the health education area such articles as microscopes, mannequins, test materials, laboratory equipment, and audiovisual equipment will be needed. In the health service area there will be a need for such items as equipment for screening vision and hearing, first-aid supplies, scales, examining table, dental equipment and supplies, beds, towels, and sheets. In the physical education area, of course, all types of balls, apparatus, uniforms, timers, and racks will be needed if individual, team, formal, aquatic, dance, and other activities are to be offered. Different types of materials will be required for the interschool and intercollegiate athletic programs, the intramural and extramural programs, the adapted programs, and the class programs. Many decisions in the purchasing of equipment and supplies will depend upon the objectives being sought by the administration.

In general, however, the administration is interested in:

1. Trying to standardize supplies and equipment as much as possible
2. Supervising the entire process of selection, purchase, storage, and maintenance
3. Maintaining a list of sources of materials
4. Preparing specifications for various items that are to be purchased
5. Securing bids for large purchases and those required by law
6. Deciding upon or recommending organizations where materials are to be purchased
7. Testing products to see that specifications are satisfactorily met
8. Checking supplies and equipment to determine if all that were ordered have been delivered
9. Expediting the delivery of purchases so that materials are available as needed

10. Continually seeking new products that meet needs of program
11. Providing overall supervision of purchase, care, and use of supplies and equipment

SELECTION OF SUPPLIES AND EQUIPMENT

A discussion of some of the principles that should be observed in the selection of supplies and equipment for school and college health and physical education programs, including athletics, follows.

Selection should be based upon local needs

Supplies and equipment should be selected because they are needed in a particular school or college situation and by a particular group of students. Items should be selected that represent materials needed to carry out the program as outlined in the course of study and that represent essentials to fulfilling program objectives.

Selection should be based upon quality

In the long run, the item of good quality is the cheapest and the safest. Bargains too often represent inferior materials that wear out much earlier. Only the best grade of football equipment should be purchased. I did a study of football deaths that occurred during a 25-year period and found that many of these deaths had resulted from use of inferior helmets and other poor equipment. What is true of football is also true of other activities.

Selection should be made by competent personnel

The persons carrying out the assignment of selecting the supplies and equipment needed in health and physical education programs should be competent to assume such a responsibility. To perform such a job efficiently means examining many types and makes of products, conducting experiments to determine such qualities as

economy and durability, listing and weighing the advantages and disadvantages of different items, and knowing how each item is going to be used. The person selecting supplies and equipment should be interested in this responsibility, have the time to do the job, and possess those qualities needed to perform the function in an efficient manner. Some schools and colleges have purchasing agents who are specially trained in these matters. In small organizations the chairman, director, or coach frequently performs this responsibility. One other point is important: regardless of who the responsible person may be, the staff member who utilizes these supplies and equipment in his or her particular facet of the total program should have a great deal to say about the specific items chosen. He or she is the one who understands the functional use of the merchandise.

Selection should be continuous

A product that ranks as the "best" available this year may not necessarily be the "best" next year. Manufacturers are constantly conducting research in order to come out with something better. There is keen competition among them. The administration, therefore, cannot be complacent and apathetic, thinking that because a certain product has served them so well in the past, it is the best buy for the future. Instead, there must be a continual search for the best product available.

Selection should take into consideration service and replacement needs

Items of supplies and equipment may be difficult to obtain in volume. Upon receipt of merchandise, sizes of uniforms may be wrong and colors may be mixed up. Additional materials may be needed on short notice. Such facts mean that in the selection process consideration should be given to selecting items that will be available in volume, if needed, and that con-

KEY TO FIGURES

1. CHEST. Be sure the tape is snug under the arms and over the shoulder blades.

2. WAIST. Place the tape above the hips around waist like a belt to determine waist measurements.

3. HIPS. Measure hips around the widest part.

4. INSEAM. Measure inseam from close up the crotch to top of the heel of the shoe when full-length pants are ordered. For shorter pants, like baseball and football pants, check on the measurement recommendations of the manufacturer of the clothing you select.

5. OUTSEAM. Measure from the waistline to top of heel of shoe for full-length pants. For baseball, football, and shorter pants check the measurement recommendations of the particular manufacturer involved.

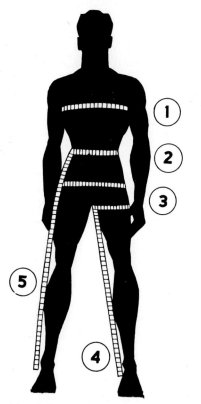

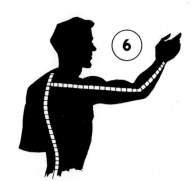

6. SLEEVE. Take measurments from center of back over elbow to wrist. Keep elbow bent, straight out from shoulder.

HEAD. (Not shown in diagram). The tape should run across forehead about 1½ inches above eyebrows and back around the large part of the head.

How to measure for athletic equipment. Correct measurement is essential for proper sizing of athletic equipment to ensure the comfort of the wearer, durability of equipment, proper protection, and appearance on the field. This illustration may be used as a measuring guide to ensure the proper fit of uniforms, jerseys, protective equipment, and warmup suits. This is a basic measuring guide for most types of athletic equipment. For a perfect fit it is also recommended that you state height, weight, and any special irregularities of build. See also p. 489. (From How to budget, select, and order athletic equipment, Chicago, 1962, The Athletic Institute.)

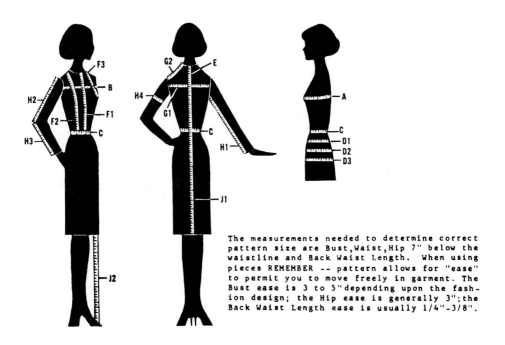

The measurements needed to determine correct pattern size are Bust, Waist, Hip 7" below the waistline and Back Waist Length. When using pieces REMEMBER -- pattern allows for "ease" to permit you to move freely in garment. The Bust ease is 3 to 5" depending upon the fashion design; the Hip ease is generally 3"; the Back Waist Length ease is usually 1/4"-3/8".

NAME ....   DATE ....

A. BUST...................................... **in.** — Measure around fullest part — a little higher in back
B. CHEST .... **in.** — Measure straight across front from seam to seam
C. WAIST .... **in.** — Put string or elastic around waist to locate natural waistline.
D. HIP   1.................................. **in.** — Measure 3" below natural waistline
        2.................................. **in.** — Measure 7" below natural waistline
        3.................................. **in.** — Measure 9" below natural waistline
E. BACK WAIST LENGTH .... **in.** — Nape of neck to waistline
F. FRONT WAIST LENGTH   1.......... **in.** — Neck to waistline at Center Front
                        2.......... **in.** — Mid-shoulder to waist over bust
                        3.......... **in.** — Base of neck at shoulder seamline to tip of bust
G. SHOULDERS   1....................... **in.** — Seam to seam across back 4" below neckline
                2....................... **in.** — One shoulder from base of neck to seamline
H. SLEEVE   1............................. **in.** — Underarm to wrist
            2............................. **in.** — Shoulder to elbow
            3............................. **in.** — Elbow to wrist
            4............................. **in.** — Around upper arm
J. LENGTH   1............................. **in.** — Waist to hemline at Center Back
            2............................. **in.** — From floor to hemline

                                                            printed in u. s. a.

How to take a girl's measurements. (Courtesy McCall's Patterns.)

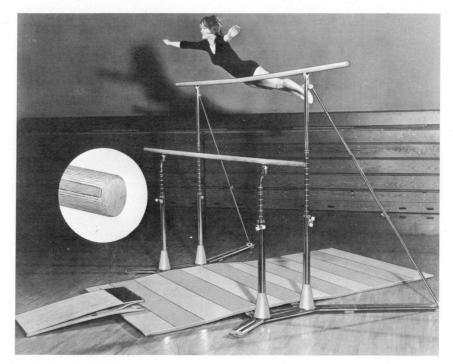

Gymnastic equipment courtesy Nissen Corporation, Cedar Rapids, Iowa.

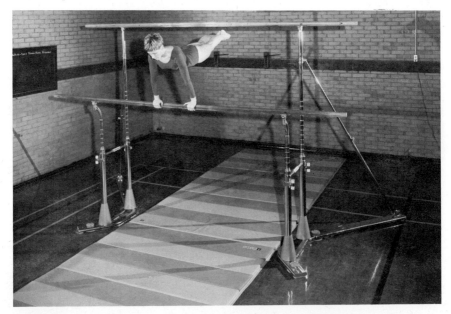

Gymnastic equipment courtesy Nissen Corporation, Cedar Rapids, Iowa.

sideration should be given to dealing with a business firm that will service and replace materials and take care of emergencies without delay and controversy.

PURCHASING SUPPLIES AND EQUIPMENT

A discussion of several important considerations in making purchases of supplies and equipment follows.

Purchases should meet the requirements established by the educational system and have administrative approval

Each educational system has its own policy providing for the purchase of supplies and equipment. It is essential that the prescribed pattern be followed and that proper administrative approval be obtained. Requisition forms that contain such information as description of items, amounts, and costs; purchase orders that place the buying procedure on a written or contract basis; and voucher forms that show receipt of materials should all be utilized as prescribed by school or college regulations. The health and physical education administrator and staff should be familiar with and follow local purchasing policies.

Below are listed a series of steps that one school system uses in purchasing equipment:

1. Initiation—A request is made by the teacher for equipment to fulfill, augment, supplement, or improve the curriculum.
2. Review of request—The building principal and central administration approve or disapprove request after careful consideration of need.
3. Review of budget allocation—A budget code number is assigned after availability of funds in that category has been determined.
4. Preparation of specifications—Specifications are prepared in detail, giving exact quality requirements,

and made available to prospective contractors or vendors.

5. Receipt of bids—Contractors or vendors submit price quotations.
6. Comparison of bids to specifications—Careful evaluation is made to determine exact fulfillment of quality requirements.
7. Recommendations to the board of education—The business administrator prepares comparisons for the board of education, with specific recommendations for their approval.
8. Purchase order to supplier—After board of education approval, a purchase is made that fulfills the requirements at a competitive price.

Purchasing should be done in advance of need

The main and bulk purchases of supplies and equipment for programs of health and physical education should be completed well in advance of the time that the materials will be utilized. Late orders, rushed through at the last moment, may mean mistakes or substitutions on the part of the manufacturer. When purchase orders are placed early, manufacturers have more time to do their jobs and can carry out their responsibilities more efficiently. Goods that do not meet specifications can be returned and replaced, and many other advantages result. Items that are needed in the fall should be ordered not later than the preceding spring, and items desired for spring use should be ordered not later than the preceding fall.

Supplies and equipment should be standardized as far as possible and practical

Ease of ordering is accomplished and larger quantities of materials can be purchased at a saving when standardized items of supplies and equipment are used. Standardization means that certain colors,

ORIGINAL
(To Superintendent's Office)

BOARD OF EDUCATION
————— , NEW YORK

REQUISITION FORM

DATE_____

The following supplies, equipment, or services are required for the use of

_____

Teacher or Department

Signed

Quantity	Description—give complete information	Purpose	Cost Unit	Total

PURCHASE REQUISITION

Comment:

Purchase requisitions are generally initiated by a school or department to cover requirements which are needed during the school year and which are to be purchased from a supplier. Requisition should be made out in duplicate:

1. Original sent to business office for processing

2. Duplicate retained in initiating school or department

APPROVED

_____

Superintendent of Schools

BOARD OF EDUCATION
——————— , New York
DEPARTMENT OF PURCHASE AND SUPPLIES

Req. No. ....

For ....

TO.....................................   School   Department

....   Date ....

....   Return to be made by ....

THIS IS NOT AN ORDER

Gentlemen:

Kindly fill in **the quotations** requested below. If unable to quote, please note and return blank.
Be sure to quote unit price and total amount. **This form must be returned.**

——————————— **Purchasing Agent**

Notice: **Resolution of the Board of Education of the city of**   prohibits the purchase of materials, supplies,
and/or services, produced by child labor, and the provisions thereof are made a part hereof.
The Board of Education is exempt from paying manufacturers' excise, floor, or sales tax. Tax exemption
certificate will be issued when requested.

Approximate number wanted	Articles and description	Vendor's description (Give manufacturer's name and number, when not as per our description)	Unit price	Total

QUOTATION FORM

Comment:

    This form is made out in the purchasing office and sent to

a vendor to obtain prices on items specified. If sent to the

vendor in duplicate, it permits the vendor to fill out the form,

indicating what he proposes to furnish and the price, and also

gives him a copy for his files. On receipt of the various

quotations covering the transaction, a summary may be made for

use of the purchasing official.

IMPORTANT - Please Specify Delivery Date   Extend total cash of each item

The following terms will be expected unless
otherwise specified:
   Cash discount 2% - 30 days   Vendor ....
   Quotations will be f. o. b. point of delivery,
     with all charges paid.   Signature ....
   Prompt delivery

ORIGINAL		
(1) Copy to vendor	**PURCHASE ORDER** **BOARD OF EDUCATION**	N⁰ 100

To:

Please enter our order for the following goods:

All claims must be mailed in duplicate to Clerk's office at the above address

Date of order ....
Quotation Bid No. ....
Requisition No........................
DELIVERY INSTRUCTIONS
WHEN WANTED
Send to
At
Via   Terms

Quantity and unit	Description	Unit price	Total amount	✓	Delivery checked by	Code

PURCHASE ORDER

Comment:

It is a generally accepted practice to make four copies of the purchase order form. In this case, the disposition might be as follows:

1. Original copy to vendor

2. One copy for purchasing department files

3. One copy to finance or auditing division

4. One copy to requisitioner which may become the receipt copy and returned to business office when goods called for have been received

If shipment cannot be made as requested, notify us at once.

CONDITIONS — READ CAREFULLY

1 Please acknowledge receipt of this order by return mail.
2 Make invoice in duplicate; send one with goods and mail the other to the purchasing agent.
3 Each shipment should be covered by a separate invoice.
4 The right is reserved to cancel this order if it is not filled within the contract time.
5 The conditions of this order are not to be modified by any verbal understanding.
6 Charges for boxing and cartage will not be allowed unless previously agreed upon.
7 If the price is stated in the order, material must not be billed at a higher price.
8 Acceptance of this order includes acceptance of all terms, prices, delivery instructions, specifications, and conditions stated.

There is a balance to credit of proper appropriation or fund to meet the expenditure covered by this purchase.

....
Clerk

....
School Purchasing Agent

styles, and types of material are ordered consistently. This procedure can be followed after careful research to determine what is the best, most reliable, and most serviceable product for the money. However, standardization of supplies and equipment should never mean that further study and research to find the best materials in the light of program objectives is terminated.

Specifications should be clearly set forth when making purchases

The trademark, item number, catalogue number, type of material, and other important specifications should be clearly stated when purchasing material so as to avoid any misunderstanding as to what it wanted and is being ordered. This procedure en-

sures that quality merchandise will be received when it is ordered. It also makes it possible to compare bids of competing business firms in a more meaningful manner.

Cost should be kept at the lowest figure possible without loss of quality

Quality of materials is a major consideration. However, among various manufacturers and business concerns, prices vary for products of equal quality. Since supplies and equipment are usually purchased in considerable volume, a few cents on each unit of purchase could represent a saving of many hundreds of dollars to taxpayers. Therefore, if quality can be maintained, materials should be purchased at the lowest cost figure.

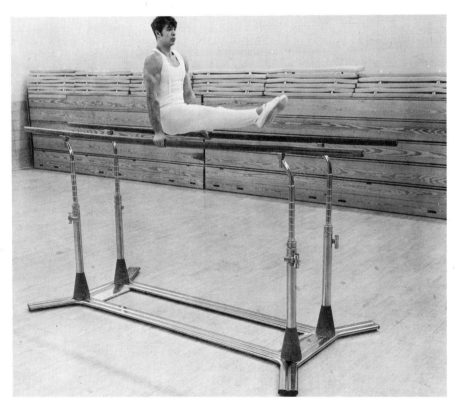

Gymnastic equipment courtesy Nissen Corporation, Cedar Rapids, Iowa.

MONTH	TYPE OF ATHLETIC EQUIPMENT			
	FOOTBALL	BASEBALL	BASKETBALL	TRACK
JANUARY	ORDER NEW EQUIPMENT	ORDER NEW EQUIPMENT	PRACTICE FREE THROWS DURING STUDY HALL	ORDER NEW EQUIPMENT
FEBRUARY	ORDER NEW EQUIPMENT	TIME IS RUNNING OUT		TIME IS RUNNING OUT
MARCH	ORDER NEW EQUIPMENT	DELIVERY	TAKE INVENTORY	MAKE PLANS FOR VACATION
APRIL	TIME IS RUNNING OUT	MARK EQUIPMENT	ORDER NEW EQUIPMENT	GO FISHING
MAY	MOW PRINCIPAL'S LAWN		ORDER NEW EQUIPMENT	
JUNE	GO TO SCHOOL BOARD PICNIC	TAKE INVENTORY	ORDER NEW EQUIPMENT	TAKE INVENTORY
JULY	DELIVERY		ORDER NEW EQUIPMENT	
AUGUST	MARK EQUIPMENT	ATTEND COUNTY FAIR	TIME IS RUNNING OUT	
SEPTEMBER			DELIVERY	DELIVERY
OCTOBER		ORDER NEW EQUIPMENT	MARK EQUIPMENT	MARK EQUIPMENT
NOVEMBER	TAKE INVENTORY	ORDER NEW EQUIPMENT		ORDER NEW EQUIPMENT
DECEMBER	ORDER NEW EQUIPMENT	ORDER NEW EQUIPMENT		ORDER NEW EQUIPMENT

ORDER NEW EQUIPMENT   TIME IS RUNNING OUT   YOU MAY BE TOO LATE

Athletic equipment buyers' almanac. (From How to budget, select, and order athletic equipment, Chicago, 1962, The Athletic Institute.)

Purchases should be made from reputable business firms

In some cases the decision concerning the firm from which supplies and equipment are to be purchased may be determined by the local board of education or college authorities. In the event of such a procedure, this principle is academic. However, where the business firm from which purchases will be made is determined by health and physical education personnel, it is wise to deal with established, reputable businesses that are known to have reasonable prices, reliable materials, and good service. In the long run this is the best and safest procedure to follow.

Local firms should be considered

The administration's main concern is to obtain good value for money expended. If local firms can offer equal values, render equal or better service for the same money, and are reliable, then preference should probably be given to local dealers. If such conditions cannot be met, however, a question can be raised as to the wisdom of such a procedure. In some cases it is advantageous to use local dealers, since they are more readily accessible and can provide quicker and better service than firms located farther away.

Bids should be obtained

A good administrative procedure that helps to eliminate any accusation of favoritism and that assists also in obtaining the best price available is use of competitive bidding. This procedure requires that special forms be distributed to many dealers who handle the supplies and equipment

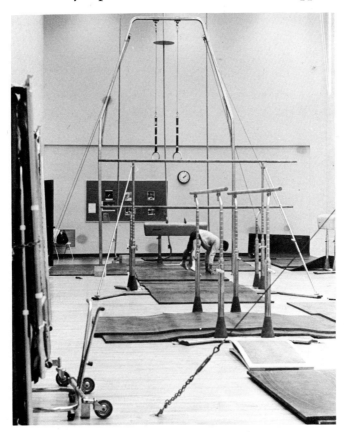

Gymnastic room with equipment. (University of California at Irvine.)

desired. In such cases, the specifics in regard to the kind, amount, and quality of articles desired should be clearly stated. After bids have been obtained the choice can be made. Low bids do not have to be accepted. However, where they are not honored, proper justification should be set forth.

Gifts or favors should not be accepted from dealers

Some dealers and salesmen are happy to present an administrator or staff member with a new rifle, set of golf clubs, tennis racquet, or other gift if, in so doing, they believe it is possible to get a school or college on their account. It is poor policy to accept such gifts or favors. This places a person under obligation to an individual or firm and can only result in difficulties and harm to the program. An administrator or staff member should never profit personally from any materials that are purchased for use in his or her programs.

A complete inventory analysis is essential before purchasing

Before purchases are made such information should be available as the amount of supplies and equipment on hand and the condition of these items. This knowledge prevents overbuying and large stockpiles of materials that may be outdated when they become needed.

CHECKING, ISSUING, AND MAINTAINING SUPPLIES AND EQUIPMENT

Some guidelines for checking, issuing, and maintaining supplies and equipment are discussed in the following paragraphs.

All supplies and equipment should be carefully checked upon receipt

Equipment and supplies that have been ordered should not be paid for until they have been checked as to amount, type, quality, size, and other specifications that were listed on the purchase order. If any discrepancies are noted, they should be corrected before payment is made. This represents a very important procedure and responsibility and should be carefully followed. It represents good business practice in a matter requiring good business sense.

Supplies and equipment requiring organization identification should be labeled

Equipment and supplies are often moved from location to location within the school plant and also are issued to students and to staff members on a temporary basis. It is a good procedure to stencil or stamp the school or college identification in some appropriate location in order to have a check on such material, to help trace missing articles, to discourage misappropriation of such items, and to know what is and what is not departmental property.

Procedures should be established for issuing and checking in supplies and equipment

There can be considerable loss of material if poor accounting procedures are followed. Procedures should be established so that items are issued in a prescribed manner, proper forms are completed, records are maintained, and there is a clear understanding at all times as to where the material is located. Articles should be listed on the records according to various specifications of amount, size, or color, together with the name of the person to whom the item is issued. The individual's record should be classified according to name, street address, telephone, locker number, or other information important for identification purposes. In all cases the person or persons to whom the supplies and equipment are issued should be held accountable.

Text continued on p. 505.

NOTICE TO BIDDERS

(For use in advertising)

The board of education of ___(legal name)___ School District

No. ____ of the Town(s) of _____ popularly known

as _____ , (in accordance with Section 103 of

Article 5-A of the General Municipal Law) hereby invites the sub-

mission of sealed bids on_____ for use in the

schools of the district. Bids will be received until _____ on the
                                                        (hour)

_____ day of _____ , 19 ____, at _____
  (date)   (month)   (place of bid

_____, at which time and place all bids will be publicly opened.
 opening)

Specifications and bid form may be obtained at the same office. The

board of education reserves the right to reject all bids. Any bid

submitted will be binding for _____ days subsequent to the date of

bid opening.

Board of Education

_____ School District No. ____

of the Town(s) of _____

County(ies) of _____

_____
           (Address)

By _____
           (Purchasing Agent)

_____
  (Date)

Note: The hour should indicate whether it is Eastern Standard or
Eastern Daylight Saving Time.

Sample notice to bidders form. (From School Business Management Handbook Number 5, The University of the State of New York, Albany, N. Y.)

	INVENTORY						
Date	Manufacturer	Dealer	Cat. No.	Total on Hand	Number Purchased	Cost	Comment

Year	New	Good	Fair	Obs.	Total	Numbers or Sizes							

Inventory form.

EQUIPMENT RECORD CARD
TO BE RETURNED TODAY

Name_____Teacher_____Period_____

No.	Article	No.	Article	No.	Article
	Archery, Arm Guard		Handball		Sponge Ball
	Archery, Arrow		Hockey Ball		Tape Measure
	Archery, Bow		Hockey Sticks		Table Tennis Net
	Archery, Glove		Jacks - Ball		Tennis Ball
	Badminton Racket		Jump Rope		Tether Ball
	Badminton Shuttlecock		Marbles		Timer (Stop Watch)
	Basketball		Pick-up Sticks		Whistle
	Bean Bag		Ping Pong Ball		
	Checkerboard		Ping Pong Paddle		
	Checker Men		Playground Ball		
	Chest Protector		10" 16"		
	Chinese Checkers		Quoits		
	Clip Board		Softball		
	Darts		Softball Bat		
	Deck Tennis Rings		Shin Guards		
	Dominoes		Shuffleboard Cue		
	Eye-glasses Guard		Shuffleboard Disc		
	Goal Guards		Shuttlecock		
	Golf Ball		Shuttle Loop		
	Golf Club		Soccer Ball		

Equipment record form. (From Bucher, C. A., Koenig, C. R., and Barnhard, M.: Methods and materials in secondary school physical education, ed. 3, St. Louis, 1970, The C. V. Mosby Co.)

EQUIPMENT ISSUE

Date...

I .... have

accepted school property ....

.... (write in article and its number)

and agree to return it clean and in good condition or pay for said uniform.

Signed ....

H. R. #

Home Phone #   Home Address...

Equipment issue form. (From Bucher, C. A., Koenig, C. R., and Barnhard, M.: Methods and materials in secondary school physical education, ed. 3, St. Louis, 1970, The C. V. Mosby Co.

DEPARTMENT OF HEALTH AND PHYSICAL EDUCATION

Re: Lost Property Report

Student owner_____ H.R._____ R___ S___

Date of loss_____ Time_____ Period_____

List missing articles:

Description of known details:

Instructor's follow-up:

(Signed)___ _____

(Use reverse side if additional space is necessary.)

Lost property report. (From Bucher, C. A., Koenig, C. R., and Barnhard, M.: Methods and materials in secondary school physical education, ed. 3, St. Louis, 1970, The C. V. Mosby Co.)

EQUIPMENT CHECKOUT RECORD

Player_____ Home Room_____

Address_____ Phone_____

Class_____ Height_____ Weight_____ Age_____

Parents Waiver_____ Examination_____ Insurance_____

Football   Cross Country   Basketball   Swimming   Wrestling

Baseball   Track   Tennis   Golf

	Out	In	Game Equipment	Out	In
Blocking pads			White jersey		
Shoulder pads			Maroon jersey		
Hip pads			White pants		
Thigh pads			Maroon pants		
Knee pads			Warm-up pants		
Helmet			Warm-up jacket		
Shoes			Stockings		
Practice pants					
Practice jersey					

I hereby certify that I have received the above-listed athletic equipment and will return same not later than the day following the last game of the season for the sport checked.

Signature_____

Equipment checkout record. (From Bucher, C. A., Koenig, C. R., and Barnhard, M.: Methods and materials in secondary school physical education, ed. 3, St. Louis, 1970, The C. V. Mosby Co.)

BOYS' PHYSICAL EDUCATION DEPARTMENT

Equipment Inspection

Please write on this sheet the names of boys not wearing clean gym clothing. Also give the advisers' names. Thank you.

Inspection may involve any day with special emphasis on each MONDAY. The
instructor should place his initials following the date of each recording.

Date	Instr. Init.	Boy's Name	Adviser	Dirty Clothes	Partial Equipment	Torn Clothing	*Borrowed Equipment

*Borrowed equipment with or without owner's consent should always be
followed up with a discipline note.

Equipment inspection form. (Courtesy Boys' Physical Education Department, New Trier
Township High School, Winnetka, Ill.; from Bucher, C. A., Koenig, C. R., and Barnhard, M.:
Methods and materials in secondary school physical education, ed. 3, St. Louis, 1970, The
C. V. Mosby Co.)

Equipment should be in a state of constant repair

Equipment should always be maintained in a serviceable condition. Procedures for caring for equipment should be routinized so that repairs are provided as needed. All used equipment should be checked and then repaired, replaced, or serviced as is needed. Repair can be justified, however, only when the cost for such is within reason. Supplies should be replaced when they have been expended.

Equipment and supplies should be stored properly

Supplies and equipment should be handled efficiently so that space has been properly organized for storing, a procedure has been established for ease of location, and proper safeguards have been taken against fire and theft. Proper shovels, bins, hangers, and other accessories should be available. Temperature, humidity, and ventilation are also important considera-

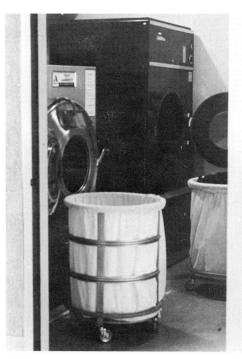

Laundry for washable supplies. (University of California at Irvine.)

ADMINISTRATOR'S CODE OF ETHICS FOR PERSONNEL INVOLVED IN PURCHASING*

1. To consider first the interests of the school district or college and the betterment of the educational program.
2. To be receptive to advice and suggestions of colleagues, both in the department and in the field of business administration, and others insofar as advice is compatible with legal and moral requirements.
3. To endeavor to obtain the greatest value for every dollar spent.
4. To strive to develop an expertise and knowledge of supplies and equipment that ensure recommendations for purchases of greatest value.
5. To insist on honesty in the sales representation of every product submitted for consideration for purchase.
6. To give all responsible bidders equal consideration in determining whether their product meets specifications and the educational needs of your program.
7. To discourage and to decline gifts that in any way might influence a purchase.
8. To provide a courteous reception for all persons who may call on legitimate business missions regarding supplies and equipment.
9. To counsel and help other educators involved in purchasing.
10. To cooperate with governmental or other organizations or persons and help in the development of sound business methods in the procurement of school and college equipment and supplies.

*Adapted from the New York State Association of School Business Officials: Code of ethics for school purchasing officials.

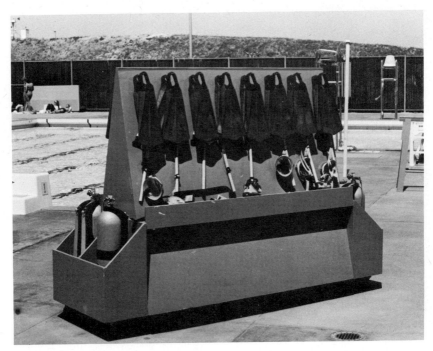

Rolling equipment cart, one of several designed for specific classes of the physical education program. These are stored in the equipment room and transported to activity areas by student helpers. (University of California at Irvine.)

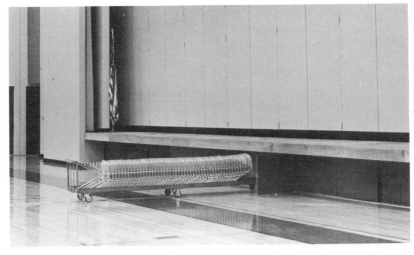

Storage cart for folding chairs. This is an interesting and functional system for storing over 1,000 chairs. Lightweight carts roll into compartments under the stage. (University of California at Irvine.)

tions. Items going into the storeroom should be properly checked as to quality and quantity. An inventory should be constantly available as to all items on hand in the storeroom. Every precaution should be taken to provide for the adequate care of the material so that a wise investment has been made.

Appendix A contains much useful information applicable to the purchase and care of supplies and equipment for health and physical education programs.

AUDIOVISUAL MATERIALS

Audiovisual aids and materials have become such an important part of health and physical education programs that space is provided for a discussion of the use, types, and guidelines for such supplies and equipment.

A recent survey among 100 schools and colleges found that more than one-half of them used some form of visual or audio aid in their programs. All of the persons surveyed felt that audiovisual media served as a valuable supplement to instruction in the learning of motor skills. The survey also found that videotaping is on the increase as an instructional tool. The audiovisual media used with the most frequency by those persons surveyed included cartridge films, loopfilms, 16- and 8-mm. films, wall charts, slide films, film strips, and instructional television.

Reasons for increased use of audiovisual materials

There are several reasons why there is an increased use of audiovisual materials in health education and physical education programs. Some of these are:

1. *They enable the student to better understand concepts and the performance of a skill, events, and other experiences.* The old cliché, "One picture is worth a thousand words," has much truth. The use of a film, pictures, or other materials gives a clearer idea of the subject being taught, whether it is how a heart functions or how to perfect a golf swing.

2. *They help to provide a variety to teaching.* There is increased motivation, the attention span of children is prolonged, and the subject matter of a course is much more exciting when audiovisual aids are used in addition to other teaching techniques.

3. *They increase motivation on the part of the student.* To see a game played, a skill performed, or an experiment conducted in clear, understandable, illustrated form helps to motivate the student to engage in a game, perform a skill more effectively, or want to know more about the relation of exercise to health. This is particularly true in video replay, for example, where a student can actually see how he performs a skill and then can compare his performance to what should be done.

4. *They provide for an extension of what can normally be taught in a classroom, gymnasium, or playground.* Audiovisual aids enable the student to be taken to other countries, to experience sporting events that occur in other parts of the United States, and to witness events that are significant to health. All of these are important to health and physical education programs and the instructional program for students.

5. *They provide a historical reference for the fields of health and physical education.* Outstanding events in sports, physical education, and health that have occurred in past years can be brought to life before students' eyes. In this way the student obtains a better understanding of these fields and the important role they play in our society and other cultures of the world.

Selected types of audiovisual aids

A partial list of audiovisual materials that are commonly used today by health and physical education teachers follows.

Visual aids (audiovisual in some cases)

Reading materials—books, magazines, encyclopedias, and almanacs

Chalkboards—for recording plays, thoughts, and ideas

Wall charts—of self-explanatory terms

Flat pictures, cartoons, posters, photographs

Graphs—bar, circle, line, and other types

Maps and globes

Bulletin boards—for posting materials pertaining to program

Models and specimens—the human body, skeleton, animals, insects, and others

Opaque projector—used to display on a screen an enlarged picture that is too small in the original for all students to readily see and understand its message

Overhead projector—a compact, lightweight machine that can be operated with ease and used to project materials on a screen. The material projected is in the form of a transparency, made of film that can either be purchased or made

Stereoscopes—machines that project a picture in three dimensions and thus give a better understanding of space relationships

Silent films

Slides—three types, generally speaking: 35-mm. individual slide encased in a cardboard holder; the larger lantern slide usually 3¼ by 4 inches, and the lantern slide that may be prepared for immediate use by a Polaroid transparency film

Filmstrips

Loop films—available in cartridges that can be inserted into a projector and shown with comparative ease. There are three types: a free 8-mm. loop film that can be shown in an 8-mm. projector; an 8-mm. cartridge film encased in a plastic cartridge that requires a special projector; and the super-8-mm. film encased in a plastic cartridge that requires a still different type of projection.

Motion pictures—usually in 8-, 16-, and 35-mm. sizes

Television—educational and closed circuit television and the kinescope recorder. Video-tape recording that enables a student to actually see how he performs a particular skill, for example, has proved effective as an instructional medium.

Audio aids

Radio—educational and commercial programs

Records and transcriptions—of important events, speeches, musical productions, and music for dances

Tape recordings—special events are recorded and used to appraise student progress in conduct, skills, concepts, and appreciation and to cover current happenings pertinent to health and physical education

Administrative guidelines for the selection and use of audiovisual aids

1. *Audiovisual materials should be carefully selected and screened before using.* Such items as appropriateness for age and grade level of students, adequacy of subject matter, technical qualities, inclusion of current information, cost, and other factors are important to know when selecting audiovisual materials to be used.

2. *The presentation of materials should be carefully planned to provide continuity in the subject being taught.* Materials should be selected and used that amplify and illustrate some important part of the material being covered in a particular course. Furthermore, they should be used at a time that logically fits into the presentation of certain material and concepts.

3. *The materials should be carefully evaluated after they have been used.* Whether or not materials are used a second time should be determined on the basis of their worth the first time they were used. Therefore, a careful evaluation should take place after their use. Records of evaluation should be maintained.

4. *Slow-motion and stop-action projections are best when a pattern of coordination of movements in a skill is to be taught.* When teaching a skill the teacher usually likes to analyze the various parts of the whole and also to stop and discuss various aspects of the skill with the students.

5. *Proper maintenance and preparation of equipment should be done.* Projectors, record players, television equipment, and other materials need to be kept in good operating condition and operated by qualified personnel in order to have an effective audiovisual program.

CHECKLIST FOR SPORTS AND OTHER PHYSICAL EDUCATION EQUIPMENT AND SUPPLIES

Anthropometric apparatus

Anthropometric tape
Chest depth caliper
Dynamometer
Manuometer
Scale
Shoulder breadth
caliper
Stadiometer
Wet spirometer

Aquatics

Clocks
Diving boards
Boards
1-meter
3-meter
Diving tramp
Ear plugs
Fins
Guns
Kickboards
Lane markers
Life buoys
15-inch diameter
18-inch diameter
Lifeguard chair
Noseclips
Pool cleaning
equipment
Pool ladders
2 foot   4 foot
3 foot   5 foot
Regulators
(breathing tank)
Robe
Snorkles
Swim caps
Swim suits
Men's
Tanks (air)
Underwater masks
Women's
Warmups
Jacket
Pants
Water basketball
(backboard and
goal)

Aquatics—cont'd
Water polo balls
Water polo goals
Water polo nets
Water slides
Weight belt
Wet suit
Boots
Gloves

Archery
Arrow points
Arrows
Field
Hunting
Target
Backstop net
Bow case
Bow sight
Bow strings
Bows
Feathers
Finger tabs
Fletching tool
Forearm guards
Gloves
Nocks
Quivers
Sets
Target face
Target standards
Targets

Audiovisual aids
Administrative aids
Coaching aids
Dance records
Film
Loudspeakers

Badminton
Net
Racquet press
Racquets
Sets
Shuttlecocks
Standards

Baseball
Backstop
Ball bag
Balls
Bases

Baseball—cont'd
Bats
Baseball
Fungo
Little League
Pony and Babe
Ruth League
Bat bag
Batting cage
Batting tee
Belts
Caps
Catcher's mask
Chest protector
Gloves
Catcher's mitt
Fielder's
First baseman's
Home plate
Leg guards
Pants
Pitcher's plate
Pitching machine
Protective helmets
Rosin
Rule book
Score book
Shirts
Shoes
Sliding pads
Socks
Umpire's body
protector
Umpire's indicator
Umpire's leg guards
Umpire's mask
Uniforms (complete)
Warmup jackets

Basketball
Backboards
Ball return
Balls
Goals
Nets
Pants
Rebound ring
Shirts
Shoes
Target socks
Warmups

Bowling
Ball bag
Balls
Shirts
Shoes

Boxing
Bag bladder
Bag gloves
Bag platforms
Corner pillows
Ear protectors
Gloves
Hand wrappings
Head protectors
Platform rings
Ring canvas
Ring ropes
Robes
Rope wrappings
Shoes
Skip ropes
Speed bag
Striking bag swivel
Teeth protector
Training bags
Trunks

Cheerleading
Briefs
Majorette boots
Skirts
Sweaters

Crew
Oars
Sculls
Shells

Exercise equipment
Abdominal board
Body weights
Dumbbells
Exerciser sets
Isogyms
Isometric kits
Leg press machine
Multipurpose weight
bench
Pulley weights
Squat stands
Weight sets
Weight shoes

Continued.

CHECKLIST FOR SPORTS AND OTHER PHYSICAL EDUCATION EQUIPMENT AND SUPPLIES—cont'd

Fencing
Chest protector
Woman's protector
Electrical equipment
Foils
Epees
Gloves
Jackets
Masks
Rubber tips
Scoring device
Shoes
Trousers
Weapons
Epees
Foils
Sabers

Field hockey
Balls
Goal
Net
Shin guards
Shoes
Sticks

Football
Ankle wraps
Balls
Belts
Bladders
Blocking sleds
2-man
5-man
7-man
Capes
Cervical neck pad
Chin straps
Cleats
Downs marker
Dummies
Face guards
Flags (corner)
Helmet racks
Helmets
Hip pads
Jerseys
Kicking tee
Knee pads
Mouth guards
Pants
Rib pads

Football—cont'd
Scrimmage vests
Shoes
Shoulder pad rack
Shoulder pads
Socks
Thigh guards

Golf
Bags (club)
Balls
Cage (practice)
Club cart
Clubs
Irons
Putters
Woods
Gloves
Head covers
Rubber driving mat
Shoes
Tees

Gymnastics
Balance beam
Low beam
Buck (vaulting)
Chalk
Chalk holder
Hand guards
Horizontal bar
Parallel bars
Low bars
Rings
Ropes (climbing)
Safety belts
Side horse
Springing and jumping
apparatus
Beat board
Reuther board
Spring board
Trampolet
Tambourine
Trampoline
Trapeze
Uneven bars
Conversion kit
Uniform
Pants
Shirts
Shoes

Gymnastics—cont'd
Uniform—cont'd
Warmups
Pants
Shirts
Vaulting box

Handball
Balls
Gloves

Ice hockey
Goal
Net
Skates
Uniform
Jerseys
Pants
Socks

Instructor's equipment
Cap
Jacket
Pants
Shirts
Shoes
Women's tunic

Judo and karate
Punching board
Uniforms
Judo
Karate

Lacrosse
Balls
Body protectors
Goal
Net
Shoes
Sticks

Paddle tennis
Balls
Net
Paddles

**Physical Education
equipment**
Basket holder
Baskets
Bicycle trainer
Bleachers
4-row
Seats 50

**Physical education
equipment—cont'd**
Seats 400
Seats 750
Goal posts
Football
Soccer and field
hockey com-
bination
Soccer and football
combination
Heat lamp
Laundry equipment
hamper
Line markers
Lockers
Box type
Double tier
Single tier
Mat hangers
Mat trucks
Peg boards
Scoreboards
Stall bars
Steam cabinet
Wall ladder
Whirlpool bath

**Physical education
supplies**
Athletic supporters
Awards
Ball carriers
Balls
Cage
Medicine
Playground
Cups (protective)
Foot baths
Game standards
(combination)
Indian clubs
Jump ropes
Locks
Mat envelope covers
Mats
Pinnies
Shower sandals
Soap
Spike wrench kit
Stop clocks
Table inflators

CHECKLIST FOR SPORTS AND OTHER PHYSICAL EDUCATION EQUIPMENT AND SUPPLIES—cont'd

Physical education supplies — cont'd
Towels
Tug-of-war ropes
Uniform hangers
Uniforms (physical education)
  Boy's
  Girl's
Whistles

Playground equipment
Benches
Bicycle racks
Castle towers
Cooking grill
Flag poles
Flying rings
Horizontal bar
Horizontal ladders
Merry-go-round
Picnic table
Seesaws
  3 Seesaws
  4 Seesaws
  6 Seesaws
Slides
Swing seats
  Nursery seat
  Rubber seat
  Belt seat
  Wood seat
Swings
  2 Swings
  4 Swings
  6 Swings
  8 Swings
Trapeze bar

Soccer
Balls

Soccer—cont'd
Goals
Net
Shin guards
Uniforms
  Pants
  Shirts
  Shoes
  Socks

Softball
Balls
Bases
Bat bag
Bats
Books
  Rule book
  Score book
Caps
Gloves
  Catcher's
  Fielder's
  First baseman's
Hose
Jackets
Jerseys
Masks
Protectors (body)
Shoes
Uniforms

Squash
Balls
Rackets

Tennis
Balls
Courts
Nets
Posts
Racquet jacket

Tennis—cont'd
Racquet press
Racquets
Rebound net
Tennis ball machine
Uniforms
  Shirts
  Shoes
  Shorts

Track
Batons
Circles
  Discus
  Shot
Competitors numbers
Cross bar lifter
Cross bars
Discus
Field marks
Finish line yarn
Hammer
Heel cup
High jump standards
Hurdles
Javelins
Measuring tapes
  50-foot
  100-foot
  200-foot
Pedometer
Pits (jumping and vaulting)
Pole vault box
Pole vault poles
Pole vault standards
Shoe laces
Shoes (indoor)
Shoes (outdoor)
Shot

Track — cont'd
Shot—cont'd
  Indoor
    8-pounds
    12-pounds
    16-pounds
  Outdoor
    8-pound
    12-pound
    16-pound
Spike wrench
Spikes
Starting blocks
Starting pistol
Stop watch
Takeoff board
Toe board
Track surface
Uniforms
  Pants
  Shirts
Warmups
  Pants
  Shirts

Volleyball
Balls
Net
Scorebook
Sets
Standards

Wrestling
Head guards
Knee guards
Sweat suit
Uniform
  Shirts
  Shoes
  Tights
  Trunks

Questions and exercises

1. What factors need to be taken into consideration in relation to the purchase and care of supplies and equipment?
2. List and discuss five principles that should be followed in respect to the selection of supplies and equipment. Apply these principles in the procedure involved in selecting a diving board for a swimming pool.
3. List and discuss five principles that should be followed in respect to purchasing supplies and equipment. Apply these principles to the procedure involved in purchasing a trampoline for the gymnasium.
4. Prepare a report on the various types of audiovisual aids that could be used effectively in the teaching of tennis.

5. Prepare an administrative plan that you, as a chairman of a health and physical education department, would recommend for the checking, issuing, and maintenance of physical education supplies and equipment. Be specific, pointing out the steps that should be followed and procedure implemented to ensure sound property accountability.

Reading Assignment in *Administrative Dimensions of Health and Physical Education Programs, Including Athletics:* Chapter 13, Selections 73 to 76.

Selected references

American Association for Health, Physical Education, and Recreation: Equipment and supplies for athletics, physical education and recreation, Washington, D. C., The Association. (Published annually in the Journal of Health, Physical Education, and Recreation.)

American Athletic Equipment Co., Jefferson, Iowa.

Bourguardez, V., and Heilman, C.: Sports equipment: selection, care, and repair, New York, 1950, A. S. Barnes & Co.

Care and maintenance of lacrosse sticks, Towson, Md., 1965, Bacharach Rasin Co., Inc.

Care of athletic equipment, River Grove, Ill., Wilson Sporting Goods Co.

Casey, L. M.: School business administration, New York, 1964, The Center for Applied Research in Education, Inc. (The Library of Education).

De Kieffer, R. E.: Audiovisual instruction, New York, 1965, The Center for Applied Research in Education, Inc. (The Library of Education).

How to budget, select, and order athletic equipment. Available from Athletic Goods Manufacturers Association, Merchandise Mart, Chicago, Ill., also through MacGregor & Rawlings Sporting Goods.

Irwin, A.: Put your equipment on wheels, Scholastic Coach 35:10, 1966.

Meyer, K.: Purchase, care, and repair of athletic equipment, St. Louis, 1948, Educational Publishers, Inc.

Murray, F.: Perpetual inventory, Scholastic Coach 31:20, 1962.

Participants in National Facilities Conference: Planning areas and facilities for health, physical education, and recreation, Chicago, 1965. The Athletic Institute, Inc.

Selway, C. P.: Efficiency in the equipment and laundry rooms, Scholastic Coach 34:30, 1965.

CHAPTER 18 LEGAL LIABILITY AND INSURANCE MANAGEMENT

The growth of school and college health and physical education programs, including athletics, in this country has brought with it many problems in the field of administration. One of these problems is legal liability and insurance management. This is especially pertinent to these specialized areas because of the danger of accidents while engaging in the various activities that comprise the programs. Furthermore, the nature of these areas involves the use of special apparatus, excursions and trips, living in camps, utilizing first-aid practices, and other items that have implications for liability.

According to Bouvier's *Law Dictionary*, liability is "the responsibility, the state of one who is bound in law and justice to do something which may be enforced by action." Another definition states: "Liability is the condition of affairs which gives rise to an obligation to do a particular thing to be enforced by court action."

Leaders in the fields of health and physical education should know how far they can go with various aspects of their programs and what precautions are necessary in order not to be held legally liable in the event of an accident. The fact that approximately 67% of all school jurisdiction accidents involving boys and 59% involving girls occur in physical education and recreation programs has implications for these specialized fields. Furthermore, the fact that an estimated 3 million boys and girls participate in interscholastic athletic programs alone indicates a further administrative concern for physical education programs.

The administration, which in the final analysis is responsible for the program, should clearly understand the implications of their work in this respect. Fear of personal liability can thwart an otherwise good educational program.

When an accident resulting in personal injury occurs on school property, the question often arises as to whether damages can be recovered. The National Commission on Safety Education points out that all school employees run the risk of suit by injured pupils on the basis of alleged negligence that causes bodily injury to pupils. Such injuries occur on playgrounds, on athletic fields, in science laboratories, in shop classes, or in any place where students congregate.

The legal rights of the individuals involved in such cases are worthy of study. Although the law varies from state to state, it is possible to discuss liability in a general way that has implications for all sections of the country. First, it is important to understand the legal basis for health, physical education, and allied areas.

THE LEGAL BASIS FOR HEALTH EDUCATION, PHYSICAL EDUCATION, AND ALLIED AREAS*

All fifty states, the District of Columbia, and Puerto Rico have laws requiring or permitting the teaching of health, physical

---

*State school laws and regulations for health, safety, driver, outdoor, physical education, Washington, D. C., 1964, Office of Education, Department of Health, Education and Welfare.

education, safety education, driver education, and outdoor education. In addition to such laws, thirty-seven states, the District of Columbia, Puerto Rico, and the Canal Zone have a total of eighty-eight regulations regarding the teaching of these subjects.

Physical education, either as a separate subject or in combination with health education, is a matter of law and/or regulation in forty-eight states, the District of Columbia, Canal Zone, Puerto Rico, and the Virgin Islands.

Health education, as a separate subject or in combination with physical education, is a matter of law and/or regulation in forty-one states, the District of Columbia, Canal Zone, Puerto Rico, and the Virgin Islands.

Safety education, as a separate subject, is a matter of law and/or regulation in thirteen states.

Driver education is a matter of law and/or regulation in thirty-six states.

Outdoor education is a matter of law in six states.

Health, physical, safety, and outdoor education are a matter of law and regulations at the elementary school level in all fifty states, the District of Columbia, Canal Zone, Puerto Rico, and the Virgin Islands.

Physical education is a required daily experience for 4 years in three states at the secondary level, and health and physical education in varying amounts is a required daily experience in fifteen other states at the same educational level.

Thirty-two states require health and physical education for graduation from school: 4 years, twelve states; 3 years, two states; 2 years, two states; 1 or 2 years, two states; 1 year, three states, and as a requirement other than length of time listed, eleven states.

Two states do not have laws or regulations requiring teaching of physical education.

Included in Appendix C is a state-by-state analysis of school laws and regulations concerning the teaching of health, physical education, and allied areas.

LEGAL IMPLICATIONS FOR REQUIRING PHYSICAL EDUCATION

Shroyer* made a study of the legal implications of requiring pupils to enroll in physical education classes and found that the courts have handed down decisions from which the following conclusions may be drawn:

1. Students may be required to take physical education. However, there should be some flexibility to provide for those cases where an individual's constitutional rights might be violated if such activities are against his principles, for example, dancing.
2. Where reasonable parental demands for deviation from the physical education requirement are called for, every effort should be made to comply with the parent's wishes. However, unreasonable demands should not result in acquiescence.
3. Where rules and regulations may be questioned, the board of education should provide for a review of the rationale behind the rule or regulation and why the policy is needed.
4. A student may be denied the right to graduate and receive a diploma when a required course such as physical education is not taken.

LEGAL LIABILITY

Some years ago the courts recognized the hazards involved in the play activities that are a part of the educational program. An injury occurred to a boy while he was playing tag. The court recognized the possibility and risk of some injury in

---

*Shroyer, G. F.: Legal implications of requiring pupils to enroll in physical education, Journal of Health, Physical Education, and Recreation **35:** 51, 1964.

physical education programs and would not award damages. However, it pointed out that care must be taken by both the participant and the authorities in charge. It further implied that the benefits derived from participating in physical education activities such as tag offset the occasional injury that might occur.

The cited decision regarding the benefits derived from participating in physical education programs was handed down at a time when the attitude of the law was that no government agency, which would include the school, could be held liable for the acts of its employees unless it so consented. Since that time a changing attitude

in the courts has been in evidence. As more accidents occurred, the courts frequently decided in favor of the injured party when negligence could be shown. The immunity derived from the old common-law rule that a government agency cannot be sued without its consent is slowly changing in the eyes of the courts so that both federal government and state may be sued.

Those elements of a school curriculum that are compulsory, such as physical education, prompt courts to decide on the basis of what is in the best interests of the public. Instead of being merely a moral responsibility, safety has become a legal

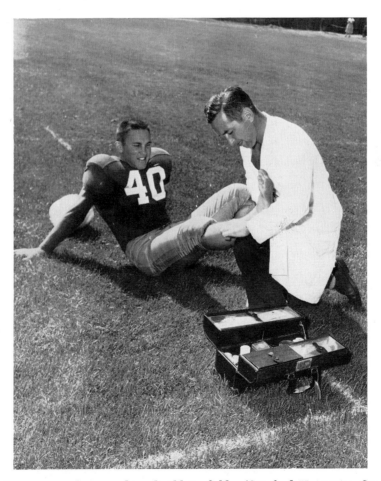

Many accidents occur on playgrounds and athletic fields. (Stanford University, Stanford, Calif.)

responsibility. Those who uphold the doctrine that a government agency should be immune from liability maintain that payments for injury to constituents is a misapplication of public funds. On the other hand, the liberal thinkers feel it is wrong for the cost of injuries to fall on one or a few persons and, instead, should be shared by all. To further their case these liberals cite the constitutional provision that compensation must be given for the taking or damaging of private property. They argue that it is inconsistent that the government cannot take or damage private property without just compensation on the one hand, yet on the other can injure or destroy the life of a person without liability for compensation. The liberal view is being used more and more by the courts.

The rule of immunity (since school districts are instrumentalities of the state, and the state is immune from suit unless it consents, the state's immunity extends to the districts) is the law, with a few exceptions, in almost all the states. Some exceptions are California, Washington, and New York. However, as has been pointed out above, the doctrine of immunity is starting to crumble. The case *Bingham v. Board of Education of Oregon City*, 223 P2d 432, handed down by the Supreme Court in Utah in October, 1950, involved a 3-year-old child who, while riding her tricycle on the school grounds, fell into some burning embers left on the grounds and suffered severe burns. The school maintained an incinerator adjacent to the playground area in which rubbish was burned. From time to time embers and ashes were removed and scattered around the adjoining area. The parents sued to recover damages and the court held the district was not liable. Judge Latimer, who wrote the court's opinion, said: "While the law writers, editors, and judges have criticized and disapproved the foregoing doctrine of government immunity as illogical and unjust, the weight of precedent of decided cases supports the general rule and we prefer not to disregard a principle so well established without statutory authority. We, therefore, adopt the rule of the majority and hold that school boards cannot be held liable for ordinary negligent acts."

The importance of this case lies in the fact that two judges dissented. The dissenting opinion pointed out: "I prefer to regard said principle for the purpose of overruling it. I would not wait for the dim distant future in never-never land when the legislature may act." It was also pointed out that the rule rests upon the "immortal and indefensible doctrine" that "the king (sovereign) can do no wrong" and that a state should not be allowed to use this as a shield.

There has been considerable court activity in regard to the principle of governmental immunity. In 1959 the Illinois Supreme Court (*Molitor v. Kaneland Community Unit*, District No. 302, 163 N.E. 2d 89) overruled the immunity doctrine. The supreme courts of Wisconsin, Arizona, and Minnesota followed suit, but in 1963 the Minnesota legislature restored the rule but provided that where school districts had liability insurance they were responsible for damages up to the extent of the coverage. The principle of governmental immunity has also recently been put to the test in courts in such states as Colorado, Iowa, Kansas, Oregon, Pennsylvania, and Utah. However, the courts in these states are hesitant to depart from the precedent that has been set and furthermore insist that it is the legislature of the state rather than the courts that should waive the rule.*

In thirty-nine of fifty states school districts have governmental immunity, which means that as long as they are engaging in a governmental function they cannot be sued, even though negligence has been

---

*Shapiro, F. S.: Your liability for student accidents, National Education Association Journal **54**: 46, 1965.

determined. In eleven states governmental immunity has been annulled either by legislation or judicial decision. In some states schools may legally purchase liability insurance (California requires and twenty-two other states expressly authorize school districts to carry liability insurance) protecting school districts that may become involved in lawsuits, although this does not necessarily mean that governmental immunity has been waived. Of course, in the absence of insurance and "save harmless" laws, which require that school districts assume the liability of the teacher, negligence, proved or not, any judgment rendered against a school district must be met out of personal funds. School districts in Connecticut, Massachusetts, New Jersey, and New York have "save harmless" laws. Wyoming permits school districts to idemnify employees.

School districts that still enjoy governmental immunity usually are either required or permitted to carry liability insurance that specifically covers the operation of school buses.

There is a strong feeling among educators and many in the legal profession that the doctrine of sovereign immunity should be abandoned. In fourteen states students injured as a result of negligence are assured recompense for damages directly or indirectly, either because governmental immunity has been abrogated or because school districts are legally required to indemnify school employees against financial loss. In eighteen other states, if liability insurance has been secured, there is a possibility that students may recover damages incurred.

Although school districts have been granted immunity in many states, teachers do not have such immunity. A decision of an Iowa court in 1938 provides some of the thinking in regard to the teacher's responsibility for his own actions (*Montanick v. McMillin,* 225 Iowa 442, 452-453, 458, 280 N.W. 608, 1938).

[The employee's liability] is not predicated upon any relationship growing out of his employment, but is based upon the fundamental and underlying law of torts, that he who does injury to the person or property of another is civilly liable in damages for the injuries inflicted. . . . The doctrine of *respondeat superior,* literally, "let the principal answer," is an extension of the fundamental principle of torts, and an added remedy to the injured party, under which a party injured by some act of misfeasance may hold both the servant and the master. The exemption of governmental bodies and their officers from liability under the doctrine of *respondeat superior* is a limitation of exception to the rule of *respondeat superior* and in no way affects the fundamental principle of torts that one who wrongfully inflicts injury upon another is liable to the injured person for damages. . . . An act of misfeasance is a positive wrong, and every employee, whether employed by a private person or a municipal corporation owes a duty not to injure another by a negligent act of commission. . . .

Tort

A tort is a legal wrong resulting in direct or indirect injury to another individual or to property. A tortious act is a wrongful act and damages can be collected through court action. Tort can be committed through an act of *omission* or *commission.* An act of omission results when the accident occurs during failure to perform a legal duty, such as when a teacher fails to obey a fire alarm after she has been informed of the procedure to be followed. An act of commission results when the accident occurs while an unlawful act is being performed, such as assault on a student.

The National Education Association points out that "A tort may arise out of the following acts: (a) an act which without lawful justification or excuse is intended by a person to cause harm and does cause the harm complained of; (b) an act in itself contrary to law or an omission of specific legal duty, which causes harm not intended by the person so acting or omitting; (c) an act or omission causing harm which the person so acting or omitting did not intend to cause, but which might and should, with due diligence, have been foreseen and prevented."[*] The teacher, leader, or other individual not only has a legal responsibility as described by law but also is responsible for preventing injury. This means that in addition to complying with certain legal regulations, such as proper facilities, there must be compliance with the principle that children should be taught without injury to them and that prudent care, such as a parent would give, must be exercised. The term *legal duty* does not mean only those duties imposed by law but also the duty that is owed to society to prevent injury to others. A duty imposed by law would be one such as complying with housing regulations and traffic regulations. A duty that teachers owe to society in general consists of teaching children without injury to them. For example, it was stated in one case (*Hoose v. Drumm*, 281 N.Y. 54): "Teachers have watched over the play of their pupils time out of mind. At recess periods, not less than in the classroom, a teacher owes it to his charges to exercise such care of them as a parent of ordinary prudence would observe in comparable circumstances."

It is important to understand the legal meaning of the word *accident* in relation to the topic under discussion. According to Black's *Law Dictionary*, accident is defined as follows: "An accident is an unforeseen event occurring without the will or design of the person whose mere act causes it. In its proper use the term excludes negligence. It is an event which occurs without fault, carelessness, or want of proper circumspection for the person affected, or which could not have been avoided by the use of that kind and degree of care necessary to the exigency and

in the circumstance in which he was placed." The case of *Lee v. Board of Education of City of New York* in 1941, for example, showed that prudent care was not exercised, and the defendant was liable for negligence. A boy was hit by a car while playing football in the street as a part of the physical education program. The street had not been completely closed off to traffic. The board of education and the teacher were found negligent.

Negligence

Questions of liability and negligence occupy a very prominent position in connection with the actions of teachers and leaders in school health and physical education programs.

The law in America pertaining to negligence is based upon common law, previous judicial rulings, or established legal procedure. This type of law differs from that which has been written into the statutes by lawmaking bodies and is called statutory law.

Negligence implies that someone has not fulfilled his legal duty or has failed to do something that according to common-sense reasoning should have been done. Negligence can be avoided if there are common knowledge of basic legal principles and proper vigilance. One of the first things that must be determined in event of accident is whether there has been negligence.

Rosenfield[*] defines negligence as follows: "Negligence consists in the failure to act as a reasonably prudent and careful person would under the circumstances involved." The National Education Association's report elaborates further: "Negligence is any conduct which falls below the standard established by law for the protection of others against unreasonable risk of harm. In general, such conduct may be of two types: (a) an act which a reason-

---

[*]National Education Research Division for the National Commission on Safety Education: Who is liable for pupil injuries? Washington, D. C., 1950, National Education Association, p. 5.

[*]Rosenfield, H. N.: Liability for school accident, New York, 1940, Harper & Row, Publishers.

able man would have realized involved an unreasonable risk of injury to others, and (b) failure to do an act which is necessary for the protection or assistance of another and which one is under a duty to do.*

According to Garber, a school employee may be negligent because of the following reasons:

1. He did not take appropriate care
2. Although he used due care, he acted in circumstances which created risks
3. His acts created an unreasonable risk of direct and immediate injury to others
4. He set in motion a force which was unreasonably hazardous to others
5. He created a situation in which third persons, such as pupils, or inanimate forces, such as shop machinery, may reasonably have been expected to injure others
6. He allowed pupils to use dangerous devices although they were incompetent to use them
7. He did not control a third person, such as an abnormal pupil, whom he knew to be likely to inflict intended injury on others because of some incapacity or abnormality
8. He did not give adequate warning
9. He did not look out for persons, such as pupils, who were in danger
10. He acted without sufficient skill
11. He did not make sufficient preparation to avoid an injury to pupils before beginning an activity where such preparation is reasonably necessary
12. He failed to inspect and repair mechanical devices to be used by pupils
13. He prevented someone, such as another teacher, from assisting a pupil who was endangered, although the pupil's peril was not caused by his negligence†

The National Education Association report includes the following additional comment:

The law prohibits careless action; whatever is done must be done well and with reasonable caution. Failure to employ care not to harm others is a misfeasance. For example, an Oregon school

bus driver who parked the bus across a driveway when he knew the pupils were coasting down the hill was held liable for injuries sustained by a pupil who coasted into the bus. (*Fahlstrom v. Denk,* 1933.)*

Negligence may be claimed when the plaintiff has suffered injury either to himself or to his property, when the defendant has not performed his legal duty and has been negligent, and when the plaintiff has constitutional rights and is not guilty of contributory negligence. The teacher or leader for children in such cases is regarded as *in loco parentis,* that is, acting in the place of the parent in relation to the child.

Since negligence implies failure to act as a reasonably prudent and careful person, necessary precautions should be taken, danger should be anticipated, and common sense should be used. For example, if a teacher permits a group of very young children to go up a high slide alone and without supervision, she is not acting as a prudent person would act. If the teacher of health education, after giving a demonstration, leaves a deadly drug on her desk and it later results in the death of a child, she is not acting as a careful person should act. In the case previously cited of *Lee v. Board of Education of City of New York,* when the physical education class was held in a street where cars were also allowed to pass, negligence existed.

A verdict by the jury in a California district court points up negligence in the sport of football. Press dispatches indicated that the high school athlete who suffered a disabling football injury was brought into court on a stretcher. The award was $325,000 (against the school district) in a suit in which the parent charged that the coach "was negligent in having the boy moved to the sidelines *too*

---

*National Education Research Division for the National Commission on Safety Education, op. cit., p. 6.

†Garber, L. O.: Law and the school business manager, Danville, Ill., 1957, Interstate Printers & Publishers, Inc., pp. 205-206.

---

*National Education Research Division for the National Commission on Safety Education, op. cit., p. 6.

soon after he was injured." The newspaper report seemed to infer that the negligence was involved not in the *method* of moving the boy from the field, but rather in the *time* at which he was moved.

An interesting case where the court ruled negligence occurred in New Jersey. In 1962 a student in the Chatham Junior High School was severely injured in an accident while participating in physical education. The testimony brought out that the physical education teacher was not present when the accident occurred but was treating another child for a rope burn. However, he had continually warned his class not to use the springboard at any time he was out of the room. (The student was trying to perform the exercise where he would dive from a springboard over an obstacle and finish with a forward roll.) The prosecution argued that the warning had not been stressed sufficiently and that the teacher's absence from the gymnasium, leaving student aides in charge, was an act of negligence. The court ruled negligence and in 1964 awarded the boy $1.2 million dollars for injuries. His parents were awarded $35,140. Upon an appeal, the award to the boy was reduced to $300,000, but the award to the parents remained the same. It is interesting to note that in this case the board of education felt there was no negligence on the part of the physical education teacher.

In respect to negligence, considerable weight is given in the law to the *foreseeability of danger.* One authority points out that "if a danger is obvious and a reasonably prudent person could have foreseen it and could have avoided the resulting harm by care and caution, the person who did not foresee or failed to prevent a foreseeable injury is liable for a tort on account of negligence."* If a teacher fails to take the needed precautions and care,

negligence is constituted. However, it must be established upon the basis of facts in the case. It cannot be based upon mere conjecture.

Teachers and leaders must realize that children will behave in certain ways, that certain juvenile acts will cause injuries unless properly supervised, that hazards must be anticipated, reported, and eliminated. The question that will be raised by most courts of law is: "Should the teacher or leader have had prudence enough to foresee the possible dangers or occurrence of an act?"

Two court actions point up legal reasoning on negligence as interpreted in one state. In the case of *Lane v. City of Buffalo* in 1931, the board of education was found not liable. In this case a child fell from a piece of apparatus in the schoolyard. It was found that the apparatus was in good condition and that proper supervision was present. In the case of *Cambareri v. Board of Albany,* the defendant was found liable. The City of Buffalo owned a park that was supervised by the park department. While skating on the lake in the park a boy playing "crack the whip" hit a 12-year-old boy who was also skating. Workers and a policeman had been assigned to supervise activity and had been instructed not to allow games that were rough or dangerous.

Although there are no absolute, factual standards for determining negligence, certain guides have been established that should be familiar to teachers and others engaged in the work under consideration in this book. Attorney Cymrot, in discussing negligence at a conference in New York City, suggested the following:

1. The teacher must be acting within the scope of his employment and in the discharge of his duties in order to obtain the benefits of the statute.
2. There must be a breach of a recognized duty owed to the child.
3. There must be a negligent breach of such duty.

---

*National Education Research Division for National Commission on Safety Education, op. cit., p. 6.

4. The accident and resulting injuries must be the natural and foreseeable consequence of the teacher's negligence arising from a negligent breach of duty.
5. The child must be a participant in an activity under the control of the teacher or, put in another way, the accident must have occurred under circumstances where the teacher owes a duty of care to the pupil.
6. A child's contributory negligence, however modified, will bar his recovery for damages.
7. The plaintiff must establish the negligence of the teacher and his own freedom from contributory negligence by a fair preponderance of evidence. The burden of proof on both issues is on the plaintiff.
8. Generally speaking, the board of education alone is responsible for accidents caused by the faulty maintenance of plants (schools) and equipment.*

Some states have a "save harmless" law. For example in New Jersey the law reads:

Chapter 311, P. L. 1938. Boards assume liability of teachers. It shall be the duty of each board of education in any school district to save harmless and protect all teachers and members of supervisory and administrative staff from financial loss arising out of any claim, demand, suit or judgment by reason of alleged negligence or other act resulting in accidental bodily injury to any person within or without the school building; provided, such teacher or member of the supervisory or administrative staff at the time of the accident or injury was acting in the discharge of his duties within the scope of his employment and/or under the direction of said board of education; and said board of education may arrange for and maintain appropriate insurance with any company created by or under the laws of this state, or in any insurance company authorized by law to transact business in this state, or such board may elect to act as self-insurers to maintain the aforesaid protection.

Defenses against negligence

Despite the fact that an individual is negligent, to collect damages one must show that the negligence resulted in or was closely connected with the injury. The

legal question in such a case is whether or not the negligence was the "proximate cause" (legal cause) of the injury. Furthermore, even though it be determined that negligence is the "proximate cause" of the injury, there are still certain defenses upon which a defendant may base his case.

Proximate cause. The negligence of the defendant may not have been the proximate cause of the plaintiff's injury.

Example: In the case of *Ohmon v. Board of Education of the City of New York*, 88 N.Y.S.2d 273 (1949), it was declared that when a 13-year-old pupil in public school was struck in the eye by a pencil thrown in classroom by another pupil to a third pupil, who stepped aside, the proximate cause of injury was an unforeseen act of the pupil who threw the pencil and that absence of the teacher (who was stacking supplies in a closet nearby the classroom) was not proximate cause of injury so as to impose liability for the injury on the board of education.

Act of God. An act of God is a situation that exists because of certain conditions that are beyond the control of human beings. For example, a flash of lightning, a gust of wind, a cloudburst, and other such factors may result in injury. However, this assumption applies only in cases where injury would not have occurred had prudent action been taken.

Assumption of risk. This legal defense is especially pertinent to games, sports, and other phases of the program in health education and physical education. It is assumed that an individual takes a certain risk when engaging in various games and sports where bodies are coming in contact with each other and where balls and apparatus are used. Participation in such activity indicates that the person assumes a normal risk.

Example: In the case of *Scala v. City of New York*, 102 N.Y.S.2d 709, where the plaintiff when playing softball on a public playground was aware of the risks caused by curbing and concrete benches near the

---

*Proceedings of the City Wide Conference with Principal's Representatives and Men and Women Chairmen of Health Education, City of New York Board of Education, Brooklyn, N. Y., 1953, Bureau of Health Education.

playing fields, it was decided that the plaintiff must be held to have voluntarily and fully assumed the dangers and, having done so, must abide by the consequences.

Example: In an action by Albert Maltz (*Maltz v. Board of Education of New York City,* 114 N.Y.S.2d 856, 1952) against the Board of Education of the City of New York for injuries, the court held that a 19-year-old boy who was injured when he collided with a doorjamb in a brick wall 2 feet from the backboard and basket in a public school basketball court and who had played on that same court several times prior to the accident knew the basket and backboard were but 2 feet from the wall, had previously hit the wall or gone through the door without injury, was not a student at the school but a voluntary member of a team that engaged in basketball tournaments with other clubs, knew or should have known the danger, and thus assumed the risk of injury.

Contributory negligence. Another legal defense is contributory negligence. A person who does not act as would a normal individual of similar age and nature thereby contributes to the injury. In such cases negligence on the part of the defendant might be ruled out. Individuals are subject to contributory negligence if they expose themselves unnecessarily to dangers. The main consideration that seems to turn the tide in such cases is the age of the individual and the nature of the activity in which he engaged.

The National Education Association's report makes this statement in regard to contributory negligence:

Contributory negligence is defined in law as conduct on the part of the injured person which falls below the standard to which he should conform for his own protection and which is legally contributing cause, cooperating with the negligence of the defendant in bringing about the plaintiff's harm. Reasonable self-protection is to be expected of all sane adults. With some few exceptions, contributory negligence bars recovery against the defendant whose negligent conduct would otherwise make him liable to the plaintiff for the harm sustained by him. Both parties being in fault, neither can recover from the other for resulting harm. When there is mutual wrong and negligence on both sides, the law will not attempt to apportion the wrong between them.

Contributory negligence is usually a matter of defense, and the burden of proof is put upon the defendant to convince the jury of the plaintiff's fault and of its causal connection with the harm sustained. Minors are not held to the same degree of care as is demanded of adults.*

Contributory negligence has implications for a difference in the responsibility of elementary school teachers as contrasted with high school teachers. The elementary school teacher, because the children are immature, has to assume greater responsibility for the safety of the child. That is, accidents in which an elementary school child is injured are not held in the same light from the standpoint of negligence as those involving high school students who are more mature. The courts might say that a high school student was mature enough to avoid doing the thing causing him to be injured, whereas if the same thing occurred with an elementary school child, the courts could say the child was too immature and that the teacher should have prevented or protected the child from doing the act from which he was injured.

Sudden emergency. This legal defense is pertinent in cases where the exigencies of the situation require immediate action on the part of a teacher and, as a result, an accident occurs. For example, an instructor in a swimming pool is suddenly alerted to the fact that a child is drowning in the water. The teacher's immediate objective is to save the child. He runs to the assistance of the drowning person and in doing so knocks down another student who is watching from the side of the pool. The student who is knocked down hits his head on the tile floor and is injured. This would

---

*National Education Research Division for the National Commission on Safety Education, op. cit., p. 9.

be a case of sudden emergency and, if legal action is taken, the defense could be based on this premise.

Nuisance

Action can be instituted for nuisance when the circumstances surrounding the act are dangerous to life or health, result in offense to the senses, are in violation of the laws of decency, or cause an obstruction to the reasonable use of property.

An authentic source states in regard to a nuisance:

There are some conditions which are naturally dangerous and the danger is a continuing one. An inherent danger of this sort is called at law a "nuisance"; the one responsible is liable for maintaining a nuisance. His liability may be predicated upon negligence in permitting the continuing danger to exist, but even without a showing of negligence the mere fact that a nuisance does exist is usually sufficient to justify a determination of liability. For example, a junk pile in the corner of the grounds of a country school was considered a nuisance for which the district was liable when a pupil stumbled over a piece of junk and fell while playing at recess (*Popow v. Central School District No. 1, Towns of Hillsdale et al., New York*, 1938). Dangerous playground equipment available for use by pupils of all ages and degrees of skill has also been determined to be a nuisance (*Bush v. City of Norwalk, Connecticut*, 1937).

On the other hand, allegations that the district has maintained a nuisance have been denied in some cases; for example, when a small child fell into a natural ditch near the schoolyard not guarded by a fence, the ditch was held not to be a nuisance for which the district would be liable (*Whitfield v. East Baton Rouge Parish School Board, Louisiana*, 1949). The court said this ditch did not constitute a nuisance; nor did the principle of *res ipsa loquitur* apply. Under this principle the thing which causes the injury is under the management of the defendant and the accident is such that in the ordinary course of events, it would not have happened if the defendant had used proper care.[*]

Mr. Cymrot, attorney at law, in address-

ing the Health Education Division of the New York City Schools had the following to say about an "attractive nuisance":

Teachers need to be aware of decisions of the courts pertaining to "attractive nuisance," . . . an attractive contrivance which is maintained, alluring to children but inherently dangerous to them. This constitutes neglect. But it is not every contrivance or apparatus that a jury may treat as an "attractive nuisance." Before liability may be imposed, there must always be something in the evidence tending to show that the device was something of a new or uncommon nature with which children might be supposed to be unfamiliar or not know of its danger. Many courts have held, however, that for children above the age of 10 years the doctrine of "attractive nuisance" does not hold. Other children are expected to exercise such prudence as those of their age may be expected to possess.[*]

The following cases point up some court rulings in respect to "nuisance."

In the case of *Texas v. Reinhardt* in 1913, it was ruled that ball games with their noises and conduct were not a "nuisance" in the particular case in question and an injunction should not be issued stopping such activity.

In the case of *Iacono v. Fitzpatrick* in Rhode Island in 1938, a boy 17 years old, while playing touch football on a playground, received an injury that later resulted in his death. He was attempting to catch a pass and in so doing crashed into a piece of apparatus. The court held that the apparatus was in evidence and the deceased knew of its presence. It further stated the city had not created or maintained a nuisance.

In the case of *Schwarz v. City of Cincinnati, Ohio*, the city had permitted an organization to have fireworks in one of its public parks. Next day a 12-year-old boy was injured after lighting an unexploded

---

[*]National Education Research Division for the National Commission on Safety Education, op. cit., p. 6.

[*]Proceedings of the City Wide Conference with Principals' Representatives and Men and Women Chairmen of Health Education, City of New York Board of Education, Brooklyn, N. Y., March, 1953, Bureau of Health Education.

bomb that he found. The court ruled that the permit granted the association was "... not authority to create a nuisance ... not authority to leave an unexploded bomb in the park." The city, which was the defendant in the case, was not held liable.

Governmental versus proprietary functions

The government in a legal sense is engaged in two types of activity: (1) governmental in nature and (2) proprietary in nature.

The *governmental function* refers to those particular activities that are of a sovereign nature. This theory dates back to the time when kings ruled under the divine right theory, were absolute in their power, and "could do no wrong." As such the sovereign was granted immunity and could not be sued without his consent for failing to exercise governmental powers or for negligence. Furthermore, a subordinate agency of the sovereign could not be sued. The municipality, according to this interpretation, acts as an agent of the state in a governmental capacity. The logic behind this reasoning is that the municipality is helping the state to govern the people who live within its geographic limits.

Many activities are classified under the *governmental function* interpretation. Such functions as education, police protection, and public health fall in this category.

In regard to public education, the courts hold that this is a governmental function and, therefore, entitled to state's immunity from liability for its own negligence. However, as has previously been pointed out, the attitude of the courts has changed and has taken on a broader social outlook that allows in some cases for the reimbursement of the injured.

Proprietary function pertains to government functions that are similar to those of a business enterprise. Such functions are for the benefit of the constituents within the corporate limits of the governmental agency. An example of this would be the manufacture, distribution, and sale of some product to the public. A cafeteria conducted for profit in a school is a proprietary function. In functions that are proprietary in nature a governmental agency is held liable in the same manner as an individual or a private corporation would be held liable.

In the case *Watson v. School District of Bay City*, 324 Mich. 1, 36 N.W.2d 195, a decision was handed down by the supreme court of Michigan in February, 1949. In this case a 15-year-old child attended a high school night football game. In going to her car she was required to walk around a concrete wall. As she attempted to do this, she fell over the wall and onto a ramp. She suffered paralysis and died 8 months later. The parking area was very poorly lighted. The supreme court held that staging a high school football game was a governmental function and refused to impose liability upon the district.

From this discussion it can be seen that education, recreation, and health are governmental functions. While this distinction between governmental and proprietary functions precludes a recovery from the governmental agency if the function was governmental in nature, the federal government and some of the states by legislation have eliminated this distinction.

Fees

Most public recreation activities, facilities, and the like are offered free of charge to the public. However, there are certain activities that, because of the expenses involved, necessitate a fee in order that such activities may continue. For example, golf courses are expensive and charges are usually made so that they may be maintained. This is sometimes true also of such facilities as camps, bathing beaches, and swimming pools.

The fees charged have a bearing upon whether recreation is a governmental or a proprietary function. The courts in most states have upheld recreation as a governmental function, because of its contribution to public health and welfare and also because its devices are free to the public at large. When fees are charged, however, the whole picture takes on a different aspect.

The attitude of the courts has been that the amount of the fee and whether or not the activity was profit-making in nature are considerations in determining whether recreation is a governmental or a proprietary function. Incidental fees that are used in the conduct of the enterprise do not usually change the nature of the enterprise. However, if the enterprise is run for profit, the function changes from governmental to proprietary in nature.

Liability of the municipality

It has been previously pointed out that a municipality as a governmental agency performs both governmental and proprietary functions.

When the municipality is performing a governmental function, it is acting in the interests of the state, receives no profit or advantage, and is not liable for negligence on the part of its employees or for failure to perform these functions. However, this would not hold if there were a specific statute imposing liability for negligence. When the municipality is performing a proprietary function—some function for profit or advantage of the agency or people who comprise it—rather than the public in general, it is liable for negligence of those who are carrying out the function.

This discussion readily shows the importance of conducting recreation as a governmental function.

Liability of the school district

As a general rule the school district is not held liable for acts of negligence on the part of its officers or employees, provided a state statute does not exist to the con-

trary. The reasoning behind this is that the school district or district school board in maintaining public schools acts as an agent of the state. It performs a purely public or governmental duty imposed upon it by law for the benefit of the public and for the performance of which it receives no profit or advantage.

Some state laws, however, provide that the state may be sued in cases of negligence in the performance of certain duties, such as providing for a safe environment and competent leadership. Furthermore, the school district's immunity in many cases does not cover such acts as those that bring damage or injury through trespass of another's premises or where a nuisance exists on a school district's property, resulting in damage to other property.

Liability of school, park, and recreation board members

Generally speaking, members are not personally liable for any duties in their corporate capacities as board members that they perform negligently. Furthermore, they cannot be held personally liable for acts of employees of the district or organization over which they have jurisdiction on the theory of *respondeat superior* (let the master pay for the servant). Board members act in a corporate capacity and do not act for themselves. For example, in the state of Oregon the general rule as to the personal liability of members of district school boards is stated in 56C.J., page 348, section 223, as follows:

School officers, or members of the board of education, or directors, trustees, or the like, of a school district or other local school organization are not personally liable for the negligence of persons rightfully employed by them in behalf of the district, and not under the direct personal supervision or control of such officer or member in doing the negligent act, since such employee is a servant of the district and not of the officer or board members, and the doctrine of *respondeat superior* accordingly has no application; and members of a district board are not personally liable for the negligence or other wrong of the board as such. A school officer or member of a district board is, however, personally liable for his own negligence or other tort, or that of an agent or employee of the district when acting directly under his supervision or by his direction.

However, a board member can be held liable for a *ministerial* act even though he cannot be held for the exercise of discretion as a member of the board. If the board acts in bad faith and with unworthy motives, and this can be shown, it can also be held liable.

Liability of teachers and leaders

The individual is responsible for negligence of his own acts. With the exception of certain specific immunity, the teacher or leader in programs of health, physical education, and recreation is responsible for what he or she does. The Supreme Court of the United States has reaffirmed this principle and all should recognize the important implications it has. Immunity of the governmental agency such as a state, school district, or board does not release the teacher or leader from liability for his or her own negligent acts.

In New York a physical education teacher was held personally liable when he sat in the bleachers while two strong boys, untrained in boxing, were permitted by the instructor to fight through nearly two rounds. The plaintiff was hit in the temple and suffered a cerebral hemorrhage. The court said: "It is the duty of a teacher to exercise reasonable care to prevent injuries. Pupils should be warned before being permitted to engage in a dangerous and hazardous exercise. Skilled boxers at times are injured, and . . . these young men should have been taught the principles of defense if indeed it was a reasonable thing to permit a slugging match of the kind which the testimony shows this contest was. The testimony indicates that the teacher failed in his duties in this regard and that he was negligent, and the plaintiff is entitled to recover." (*LaValley*

v. Stanford, 272 App. Div. 183, 70 N.Y.S. 2d 460.)

In New York (*Keesee v. Board of Education of City of New York,* 5 N.Y.S.2d 300, 1962) a junior high school girl was injured while playing line soccer. She was kicked by another player. The board of education syllabus listed line soccer as a game for boys and stated that "after sufficient skill has been acquired two or more forwards may be selected from each team." The syllabus called for ten to twenty players on each team and required a space of 30 to 40 feet. The physical education teacher divided into two teams some forty to forty-five girls who had not had any experience in soccer. A witness who was an expert in such matters testified that in order to avoid accidents no more than two people should be on the ball at any time and criticized the board syllabus for permitting the use of more than two forwards. The expert also testified that pupils should have experience in kicking, dribbling, and passing before being permitted to play line soccer. The evidence showed that the teacher permitted six to eight inexperienced girls to be on the ball at one time. The court held that possible injury was at least reasonably foreseeable under such conditions and that the teacher had been negligent and that the teacher's negligence was the cause of the pupil being injured.*

Teachers and leaders are expected to conduct their various activities in a careful and prudent manner. If this is not done, they are exposing themselves to lawsuits for their own negligence. As respects administrators, the National Education Association's report has the following to say:

The fact that administrators (speaking mainly of principals and superintendents) are rarely made

---

*School Law Series: The pupil's day in court: review of 1963, Washington, D. C., 1964, Research Division, National Education Association, p. 43.

defendants in pupil-injury cases seems unjust to the teachers who are found negligent because of inadequate supervision, and unjust also to the school boards who are required to defend themselves in such suits. When the injury is caused by defective equipment, it is the building principal who should have actual or constructive notice of the defect; when the injury is caused by inadequate playground supervision, the inadequacy of the supervision frequently exists because of arrangements made by the building principal. For example, a teacher in charge of one playground was required to stay in the building to teach a make-up class; another teacher was required to supervise large grounds on which 150 pupils were playing; another teacher neglected the playground to answer the telephone. All of these inadequacies in playground supervision were morally chargeable to administrators; in none of these instances did the court action direct a charge of responsibility to the administrator. Whether the administrator in such cases would have been held liable, if charged with negligence, is problematical. The issue has not been decided, since the administrator's legal responsibility for pupil injuries has never been discussed by the courts to an extent that would make possible the elucidation of general principles; the administrator's moral responsibilities must be conceded.*

Accident-prone settings

Since many accidents occur on the playgrounds, during recess periods, in physical education classes, and at sports events, some very pertinent remarks are included here that have been stated in the National Education Association's report:

Playground and recess games

. . . [T]he unorganized games during recess and noon intermissions are more likely to result in pupil injuries than the organized games of physical education classes. Playground injuries may be pure accidents, such as when a pupil ran against the flagpole while playing (*Hough v. Orleans Elementary School District of Humboldt County, California*, 1943), or when a pupil was hit by a ball (*Graff v. Board of Education of New York City, New York*, 1940), or by a stone batted by another pupil (*Wilbur v. City of Binghamton, New York*, 1946). The courts have said in connec-

tion with this type of injury that every act of every pupil cannot be anticipated. However, the school district should make rules and regulations for pupils' conduct on playgrounds so as to minimize dangers. For example, it was held to be negligence to permit pupils to ride bicycles on the playground while other pupils were playing. (*Buzzard v. East Lake School District of Lake County, California*, 1939.)

Playgrounds should be supervised during unorganized play and such supervision should be adequate. One teacher cannot supervise a large playground with over a hundred pupils playing (*Charonnat v. San Francisco Unified School District, California*, 1943), and when the supervision is either lacking or inadequate districts which are not immune are liable for negligence in not providing adequate supervision (*Forgnone v. Salvadore Union Elementary School District, California*, 1940). Pupils are known to engage in fights and may be expected to be injured in fights; it is the responsibility of the school authorities to attempt to prevent such injuries. The misconduct of other pupils could be an intervening cause to break the chain of causation if the supervision is adequate; but when the supervision is not adequate, misconduct of other pupils is not an intervening superseding cause of the injury.

If a pupil wanders away from the group during playground games and is injured by a dangerous condition into which he places himself, the teacher in charge of the playground may be liable for negligence in pupil supervision (*Miller v. Board of Education, Union Free School District, New York*, 1943), although the district would not be liable in common-law state because of its immunity (*Whitfield v. East Baton Rouge Parish School Board, Louisiana*, 1949).

Supervision of unorganized play at recess or noon intermissions should be by competent personnel. A school janitor is not qualified to supervise play. (*Garber v. Central School District No. 1 of Town of Sharon, New York*, 1937.)

All injuries sustained by pupils on playground equipment are excluded in the Washington statute imposing liability for certain other kinds of accidents. Injuries may occur because playground equipment is in a defective condition. The New York courts have not been consistent in their rulings on this point. In one New York case the district was not liable for injury caused by a defect in a slide because there was no evidence that the defect had existed a sufficient length of time for the school authorities to have knowledge of it (*Handy v. Hadley-Luzerne Union Free School District No. 1, New York*, 1938), but another district in New York was held liable for a defect

---

*National Education Research Division for the National Commission on Safety Education, op. cit., p. 14.

in a slide (*Howell v. Union Free School District No. 1, New York,* 1937).

Nor have the New York courts been consistent in fixing liability when the injury was sustained on playground equipment which was not defective but was dangerous for the individual pupil who played on it. One pupil who fell off a monkey bar was unable to collect damages because the court held specific supervision of each game and each piece of playground equipment would be an unreasonable requirement. The pupil merely met with an accident which was not the fault of the playground supervisor. (*Miller v. Board of Education of Union Free School District No. 1, Town of Oyster Bay, New York,* 1936.) However, another district was declared liable for injuries sustained by a pupil who fell from a ramp during recess, the court holding that liability rested upon the maintenance of a dangerous piece of playground equipment. This ramp had been constructed for the use of older boys and even they were to use it only under supervision; the injured pupil was a small child. (*Sullivan v. City of Binghamton, New York,* 1946.)

Where children of all ages share a playground extra precautions should be taken to prevent accidents, since some children are more adept in using equipment than others and some playground equipment is dangerous to the unskilled.

Physical education and sports events

Pupil injuries in this area occur when playground or gymnasium equipment is defective, when pupils attempt an exercise or sport for which they have not been sufficiently trained, when there is inadequate supervision of the exercise, when other pupils conduct themselves in a negligent manner, and even when the pupils are mere spectators at sports events.

It has been held that physical education teachers, or the school district in States where the district is subject to liability, are responsible for injuries caused by defective equipment. For example, there was liability for the injury to a pupil who was injured in a tumbling race when the mat, not firmly fixed, slipped on the slippery floor. (*Cambareri v. Board of Education of Albany, New York,* 1940.)

Defects in equipment should be known to the physical education instructor. There may be what is called actual or constructive notice of the defect. Actual knowledge is understandable; constructive notice means that the defect has existed for a sufficient time so that the instructor should have known of its existence, whether he did or not. Teachers of physical education should make periodic examination of all equipment at rather frequent intervals; otherwise they may be charged with negligence in not having corrected defects in equipment which have existed for a sufficient time that ignorance of the defect is a presumption of negligence.

Physical education teachers may be liable also for injuries which occur to pupils who attempt to do an exercise which is beyond their skills. A running-jump somersault is one such instance (*Govel v. Board of Education of Albany, New York,* 1944); boxing is another (*LaValley v. Stanford, New York,* 1947); and a headstand exercise is another (*Gardner v. State of New York, New York,* 1939). All of these exercises were found to be inherently dangerous by the courts, and the evidence showed that previous instruction had been inadequate and the pupils had not been warned of the dangers. However, where the previous instruction and the supervision during the exercise are both adequate, there is no liability so long as it cannot be proved that the teacher is generally incompetent (*Kolar v. Union Free School District No. 9, Town of Lenox, New York,* 1939). These cases suggest that teachers should not permit pupils to attempt exercises for which they have not been fully prepared by warnings of the dangers and preliminary exercises to develop the required skills.

As in other types of pupil injuries, the physical education teacher is not liable if the injury occurred without his negligence. If caused by the negligence of another pupil, the teacher will likely be relieved of liability if the other pupil's misconduct was not foreseeable. Pure accidents occur in sports also and if there is no negligence there is no liability (*Mauer v. Board of Education of New York City, New York,* 1945).

Sports events to which nonparticipating pupils and even the public are invited raise other problems of liability for the district or the physical education teacher in charge. If the locality is in a common-law State where the district is immune, the charge of an admission fee does not nullify the district's immunity or make the activity a proprietary function as an exception to the immunity rule (*Watson v. School District of Bay City, Michigan,* 1949). If the accident occurs in a State where the district is liable for at least certain kinds of injuries, such as California, the invitation to attend a sports event includes an invitation to use the nearby grounds and equipment, imposing liability for injury from hidden glass or other dangers (*Brown v. City of Oakland, California,* 1942). If a spectator is accidentally hit by a ball, however, there is no liability; even when a pupil was injured by being hit by a bottle at a game there was no liability because the misconduct of the other spectator was not foreseeable (*Weldy v. Oakland High School District of Alameda County, California*, 1937).*

Common areas of negligence

Common areas of negligence in health and physical education activities listed by Begley† in a New York University publication are situations involving poor selection of activities, failure to take protective procedures, hazardous conditions of buildings or grounds, faulty equipment, inadequate supervision, and poor selection of play area. Cases involving each of these common areas of negligence are as follows.

Poor selection of activities. The activity must be suitable to the child or youth. In *Rook v. New York*, 4 N.Y.S.2d 116 (1930), the court ruled that tossing a child in a blanket constituted a dangerous activity.

Failure to take protective measures. The element of "foreseeability" enters here and proper protective measures must be taken to provide a safe place for children and youth to play. In *Roth v. New York*, 262 App. Div. 370, 29 N.Y.S.2d 442 (1941), inadequate provisions were made to prevent bathers from stepping into deep water. When a bather drowned, the court held the state was liable.

Hazardous conditions of buildings or grounds. Buildings and grounds must be safe. Construction of facilities and their continual repair must have as one objective the elimination of hazards. In the case of *Novak et al. v. Borough of Ford City*, 141 Atl. 496 (Pa., 1928), unsafe conditions were caused by an electric wire over the play area. In the case of *Honaman v. City of Philadelphia*, 185 Atl. 750 (Pa., 1936), unsafe conditions were caused by failure to erect a backstop.

---

*National Education Research Division for the National Commission on Safety Education, op. cit., pp. 18-20.

†Begley, R. F.: Legal liability in organized recreational playground areas, Safety Education Digest, 1955.

Faulty equipment. All play and other equipment must be in good condition at all times. In the case of *Van Dyke v. Utica*, 203 App. Div. 26, 196 N.Y. Supp. 277 (1922), concerning a slide that fell over on a child and killed him, the court ruled that the slide was in a defective condition.

Inadequate supervision. There must be qualified supervision in charge of all play activities. In the case of *Garber v. Central School District No. 1, Town of Sharon, N.Y.*, 251 App. Div. 214, 295 N.Y. Supp. 850, the court held that a school janitor was not qualified to supervise school children playing in a gymnasium during the lunch hour.

Poor selection of play area. The setting for games and sports should be selected with a view to the safety of the participants. In the case *Morse v. New York*, 262 App. Div. 324, 29 N.Y.S.2d 34 (1941), when sledding and skiing were permitted on the same hill without adequate barriers to prevent participants in each activity from colliding with each other, the court held that the state was liable for negligence.

Supervision

Children are entrusted by parents to recreation, health, and physical education programs, and it is expected that adequate supervision will be provided so as to reduce to a minimum the possibility of accidents.

Questions of liability in regard to supervision pertain to two points: (1) the extent of the supervision and (2) the quality of the supervision.

Regarding the first point, the question would be raised as to whether adequate supervision was provided. This is a difficult question to answer because it would vary from situation to situation. However, the answers to these questions: "Would additional supervision have eliminated the accident?" and "Is it reasonable to expect that additional supervision should have been provided?" will help to determine this.

In regard to the quality of the supervision, it is expected that competent personnel will handle specialized programs in health, physical education, and recreation. If the supervisors of such activities do not possess proper training in such work, the question of negligence can be raised.

Waivers and consent slips

Waivers and consent slips are not synonymous. A waiver is an agreement whereby one party waives a particular right. A consent slip is an authorization, usually signed by the parent, permitting a child to take part in some activity.

In respect to a waiver, a parent cannot waive the rights of a child who is under 21 years of age. When a parent signs such a slip, he is merely waiving his or her right to sue for damages. A parent can sue in two ways, from the standpoint of his rights as the parent and from the standpoint of the child's own rights that he has as an individual, irrespective of the parent. A parent cannot waive the right of the child to sue as an individual.

Consent slips offer protection from the standpoint of showing that the child has the parent's permission to engage in an activity.

SAFETY

It is important to take every precaution possible to prevent accidents by providing for the safety of students and other individuals who participate in programs of health education, physical education, and recreation. If such precautions are taken, the likelihood of a lawsuit will diminish and the question of negligence will be eliminated. A few of the precautions that the leader or teacher should make provision for are as follows:

1. Instructor should be properly trained and qualified to perform specialized work.

2. Instructor should be present at all organized activities in the program.

3. Classes should be organized properly according to size, activity, physical condi-

---

Gen. No. 1 100M-1-54-3181   **WAIVER FORM**   Long Beach, California
LONG BEACH PUBLIC SCHOOLS   Date_____

We,_____, are the parents or guardians
of_____, and in consideration of the special benefits
of the extracurricular activity being afforded the student by the Long Beach Board of Education and the school districts whose school the aforementioned child attends, hereby permit_____
_____to participate in_____
_____

and we hereby release and discharge the said Long Beach Board of Education, the said school district, and each and all their agents and employees from any liability whatever to the undersigned resulting from or in any manner arising out of any injury or damage which may be sustained by the said_____, on account of his participation in

_____or in the transportation in connection therewith.
We further agree that in case of any action being brought for, or on behalf of the aforementioned child on account of any injury received during his participation in the above mentioned events, or in the transportation connected therewith, that we will be personally responsible to the school district, the Board of Education, and any of its officials or agents concerned, and will repay to them and hold them harmless against any judgment recovered in any such action against them or either of them.
Signed this_____day of_____, 195_____

_____   _____
Signature of Parent or Guardian   Address

_____   _____
Signature of Parent or Guardian   Address
NOTE: Parents or Guardians, read the reverse side of this form.

tion, and other factors that have a bearing on safety and health of the individual.

4. Health examinations should be given to all pupils.

5. A planned, written program for proper disposition of students who are injured or become sick should be followed.

6. Regular inspections should be made of such items as equipment, apparatus, ropes, or chains, placing extra pressure upon them and taking other precautions to make sure they are safe. They should also be checked for deterioration, looseness, fraying, splinters, and so on.

7. Overcrowding athletic and other events should be avoided, building codes and fire regulations should be adhered to, and adequate lighting for all facilities should be provided.

8. Protective equipment such as mats should be utilized wherever possible. Any hazards such as projections or obstacles in an area where activity is taking place should be eliminated. Floors should not be slippery. Shower rooms should have surfaces conducive to secure footing.

9. Sneakers should be worn on gymnasium floors and adequate space provided for each activity.

10. Activities should be adapted to the age and maturity of the participants, proper and competent supervision should be provided, and spotters should be utilized in apparatus and other similar activities.

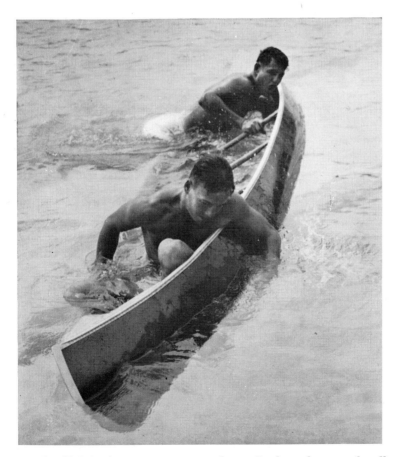

Every precaution should be taken to prevent accidents. Students learn to handle a canoe in water safety course. (University of Florida, Gainesville, Fla.)

11. Students should be instructed in the correct methods of using apparatus and performing in physical activities. Any misuse of equipment should be prohibited.

12. The buildings and other facilities used should be inspected regularly for safety hazards such as loose tiles, broken fences, cracked glass, and uneven pavement. Defects should be reported immediately to responsible persons and necessary precautions be taken.

13. In planning play and other instructional areas the following precautions should be taken:

a. There should be sufficient space for all games.

b. Games that utilize balls and other equipment that can cause damage should be conducted in areas where there is minimum danger of injuring someone.

c. Quiet games and activities that require working at benches, such as arts and crafts, should be in places that are well protected.

14. Truesdale lists certain questionable practices in which teachers, coaches, nurses, and trainers sometimes engage:

1. Supply "pills" for headaches or as laxatives or for menstrual discomfort.
2. Examine and diagnose by the stethoscope.
3. Prescribe anticold pills or capsules.
4. Strap joint injuries under supposition of sprain without expert assessment for possible fracture.
5. Permit return to play of a player with a head injury.
6. Play injured players not medically certified.
7. Permit return of students without medical certification to class, or particularly to activity, after illness.
8. Prescribe gargles or swabs for sore throats.
9. Use cutting tools (knives or razor blades) on calluses, corns, blisters, ingrown nails, etc.
10. Administer local anaesthesia to permit play after injury.
11. Employ physical forces such as heat or electric current to produce tissue change and decongestion and repair without medical order, or by unqualified persons.
12. Possibly further damage unconscious players

by dashing water in the face, by slapping the face or by unwarranted use of aromatic spirits of ammonia to "bring them to."[*]

Truesdale also points out that "it is the duty of adults engaged in education not only to know of and be skillful in the proper techniques for protecting persons against injury, or protecting injured persons against aggravation, but also to know the limits beyond which the untrained or the partially trained person may not go."

15. In the event of accident the following or a similar procedure should be followed:

a. The nearest teacher or leader should proceed to the scene of the accident immediately, notifying the person in charge and nurse, if available, by messenger. Also, a doctor should be called at once if one is necessary.

b. A hurried examination of the injured person will give some idea as to the nature and extent of the injury and the emergency of the situation.

c. If the teacher or leader is well versed in first aid, assistance should be given (a qualified first-aid certificate will usually absolve the teacher of negligence). Every teacher or leader who works in these specialized areas should and is expected to know first-aid procedures. In any event everything should be done to make the injured person comfortable and reassure the injured until the services of a physician can be secured.

d. If the injury is serious an ambulance should be called.

e. After the injured person has been provided for, the person in charge should fill out the accident forms and take the statements of witnesses and file for future reference. Reports of accidents should be prepared promptly and sent to proper persons. They should be accurate as to detail

[*]Truesdale, J. C.: So you're a good samaritan! Journal of the American Association for Health, Physical Education, and Recreation **25**:25, 1954.

STANDARD STUDENT ACCIDENT REPORT FORM
Part A. Information on ALL Accidents

1. Name: _____ Home Address. _____
2. School _____ Sex M ☐; F ☐. Age: _____ Grade or classification· _____
3. Time accident occurred Hour _____ A.M., _____ P.M. Date· _____
4. Place of Accident   School Building ☐   School Grounds ☐   To or from School ☐   Home ☐   Elsewhere ☐

5. NATURE OF INJURY				DESCRIPTION OF THE ACCIDENT
Abrasion	____	Fracture	____	How did accident happen? What was student doing? Where was student? List specifically unsafe acts and unsafe conditions existing. Specify any tool, machine or equipment involved. _____
Amputation	____	Laceration	____	
Asphyxiation	____	Poisoning	____	
Bite	____	Puncture	____	
Bruise	____	Scalds	____	
Burn	____	Scratches	____	
Concussion	____	Shock (el.)	____	
Cut	____	Sprain	____	
Dislocation	____			
Other (specify) _____				

PART OF BODY INJURED				
Abdomen	____	Foot	____	
Ankle	____	Hand	____	
Arm	____	Head	____	
Back	____	Knee	____	
Chest	____	Leg	____	
Ear	____	Mouth	____	
Elbow	____	Nose	____	
Eye	____	Scalp	____	
Face	____	Tooth	____	
Finger	____	Wrist	____	
Other (specify) _____				

6. Degree of Injury. Death ☐ Permanent Impairment ☐ Temporary Disability ☐ Nondisabling ☐
7. Total number of days lost from school: _____ (To be filled in when student returns to school)

Part B. Additional Information on School Jurisdiction Accidents
8. Teacher in charge when accident occurred (Enter name) ._____
Present at scene of accident: No _____ Yes· _____

9. IMMEDIATE ACTION TAKEN

First-aid treatment _____ By (Name) ._____
Sent to school nurse _____ By (Name) :_____
Sent home _____ By (Name) :_____
Sent to physician _____ By (Name) :_____
Physician's Name:_____
Sent to hospital _____ By (Name) :_____
Name of hospital:_____

10. Was a parent or other individual notified? No.__ Yes.__ When._____ How· _____
Name of individual notified· _____
By whom? (Enter name) . _____
11. Witnesses· 1. Name· _____ Address: _____
  2. Name· _____ Address: _____

12. LOCATION

	Specify Activity		Specify Activity	Remarks
Athletic field	_____	Locker	_____	What recommendations do you have for preventing other accidents of this type? _____
Auditorium	_____	Pool	_____	
Cafeteria	_____	Sch. grounds	_____	
Classroom	_____	____ shop	_____	
Corridor	_____	Showers	_____	
Dressing room	_____	Stairs	_____	
Gymnasium	_____	Toilets and		
Home Econ.	_____	washrooms	_____	
Laboratories	_____	Other (specify)	_____	

Signed: Principal: _____ Teacher: _____

(National Safety Council—Form School 1)   Printed in U.S.A. Rep. 200M—25302

Form recommended by National Safety Council.

and complete as to information. Among other things they should contain information about:

Name and address of injured person
Activity engaged in
Date, hour, and place
Person in charge
Witnesses
Cause and extent of injury
Medical attention given
Circumstances surrounding incident

f. There should be a complete followup of the accident, an analysis of the situation, and an eradication of any hazards that exist.

Herman Rosenthal, Assistant to the Law

GROVER CLEVELAND HIGH SCHOOL
HIMROD & GRANDVIEW AVE.
Ridgewood, New York

STATEMENT BY WITNESS
(Write in Ink)

Witness..Address..

Age...Rank..Class....................................

Name of one injured...........................Injured's Official Class.............Age of Injured...............

Date of accident...........................Time..............................Day of week...............................

A. Circumstances of Accident

1. Locate the position from which you witnessed the accident, using such phrases as, in front of, as I entered, standing on the, in back of, etc...

....

....

2. Locate the position where the accident occurred, using such phrases as, on the landing, exit 8 up, on the horizontal bar, etc..

....

....

3. Tell what you saw..

....

....

....

B. Additional remarks, if any..

....

C. Signature of Witness...

Statement by witness to accident. (Grover Cleveland High School, Ridgewood, N. Y.)

Secretary, City of New York, in addressing a health education conference in New York City, pointed up the following remarks in respect to reporting accidents:

Reports should be complete, full and in detail. He advised that where a case does go into litigation, there is a delay in the court calendar of 2 to 3 years before the case is tried. A complete and detailed report is always better than a teacher's or a child's memory. He pointed out that the completion of accident reports was the function and duty of the teacher and in no case should a child be expected to prepare the report. Reports in the handwriting of children, he said, should be limited only to the statements and signatures of the injured and of the witnesses to the accident. He emphasized that should an injured child at the time of the accident be unable to prepare a written statement or affix his signature to a report, the teacher should prepare the necessary statement and signature and indicate the reasons for so doing. He further focused attention on the fact that teachers should not attempt to color or distort facts in order to protect the school or the child, because such a practice does more harm than good. An extremely important point, he said, was the need to report where the teacher was at the time of the accident, the extent of the supervision, and the teacher control of the activity at the time of the accident. Also, he said that with few exceptions reports should be submitted within 24 hours of the time of the accident. He explained that in some cases this might not be possible, but in such cases no report need be delayed more than 48 hours.*

g. Thelma Reed, Chairman of Standard Student Accident Report Committee of the National Safety Council, listed the reasons why detailed injury reports are important for school authorities:

1. Aid in protecting the school personnel and district from unfortunate publicity and from liability suits growing out of student injury cases;
2. Aid in evaluating the relative importance of the various safety areas and the time each merits in the total school safety effort;
3. Suggest modifications in the structure, use,

and maintenance of buildings, grounds, and equipment;
4. Suggest curriculum adjustments to meet immediate student needs;
5. Provide significant data for individual student guidance;
6. Give substance to the school administrators' appeal for community support of the school safety program;
7. Aid the school administration in guiding the school safety activities of individual patrons and patrons' groups.

Some suggestions to help reduce injuries on the gridiron

Approximately 700 American boys have been killed directly or indirectly playing football in the last quarter century. Studies show that football is by far the most dangerous part of the educational program. According to the National Safety Council, in a recent year football accounted for one out of every five accidents occurring under the school's jurisdiction to students in the sophomore year, one out of every four to junior-year students, and one out of every three to seniors. By contrast baseball accounted for one out of twenty-six to sophomore students, one out of twenty-nine to the juniors, and one of thirty-three to the seniors.

Football can be made a much safer game. Many times chances are taken, players are urged to participate when not in the best of physical condition, the safest type of uniforms and equipment are not used, and the necessary precautions are not taken. In some cases there is negligence on the part of school authorities. Some suggestions to help make football a safer game are as follows:

1. A qualified coaching staff and a qualified trainer should be hired.
2. The best equipment that money can buy should be purchased.
3. Qualified officials should be present for all games and scrimmages.
4. Safe facilities, such as good turf, adequate space, and elimination of all hazards should be required.

*Proceedings of the City Wide Conference with Principals' Representatives and Men and Women Chairmen of Health Education, City of New York Board of Education, Brooklyn, N. Y., 1953, Bureau of Health Education.

5. A doctor should be present at all games and at all scrimmages.

6. A thorough physical examination before the season starts and again at mid-season is a *must*. It should include a detailed study of the health history of each player. If health history shows heart abnormalities or other defects that might be aggravated, the boy should not be permitted to play.

7. Provisions should be available for such essentials as an x-ray study, encephalogram, physical therapy, and bandaging.

8. Accident insurance to cover full cost of diagnosis and treatment of all injuries should be obtained.

9. No boy should be allowed to return to a game after a head injury until an x-ray film has been taken and a doctor has approved return to action. If injury is diagnosed as severe concussion, he should never be allowed to participate in gridiron activities again.

10. The temptation to send in the star who insists that he is not hurt and wants to return to play should be resisted. Decision to return to play should not be permitted unless approved by the doctor in writing.

11. Each school should play only schools of its own size and teams of its own stature.

12. More stress should be placed on training and conditioning: at least twenty practices spaced over a 3-week period before the first game for each player, longer warmups for reserves sitting on the bench and for all players at halftime of the game, and greater emphasis on fundamentals, such as blocking, tackling, and techniques of play.

13. If the rules could be changed as follows, injuries could be reduced:

a. Eliminate second-half kickoff.

b. Increase the penalty for piling on. Ban from the game the player who persists in ignoring this rule.

c. Allow for substitutions to the ex-tent that exhausted players will not be in the game.

d. Provide 5 minutes longer between halves of the game, with specific stipulation that this time is to be used for warm-up.

Safety code for the physical education teacher

The following safety code should be followed by the physical education teacher:

1. Have a proper teacher's certificate in full force and effect.
2. Operate and teach at all times, within the scope of his employment as delimited and defined by the rules and regulations of the employing board of education and within the statutory limitations imposed by the state.
3. Provide the safeguards designed to minimize the dangers inherent in a particular activity.
4. Provide the amount of supervision for each activity required to ensure the maximum safety of all the pupils.
5. Inspect equipment and facilities periodically to determine whether or not they are safe for use.
6. Notify the proper authorities forthwith concerning the existence of any dangerous condition as it continues to exist.
7. Provide sufficient instruction in the performance of any activity before exposing pupils to its hazards.
8. Be certain that the task is one approved by the employing board of education for the age and attainments of the pupils involved.
9. Not force a pupil to perform a physical feat which the pupil obviously feels he is incapable of performing.
10. Act promptly and use discretion in giving first aid to an injured pupil, but nothing more.
11. Exercise due care in practicing his profession.
12. Act as a reasonably prudent person would under the given circumstances.
13. Anticipate the dangers which should be apparent to a trained, intelligent person (a legal principle known as "foreseeability").*

---

*Munize, A. J.: The teacher, pupil injury, and legal liability, Journal of Health, Physical Education, and Recreation 33:28, 1962.

INSURANCE MANAGEMENT

There are three major types of insurance management that school districts utilize to protect themselves against loss. The first type is insurance for *property*, owned by the school district. The second type is insurance for *liability protection*, where there might be financial loss arising from personal injury or property damage for which the school district is liable. The third type is insurance for *crime protection* against a financial loss that might be incurred as a result of theft or other illegal act. This section on insurance management is primarily concerned with the second type of insurance, namely, liability protection.

A definite trend can be seen in school districts toward having some form of school accident insurance to protect students against injury. School administrators and boards of education in many communities feel this is one additional and important way of giving service to its school population. Along with this trend can be seen the impact upon casualty and life insurance companies that offer insurance policies for school children and staff. The premium costs of school accident policies vary from community to community and also in accordance with age of insured and type of plan offered. The area of interscholastic athletics has been responsible for the development of many state athletic protection plans as well as the issuance of special policies by commercial insurance companies. When it is realized that accidents are the chief cause of death among students between the ages of 5 and 18, it can readily be seen that some protection is needed.

Common features of insurance management plans

Some common features of insurance management plans across the United States are as follows:

1. Premiums are paid for by the school, by the parent, or jointly by the school and parent.

2. Schools obtain their money for payment of premiums from the board of education, general organization fund, or a pooling of funds for many schools taken from gate receipts in league games.

3. Schools place the responsibility upon the parents to pay for any injuries incurred.

4. The blanket type coverage is a very common policy for insurance companies to offer.

5. Insurance companies frequently offer insurance coverage for athletic injuries as part of a package plan that also includes an accident plan for all students.

6. Most schools have insurance plans for the protection of athletes.

7. Most schools seek insurance coverage that provides for benefits whether x-ray films are positive or negative.

8. Hospitalization, x-ray films, and medical fees and dental fees are increasingly becoming part of the insurance coverage in schools.

Some school boards have found it a good policy to pay the premium on insurance policies because the full coverage of students provides peace of mind for both parents and teachers. Furthermore, it has been noted by some educators that many liability suits have been avoided in this manner.

Other school officials investigate the various insurance plans available and then recommend a particular plan and the parents deal directly with the company. Such parent-paid plans are frequently divided into two options: (1) they provide coverage for the student on a door-to-door basis (to and from school, while at school, and in school-sponsored activities) and (2) they provide 24-hour accident coverage with premiums usually running to four times higher than the "school only" policy. The "school only" policy rates are based upon age with rates for children in the elementary grades less than those in the higher grades. These policies also usually run only for the school year.

Student accident insurance provides coverage for all accidents regardless of whether the insured is hospitalized or treated in a doctor's office. Such medical plans as Blue Cross and Blue Shield are limited in the payments they make. Student accident insurance policies, as a general rule, offer reasonable rates and are a good investment for all concerned. Parents should be encouraged, however, to examine their existing family policies before taking out such policies to avoid overlapping coverage.

A survey of nine school districts in Ohio a few years ago indicated some practices and problems concerned with answering the question: "What to look for in selecting an insurance policy for athletics?"* These facts were disclosed by this survey:

1. The chief school administrator was the person who usually selected the insurance company from whom the policy would be purchased.
2. Medical coverage on policies purchased ranged from $30 to $5,000 and dental coverage from nothing to $500.
3. The claims collected for one particular type of injury ranged from nothing to $792.30.
4. Companies did not follow through at all times in paying the amount for which the claim was made.
5. Most insurance companies writing athletic policies have scheduled benefit plans.
6. Catastrophe clauses were absent from all policies.
7. Athletes covered ranged from 80% to 100%.
8. In most cases part of each athlete's premium was paid for from a school athletic fund.

---

*Rockhold, J.: How to buy athletic insurance, The Ohio High School Athlete 23:169 1964.

9. Football was covered in separate policies.

As a result of this survey the following recommendations were made:

1. Some person or group of persons should be delegated to explore insurance policies and, after developing a set of criteria, to purchase the best one possible.
2. Where feasible, cooperative plans with other schools on a county or other basis should be encouraged in order to obtain less expensive group rates.
3. Criteria for the selection of an insurance policy should, in addition to cost, relate to such important benefits as maximum medical, excluded benefits, maximum dental, hospital, death or dismemberment, surgical, and x-ray.
4. The greatest possible coverage for cost involved should be an important basis for the selection of policy.
5. In light of football programs especially, the catastrophe clause should be investigated as possible additional coverage.
6. Deductible clause policies should not be purchased.
7. Dental injury benefits are an important consideration.
8. Determine what claims the insurance company will and will not pay.
9. The school should insist on 100% enrollment in the athletic insurance program.
10. Schools should have a central location for keeping insurance records, and there should be an annual survey to ascertain all the pertinent facts about the cost and effectiveness of such coverage.

Procedure for insurance management

Every school should be covered by insurance. There are five types of accident insurance that can be used: "(1) commercial insurance policies written on an individual basis; (2) student medical benefit plans written on a group basis by commercial insurers; (3) state high school athletic association benefit plans; (4) medical benefit plans operated by specific city school systems; and (5) self-insurance."* Before adoption by any school each type of insurance should be carefully weighed so that best coverage is obtained for the type of program sponsored.

A suggested procedure to be followed as a guide for the administration of an insurance program follows:

(1) the entire school should be organized to study the insurance problems and needs, (2) a survey should be made to ascertain the need for insurance before it is purchased, (3) after the need has been established, specifications should be constructed indicating the kind and amount of insurance needed, (4) the specifications should be presented to several insurers to obtain estimates of coverage and costs, (5) the plans presented to the school by the several insurers should be studied, and the one best suited to that particular situation should be selected, (6) parents should be given full information about the insurance, (7) workable and harmonious relations should be established with the insurer selected (8) continuous evaluation of the insurance program should be carried out, and (9) records should be carefully kept of costs, accidents, claims payments, and other pertinent data.

School administrators should insist upon the following conditions and requirements when purchasing accident insurance: (1) the coverage should include all school activities and provide up to $500 [more today] for each injury to each pupil, (2) the medical services should include (a) cost of professional services of physician or surgeon, (b) cost of hospital care and service, (c) cost of a trained nurse, (d) cost of ambulance, surgical appliances, dressings, x-rays, etc., and (e) cost of repair and care of natural teeth, (3) the policy should be tailor-made to fit the needs of the school, (4) the coverage should be maximum for minimum cost, (5) all pupils as well as all teachers, should be included, (6) a deductible clause should be avoided unless it reduces the premium substantially and the policy still fulfills its purpose, (7) blanket rather than schedule type coverage should be selected, and (8) claims payment must be simple, certain, and fast.†

School athletic insurance*

According to Grimes, prior to 1930 there was very little accident insurance carried by school districts to protect their athletes, and there was little activity on the part of commercial insurance companies in this area. Only a very few schools were self-insured, and if they were it was primarily for football. Grimes further relates that the Wisconsin High School Athletic Association provided the first movement in school athletic insurance coverage when it established its plan in 1930 and made it available to member schools. Thereafter, many other states followed the example set by Wisconsin, and athletic associations established their own athletic insurance plans. The practice grew and by the 1940's, twenty-five states had such plans. By the 1950's commercial insurance companies, recognizing the possibilities in this area, started to penetrate the high school athletic field and provided special policies to cover athletes in various sports. The commercial insurance companies became so competitive that they made deep inroads into the nonprofit state athletic association plans. Also, according to Grimes, as a result of the commercial insurance company inroads, insurance plans became more comprehensive and coverage was extended to pupils for all school activities for all grades. Today, only eight high school athletic associations sponsor their own insurance plans. These plans stay in business largely because they have adopted many of the features of commercial insurance plans, such as nonallocated benefits, catastrophic coverage, group coverage, nonduplication of benefits, and varying premium rates.

Athletic protection funds usually have these characteristics: they are a nonprofit

---

*Joint Committee: Administrative problems in health education, physical education and recreation, Washington, D. C., 1953, American Association for Health, Physical Education, and Recreation, p. 105.

†Joint Committee, op. cit., p. 106.

---

*From Grimes, L. W.: Trends in school athletic insurance. In Secondary school athletic administration—a new look, Washington, D. C., 1969, The American Association for Health, Physical Education, and Recreation.

venture, they are not compulsory, a specific fee is charged each person registered with the plan, and there is provision for recovery for specific injuries. Generally the money is not paid out of tax funds but instead is paid either by the participants themselves or by the school or other agency.

In connection with such plans, it should be recognized that an individual, after receiving benefits, could in most states still bring action against the coach or other

---

CLAIM NO.

To be filled in by School

REQUEST FOR ACCIDENT BENEFIT
INTERSCHOLASTIC

SPORT_____

Dr._____
X-Ray_____
Total_____

DO NOT WRITE
IN ABOVE SPACE

1. School _____   4. Grade _____
2. Name _____   5. Age _____
3. Date and Time of Injury _____   6. No. of years of competition _____

7. Game_____	8. Type of play at time of injury	9. Boy activity at time of injury
Practice_____	Offense____ Run____	Block_____
Scrimmage_____	Defense____ Pass____	Tackle_____
Skills_____	Rebound____ Kick____	Shooting_____
Night Football Game_____	Etc.____	Etc._____

10. Explain exactly where and how the injury occurred _____

11. Name of the doctor who first attended or examined your injury_____
Date and hour?_____**STATE DATES** of treatment_____
12. After the injury I returned to the squad on ____ (date), was not in school for ____days.
13. Does the parent have other insurance to cover this expense_____

I, Principal of_____High School, have examined the above statements, and the statements of the Doctor or Dentist who attended this student. The statements are true to the best of my knowledge and I believe this claim to be just.

(Date)_____   (Principal)_____

(Signature of Claimant)
This boy was given a Physical Examination on
(DATE)____ at the beginning of **THIS SPORTS SEASON**, which was recorded on the regulation Physical Examination Card which is on file in the school.

(Signature of Coach present at time of injury)

AFFIDAVIT OF ATTENDING PHYSICIAN

1. Date of first treatment _____   2. Diagnosis _____

(Here state the nature, character and extent of injury to claimant)

3. X-RAY READING REPORT MUST ACCOMPANY ALL CLAIMS FOR INDEMNITY FOR FRACTURE OR DISLOCATION.

4. In your opinion was there any predisposing factor contributory to the injury? _____
5. Give name of any consulting or assistant physician _____
6. Describe your treatment and **State Dates** of examination or treatment _____

7. Prognosis and General Remarks_____

Facsimile of Physician's Fees	
( ) Office Calls @ $3.00	$____
( ) Home Calls @ $4.00	$____
( ) Operation	$____
( ) X-ray	$____
	$____
Total	$____

X-RAY not taken by you — attach official copy of report and statement for charge.

SINCE THE PROTECTION PLAN IS A NON-PROFIT ORGANIZATION ESTABLISHED TO SERVE THE SCHOOLS, THE MAXIMUM SCHEDULED INDEMNITY IS NOT TO BE CLAIMED UNLESS ITEMIZED PROFESSIONAL SERVICES JUSTIFY THAT AMOUNT AS LISTED ON REVERSE SIDE.

8. The above named student is again able to PARTICIPATE in athletics and physical education on _____
date

9. Patient discharged from my care on _____
date

I, a Duly Licensed Physician, personally performed the above services.
Signature of Physician: _____ M. D.
Address _____

Form No. 3
25M—5-62

PHYSICIAN: RETURN FORM TO SCHOOL WITH STUDENT ON LAST VISIT
All Bills Must Be Presented Within 90 Days of Accident If Claims Are To Be Paid

Request for accident benefit form. (New York State High School Athletic Protection Plan, Inc.)

leader whose negligence contributed to the injury.

In respect to paying for liability and accident insurance out of public tax funds, the states vary as to their practices. Some states do not permit tax money to be used for liability or accident insurance to cover students in physical education activities. On the other hand, the state legislature of Oregon permits school districts to carry liability insurance. This section is stated as follows in the revised code, O.R.S.:

332.180 Liability insurance; medical and hospital benefits insurance. Any district school board may enter into contracts of insurance for liability coverage all activities engaged in by the district, for medical and hospital benefits for students engaging in athletic contests and for public liability and property damage covering motor vehicles operated by the district, and may pay the necessary premiums thereon. Failure to procure such insurance shall in no case be construed as negligence or lack of diligence on the part of the district school board or the members thereof.

Some athletic insurance plans in use in the schools today are entirely inadequate. These plans indicate a certain amount of money as the maximum that can be collected. For example, a boy may lose the sight of an eye. According to the athletic protection. fund, the loss of an eye will draw, say, $1,500. This amount does not come even remotely close to paying for such a serious injury. In this case a hypothetical example could be taken by saying that the parents sue the athletic protection fund and the teacher for $30,000. In some states if the case is lost, the athletic fund will pay the $1,500 and the teacher the other $28,500. It can be seen that some of these insurance plans do not give complete and adequate coverage.

In many states teachers need additional protection against being sued for accidental injury to students. Legislation is needed permitting school funds to be used as protection against student injuries. In this way a school would be legally permitted to and could be required to purchase liability insurance to cover all pupils.

Questions and exercises

1. Consult the legal files in your local governmental unit to determine any court cases on record that have implications for the fields of health education, physical education, and/or recreation. Describe the circumstances surrounding each.
2. Arrange a mock trial in your class. Have a jury, prosecutor, defendant, witnesses, and other features characteristic of a regular court trial. Your instructor will state the case before the court.
3. Why is it important that leaders in health, physical education, and recreation have knowledge in respect to legal liability?
4. Define and illustrate each of the following: (a) liability, (b) tort, (c) negligence, (d) in loco parentis, (e) plaintiff, (f) nuisance, (g) misfeasance, (h) respondeat superior, and (i) proximate cause.
5. What are the defenses against negligence? Illustrate each.
6. What is the difference between governmental and proprietary functions? Illustrate each.
7. How does the charging of fees affect liability?
8. What is the extent of liability of (a) municipality, (b) school district, (c) board member, and (d) coach?
9. What are some safety procedures that should be followed by every physical education teacher?
10. Prepare a form to be used for the reporting of accidents.
11. What are the advantages of waivers and consent slips?
   Reading assignment in *Administrative Dimensions of Health and Physical Education Programs, Including Athletics:* Chapter 14, Selections 77 to 82.

Selected references

American Association for Health, Physical Education, and Recreation, National Association of Secondary School Principals, and National Commission on Safety Education: The physical education instructor and safety, Washington, D. C., 1948, National Education Association.

American Association for Health, Physical Education, and Recreation: Secondary school athletic administration—a new look, Washington, D. C., 1969, The Association.

Bucher, C. A.: Football can be made safer, New

York World-Telegram and Sun, Saturday Feature Magazine, Sept. 1, 1956.

Casey, L. M.: School business administration, New York, 1964, The Center for Applied Research in Education, Inc. (The Library of Education).

Curtis, P.: Safety and fun synonymous, Chicago, 1955, National Safety Council.

Doscher, N., and Walke, N.: The status of liability for school physical education accidents and its relationship to the health program, The Research Quarterly 23:280, 1952.

Dyer, D. B., and Lichtig, J. G.: Liability in public recreation, Milwaukee, 1949, C. C. Nelson Publishing Co.

Elkow, D.: Safety for recreation areas and playgrounds, Safety Education Digest, 1955 (entire issue).

Foraker, T., and others: School insurance, School and Community, p. 28, October, 1967.

Garber, L. O.: Tort and contractual liability of school districts, Danville, Ill., 1963, The Interstate Printers & Publishers, Inc.

Garber, L. O.: Yearbook of school law, Danville, Ill., 1963, The Interstate Printers & Publishers, Inc.

Gauerke, W. E.: School law, New York, 1965, The Center for Applied Research in Education, Inc. (The Library of Education).

Grieve, A.: Legal aspects of spectator injuries, The Athletic Journal 47:74, 1967.

Guenther, D.: Problems involving legal liability in schools, Journal of the American Association for Health, Physical Education, and Recreation 20:511, 1949.

Hamilton, R. R.: School liability, Chicago, 1952, National Safety Council.

Kurtzman, J.: Legal liability and physical education, The Physical Educator 24:20, 1967.

Liebee, H. C.: Liability for accidents in physical education, athletics, recreation, Ann Arbor, Mich., 1952, Ann Arbor Publishers.

National Education Association, Research Division: School laws and teacher negligence: summary of who is responsible for pupil injuries, National Education Association Research Bulletin 40:75, 1962.

National Education Association: The pupil's day in court: review of 1968, Washington, D. C., 1969, The Association.

National Education Association: Tort liability and liability insurance, School Law Summaries, NEA Research Division, March, 1969.

Proceedings of the City Wide Conference with Principals' Representatives and Men and Women Chairmen of Health Education, City of New York Board of Education, Bureau of Health Education, 1953.

Research Division for the National Commission on Safety Education: Who is liable for pupil injuries? Washington, D. C., 1950, National Education Association.

Rosenfield, H. N.: Liability for school accidents, New York, 1940, Harper & Row, Publishers.

Shroyer, G. F.: Coach's legal liability for athletic injuries, Scholastic Coach 34:18, 1964.

State school laws and regulations for health, safety, driver, outdoor, and physical education, Washington, D. C., 1964, Department of Health, Education, and Welfare.

Truesdale, J. C.: So you're a good samaritan! Journal of the American Association for Health, Physical Education, and Recreation 25:25, 1954.

CHAPTER 19 CURRICULUM DEVELOPMENT

One of the most striking changes to be observed in education during the last few years is the national curriculum reform movement. There is a new mathematics, a new physics, a new English, and a new social studies. Many of the approximately 85,000 public elementary and 24,000 public secondary schools have felt the impact of change, with the movement being most pronounced in suburban schools. A recent study conducted by the Educational Testing Service of Princeton, New Jersey, covered 38,000 students from more than 7,500 academic high schools. It reported that curriculum innovations had a substantial effect in the teaching of school subjects.

In curriculum development, tradition and other pressures are difficult to overcome. Proposals for change encounter obstacles in trying to penetrate the school and college structures in many communities and campuses. Yet the explosion of knowledge, the growth of education in America, the complexity of society, and the impact of social change make it imperative that educators and the public alike examine what they have been doing in the past, evaluate what they are doing now, and plan for the future.

Each subject matter field must relate to and help each student approach self-realization and effective social behavior through an involvement of pertinent ideas, people, and activities. Individual differences must be provided for. Each school system's program must reflect the fact that learning is a continuous and individual process that proceeds at various rates and to various degrees in the attainment of each student's maximum potential.

The curriculum in health education or physical education represents the experiences that are provided children and young people so that the objectives of the profession may be met. The curriculum functions as the vehicle for achieving such objectives as organic development, skill development, mental development, and social development. It provides for experiences in terms of courses, subject matter, and activities that will best approach those goals. It creates the environment that will enable sound and meaningful education to take place. The experiences provided are means to an end—that end being the realization of the broad goals that we have established as a profession and that enrich human living. Each student is, through the experiences provided, helped to develop his abilities and to realize his full potential.

IMPORTANCE OF CURRICULUM DEVELOPMENT AND ROLE OF ADMINISTRATION

Curriculum development is important as a service to the student. It should be concerned with matching the experience and the student; it must meet the needs of boys and girls. Since no two students are exactly alike, there is great need for flexibility and for a wide range of experiences that meet the requirements of all pupils. Continuous curriculum development is a way of determining what needs to be learned and of providing the means for seeing that it is accomplished.

The administration plays a very important part in curriculum planning. The end result of all administrative effort is to provide better instructional services, better programs, better learning situations, and better experiences to achieve the objectives that have been established. Since new problems constantly arise and since unmet needs continue to exist or go unrecognized, there is an urgent need for continuous curriculum planning. It is the administrator who provides the required leadership. The educational philosophy that represents the foundation of curriculum development should reflect faculty thinking as determined by their study of pupil needs. If an administrator possesses what he considers to be a better philosophy, he should discuss this with the faculty, bringing forth facts, good reasoning, and logic to support his concept. If it is then accepted by the faculty, it can be utilized. Otherwise, it will not receive extensive practical application because it is not understood or accepted.

Curriculum construction requires the selection, guidance, and evaluation of experiences in the light of both long-term and more immediate goals. It provides for an orderly periodic evaluation of the total program, both the inclass and the out-of-class, with changes being made whenever necessary. It takes into consideration such factors as students, total community, existing facilities, personnel, time allotments, national trends, and state rules and regulations. It sets up a framework for orderly progression from the kindergarten through college. It offers a guide to health education and physical education teachers so that they are better able to achieve educational goals.

Curriculum development is very important and school administrators have the responsibility for making the necessary provisions to see that it is accomplished.

CATALYSTS THAT BRING ABOUT CURRICULUM CHANGE

Changes occur in health education and physical education curricula as they do in other areas of the school offering. There is usually a continuous list of myriad proposals for change. Each proposal should be considered on its own merits and put to the test of whether or not it has value.

What are the influencing factors in regard to change? A few associations, agencies, and individuals who produce change in health and physical education are discussed in the following paragraphs.

National associations and agencies

The President's Council on Physical Fitness and Sports is an outstanding example of one national governmental agency that brought about much change in programs of health, physical education, and recreation throughout the United States and the world. Through their speakers, publications, and communication media pronouncements, many changes have taken place in the schools and colleges of this nation. Physical fitness in some communities has become the overriding purpose of programs of health education and physical education, sometimes at the expense of the other objectives of these fields and a well-balanced program of activities.

Examples of other national associations and agencies that play a part in curriculum change are the National Education Association, the American Association for Health, Physical Education, and Recreation, the United States Office of Education, the Association for Supervision and Curriculum Development, and The American Medical Association.

State associations and agencies

As national organizations influence the curricula of our schools and colleges, so do state organizations. State boards of education or departments of public instruction, state bureaus, departments or divisions of health and physical education, state education associations, citizens committees, teachers associations, and associations for health, physical education, and recreation are a few examples of organizations that influence curricula. Through the publication of syllabi, sponsorship of legislation, enactment of rules and regulations, exercise of supervisory powers, allocation of funds, and initiation of projects, organizations promote certain ideas and programs that initiate changes in schools and colleges.

Research

Research brings about change. As new knowledge is uncovered, more information is known about the learning process, new techniques are developed, and other research is conducted. Change eventually ensues if the research is significant, but the change may be slow in coming. It usually takes a long period of time for the creation of knowledge to penetrate to the grass roots, where it becomes part of an action program.

In the fields of health education and physical education, research on motor learning, the relationship of health and physical fitness to academic achievement, movement education, cognitive learning, physiologic changes that occur in the body through exercise, smoking, ecology, and the relationship of mental health and physical activity represent a few examples of research that have or will have a bearing upon programs of health education and physical education throughout the country.

College and university faculties

The leaders in education from the campuses of this nation who serve as consultants, write textbooks, make speeches, and are active in professional associations, help to bring about changes in education in general and in the special fields of health education and physical education.

Social forces

Such social forces in the American culture as the civil rights movement, automation, mass communication, student acti-

vism, black studies, sports promotion, and collective bargaining through unions are a few of the movements sweeping the nation that have implications for curricula in schools and colleges. In addition, the social trends of the times involving attitudes toward sex, driving, alcohol, tobacco, and narcotics bring about curricula change. Times change, customs change, the habits of people change, and with such change the role of educational institutions and their responsibilities to their society frequently change.

THE HEALTH EDUCATOR AND PHYSICAL EDUCATOR AND CURRICULUM CHANGE

Since there are so many factors that continually influence curricula, it is important for the health educator and physical educator to assess the recommended changes so that informed and wise decisions may be made. Four questions that administrators and teachers might ask themselves in rationalizing the importance of suggested changes are as follows:

1. *What are the functions of the schools and colleges?* To what extent is the suggested change in conformance with the philosophy and purpose of education in the American society? How will it better help the students?

2. *Am I sufficiently well informed so that I can make an intelligent decision?* Teachers and administrators will need to be knowledgeable about the learning process, the patterns of human growth and development, current program needs, and such matters as the needs and interests of the people in the local community who are served by the educational institution. The responsibility rests with administrators and teachers to be well informed in the areas pertinent to the decisions that need to be made.

3. *How does the change relate to staff, plant, budget, and other important administrative items?* The change must be prac-

tical of implementation and the best use of staff, plant, and other items taken into consideration in making the decision.

4. *What do the experts say?* What is the thinking of professionals who have done research, studied the problem intensively, and tested the proposal on a wide scale? Expert opinion may be of help as an additional source of information for making a wise curriculum decision.

PROCEDURAL CONSIDERATIONS FOR CURRICULUM CHANGE

Curricular revision cannot occur without taking into consideration an investigation into such procedural matters as the following:

1. *Students.* The number of students, their characteristics and needs, and their socioeconomic backgrounds and interests need to be considered prior to initiating any pertinent curriculum change.

2. *Faculty.* The members of the staff play a key role in curricular revision. For example, the attitude of faculty toward change, present teaching loads, comprehension of goals of the school, attitudes toward inclass and out-of-class programs, competencies in areas of curriculum revision, and past training and experience are a few important considerations. Change in curriculum might well mean new members being added to the faculty or a different type of competency being represented on the staff.

3. *Physical plant.* Information in regard to the adequacy of the physical plant for present and future programs must be considered. Information should be available on capabilities and limitations of the present plant. There may be new demands placed upon facilities through a curricular revision that brings about changes in such matters as class size.

4. *Budget.* The financial plan is another important consideration in curriculum change. What will the new program cost? What are the sources of support? Before the faculty expends large amounts of time and effort in a study of curriculum change, there should be a reasonable assurance that proposed changes are economically feasible.

5. *Curriculum.* Since any new curricular proposal is likely to reflect present practices to some degree, it seems logical that the present curriculum needs careful scrutiny to determine what has happened over the years, the degree to which the faculty has brought about change, and the general direction in which the institution is moving.

6. *Administration.* It is important for the faculty to take a hard look at the administrative leadership of the school or college, including the principals, superintendents, deans, and presidents, as well as the boards of education and boards of trustees. The philosophy of the administration and its views toward change should be carefully weighed. Administrators will need to approve budgetary allocations and necessary expenditures as well as, in many cases, pass upon the proposed changes.

PEOPLE INVOLVED IN CURRICULUM DEVELOPMENT

Curriculum planning should be characterized by broad participation on the part of many people. The consideration of administrators, teachers, state groups, students, parents, and other individuals is important.

Administrators

Administrators—whether the college president in the field of higher education, the superintendent of schools or principal of an elementary, middle, junior high, or senior high school, or the chairman or director of the health and physical education department—are key personnel in curriculum planning. These individuals serve as the catalytic forces that set curriculum studies into motion; as the leadership that encourages and stimulates interest in providing better learning experiences for students; as the obstacle clearers who provide the time, place, and materials for doing an effective job; and as the implementors who help to see that the fruits of such studies are actually put into practice.

Teachers

Teachers, because they are the persons representing the grass-roots level of the curriculum enterprise, are the ones who actually know what is feasible and what will or will not work. They mingle daily with the pupils and they play a key role in curriculum planning. In smaller school systems each member of the health education and physical education staff should take part in curriculum planning. In larger school systems volunteers or representatives from the various schools might make up the study group.

The teacher's role in active curriculum development can involve contributing his or her experiences and knowledge and presenting data to support recommendations of desired changes. An effective way to utilize faculty groups is the committee system. Committees can be established for the study of such considerations as school philosophy, specific instructional areas, pertinent case studies, immediate and specific objectives for each grade level, needs of children, student readiness for various activities, experiences to satisfy the needs

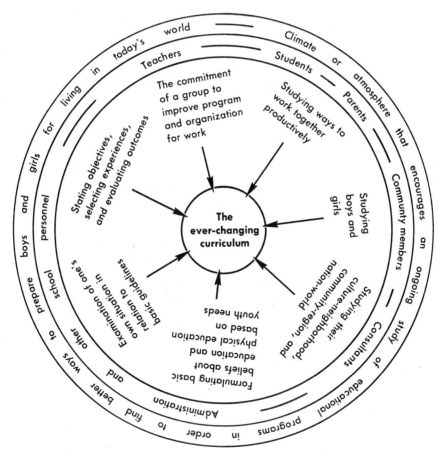

The curriculum merry-go-round. (From Cassidy, R.: Curriculum development in physical education, New York, 1954, Harper & Row, Publishers.)

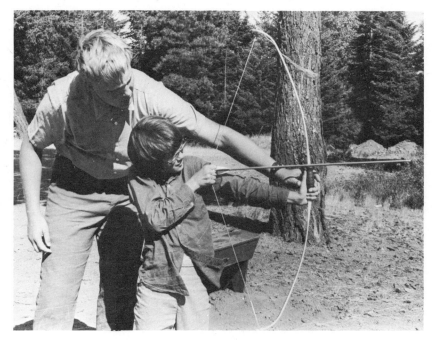

The curriculum must take into consideration the needs of each student. A camp junior counselor helps a special education (handicapped) student with a bow and arrow. Archery is one of many activities offered the special education students during a week-long summer camp near Ellensburg, Wash., as part of the Broadfront Program.

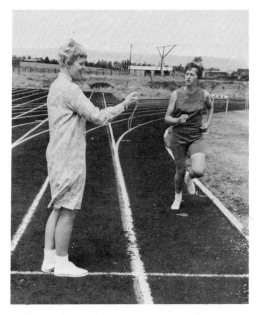

High school physical education instructor Sherry Ortman checks the stopwatch as a student finishes a jog around the track, as part of the Broadfront Program.

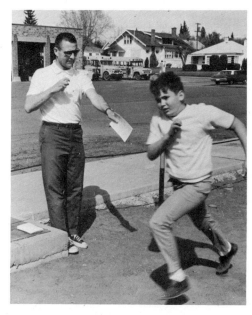

Broadfront Project physical education specialist Clyde Buehler times a sixth-grade student in a 50-yard dash, one of the physical fitness test items administered in the fall and spring.

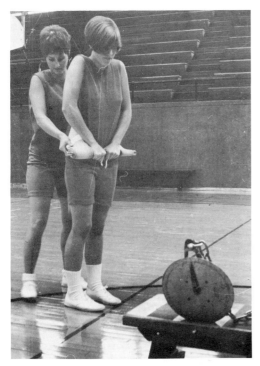

Junior high school physical education instructor Sue Kennedy readies a student for a leg-lift test, using a dynamometer. The leg-lift is one of the physical fitness tests administered in the fall and spring, as part of the Broadfront Program.

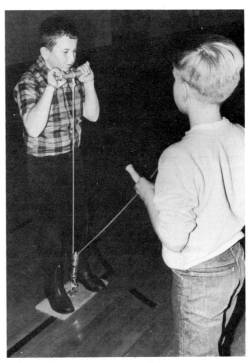

Two students work with the "Exer-Genie" exerciser as part of their developmental physical education program, a part of the Broadfront Program. The developmental program is aimed at improving students with low fitness ability.

of children, means of implementing curriculum changes, and the program of evaluation.

Each teacher in the school should be regarded as a curriculum planner in regard to his or her own instructional offering and, in addition, as a contributor to the total departmental and all-school educational program.

State groups

Throughout most states are located many people and agencies that can help in health and physical education curriculum planning. These include the state department of public instruction or education, the state department of health, colleges and universities, and voluntary health agencies. These groups may provide curriculum guides, courses of study, advice, teaching aids, other materials, and help that will prove invaluable in curriculum planning.

Students

Students can play a part in curriculum development. As a result of an indication of their thinking in regard to such items as their interests, significant learning experiences, obstacles to desirable learning, and learning experiences recommended in the out-of-class program, guides may be provided that will help in curriculum development. The suggestions and ideas of students can be taken and evaluated by adults, in the light of their own thinking; it may be that the adults will find much merit and substance in the thinking of students.

Parents and community leaders

Discussions with parents and other interested citizens can sometimes help in curriculum development. Since the home plays such an important part in a child's learning and since parents are in essence one-half of the teaching team, there is an opportunity present, in group planning, to communicate to the public what the school is trying to achieve and how it can best be accomplished. Mothers and fathers and other community-minded people can also make significant contributions in evaluating students' behavior in terms of desired outcomes, as established and delineated by the schools.

Other individuals from specialized areas

Curriculum development should utilize the services of individuals who are interested and who can make a worthwhile contribution. For example, such persons as doctors, nurses, and recreation leaders should not be overlooked. It is desirable to look at the curriculum from all sides and all angles, to look at it right side up and upside down, to look at it from the student's as well as the teacher's point of view, and from the parent's as well as the administrator's. Desirable results will flow from a continuous appraisal of the curriculum, made by many persons whose efforts, resources, qualifications, and interests are utilized in a meaningful manner.

STEPS IN CURRICULUM DEVELOPMENT

Krug,* in discussing curriculum development from the general educator's point of view, classifies the following steps involved in curriculum planning: determining the purposes of education, translating the pur-

---

*Krug, E. A.: Curriculum planning, New York, 1950, Harper & Row, Publishers.

poses into an all-school program, translating the purposes into specific subject matter areas, providing curriculum guides and instructional aids and materials, and carrying on the teaching-learning process. These appear below in adapted form.

Determining the purposes of education

This step involves studying the various factors that contribute to and result in the formulation of objectives, such as the nature of society, the learning process, and the needs of children and youth. After consideration has been given to such important factors by a faculty or presentations have been made by curriculum specialists, educational objectives can be more clearly formulated.

Translating the purposes into an all-school program

Having determined the objectives of education as a whole and knowing the characteristics of children of different grade levels, those persons developing a curriculum can focus attention on outlining and analyzing broad categories of learning experiences and assigning relative emphases to the various phases of the educational process. The specialized fields of health and physical education should be viewed as part of the total educational program. Consequently, their specific objectives should relate to the overall educational objectives.

Translating the purposes into specific subject matter areas

The next step is to focus attention on subject matter and the activities of the teaching-learning process. Relating this to one phase of the physical education program, for example, it is obvious that the physiologic needs of children would necessitate provision of ample opportunities for a wide range of physical movements involving the large muscles. Growth and development characteristics of children,

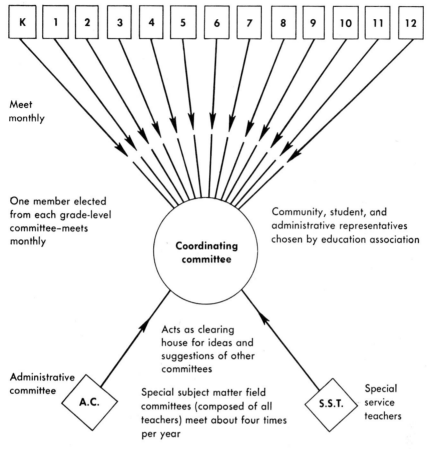

Grade-level committees. Purpose of program is to ascertain the needs of children and to devise means of meeting those needs. (From Oliver, A. I.: Curriculum improvement—a guide to problems, principles, and procedures, New York, 1965, Dodd, Mead & Co.)

physical capacities and abilities, and other considerations also would need to be studied.

Providing curriculum guides and instructional aids and materials

Curriculum guides and instructional aids such as textbooks, visual aids, and other materials are an important consideration in curriculum development. An opportunity is presented here to utilize educationally sound materials that will assist the teacher in exploiting the educational environmental situation most effectively so that desirable learnings will take place and objectives will be accomplished.

Carrying on the teaching-learning process

This step represents the culmination of the curriculum development process—what actually takes place in the classroom, gymnasium, playfield, or swimming pool. The effectiveness with which learning takes place, the aids and materials utilized, the good methods used, and the desirable outcomes accomplished determine the success or the failure of curriculum development.

Cassidy, discussing steps in curriculum development from the point of view of physical education, lists the following as the most effective in curriculum building in the process of cooperative program planning:

1. The commitment of a group of individuals to the importance of the task and organization of the group to work cooperatively in the study and formulation of program experiences which include both methods and materials.
2. Formulation of a philosophy of education and of physical education or a set of guiding principles or basic beliefs which will serve to give direction in program making and in evaluation.
3. In order to complete step 2, the group must study foundation facts concerning the needs of youth—this includes the demands of the culture and the developmental tasks required of youth by that culture.
4. Clarification of the objectives of education and of physical education.
5. Study of one's own students, the school and community situation, relationships, values, attitudes, program, and facilities in the light of stated principles.
6. Statement of objectives based on student needs, consistent with the basic point of view of the group and the situation in which the program must operate.
7. Selection of units of activity or experiences to accomplish these objectives.
8. Development of the materials of instruction—the resource and the teaching units.
9. Development of tools for evaluating the progress toward the stated objectives.
10. Provision for ongoing machinery to assure the continuance of such study.*

A CONCEPTUAL APPROACH TO PHYSICAL EDUCATION

The goal of education is to help boys and girls to become mature adults, possess ability to make wise decisions, and be capable of intelligent self-direction.

Physical education, as a part of education, should provide each boy and girl with carefully planned experiences that result in knowledge about the value of physical activity, essential motor skills, strength, stamina, and other essential physical characteristics and about the social qualities that make for effective citizenship.

*Cassidy, R.: Curriculum development in physical education, New York, 1954, Harper & Row, Publishers, pp. 12-14.

Over the years physical educators in many of our schools have attempted to achieve these goals in a dedicated and conscientious manner. However, most physical educators will agree there is still much room for improvement. Those persons who advocate change cite educational systems where there is lack of progression, sequential treatment of subject matter, and an orderly developmental pattern for teaching motor skills. Furthermore, they say, physical education curricula vary from school to school and state to state without any degree of uniformity. As a result of these conditions, they lament, students are not becoming as physically educated as they could be, and, also, physical education is not gaining the respectability in the educational process it justly deserves.

A new development that has won the acclaim of educators in recent years is the concept approach to curriculum planning. This innovation may have possibilities for helping physical education to achieve a more important and respected place in the schools of this nation.

Each subject matter field has objectives toward which they teach and that represent the worth of the field for the students. Physical education has traditionally advocated the four objectives of organic development, neuromuscular development, mental development, and social development. These goals have proved valuable as targets toward which both the teacher and student strive. At the same time, they are rather general in nature and may not provide the best basis for the most effective structural organization of physical education.

The student should be aware of the general objectives of physical education but, in addition, as a result of his school experiences, should be sensitive to, understand, and know the framework that constitutes the field of physical education. He should be aware of the unity, the wholeness, and the interrelatedness of the many activities in which he engages from kindergarten through college. He should even think at times as a physical educator might think, particularly from the standpoint of recognizing the importance and value of such course experiences to human beings. He should understand what constitutes the master plan of education and the structure of physical education as it fits into this master plan.

In creating this structure of physical education, one might draw an analogy between our field and the construction of a house. Just as there are key pillars and beams that give the house form and support, so the key unifying elements within physical education that give it a strong foundational framework and hold it together as a valuable educational experience for every boy and girl should be identified. These unifying threads would tie together the various parts of the discipline into a meaningful and cohesive learning package.

These unifying threads would be the *concepts* and, as such, would represent the basic structure of physical education in the school program. They would be the *key ideas, principles, skills, values,* or *attitudes* that represent points upon which we as physical educators should focus our efforts throughout the school life of the child. They would be part of both the teacher's and student's thinking and would range from very simple ideas to high-level abstractions. They would start with simple, elementary, fundamental experiences and in a sequential, progressive, and developmental pattern gain depth and comprehensiveness over the years as schooling progresses and the student matures. They would as unifying threads define the domain of physical education.

Concepts in physical education would not be memorized by the students. Rather, they would be ideas—analytic generalizations that would emerge and be understood by the student as a result of his school experiences in physical education. They

would also provide him with a reservoir of information, skills, and understandings that would help him to meet new problems and situations.

The concepts, of course, would need to be carefully selected according to acceptable criteria and be scientifically sound. Furthermore, after the concepts had been identified, there would be need for extensive testing of their validity by many experts, including teachers in the field and specialists in curriculum development.

To implement the concepts within the physical education structure, there would be a need to delineate the identified concepts into meaningful units and topics that would be progressive in nature and reinforce the concepts that had been identified. The subdivisions of concepts in the structure would represent basic elements needed to develop a meaningful course of study and bring about desirable behavior. Furthermore, they would emanate and flow from the key concepts and would help to give greater meaning and understanding to them. As the conceptual, unifying threads were developed at each ascending grade and educational level, the student would be provided with new challenges, where the information, skills, and understanding he has acquired could be applied. The result would be that finally the student would reach a point where he could on his own arrive at valid answers and make wise decisions in the area of physical education.

As a result of the concept approach, students would have a greater mastery of the field of physical education, increased understanding and power in dealing with problems related to their physical self that are new and unfamiliar, and motivation to want to become physically educated in the true sense of the term. The approach would provide a stable system of knowledge and provide guideposts for thinking intelligently about physical education.

The concept approach would have par-

GENERAL SEQUENCE OF PROCEDURE

Recognition of the Need

↓

Tentative Philosophy

↓

Criteria for Selecting the Body of Knowledge

↓

Identification of the Body of Knowledge

↓

Revision of Philosophy

↓

Master Plan

↓

Scope and Sequence

↓

Organizing Ideas

↓

Content Units

↓

Sequential Lessons

IDENTIFICATION OF THE BODY OF KNOWLEDGE
Example of Theme Format

Theme II Human development is characterized by an orderly progression, but the age of onset and the rates of progress within each phase are unique to the individual.

    KEY Fundamental patterns or common elements of movement are combined to form complex patterns of movement which make up the skills of sports and dance.

      SUBKEY All specialized activities have elements of movement which are common to other activities.

        STATEMENT Complex skills are composed primarily of familiar patterns which require some specific adjustment to meet the demands of the new activity.

          SUBSTATEMENT All sports, games and dances involve propelling the body and/or other objects. (84)

            To meet new motor activities with success an individual must have mastered a variety of fundamental motor patterns. (85)

MASTER PLAN OUTLINE
Outcome and Major Behavioral Objectives

GENERAL OBJECTIVE I: Acquisition of motor skills and knowledge of their practice.

    OUTCOME: To be proficient in a variety of motor skills.

    MAJOR BEHAVIORAL OBJECTIVES:

      To acquire proficiency in a wide range of sports, games and dances.

      To be able to move the body efficiently in all fundamental skills.

      To be able to combine the fundamental skills into complex patterns of sports, games and dances.

      To know the rules, strategy and ethics of various sports, games and dances.

      To understand role of gross motor activity in intellectual development.

MASTER PLAN OUTLINE
GENERAL PROGRAM OBJECTIVES

| # 1 | # 2 | # 3 | # 4 |

OUTCOMES

MAJOR BEHAVIORAL OBJECTIVES

RELATIVE EMPHASIS OF ORGANIZING IDEAS

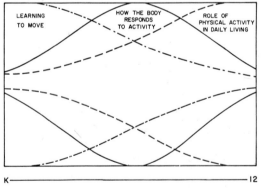

| LEARNING TO MOVE | HOW THE BODY RESPONDS TO ACTIVITY | ROLE OF PHYSICAL ACTIVITY IN DAILY LIVING |

K ———————————————————— 12

SCOPE AND SEQUENCE
Development of Specific Behavioral Objectives

CRITERIA

Specific Behavioral Objectives

Developmental Characteristics

Performance Standards

Current Practices

Associated Concepts

Taxonomy of Educational Objectives

Major Behavioral Objectives

To be able to move the body efficiently in all fundamental skills

K   To be able to gallop
    To be able to skip

1   To be able to change direction, change configuration in basic locomotor activities.

2   To be able to execute a basic locomotor activity on signal, change direction and activity without hesitation.

UNIT I

| EPISODE 1 |

1. SEGMENTS
2.
3.

→

| EPISODE 2 |

1. SEGMENTS
2.
3.
4.

| EPISODE 3 |

1. SEGMENTS
2.
3.

UNIT 2

FORMAT OF UNIT CONTENT

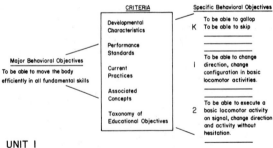

	CONCEPTS	ASSOCIATED CONCEPTS	SPECIFIC BEHAVIORAL OBJECTIVES	LEARNING ACTIVITIES
SEGMENT # 1				
SEGMENT # 2				
SEGMENT # 3				

FORMAT OF UNIT CONTENT

UNIT I LEARNING TO MOVE

  EPISODE A: Body Awareness
    SEGMENT I. Identification of Body Parts

  EPISODE B: Concepts of Space, Force, Time, Direction, Form
    SEGMENT I. Direction in Space

UNIT II LEARNING ABOUT PHYSICAL CHANGES AND DIFFERENCES

ASSOC. CONCEPTS	CONCEPTS	SPECIFIC BEHAVIORAL OBJECTIVES	LEARNING ACTIVITIES
Muscle Skeleton Bone Together Separate Segment Extremity	Head Trunk Arms Legs	To identify various parts of the body. To move specific parts of the body in various ways.	Problem Solving Movement Exploration Games: Simon Says Hokey Pokey
Space Direction Position	Toward – Away Up – Down Right – Left Over - Under Through	To move toward an object. To move through an object.	Obstacle Course Problem Solving

The Battle Creek Physical Education Curriculum Project. (Battle Creek, Mich.)

ticular value to physical education because of such things as the great breadth of skills, knowledge, and values that make up this field of endeavor. It would provide a logical and systematic means for identifying among the many elements those that give form and structure to the type of physical education program professionals want taught in schools. The identified concepts would have permanence, and as the explosion of knowledge takes place in the years ahead through the efforts of our scholarly researchers, this new information can become part of the structure, wherever applicable. Finally, the concept approach would be readily adaptable to individual differences that exist among students as well as sufficiently flexible to provide for the many geographic types of facilities and other factors that differentiate one community or school from another.

Some physical educators might say that the subject matter, skills, and other elements of physical education are the same under the concept approach as under the traditional approach. It may be that the facts will be the same in some cases but the approach will be different. For example, in the new mathematics, as developed by one professional group in grade nine, there is still concentration upon algebra, but the emphasis is not on the solving of algebraic equations but, instead, on the behavior of numbers—a verbalization of concepts.

Under the traditional approach, the organization of courses involved topics and activities, but without sufficient regard to the relationship of the topic and activity to what had gone on previously for the student and what lies ahead. This new method would still discuss topics and conduct activities, but topics and activities would be related to key concepts that the topic and activity are designed to elaborate upon, contribute more understanding, and make the area of learning more meaningful in the life of the student.

Physical education needs a curriculum study with careful consideration being given to the concept approach. At a time when the curriculum reform movement is sweeping the nation and when there already is a new mathematics, a new physics, a new English, and a new social studies, physical education can no longer be apathetic about what it teaches and how it teaches. The concept approach is one that should be very carefully weighed for the *new physical education*.

CURRICULUM DEVELOPMENT IN PRACTICE

A noteworthy example of practical curriculum planning is the work of leaders in the Columbus, Ohio, public schools,* who developed a curriculum guide for a school health science course. The procedures for curriculum development were formulated by a committee consisting of a supervisor of health education, six health teachers, two advisory committee members, a school physician, and a director of public information. This committee consulted with curriculum authorities in health education and read literature on curriculum research. The plan involved the following eight-point process:

1. *Study of the existing program.* A review of course offerings, teaching guides, textbooks, and other curriculum materials was made.
2. *Collection and review of pertinent literature.* Thirty cities, counties, states, and professional health associations were canvassed and thirty health textbooks reviewed.
3. *Aims and objectives of guide determined.* The basic philosophy of health education as viewed by the committee was formulated.

*Cauffman, J. G.: How to develop a curriculum guide for a school health science course, Journal of Health, Physical Education, and Recreation 33:19, 1962.

4. *Needs and interests identified.* The needs and interests of the students who would represent the consumer of the teaching were studied.
5. *Judgments obtained from selected individuals.* The thinking of administrators, health teachers, nurses, counselors, parents, and health authorities was sought on problem areas of health education.
6. *Available resources screened.* Resources within the school system, within the community, and out-of-town resources were surveyed relating to selected health problem areas and what was available to help in solving problems.
7. *The organization of resource units.* After problem areas had been identified and resources screened, resource units were developed for teaching.
8. *Experimental use of guide.* The guide was used experimentally for 2 years in the Columbus schools. Evaluations were done and changes made where it was thought they were needed.

An example of one community of more than 50,000 people that made a curriculum study is White Plains, New York. The methods and materials utilized by this community have been described elsewhere* and may be of help to other communities or school districts.

The study was initiated by the director of health and physical education for the public schools after a discussion with several faculty members. The board of education allocated $750 for the study, and these funds enabled the staff to secure, as a consultant, a university professor who was well versed in the field of physical education.

The consultant and the director prepared the outline for the study group that consisted of the physical education staff. The board of education allowed the experience to be credited toward inservice education credit that was recognized on the salary increment scale. The workshop experience required that staff members meet one evening each week as a group. All administrative arrangements were handled by the director and leader. During the actual deliberations, however, the director remained in the background, allowing the staff to act on its own.

The physical education staff was divided into committees according to school level —elementary, junior high school, and senior high school. Each committee prepared its recommendations, worked with the study leader, and presented its findings to the staff as a whole. The entire faculty discussed and made suggestions to each committee. In the light of these deliberations each group then reworked its recommendations into final form.

The curriculum guide that was developed as a result of these deliberations contains the following:

1. A general statement of philosophy in regard to the curriculum guide
2. A statement of objectives for each educational level
3. A grouping of activities to meet objectives
4. The time requirement for each grade
5. The percentage of total time used for each grade activity at each grade level
6. A statement on evaluation—its purposes and its use as a basis for grading
7. A cumulative record card

The White Plains curriculum guide placed the physical education program in a more favorable light among the students, administrators, and teachers and in the community. Most important, it helped to ensure that the right experiences were pro-

*Bucher, C. A., Koenig, C., and Barnhard, M.: Methods and materials for secondary school physical education, St. Louis, 1970, The C. V. Mosby Co.

vided each school child as part of his or her education.

EVALUATION OF THE CURRICULUM

Once a curriculum has been developed, evaluation is essential. The major purpose of such an evaluation is to determine the extent to which the experiences provided are reflected in desirable learnings on the part of the students. Unless the educational outcomes are desirable and are acceptable to educators, the curriculum cannot be considered successful. Saylor and Alexander have pointed out essential characteristics of an evaluation program:

1. The integral relationship of curriculum planning and evaluation should be clearly understood by all persons who participate in planning the school program.
2. Changes in the procedure of curriculum planning and in over-all curriculum plans should be based on evaluative evidence.
3. The planning of learning experiences for all learning groups should include provisions for evaluation by the groups and their teachers of the experiences.
4. A systematic set of procedures for securing evaluative evidence should be in operation.
5. These procedures should be based on values agreed upon by all who participate in curriculum planning.
6. Evidence should be secured regarding (a) the progress of pupils during the period concerned toward specific curriculum goals; (b) the progress of pupils after completing phases of the curriculum; (c) the opinions of parents and teachers bearing on curriculum planning.[*]

Curriculum evaluation to date has used four means of determining whether or not a new program has worth.[†] One method is through observations of students who have been exposed to the new program

and the progress they have made. A second method is systematic questioning of teachers and students involved in the program. A third procedure involves testing of students periodically to determine their progress. A fourth method is the comparative testing of students under the "new" and under the "old" programs to determine progress under each.

Suggested outline

A score card or outline by which the curriculum of any school system may be checked has been developed by the Bureau of Curriculum Research of Teachers College, Columbia University. The suggested outline for evaluation follows:

A. Recognition of Basic Educational Objectives
  1. General aims or objectives
  2. Statement of objectives or aims
  3. Validity (soundness, worth) of the stated and implied objectives
  4. Degree in which objectives have been consistently carried out in the selection and organization of subject matter and methods suggested
B. What to Teach—Organization of Subject Matter
  1. Nature of subject matter
  2. Major emphasis
  3. Form of development of subjects
  4. Use made of scientific studies in selection and organization of subject matter
C. Recognition of, and Adaptation to, Pupil Needs
  1. Effective utilization of pupils' experiences
  2. Course of study so organized as to provide for individual differences in children's interests and abilities
  3. Gradation of material on basis of pupils needs for immediate use
  4. Regard for relative value of topics within a subject
  5. Suggested use of varied forms of activities
  6. Use made of scientific studies in provision for pupil needs
D. Adaptation to Teacher Needs—Suggestions as to Methods and Materials
  1. Respect for the judgment and initiative of the teacher
  2. Suggestions for correlations between subjects

---

[*]Saylor, J. G., and Alexander, W. M.: Curriculum planning for better teaching and learning, New York, 1954, Holt, Rinehart & Winston, Inc., p. 607.

[†]Goodlad, J. I.: School curriculum in the United States, New York, 1964, The Fund for the Advancement of Education, p. 59.

3. Definite suggestions for work dealing with materials and topics of local interest
4. Illustrative and type lessons given
5. Suggested standards for checking results of teaching
6. Reference to proper use of maps
7. Use of scientific studies in determining methods and materials
8. References, basic and supplemental, for children

E. Course of Study Itself—Mechanical Make-up
1. Clearness and conciseness
2. Proper methods of emphasizing important phases of work
3. Attractiveness, useableness
4. Convenience
5. Ease of revision
6. Economy of space and expense*

PRINCIPLES TO CONSIDER IN CURRICULUM DEVELOPMENT

In summary, it can be pointed out that although curriculum development will vary from school to school and from community to community, some general principles are applicable to all situations:

1. Learning experiences should be selected and developed that will be most helpful in achieving educational outcomes.

2. Curriculum development is a continuous effort rather than one that is accomplished at periodic intervals.

3. The leadership in curriculum development rests primarily with the administration and supervisory staffs.

4. The administration should utilize (wherever possible and practicable) the services of teachers, laymen, students, state consultants, and other persons who can contribute to the development of the best curriculum possible. The work should not, however, place an unreasonable demand on any person's time and effort.

5. Curriculum development is dependent upon a thorough knowledge of the needs and characteristics, developmental levels, capacities, and maturity levels of the students, as well as an understanding of the environments in which those students live.

6. Curriculum development should permit teachers to exploit sound principles of learning in the selection and development of learning experiences.

7. Curriculum development should take into account out-of-school learning experiences and integrate them with school experiences.

8. The main value of curriculum development is determined by the degree of improved instruction that results.

EDUCATIONAL INNOVATIONS AFFECTING CURRICULUM DEVELOPMENT

There are many new developments that affect the curriculum, both from the standpoint of administrative innovations that affect school organization and scheduling and what is taught and from the standpoint of new teaching techniques that influence how the subject matter is taught and the degree to which learning takes place.

Teaching machines, language laboratories, educational television, tape recorders, super-8 films, and opaque projectors are affecting school programs. Too few teachers and administrators are familiar with the "new" media that have come not from educators themselves but from individuals with vision and creativeness outside the schools. Educators need to get away from the routine administrative detail and traditional ways of teaching, at least to the point where they are familiar with and know the advantage of new ways of doing things. Although nothing has been developed as a substitute for sound teacher-student relationships, much has been introduced that can make this relationship more meaningful and productive. With the great expansion in school enrollments, teacher shortages, and international em-

---

*Reeder, W. G.: The fundamentals of public school administration, New York, 1958, The Macmillan Co., pp. 497-499.

phasis, innovations need to be evaluated for their possible use in the classroom.

Constant evaluation is, of course, necessary. The innovation must stand the test of making it possible to have higher quality education, including more individualized instruction, better learning, and freedom for the teacher to do more important work.

A few of the innovations include flexible school structures, newer audiovisual aids, programmed learning, ungraded classes, team teaching, teacher aids, hidden talent projects, paperbacks and other variations in text materials, automated data processing, language laboratories, and new approaches to grouping. Discussed in this chapter are selected administrative innovations and also some new teaching innovations with which each health educator and physical educator should be familiar.

Administrative innovations affecting curriculum development

Administrative innovations affecting curriculum planning include flexible scheduling, nongraded schools, middle school, and year-round school.

Flexible scheduling. Flexible scheduling, sometimes called modular scheduling because of the time units involved—most frequently about 20 minutes each—is a term used to describe a school schedule in which classes do not meet for the same length of time each day. Flexible scheduling uses blocks of time to build periods of different length. For example, one module might be 20 minutes in length, a double module would be 40 minutes, a triple module would be 60 minutes, and a quadruple module would be 80 minutes. Time is left between each module for purposes of organization of classes.

One advantage of flexible scheduling over the traditional pattern of fixed scheduling, or the same allotment of time per day to a subject, is that flexible scheduling enables subjects to have varying times for instruction. For example, teachers say that

usually more time is necessary in a science laboratory than for instruction in a foreign language newly introduced to students. It has been pointed out that a foreign language can be most effectively taught in shorter time periods at more frequent intervals. Flexible scheduling also provides more instructional time, more opportunity for small group instruction, and less time in study halls where learning time is not always put to the best use. With flexible scheduling it is possible to have subject matter and courses presented under optimum conditions, on an individual basis, and in smaller or larger groups, as best meets the needs of the subject and teacher. Flexible scheduling also helps the teacher by permitting more time for instruction.

It can no longer be assumed that all subject matter and all courses should be taught in the same unit of time to the same number of students. New research shows that some subjects are taught best in shorter periods of time, given more frequently, and with a smaller group of students.

The use of the computer has made flexible scheduling a reality. The principal can tell a 707 computer how many teachers he has, what courses they can teach, how many students there are, and what courses each student wants to take. Within 60 minutes the answers are provided in the form of a complete master schedule and individual schedules for each student enrolled.

Operation G.A.S.P. (Generalized Academic Simulation Programs) is one example of flexible scheduling. It was developed at the Massachusetts Institute of Technology under a grant from the Ford Foundation's Education Facilities Laboratories. As a result of G.A.S.P., time and money have been saved, flexibility in schools has been provided, and preplanning space utilization before construction blueprints are made is much more accurate and meaningful.

Form No. 1

LESSON JOB ORDER

Date needed _____

From _____
Teacher

Subject _____

Total number of modules in group	Number of groups	Class size request	Module request	Room request	Additional teacher	Method of instruction (large group, small group, individual study group, etc.)

Bulletin notice: _____

_____

_____

Approved _____
Team leader   Date

Lesson job order for flexible scheduling. (Courtesy Gardner Swenson, Principal, Brookhurst Junior High School, Anaheim Union High School District, Anaheim, Calif.)

One example of a school district where flexible scheduling is carried out is the Anaheim Union High School District in Anaheim, California (see accompanying illustrations). It has utilized the Brookhurst Plan, encompassing both team teaching and flexible scheduling. Some of the characteristics of this plan are that the faculty is organized into teams in each subject matter area, teachers submit daily job orders that include number of students desired in a group, length of time needed, facilities required, and method of instruction to be used. A master schedule is developed from the job orders, and students schedule a 14-modular day using the master schedule as a guide. The student's schedule becomes operational 3 days after the construction of the master schedule, a procedure that is completed each day throughout the year. The method of instruction is determined according to the following criteria: (1) When facts and data are presented, large group instruction is utilized. (2) When it is desired to use information presented in large group discussion as a means of developing insight and effectively using the information, small group discussion is scheduled. (3) When the goal is to help students develop study habits, use research techniques effectively, and develop self-direction, independent study is utilized.

Nongraded school. The practice of grouping students into grades according to chronologic age has been a part of American education for more than 100 years. However, this procedure has been challenged along the way. Dr. Francis W. Parker, as early as 1870, and John Dewey, in the 1930's, raised questions about this method of grouping boys and girls. Today, it is not only being questioned but the nongraded school has also become a reality in

The keysort card used in flexible scheduling at Anaheim, Calif. This is the student schedule. There are four parts to the keysort card: the original, which after being processed, becomes the student's copy; the attendance ticket section, made up of two sheets with four sections to each sheet, which goes to the teacher; and the last copy, which is used by the attendance officer. The card is coded so that specific notches may be made, indicating what has been printed on the card. Based upon achievement and ability, teacher's recommendation, as well as counselor's recommendations, the student's card is notched to indicate his class section in the required courses. The grooves on the top of the card indicate the fourteen modules of the school day. They are used in the scheduling process by the office in eliminating conflicts of time. (Courtesy Gardner Swenson, Principal, Brookhurst Junior High School, Anaheim Union High School District, Anaheim, Calif.)

many school districts from coast to coast. It is being used most extensively at the elementary level, but it finds use at the secondary level as well.

The dissatisfaction with the grouping of children according to chronologic age came about because it was thought to prevent the academic progress of many youngsters. The graded school was not in harmony with modern research and theory on human behavior and child development. Students vary in readiness to learn, ability, social and mental development, home environments, rate of achievement, and other similar factors. Studies show sharp differences in academic achievement among children entering the first grade and also in any one grade. They also show sharp differences in both physical and social development.

In the nongraded school children are grouped on the basis of age, abilities, and other pertinent factors essential to success in school, and then the child is permitted to advance at his own speed. Continuous pupil progress becomes the policy with grade names and nonpromotion policies eliminated. The chonrologic age system of grouping and promotion is abandoned and a new plan established that calls for four areas each with a 3-year span, including primary, intermediate, junior high school, and senior high school. Within each area the student may move freely and progress as rapidly as he can master the subject matter and requirements. Various phases in each 3-year span are established through which the student may move and progress. In one high school in Florida, for example, there are five phases in each subject area: (1) remedial program, (2) basic skills, (3) intermediate program for students seeking an average education, (4) depth study for students desiring depth in education, and (5) independent study and research. Students are placed in the proper phase for each subject according to the results achieved on standard achieve-

ment tests and teacher evaluations. There are opportunities for regular appraisals and frequent reclassification.

For the nongraded school to be a success there must be a cooperative and sympathetic faculty, good guidance and counseling program, and parental support. Team teaching and both large and small group instruction are also part of the nongraded program.

There are many problems associated with the nongraded schools and also many advantages. Before accepting the nongraded concept wholeheartedly, a school needs to determine how much a plan affects the child, the teachers, and the curriculum.

Physical educators and health educators must carefully weigh the value of the nongraded school as it relates to their fields of specialization. They must decide its value as it relates to skill, organic, social, and mental development. They need to ask such questions as: How should a student be scheduled in advanced skills—with his own age group or with older groups? How should a student be classified in the nongraded school where each of the objectives—social, emotional, and mental development—is a determining factor?

Middle school. The question as to what is the most desirable pattern of grade organization is the topic of many discussions among school administrators, teachers, and the lay public. One survey of 366 unified school systems with pupil enrollment of 12,000 or more, conducted by the Educational Research Service, showed that 71% of these school systems were organized on the 6-3-3 plan, 10% on the 8-4 organization, and 6% on a 6-2-4 pattern. Other patterns include 7-5, 6-6, 5-3-4, and 7-2-3.

The pattern of organization being considered by many school systems today is the middle school concept. Most simply, a middle school is for boys and girls between the elementary and high school years—grades six, seven, eight, and sometimes five. New York City, for example, the nation's largest school system, has middle schools grouped by grades five to eight or six to eight. The secondary schools have become 4-year comprehensive high schools. Other places that are embarked on the middle school pattern are Bridgewater, Massachusetts; Bedford Public Schools in Mount Kisco, New York; Sarasota County, Florida; Saginaw, Michigan; Easton, Connecticut; and Independence, Ohio.

Some of the reasons for the middle school concept are as follows:

1. There is an opportunity for more departmentalization than found in the elementary schools but less than found in the high schools, especially in such fields as science, mathematics, art, and music.

2. There is an opportunity for greater stimulation of students and better facilities and equipment, such as laboratories and shops.

3. There is an opportunity for special teachers and special programs essential for children passing through the early adolescent period.

4. Students today have subjects that were taught much later in the school program years ago. For example, in terms of the required curriculum, the fourth grader today is in advance of the sixth grader years ago. Therefore, the middle school concept is applicable to the present educational era.

5. There is a better opportunity for student grouping and meeting individual differences.

6. There is a better opportunity for guidance services to be extended into the lower grades.

7. There is better opportunity for a more personalized approach than is possible under other types of organization.

8. The ninth grade youngsters are more mature and can fit into the high school program, permitting them to take advanced courses.

9. There is better opportunity for a gradual change from self-sustained classroom to complete departmentalization.

Some of the reasons against the middle school are as follows:

1. There is lack of evidence to support its value because of its relative newness.

2. There are social adjustment problems in placing ninth graders with twelfth graders.

3. Youngsters in the middle school will be pushed too hard academically and socially.

4. Administrative techniques and procedures would need to be altered.

An example of the middle school in operation is the Saginaw Township Community Schools in Saginaw, Michigan. In Saginaw the administrative plan includes the neighborhood school (grades one to four), the middle schools (grades five to eight), and the community high school (grades nine to twelve).

Students at the middle school have a self-contained classroom environment in the fifth grade, where there is an educational climate that provides the needed security with one base and one teacher but at the same time provides for a more open school plan in which there is not complete isolation between fifth-grade classrooms. Also, fifth graders begin to learn how to operate in a more flexible pattern utilized in the succeeding grades.

The sixth grade provides for a marked transition that involves a departure from the self-contained classroom, with the teachers working in informal teams, although the student spends most of his time with one teacher in one classroom. Students assume more responsibility for their own and each other's welfare and become acquainted with several teachers and different groups of children.

In the seventh and eighth grades, students spend two periods of each school day in their homerooms but the rest of the time is spent in specialized classrooms receiving instruction from specialists in

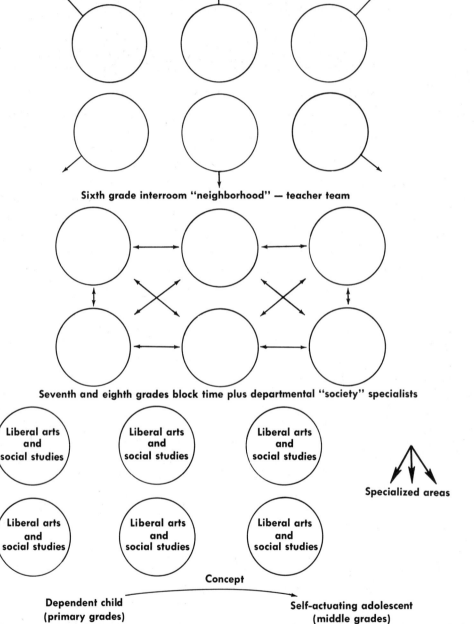

Middle school concepts—graphic representation. (Courtesy Saginaw Township Community Schools, Saginaw, Mich.)

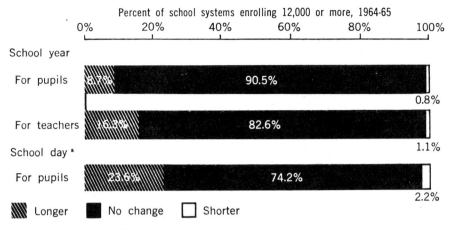

Percent of school systems enrolling 12,000 or more, 1964-65

0%   20%   40%   60%   80%   100%

School year

For pupils — 8.7% / 90.5% / 0.8%

For teachers — 16.3% / 82.6% / 1.1%

School day *

For pupils — 23.6% / 74.2% / 2.2%

▨ Longer   ■ No change   □ Shorter

* Information not available on changes in length of teachers' day.

Lengthening the school year and school day. Change during 1962 to 1967. (From NEA Research Bulletin **43**:105, 1965.)

such areas as physical education, music, arts, mathematics, and science. Students are encouraged to do more independent study in seventh and eighth grades. (See accompanying graphic representation.)

Health and physical educators will want to evaluate the middle school concept in respect to their special fields. It has many implications for the utilization of specialists, the presentation of skills and subject matter, and the organization of intramural and extramural athletic activities.

Year-round school. The need for a year-round school program is being increasingly heard whenever educational topics are discussed. Such developments as the child's becoming an economic liability in our modern industrial society, the great technologic advance that has resulted in a raising of the minimal requirements for vocational adequacy, the knowledge explosion, and the taking over of many functions of the home by other agencies and institutions have resulted in many people asking the question—why not have the children in school for a longer period of time?

The year-round school also makes sense to some educators because the school plant is idle during the summer months, although

costs for administration, insurance, and capital outlay remain constant. Also, many school-age children do not have constructive programs for the summer months, and teachers would be available in many cases.

Some of the plans suggested for extending the school year include the staggered quarter plan, in which the calendar year is divided into four quarters with pupils attending three of four quarters and having a vacation the fourth quarter. Teachers could be hired for either three or four quarters.

A second suggestion is the 48-week school year, which would be divided into four 12-week periods, with the remaining 4 weeks being used for vacation purposes. Teachers would be employed on a 12-month basis.

A third suggestion would be the voluntary summer program that students could attend if they so desired for purposes of remedial work, avocational, recreational, and enrichment type courses.

The fourth suggestion is the summer program for professional personnel plan. Under this arrangement teachers would be employed on a 12-month basis and would work 48 weeks and have a 4-week vacation. The students would go to school from

36 to 40 weeks. Teachers would spend the other weeks working on curriculum and instructional planning.

Health educators and physical educators should study the year-round school patterns and draw implications for their special fields. If school were conducted on a year-round basis, many of the objectives health and physical educators seek could be accomplished in a much better way. There would be more time for skill teaching. There could be greater relief from academic pressures, and healthful habits could be better encouraged and implemented.

New developments affecting methods and techniques of teaching

In recent years new approaches to the presentation of subject matter and other educational experiences have gained widespread recognition. These new innovations have implications—for the teacher, by utilizing special talents and saving time, and for the student, by promoting learning and recognizing individual differences and abilities. A few of the innovations that have special implications for health education and physical education are briefly cited here since they are of concern to all teachers, administrators, and leaders in these special fields.

Creativity. Creativity is a process whereby the student or individual formulates and produces new ideas, patterns of thinking, products, or something entirely new. Since creativity is designed to help each person reach his fullest development, it should be encouraged on the part of students and teachers. The teacher is a very important factor in encouraging creativity among students. By being interested in seeking new and better ways of creativeness among her students, she recognizes its value and nurtures it constantly.

Environment also plays an important part in creativity. The school must be characterized by a congenial and friendly atmosphere. Freedom must be afforded the student since creativity does not occur during a particular period or time of day. Also, the physical environment should be conducive to creativity by being cheerful, colorful, and challenging.

Courses in health education and physical education should encourage boys and girls to explore, investigate, express themselves, and experiment. Each student should be recognized for his uniqueness. Movement education, gymnastics, dance, and many other activities in physical education, as well as such experiences as problem-solving in health education, offer opportunities for creativity.

Teachers of health education and physical education should try to think up new and different approaches to subject matter presentation. By being creative in the teaching process itself, the instructor may stimulate new interests among the students in the subject matter being taught and the experiences being provided.

Movement education. Movement education is primarily concerned with the teaching of physical education through a sound understanding and application of the basic and scientific fundamentals of movement. Movement education had its origin in England, where Rudolf Laban gave it considerable thought, emphasis, and impetus. It can be the basis for teaching all forms of physical activity.

Movement education is based upon the concept that movement involves time, space, force, and flow. All sports and activities in the physical education program require basic movements for accomplishment. The student attempts to determine what he can achieve through problem-solving situations. Students try to discover why they move in a particular way, how they move differently than other persons, where they may move, and with what and with whom they may move. They become aware of body movements and how they affect not only the activities in physical education but also daily living.

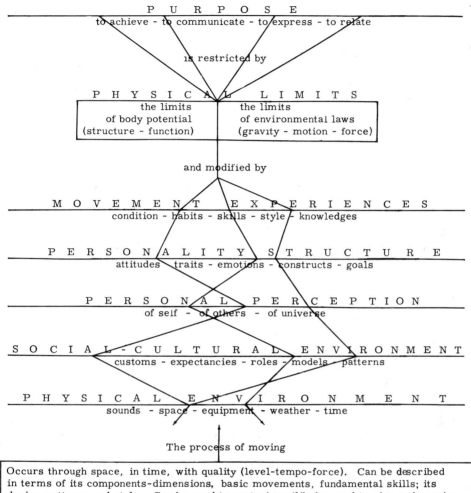

Human movement is initiated by

P   U   R   P   O   S   E
to achieve - to communicate - to express - to relate

is restricted by

P H Y S I C A L   L I M I T S

| the limits of body potential (structure - function) | the limits of environmental laws (gravity - motion - force) |

and modified by

M O V E M E N T   E X P E R I E N C E S
condition - habits - skills - style - knowledges

P E R S O N A L I T Y   S T R U C T U R E
attitudes - traits - emotions - constructs - goals

P E R S O N A L   P E R C E P T I O N
of self - of others - of universe

S O C I A L - C U L T U R A L   E N V I R O N M E N T
customs - expectancies - roles - models - patterns

P H Y S I C A L   E N V I R O N M E N T
sounds - space - equipment - weather - time

The process of moving

| Occurs through space, in time, with quality (level-tempo-force). Can be described in terms of its components-dimensions, basic movements, fundamental skills; its design-patterns and style. Can be used to control equilibrium and to give and receive impetus. May or may not be efficient in terms of mechanics and purpose. Is perceived variantly with occurrence, the mover, and observers. |

and
IS A MODIFIER OF ITS OWN DETERMINANTS

Movement education—an approach to the study of observable movement. (From Abernathy, R., and Waltz, M.: Toward a discipline: first steps first, Quest, monograph II, p. 3, April, 1964.)

Movement education may be utilized in physical education in different ways. In some cases it represents a different and separate course, whereas in other situations it may represent the basic philosophy underlying the entire program.

Team teaching. Team teaching usually refers to an arrangement in which two or more teachers cooperatively work together in planning, instructing, and evaluating one or more class groups so as to utilize the special competencies and qualifications of the team members. In some team teaching projects, the team is made up of two or more experienced and inexperienced teachers, a student teacher, a master teacher, teacher aids, consultants, and secretary.

The purpose of team teaching is to involve the talents of many teachers and specialties. As a team they formulate the program of study and plan a schedule that consists of lecture sessions for large groups of students, small study group classes for practice, review, and discussion, and independent study time or individual projects to meet the individual needs and interests of students. A student might find himself following a schedule that consisted of 40% of his time in large group instruction, 40% in smaller group discussions, and 20% in individual study or research.

Team teaching in essence means that planning is done by a team, the material is presented by a team, and the educational experiences are evaluated by a team. Some obvious advantages of team teaching are that it utilizes a teacher's talents to best advantage, individual differences are better realized, duplication of effort is avoided, and pupil self-responsibility is developed.

Educational television. Teaching with the aid of television has been introduced into health and physical education programs with considerable success. Areas of first aid and instruction in many health problems and various forms of physical activities have been successfully brought to large groups viewing televised lectures or demonstrations by specialists. Furthermore, such a technique has also permitted questions and answers on the part of students, with the entire audience benefiting from such an exchange.

One of the most impressive studies in educational television was performed by the Board of Education, Washington County, Hagerstown, Maryland, where this medium was used on a closed-circuit basis for 8 years. The results showed that pupil achievement was enhanced, the teacher's professional growth was accelerated, the curriculum was enriched and upgraded more readily, more pupils were reached, and the team teaching concept with the studio teacher and the classroom teacher was enhanced.

Programmed instruction. Programmed instruction was introduced by B. F. Skinner, a psychologist at Harvard. It is a process that arranges materials to be learned in a series of small steps designed to help the student educate himself by progressing from what he actually knows to areas of learning that are new and more complex. The student is usually checked as he progresses to determine his mastery of the material to be learned. If he is successful, he proceeds to the next material, but if he is not correct, he has to go back and review the material that he missed. The learning program represents an orderly, sequential route to the mastery of the subject.

Programs are found in two major forms —the teaching machine and the programmed textbook. However, both forms operate on the basic principles outlined in the previous paragraph. Both techniques have proved of value in supplementing classwork and in meeting individual differences.

The fields of health education and physical education are fertile territory for programmed instruction. New materials are starting to appear on the market for programmed teaching. Much more will be available in the months and years ahead. Obvious advantages to such teaching are that students will be able to learn much more on their own outside of class, the student who is absent because of illness will have a medium for making up what has been missed, and large classes may be broken down, with some of the students doing programmed instruction.

RESEARCH IN HEALTH EDUCATION AND PHYSICAL EDUCATION

There is an urgent need to advance the frontiers of knowledge in the fields of health education and physical education.

There have been too many unsupported claims for the value of physical education and health in education. There is a need to determine their worth through valid research findings—basic research that will advance knowledge and also applied research that will determine the best ways of applying this knowledge to these fields of endeavor.

There are many questions left unanswered. A few problems that need considerable investigation include the following: Why do school accidents happen? Why are health practices not followed? How much can retarded children learn? What is the value of programmed learning materials? What are the attitudes toward physical education? What should be the place of international studies in education? What are the biomechanics of human movement? What do we know about exercise physiology? What is the scientific basis for human movement? What is the relationship of personality development to motor performance? What is the relationship of scholastic achievement to physical fitness? What are the best ways to develop creativity? What social changes take place through outdoor education and camping? What is the therapeutic value of recreational activity? What are the qualities of leadership needed for working with mentally disturbed patients?

Research can help physical education and health to develop a better understanding as to the accepted body of knowledge, skills, attitudes, and practices that should be imparted through educational means and how they can best be transmitted. In so doing the status of these professions will be enhanced.

Graduate schools in particular should sponsor and encourage research. They should extend a student's range of knowledge and understanding of his field of special interest, as well as provide opportunities to engage in creative research.

There is a need for effective channels for the communication of research findings to the practitioners in the field. The *Research Quarterly* of the American Association for Health, Physical Education, and Recreation is one good outlet but offers an opportunity for only comparatively few research studies. One estimate points out that the field of medicine has more than 400 journals published monthly, as well as some published weekly, such as the *Journal of the American Medical Association.*

There is a need for the professions of health, physical education, and recreation to more clearly delineate the answers to such questions as the following:

1. What areas need research in health, physical education, and recreation?
2. What questions does research raise about present programs in health, physical education, and recreation?
3. How can research findings be disseminated and used most effectively in our professional programs?
4. What constitutes a desirable program of research for health, physical education, and recreation?
5. What are some of the problems concerning financing, misconceptions, and poor techniques in research in the professional fields of health and physical education?

STATE AND FEDERAL LEGISLATION—FINANCIAL AID TO EDUCATION PROGRAMS

State and federal legislation, philanthropic foundations, and other agencies are becoming increasingly interested in education and are providing financial help to schools and colleges.

Education and the pursuit of learning are becoming a major point of emphasis in the American culture. At the turn of the century the population was approximately 76 million and only about 6% of the nation's 17 year olds graduated from high school, and only approximately 4% of the college-age boys and girls went to college. Today, better than 70% of the 17 year olds are graduating from high school and about 30% of the college-age population is on campus. The bill for education is more than $50 billion a year and going up. There are approximately 125,000 schools, 100,000 administrators, and 2 million teachers in America's largest industry.

With the explosion in knowledge playing such a prominent role in American life, there are many concerns for the types of programs to be offered and individuals to be served. Consequently, dollars are being poured into facilities, personnel, programs, and other essentials.

The health educator and physical educator need to be conscious of these grants-in-aid monies that are being given to educational pursuits. Many of the sources of funds can be tapped for programs in the special fields of health education and physical education. Furthermore, it may be possible for specialists in these fields to influence legislation at the state and/or national level so that the bills passed include allocations for these special fields in the wording of the legislation.

Some of the specific ways in which the professions of health education and physical education may use this money might be to correct weak spots in the lack of facilities, sponsor research, hire additional personnel, offset low salaries, and purchase equipment.

A sampling of suggested projects, activities, and programs that might receive funds for research and grants-in-aid at the federal level in programs of health, physical education, recreation, and safety are as follows:

1. Employment of specialists to help in developing and implementing programs in adapted physical education
2. Inservice education programs for teachers
3. The development of curriculum guides
4. The purchase of special types of equipment, supplies, and facilities
5. The employment of specialists to work with underprivileged children who have special health problems
6. The employment of consultants who are specialists on various health and physical education problems
7. The development of health guides
8. The conduct of research for more effective teaching and better meeting the needs of children
9. The conduct of workshops
10. Immunization programs
11. The development of programs for physically underdeveloped children

Questions and exercises

1. Outline the steps you think should be followed in curriculum planning by a chairman of a health and physical education department.
2. What is the relationship between curriculum planning and objectives?
3. Examine the health and/or physical education curriculum of three high schools. What are their strong and their weak points?
4. What are three references that the teacher can use for curriculum planning?
5. How can community resources be used effectively in curriculum planning?
6. Prepare what you consider to be an outstanding curriculum for health and/or physical education at the elementary, junior high school, or senior high school level. Analyze the steps you followed in constructing this curriculum.

Reading assignment in *Administrative Dimensions of Health and Physical Education Programs, Including Athletics:* Chapter 15, Selections 83 to 86.

Selected references

Allen, D. W.: Elements of scheduling a flexible curriculum, Journal of Secondary Education **38:** 84, 1963.

Association for Supervision and Curriculum Development: Assessing and using curriculum content, Washington, D. C., 1965, The Association.

Blair, M., and Woodward, R.: Team teaching in action, Boston, 1964, Houghton Mifflin Co.

Bucher, C. A.: Foundations of physical education, ed. 5, St. Louis, 1968, The C. V. Mosby Co.

Bucher, C. A., and Reade, E.: Physical education and health in the elementary school, New York, 1971, The Macmillan Co.

Bucher, C. A., Koenig, C., and Barnhard, M.: Methods and materials for secondary school physical education, ed. 3, St. Louis, 1970, The C. V. Mosby Co.

Bush, R. N.: New design for high school education: assuming a flexible schedule, Bulletin of the National Association of Secondary-School Principals 46:30, 1962.

Cassidy, R.: Curriculum development in physical education, New York, 1954, Harper & Row Publishers.

Daniels, A. S.: The potential of physical education as an area of research and scholarly effort, Journal of Health, Physical Education, and Recreation 36:32, 1965.

Eichhorn, D. H.: The middle school, New York, 1966, The Center for Applied Research in Education, Inc. (The Library of Education).

Evaul, T. W.: The automated tutor, Journal of Health, Physical Education, and Recreation 35: 27, 1964.

Good, C. V., and Seates, D. E.: Methods of research: educational, psychological, sociological, New York, 1964, Appleton-Century-Crofts.

Goodlad, J. I.: School curriculum reform in the United States, New York, 1964, The Fund for the Advancement of Education.

Goodlad, J. I., and Anderson R. H.: The nongraded elementary school, rev. ed., New York, 1963, Harcourt, Brace & World, Inc.

Koopman, G. R.: Curriculum development, New York, 1966, The Center for Applied Research in Education, Inc. (The Library of Education).

Lloyd, F. V.: Curricular responsibilities of today's school board, Administrator's Notebook, vol. 14, October, 1965.

Meyers, K.: Administering the curriculum, The Clearing House 39:145, 1964.

Nixon, J. E., and Jewett, A. E.: Physical education curriculum, New York, 1964, The Ronald Press Co.

Nunnelley, W. A.: Physical education goes on television, Journal of Health, Physical Education, and Recreation 36:66, 1964.

Oliver, A. I.: Curriculum improvement—a guide to problems, principles, and procedures, New York, 1965, Dodd, Mead & Co.

Report of the Second National Conference on Curriculum Projects: Assessing and using curriculum content, Washington, D. C., 1964, Association for Supervision and Curriculum Development.

School Health Education Study: Health education: a conceptual approach, New York, 1965, sponsored by the Samuel Bronfman Foundation of New York City.

Sliepcevich, E.: A conceptual approach to curriculum development in health education, Journal of Health, Physical Education, and Recreation 36:12, 1965.

The University of the State of New York, The State Education Department, Bureau of Secondary Development: Physical education in the secondary schools, Albany, 1964, State Department of Education.

Wisconsin Department of Public Instruction: A guide to curriculum building in physical education—elementary schools, Curriculum Bulletin No. 28, Madison, 1963, The Department.

There are many reasons why each health and physical education program must be vitally concerned with public relations today. The increased costs of programs in these specialized areas, including allocations of funds for facilities, personnel, and other essential items, has raised many questions in the minds of the public. The changes taking place in education and in our programs have confused many persons and thus raised the need for clarification. Criticism of the schools and of such programs as athletics, physical education, sex education, sensitivity training, and others has resulted in increased public involvement in our programs.

Sometimes when the terms *public* or *professional relations* are used, the reader, administrator, physical educator, or other person frequently associates the term with radio, television, and other communications media. However, one should not forget that the most effective avenues of public and professional relations include: (1) relations with students, (2) relations with parents of students, (3) personal contacts with the public at large, (4) the leadership role exerted by physical educators and health educators in their communities, (5) contacts established with various groups in the community, and (6) communications media such as correspondence, records, and telephone conversations.

PUBLIC RELATIONS DEFINED

Public relations is a much-defined term. Some of the common definitions for this term as given by experts in this specialized field are as follows: Philip Lesly speaks of it as comprising the activities and attitudes that are used to influence, judge, and control the opinion of any individual, group, or groups of persons in the interest of some other individuals. Professor Harwood L. Childs defines it as a name for those activities and relations with others that are public and that have significance socially. J. Handly Wright and Byron H. Christian, experts in public relations, refer to it as a program that has the characteristics of careful planning and proper conduct, which in turn will result in public understanding and confidence. Edward L. Bernays, who has written widely on the subject of public relations, lists three items in his definition: first, information that is for public consumption, second, an attempt to modify the attitudes and actions of the public through persuasion, and third, the objective of attempting to integrate the attitudes and actions of the public and of the organization or people who are conducting the public relations program. Benjamin Fine, a specialist in educational public relations, defines public relations as the entire body of relationships that go to make up our impressions of an individual, an organization, or an idea.

These selected definitions of public relations help to clarify its importance for any organization, institution, or group of individuals trying to develop an enterprise, profession, or business. Public relations takes into consideration such important factors as consumer's interests, human relationships, public understanding, and good will. In business, it attempts to show the important place that specialized enterprises

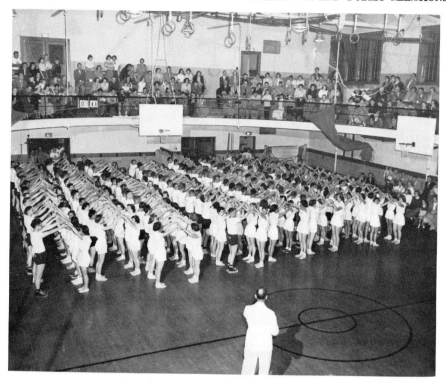

La Crosse Tribune.

One purpose of school public relations is "to inform the public about the work of the schools." (Wisconsin State College, La Crosse, Wis.)

have in society and how they exist and operate in the public interest. In education, it is concerned with public opinion, the needs of the school or college, and acquainting constituents with what is being done in the public interest. It also concerns itself with acquainting the public with the educational problems that must be considered in order to render a greater service.

The American Association of School Administrators points out these purposes of school public relations: "(a) to inform the public about the work of the schools, (b) to establish confidence in the schools, (c) to rally support for proper maintenance of the educational program, (d) to develop awareness of the importance of education in a democracy, (e) to improve the partnership concept by uniting parents and teachers in meeting the educational needs of children, (f) to integrate the home, the school, and the community in improving educational opportunities for all children, (g) to evaluate the offerings of the schools in meeting the needs of the children in the community, and (h) to correct misunderstandings as to the aims and objectives of the schools."[*]

Public relations means that the opinions of the populace must be taken into consideration. Public opinion is very powerful, and individuals, organizations, and institutions succeed or fail in terms of its influence. Therefore, in order to have good public relations the interests of human beings and what is good for people in general must be considered.

[*]American Association of School Administrators: Public relations for America's schools, Twenty-eighth Yearbook, Washington, D. C., 1952, The Association, p. 14.

The practice of public relations is pertinent to all areas of human activity: religion, education, business, politics, military, government, labor, and other affairs in which individuals engage. A good public relations program is not hit-and-miss. It is planned with considerable care, and great amounts of time and effort are necessary to produce results. Furthermore, it is not something in which only the "top brass," management, executives, or administrative officers should be interested. In order for any organization to have a good program, all members must be public relations–conscious.

The extent to which interest has grown in the field of public relations is indicated by the number of individuals specializing in this area. The *Public Relations Directory and Yearbook* lists personnel who specialize in this work. A recent edition of this publication listed more than 800 individuals who are doing work in this area on an independent basis, approximately 4,500 who were directors of public relations with business firms, approximately 1,900 who were associated with trade and professional groups, and nearly 700 who were with social organizations. In a recent Manhattan telephone directory there were over 500 names listed under the heading of "Public Relations." In contrast, in 1935, there were only ten names.

The importance of public relations is being increasingly recognized for the part it can play in educational, business, or social advancement. All need public support and understanding in order to survive. Public relations helps in obtaining these essentials.

PLANNING THE PUBLIC RELATIONS PROGRAM

Public relations programs are much more effective when they are planned by many interested and informed individuals and groups. Such individuals and groups as school boards, teachers, administrators, and citizens' committees can provide valuable assistance in certain areas of the public relations program. These people, serving in an advisory capacity to health and physical education departments, can help immeasurably in fulfilling the following specific steps that should be followed in planning a public relations program, which have been identified by McCloskey:

1. Establish a sound public-communications policy.
2. Determine what educational services and developments benefit pupils.
3. Obtain facts about what citizens do and do not know and believe about educational values and needs.
4. Decide what facts and ideas will best enable citizens to understand the benefits children obtain from good schools and what improvements will increase these benefits.
5. Make full use of effective teacher-pupil planning techniques to generate understanding and appreciation.
6. Relate cost and tax facts more closely to opportunity for boys and girls to achieve.
7. Decide who is going to perform specific communication tasks at particular times.*

McCloskey further suggests that after putting the public relations plan into operation, it is important to test and evaluate its results and then improve the educational program accordingly.

PUBLIC RELATIONS MEDIA

There are many media that can be utilized in a public relations program. Some have more significance in certain localities than others. Some are more readily accessible than others. Health and physical education persons should survey their communities to determine media that can be utilized and will be most effective in their public relations program.

It should be pointed out, however, that the *program* and the *staff* represent the best media for an effective public relations pro-

---

*McCloskey, G.: Planning the public relations program, National Education Association Journal **49**:17, 1960.

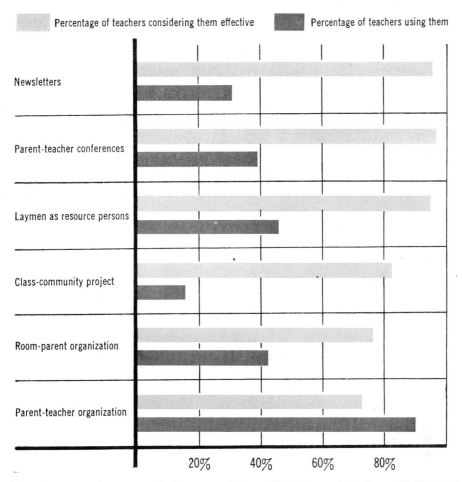

Percentage of teachers considering them effective   Percentage of teachers using them

Newsletters

Parent-teacher conferences

Laymen as resource persons

Class-community project

Room-parent organization

Parent-teacher organization

20%   40%   60%   80%

Public relations techniques and their use. (From NEA Research Bulletin **37:**39, 1959.)

gram. Through the activities and experiences provided and the leadership given, much good will may be built for any school, or college, department or profession. This should never be forgotten.

Another important consideration is that the most effective public relations is carried on through the person-to-person medium. This might be teacher to student, student to parent, or teacher to citizen. In all cases the child is a very important consideration, being really the most important means of communication between the school and the home. What is accomplished in school or college, the effectiveness of a teacher's work, and the material learned become subjects of conversation around the dinner table and other places in the home. The attitudes developed in students often become those of the parents as well.

Newspapers

The newspaper is one of the most common and useful media for disseminating information. It reaches a large audience and can be very helpful in interpreting health and physical education to the public at large. Some questions that might be asked to determine what makes a good news story are: Is the news of interest to the public? Are the facts correct? Is it direct in style, written in the third person in a layman's vocabulary, and well organized? Does it include news on individuals who are closely related to the schools or colleges? Does the article have a plan of action, and does it play a significant part in interpreting the school or college program?

When a story is submitted to a newspaper there are certain standard rules that apply in the preparation of copy:

1. Prepare all copy in typewritten form as neatly as possible, double spaced, and on one side of the paper only.

2. The name, address, and telephone number of your organization should be on page one, in the upper left-hand corner. Also at the top of page one, but below the address, should be the headline and release date for the story.

3. Paragraphs should be short, and if the story necessitates more than one page, write the word "More" at the end of each page. At the top of each additional page, list the name of the story in the upper left-hand corner. The symbols # # # should be placed at the end of the article to indicate the end.

One expert on newspapers has pointed out that the most common reasons for rejecting material includes limited reader interest, poor writing, inaccuracies, and insufficient information.

Pictures and graphic materials

Pictures represent a very effective medium for public relations. Two words should be kept in mind by the persons who take and select the pictures for publication. These words are "action" and "people." Pictures that reflect "action" are much more interesting and appealing than "still" pictures. Furthermore, pictures that have people in them are much more effective than ones that do not possess this essential ingredient. It should also be recognized that usually a few people are better than many persons. Finally, such considerations as good background, accuracy in details, clearness, and educational significance should not be forgotten.

Educational problems, such as budgets, statistical information in regard to growth of school population, information about participation in various school or college activities, and many other items can be made more interesting, intelligible, and appealing if presented through colorful and artistic charts, graphs, and diagrams.

Magazines

There are thousands of popular magazines, professional journals, trade publications, and other periodicals being published today.

Such national magazines as *Look, Life, McCall's,* and *Reader's Digest* are excellent for publicity purposes. It is, however, very difficult to get stories in such publications because of their rigid requirements and the fact that they like to cover the stories with their own staff. Many times it is better to suggest ideas to them rather than to submit a manuscript. There are other methods that may be used. One can attempt to interest the editors in some particular work being done and have them send a staff writer to cover the story. It might be possible to get a free-lance writer interested in the organization and have him develop a story. Someone on the department staff who possesses writing skill can be assigned to write a piece for magazine consumption and then submit it to various periodicals for consideration.

Public speaking

Public speaking can be a very effective medium for public relations. Through public addresses to civic and social groups in the community, public affairs, gatherings, professional meetings, and any organization or group that desires to know more about the work that is being performed, a good opportunity is afforded for interpreting one's profession to the public. However, it is very important to do a commendable job or the result can be poor rather than good public relations.

In order to make an effective speech one should observe many fundamentals. A few that may be listed are mastery of the subject, sincere interest and enthusiasm, interest in putting thoughts across to the public rather than in putting the speaker across, directness, straightforwardness, preparation, brevity, and clear and distinct enunciation.

If the organization is of sufficient size, a speakers' bureau may be an asset. This may be utilized if there are several qualified speakers within an organization. Various civic, school, college, church, and other leaders within a community can be informed of the services that the organization has to offer along this line. Then, when the requests come in, speakers can be assigned on the basis of qualifications and availability. The entire department or organization should set up facilities and make information and material available for the preparation of such speeches. If desired by the members of the organization, inservice training courses could even be worked out in conjunction with the English department or some experienced person in developing this particular phase of the public relations program.

Discussion groups

Discussion groups, forums, and similar meetings are frequently held in various communities. At such gatherings, representatives from the community, which usually include educators, industrialists, businessmen, physicians, lawyers, clergymen, union leaders, and others, discuss topics of general interest. This is an excellent setting to clarify issues, clear up misunderstandings, enlighten civic leaders on particular fields of endeavor, and discuss the pros and cons of community projects. Health and physical education persons should play a larger role in such meetings than has been the case in the past. Much good could be done for these specialized fields through this medium.

Radio and television

Radio and television are powerful media of communication because of their universal appeal. These public relations media are well worth the money spent for the purpose, if this is the only way they are available. First, however, the possibilities of obtaining free time should be thoroughly examined. The idea of public service will influence some radio and television station managers to grant free time to an organization. This may be in the nature of an item included in a newscast program, a spot announcement, or a public service program that utilizes a quarter, half, or even a full hour.

There are some radio and television stations that are reserved for educational purposes. This possibility should be examined carefully. Many schools and colleges have stations of their own that may be utilized.

Sometimes one must take advantage of these media on short notice; therefore, it is important for an organization to be prepared with written plans that can be put into operation immediately. This might make the difference between being accepted or rejected for such an assignment. The organization must also be prepared to assume the work involved in rehearsals, preparation of scenery, or other items that are essential in presenting such a program.

Radio and television offer some of the best means of reaching a very large number of people at one time. As such, organizations concerned with specialized work of health and physical education should continually utilize their imaginations to translate the story of their professions into material that can be utilized effectively by these media.

Films

Films can present dramatically and informatively such stories as an organization's services to the public and highlights in the training of its leaders. They constitute a most effective medium for presenting a story in a short period of time. A series of visual impressions will remain long in the minds of the audience.

Since such a great majority of the American people enjoy movies today, it is important to consider them in any public relations program. Movies are not only a form of entertainment but also an effective medium of information and education. Films stimulate attention, create interest, and provide a way of getting across information not inherent in printed matter.

Movies, slides, slidefilm, and other phases of these visual aids have been utilized by a number of departments of health and physical education to present their programs to the public and to interest individuals in their work. Voluntary associations, professional associations, and official agencies in these fields have also used them to advantage.

Posters, exhibits, brochures, demonstrations, miscellaneous media

Posters, exhibits, and brochures should be recognized as playing an important part in any public relations program concerned with health and physical education. Well-illustrated, brief, and attractive brochures can visually and informatively depict activities, facilities, projects, and services that a department or organization has as part of its total program.

Drawings, paintings, charts, graphs, pictures, and other aids, when placed upon posters and given proper distribution, will illustrate activities, show progress, and present information visually. These media will attract and interest public thinking.

Exhibits, when properly prepared, interestingly presented, and properly located, such as in a store window or some other prominent spot, can do much to demonstrate work being done by an organization.

Demonstrations that present the total program of an organization or profession in an entertaining and informative manner have a place in any public relations program.

Other miscellaneous media, such as correspondence in the forms of letters and messages to parents, student publications, and reports, offer opportunities to develop good relations and favorable understanding in respect to schools and colleges and the work they are doing. Every opportunity must be utilized in order to build good public relations.

THE MANY PUBLICS

In order for any public relations program to be successful, accurate facts must be presented. To establish what facts are to be given to the public, the particular public at which the program is directed must be known. Contrary to general belief there is no *one* public. There are an infinite number of publics varying according to interests, problems, and other factors that make individuals different.

A public is a group of people who are drawn together by common interests, who are located in a specific geographic area, or who are characterized by some other common feature. There are over 220 million people in the United States composing hundreds of different publics—farmers, organized laborers, unorganized workers, students, professional people, and veterans. The various publics may be national, regional, and local in scope. They can be classified according to race or nationality, age, religion, occupation, politics, sex, income, profession, economic level, or business, fraternal, and educational backgrounds. As one can readily see, there are many publics. Each organization or group that has a special interest is a public. The public relations–minded person must always think in terms of the publics with which he desires to promote understanding and how they can best be reached.

In order to have a meaningful and purposeful public relations program, it is essential to obtain some facts about these various publics. It is necessary to know their understanding of the professions, their needs and interests, their health practices and hobbies, and other essential information.

Public opinion decides whether a profession is important or not, whether it meets an essential need, whether it is making a contribution to enriched living. It determines the success or failure of a department, school, institution, or profession. Public opinion is dynamic and continually changing. Public opinion results from the interaction of people. Public opinion is king in this game of life and it behooves any group of individuals or organization that wants to survive to know as much about it as possible.

To get information on what the public thinks, why it thinks as it does, and how it reaches its conclusions, various techniques may be used. Surveys, questionnaires, opinion polls, interviews, expert opinion, discussions, and other techniques have proved valuable. Anyone interested in public relations should be acquainted with these various techniques.

Public opinion is formed to a great degree as a result of influences in early life, such as the effect of parents, home, and environment; on the basis of people's own experiences in everyday living, what they see, hear, and experience in other ways; and finally by media of communication such as newspapers, radio, and television. It is important not only to be aware of these facts but also to remember that one

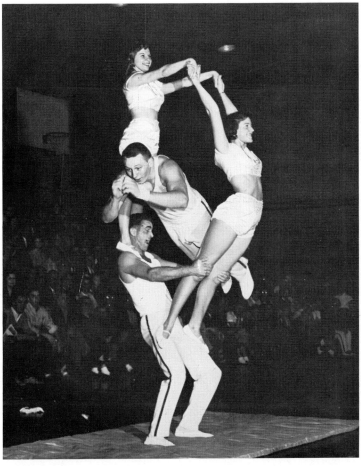

Demonstrations as part of a public relations program. Gamma Phi gym circus. (Illinois State University, Normal, Ill.)

is dealing with many different publics, each requiring a special source of research and study in order to know the most effective way to plan, organize, and administer the public relations program.

PUBLIC RELATIONS IN PRACTICE

A survey was recently conducted among eleven school systems to determine the nature and scope of their professional and public relations programs. Several questions were asked of health and physical education personnel through the personal interview technique. The information gained from these interviews is highlighted in the following paragraphs.

In respect to policies

1. The director of health and physical education was directly responsible for all public relations releases to the press.

2. All printed matter needed the approval of the director of health and physical education and the superintendent of schools before being released.

3. The coaches of interscholastic athletics were responsible for preparing all releases in regard to their programs.

4. Each staff member in the health and physical education program was urged to recognize that his or her activities were part of the professional and public relations programs of his or her school.

In respect to communication

In respect to communications media, the following were utilized:
Total physical education program
Newspaper
Posters
Films
Public speaking
School publications
Newsletter
Letters to parents
Demonstrations and exhibits
Personal contact
Pictures
Radio
Television

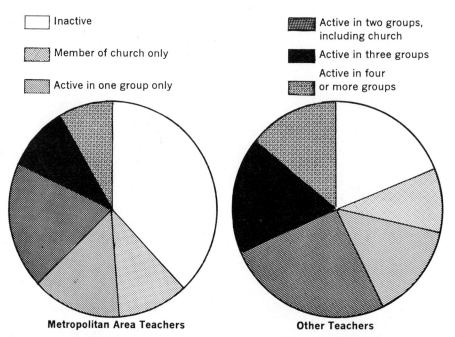

Metropolitan Area Teachers   **Other Teachers**

Inactive

Member of church only

Active in one group only

Active in two groups, including church

Active in three groups

Active in four or more groups

Metropolitan area teachers are less inclined to be joiners than are teachers in smaller districts. (From NEA Research Bulletin **40:**73, 1962.)

Window displays
Brochures
Sports days
Bulletin boards

The five media found to be most effective in their professional and public relations programs were (1) the total physical education program and the total health education program, (2) personal contact, (3) newspapers, (4) public speaking, and (5) demonstrations and exhibits.

All of the directors of health and physical education indicated that athletics received more publicity than any other phase of the physical education program. When asked why they thought this was so, some typical comments were: "The public demands it," "It is required because of public interest," and "The newspapers will only accept and print releases on athletics."

In respect to the message that was desired to be communicated to the public

When the directors were asked, "What message are you trying to convey to the public?" the following are typical answers that were given:

1. The value of the total physical education and health program
2. The importance of the program to the student
3. Recognition and achievement of all students in all areas of health and physical education, not just athletics
4. Efforts and energies being expended to give each child a worthwhile experience in health and physical education
5. The role of the health and physical education program in enhancing the health and welfare of the student
6. The aims and objectives of the total health and physical education programs

Guiding principles

In summary, the professional and public relations programs in the eleven school districts were conducted in light of the following principles:

1. Each physical education and health department recognized the importance of an active public relations program.
2. Definite policies guided the program.
3. Responsibility for public relations was shared by all members of the department, with the central authority residing with the director.
4. Many different communications media were used to interpret the program to the numerous publics.
5. The total health and physical education program was recognized as being the most effective medium of professional and public relations.
6. Efforts were made to interpret accurate facts about physical education and health to the public.
7. Considerable planning was needed for the effective utilization of public relations media.

Limitations of program of professional and public relations

Some obvious limitations of the professional and public relations programs surveyed were as follows:

1. Information had not been gained through research as to how various publics thought and felt about health and physical education—what they did and did not know concerning these special fields.
2. There was a lack of budgetary allocations to carry on a professional and public relations program.
3. No specific plans had been established to evaluate the professional and public relations programs in the various schools.
4. Communications media overemphasized the role of athletics in the total physical education program.
5. Information had not been gained through research as to what services most benefited pupils and what facts best enabled the public to understand the benefits children derive from such programs.

6. There was a lack of effective pupil-teacher planning techniques.

PRINCIPLES OF PUBLIC RELATIONS

A few of the principles that should be observed in developing a public relations program are listed:

1. Public relations should be considered internally before they are developed externally. The support of everyone within the organization, from the top administrator down to the last worker, should be procured. Furthermore, such items as purpose of program, person or persons responsible, funds available, media to be utilized, and tools to carry on the program should be primary considerations.

2. A public relations program should be outlined and put in writing, and every member of the organization should become familiar with it. The better it is known and understood, the better chance it has of succeeding.

3. The persons directly in charge of the public relations program must have complete knowledge of the professional services that are being rendered; the attitudes of those who are members of the profession and of the organization represented; and the nature, background, and reactions of the consumers and of all the "publics" that are directly or indirectly related to the job being performed.

4. After all the information has been gathered, a program should be developed that meets the needs as shown by the research that has been done.

5. There should be adequate funds available to do the job. Furthermore, the person or persons in charge of the public relations program should be given freedom in spending this money in whatever ways they feel will be most helpful and productive for the organization.

6. The formation of a public relations staff will be determined by the needs of the organization, the amount of money avail-able, the attitude of the administration, and the size of the organization. If additional staff is available, special talents should be sought so as to provide effectively for a well-rounded program.

7. Individuals assigned public relations work should modestly stay in the background instead of seeking the limelight, keep abreast of the factors that affect the program, develop a wide acquaintance, and make contacts that will be helpful.

8. In developing a public relations program, such items as the following should be checked: Is there a handbook or a newsletter to keep members of the organization informed? Is there a system for dispensing information to local radio and press outlets? Is there a booklet, flyer, or printed matter that tells the story of the organization? Do members of the organization participate regularly in community affairs? Is there provision for a speakers' bureau where civic clubs and other organizations may procure speakers on various topics? Does the organization hold open house for parents and interested persons? Does the organization have a film or other visual material that can be shown to interested groups and that explains and interprets the work?

9. A good public relations program will utilize all available resources and machinery to disseminate information to the public in order to ensure adequate coverage.

PUBLIC RELATIONS AND EDUCATION

Education is recognized as essential in present-day society. In order that knowledge and experience may be transmitted from generation to generation, education is necessary. This is the essential that gives continuity to any culture.

A major obstacle today to education is in the area of public relations. Unless the public understands the work being performed by the schools, educators cannot expect their support. Today a great segment of the American public does not

The Physical Education Department
of the
Rapid City Public Schools
PRESENTS THE
FOURTH ANNUAL

FITNESS IS FUN

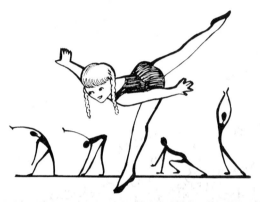

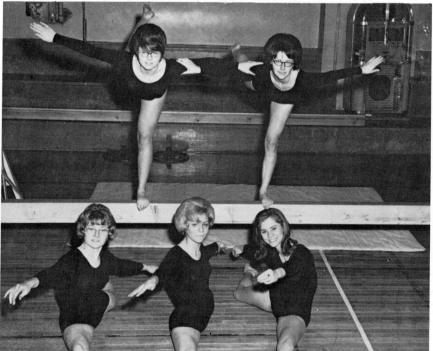

Public relations. (Rapid City Public Schools, Rapid City, S. D.)

understand and appreciate the work that is being performed in the schools and colleges.

The need for a broad public relations program is evidenced by many facts in American life. The American people spend more for tobacco each year than they do for education and twice as much for liquor. Schools and colleges are overflowing and there is a need for $10 to $20 billion for new buildings alone. Schools and colleges must absorb thousands of pupils a year, yet the necessary provisions have not been made. There is need for greater financial support, increased teachers' salaries, more buildings, and better teacher training. The necessary improvements cannot be obtained without public understanding and public support.

The National Education Association conducted a survey several years ago that included the factor of teachers' salaries. Of the persons surveyed, 33% felt that teachers' salaries were satisfactory, 2% thought they were high, and 20% did not have sufficient information on which to base an opinion.

A Gallup poll showed that 87% of the people are satisfied with the schools their children attend.

Elmer Roper conducted a poll that showed that 71.6% of the people in this country are either very satisfied or fairly well satisfied with the public school system. Less than one-half of the people indicated that teachers were underpaid and yet the poll showed that teachers received the highest percentage when the public was asked to "rank the order of importance to the community of public school teachers, clergymen, public officials, merchants, and lawyers."

The public in general is not informed in respect to education. What is true of education in general is even more true of health and physical education, which are important phases of the educational program. This has important implications for a well-organized and long-term public relations program.

Bernays, in addressing the American Association of School Administrators, listed some pertinent remarks that he felt were essential to public understanding and action on the part of the American people.

He pointed out that three forces are responsible for social change: namely, public opinion, voluntary groups, and the law, which is dependent upon public opinion. In the light of this principle, voluntary groups are needed to aid in informing the public about education. These voluntary groups should consist of leading civic leaders as well as professional educators. Lay and professional groups must coordinate their programs closely and gear their campaigns to everyone, from kindergarten to college, throughout the entire country. One of the most important considerations is that a unified front be presented to the public. All should agree on the issues and present them in the same light. If the various professional associations that are now organized and exist on national, district, state, and local levels and the various lay organizations could speak with one voice and with unison and similarity of purpose, much could be accomplished.

Bernays also recommended that a central board of strategy establish policy and goals and iron out problems so that a unified approach would be followed. Through such a board, research could be conducted to ascertain and reach a common agreement at the various levels as to what the needs of education are. It could also determine the reasons for the apathy, indifference, and misunderstanding on the part of the public. It could wage a unified battle against enemies of public education.

Another step in the overall public relations program would be a clear-cut operational program. Such a program would provide for a continuous campaign, personnel, money, utilization of mass communications media, close cooperation between school, college, and parents and between the school, college, and community in general, and a more active role for teachers in community activities.

The American Association of School Administrators lists various principles that it considers essential to school public relations:

a. School public relations must be honest in intent and execution.
b. School public relations must be intrinsic (school program should be recognized as worthwhile in itself).
c. School public relations must be continuous.
d. School public relations must be positive in approach.
e. School public relations should be comprehensive.
f. School public relations should be sensitive to its publics.
g. The ideas communicated must be simple.*

Through such a public relations program, all the people would have a better understanding of education in this country.

PUBLIC RELATIONS IN SCHOOL HEALTH AND PHYSICAL EDUCATION PROGRAMS

A definition of public relations heard some time ago stated: "Public relations is getting the *right facts* to the *right people* at the *right time* and in the *right way*."

Some of the facts that we need to get across to the public are these:

1. Physical education, health education, and recreation are closely allied but not the same. Each is separate and distinct; each needs its own specialists and deserves its own place in the educational program.

2. The professional fields of physical education, health education, and recreation are more than muscle and perspiration. Skills are not performed in a vacuum. Something happens to behavior, ethics, and mental development.

3. Athletics are an integral part of phys-

ical education, but physical education is not just athletics.

4. A well-rounded health program is an essential and integral part of modern education.

Some of the right people we must reach are the following:

1. Superintendents of public instruction, school administrators, presidents and deans of colleges and universities, mayors, and others. They are the ones who make the decisions, determine the main points of emphasis, and decide how funds will be allocated. They can help us to grow into that dynamic force for good that we are capable of becoming.

2. Other members of the faculty. The teachers of English, mathematics, industrial arts, and other disciplines are very important cogs in the educational system. We should not isolate ourselves from them. They can help us and we can help them. We are all in this business together, working toward common goals. "United we stand and divided we fall."

3. Consumers of our products and services. Let's reach those for whom we exist. And let's get to more than just the star player—let's contact the dub as well as the skilled, the girl as well as the boy, the oldster as well as the youngster. Let's reach everyone, from the cradle to the grave.

The right time is now. Now is the time when:

1. There is a "bull market" in education —enrollments are booming, budgets skyrocketing, facilities expanding. And there is tremendous interest in education, America's largest industry.

2. There is interest in the *whole* individual. The theory of dualism of mind and body has been exploded. We are interested in the physical as well as the mental, emotional, and social aspects of human beings.

3. Research is pointing up the importance of our fields of endeavor. This research shows the importance of exercise, the value of hobbies, the need for health

---

*American Association of School Administrators, op. cit., pp. 16-33.

instruction and recreation, and the contribution that sports can make in helping conquer physical and mental problems.

4. The President of the United States is interested in fitness. He places a high priority on our fields of endeavor.

5. The automation era is at hand, with its increased hours of leisure. Education also consists of knowing what to do when you have nothing to do.

6. The interest in such areas as drugs, ecology, sports, sex education, and smoking is at an all-time high.

The right facts, the right people, and the right time will lose effectiveness unless we *act in the right way:*

1. Since close national-community relationships are important, keep the lines of communication constantly open from the national organizations down to the grass roots programs. There should be a constant flow of ideas that can be translated into action.

2. Develop the best possible programs of health and physical education. Have satisfied children and youth go out from your programs.

3. Utilize every opportunity available to sell someone else on the worth of your professional field of endeavor. If you are sold, yourself, it will not be difficult to sell someone else.

4. Exploit every medium of communication to get your message across.

5. Think in positive terms—think *success,* and our chances of achieving big things will be better assured.

Questions and exercises

1. Outline what you consider to be an effective public relations plan for a school program of health or physical education.
2. Prepare a news release on some event or phase of the department program. Follow through with it for publication or broadcast.
3. Analyze the strengths and weaknesses of the present public relations program of the American Association for Health, Physical Education, and Recreation. Send a letter to headquarters on your findings.
4. After careful firsthand study, list the main features of the public relations program of some successful business concern. Show how some of the same techniques, media, and ideas may be applied to your professional field of endeavor.
5. What is meant by the fact that we are dealing in public relations with not just one but many "publics"?
6. Why is a knowledge of public relations important to teachers and administrators alike?
7. Discuss the potentialities of five public relations media in promoting physical education, health education, and recreation.
8. Prepare a speech that is to be given before a lay audience on the importance of physical education and health education to community welfare. Give the speech before class.
9. Prepare a bibliography of films that could be utilized effectively to interpret your profession to the public.
10. What qualifications would you need to become a full-time public relations person in your field?
11. List and discuss some principles that should be observed in public relations.
12. To what extent have the schools done a good public relations job?

Reading assignment in *Administrative Dimensions of Health and Physical Education Programs, Including Athletics:* Chapter 16, Selections 87 to 90.

Selected references

American Association for Health, Physical Education, and Recreation: Physical education—an interpretation, Washington, D. C., The Association.

American Association for Health, Physical Education, and Recreation, and National School Public Relations Association: Putting PR into HPER, Washington, D. C., 1953, The Association.

American Association of School Administrators: Public relations for America's schools, Twenty-eighth Yearbook, Washington, D. C., 1952, The Association.

Baughman, M. D.: The school's role in community life, School and Community **51:**9, 1969.

Bernays, E. L.: Public relations, Norman, 1952, University of Oklahoma Press.

Bucher, C. A.: Sportswriters—physical educator's nemesis, The Physical Educator **10:**51, 1953.

Chester, E. B.: School district in trouble, American School Board Journal **150:**17, 1965.

Ciernick, S.: Getting more mileage from school publications, National Education Association Journal **49:**24, 1960.

Dapper, G.: Public relations for educators, New York, 1964, The Macmillan Co.

Douglas, H. R.: Trends and issues in secondary education, New York, 1962, The Center for Applied Research, Inc. (The Library of Education).

Flesch, R.: The art of readable writing, New York, 1949, Harper & Row, Publishers.

Harral, S.: Tested public relations for schools, Norman, 1952, University of Oklahoma Press.

Humphrey, J. W.: Educators at your service, The Clearing House 38:556, 1964.

Jones, J. J.: School public relations, New York, 1966, The Center for Applied Research, Inc. (The Library of Education).

McCloskey, G.: Planning the public relations program, National Education Association Journal 59:17, 1970.

National Recreation Association: The ABC's of public relations for recreation, New York, 1946, National Recreation Association.

National School Public Relations Association: It starts in the classroom, Washington, D. C., 1951, National Education Association.

National School Public Relations Association: Print it right, Washington, D. C., 1953, National Education Association.

Scherer, D. J.: How to keep your district in the public eye, School Management 10:22, 1966.

Suttoff, J.: Local cosmopolitan orientation and participation in school affairs, Administrator's Notebook, vol. 9, No. 3, November, 1960.

Torpey, J.: Interpreting physical education for the public, The Physical Educator 24:131, 1967.

CHAPTER 21 OFFICE MANAGEMENT

The health and/or physical education office is one of the key centers for these professional fields. Too often health and physical educators give considerable attention to the development of their programs, the construction of facilities, and detailed measurement and evaluation programs but give little thought to the conduct of the office. As a result the program, facilities, public relations, and other factors often suffer. Office management is important because the office has many functions. It is the place for first impressions, center of communications, focus of administrative duties, and point of contact for administration and staff.

IMPORTANCE OF OFFICE MANAGEMENT

Colleagues, pupils, visitors, and other persons frequently have their initial contacts with departments of health and physical education in the central office. Their reception, the courtesies they are shown, the efficiency with which the office work is carried out, and other operational details leave a lasting impression upon their minds. Friends are often made or lost at this strategic point.

Center for communications

Office work, broadly conceived, is the handling and management of information. The office is usually the place where schedules are arranged and distributed, telephone calls made and received, reports typed and mimeographed, bulletins prepared and issued, conferences arranged and held, appointments made and confirmed, and greetings voiced and exchanged. The office represents the setting for a hub of activity around which revolves the efficient functioning of the work of health and physical education personnel. Unless these communications are carried out with dispatch, accurately and courteously, the entire administrative process breaks down.

Focus of administrative duties

The chief administrative personnel, secretarial assistants, and clerical help comprise the office staff. The filing system, key records, and reports are usually housed in the office. When inventories need to be examined, letters pulled from the files, or the chairman of the department consulted on important matters, the office is frequently the point of contact. Administrative responsibilities are carried out in the office, making this space a central point or focus for the entire organization.

Point of contact for administration and staff

Staff members visit the office regularly. Mailboxes are located there, and telephone calls may be taken in the office. Conferences and appointments with pupils and visitors often bring the teacher to the office. Constant communication takes place between administration and staff in this setting. High staff morale, efficiency, a friendly climate, and a feeling of working toward common goals can be imbued to a large degree through the atmosphere that exists in the office.

OFFICE SPACE

The central office for the health and/or physical education department, in accordance with its clearinghouse activities, should be located in a readily accessible position in the school or college plant. This office should be as near the entrance of the building as possible and at the same time have ready accessibility to health service offices, gymnasia, locker rooms, athletic fields, and other facilities of the department.

Most central offices for health and physical education should consist of at least three divisions: general reception area, clerical space, and private office. Other desirable features to be considered are a toilet, a storage room, and a conference room for staff and other meetings.

General reception area

The general reception office is that part of the office layout used by visitors as a waiting room or information center, for teachers and pupils who desire to get their mail, have appointments, or wish information, and for office services in general. It should be attractive, with some pictures on the wall, comfortable chairs, bulletin boards, and other items essential to carrying out the necessary administrative routines and creating a warm, friendly climate. A counter or fence should separate the general waiting room from the rest of the office facilities. This helps to ensure greater privacy and more efficient conduct of office responsibilities.

Clerical space

The clerical space should be separated from the general waiting and reception room. It should be equipped with such necessary materials as typewriters, files, tables, and telephones. It is often desirable to have a private alcove or office for one or more of the secretaries, depending upon the size of the department and office. Privacy is often needed for the typing of letters, the preparation of reports, or the convenience of visitors and other personnel. There should be ample lighting, freedom of movement, and sufficient space for the various administrative duties to be carried out with a minimum of confusion and of difficulty.

Private offices

The chairman of the department and possibly other personnel, depending upon the size of the department, should have private offices. The offices should be such that the persons in charge of administration can concentrate on their work without interruptions, have private conferences with students, faculty members, or visitors, and in general carry out their duties in the most efficient way possible. The offices should be decorated and equipped in an appropriate manner. There should be desks of sufficient working size that are neat in appearance, with calendars, schedule pads for appointments and conferences, and other essential materials. Filing cases, storage cabinets, and other equipment should be provided as needed. Faculty should also be provided with offices as much as possible.

OFFICE PERSONNEL

The number of office personnel will depend upon the size of the department. The staff could consist of secretaries, stenographers, transcribing machine operators, a receptionist, switchboard operator, and typists in a large department in a school or college. However, the usual office will probably consist of one secretary. In some small schools, student help may be all the personnel available.

The *secretary* should be a "good right arm" to the chairman and to the department as a whole. To be most helpful, she

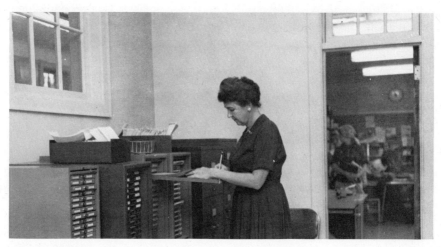

The secretary should be a "good right arm" to the administrator. (Office in senior high school, Mamaroneck, N. Y.)

will be a typist, a stenographer, and a public relations representative, will operate a dictaphone and mimeograph machine, and will see that the office runs smoothly. She will help the chairman and other staff members to remember facts, appointments, and other important information. She should know where materials are filed and be able to obtain them on a moment's notice, relieve the "boss" of minor details, and see that reports are sent out on time and that accurate records are kept.

A *stenographer* is a typist who can also take shorthand. A stenographer, however, differs from a secretary. She usually takes dictation and types letters and other material but does not have the personal relationship and confidential duties that a secretary has. Large departments frequently have stenographic "pools" wherein girls are on call to do work for any faculty member having work to be done.

A *transcribing operator* takes correspondence and other material that has been dictated and listens to a dictaphone or other playback mechanism upon which such information has been recorded. Using earphones, she sits at a typewriter and listens and types in accordance with the instructions that have been given.

A *receptionist's* position will vary with the department. In some departments a receptionist is a "greeter" who presents an attractive appearance and is polite, courteous, and helpful to callers. Some departments also assign her certain typing, filing, and telephone duties, in addition to the reception of callers.

Large departments frequently have *switchboard operators* who cover the phones for many faculty members and other personnel. Frequently staff members are not in, and messages are then relayed by the switchboard operator through the prescribed channels.

Office personnel should be selected very carefully. Experience, character, personality, looks, and ability should play important roles in the selection process. The secretary should have, as a minimum of education, a high school diploma. The achievements of a girl who has been through the commercial course and who has a good background in typewriting, bookkeeping, English, and secretarial practice will help to ensure her value to the department.

The chairman of the department and other faculty members should treat a secretary and other office personnel with respect and make them feel that they are very important parts of the work being accomplished. The staff should be patient and see that clerical help know the details of their jobs, recognize the importance of each, and appreciate the responsibilities that rest with their positions.

In smaller high schools, elementary schools, and colleges, the administrator may have to rely partially or entirely upon *students* to get some of the clerical work accomplished. Probably, senior students who have particular inclinations along this line will be most successful. Inservice education should take place for these students to see that acceptable precedures are followed in filing, typing, mimeographing, maintaining records, and performing other office duties.

EQUIPMENT AND SUPPLIES

Whether or not an office is efficient in its clerical and other responsibilities will depend upon the equipment and supplies available. It must be recognized that the materials needed will vary with the size of the school or college. In smaller schools and colleges such equipment as adding machines might readily be available in the central office but not in departmental offices. Following are some of the items that should be considered:

Adding machine	Maps of school district
Bookcases	Paper cutter
Bulletin boards	Paste
Buzzers	Pencil sharpeners
Calendars	Pencils and pens
Chairs	Reproducing machines
Clips	Rulers
Cloak racks	Safe
Clock	Scissors
Desk baskets	Scrapbooks
Desk lights	Stamps
Desk pads	Stapling machine
Desks	Stationery and paper
Dictionaries	Tables
Ditto machine	Telephone
First-aid cabinet	Typewriters
Letter trays	Umbrella rack
Magazine racks	Wardrobe cabinets
	Wastebaskets

In some large offices where many, many details are handled, data processing equipment should be available.

OFFICE WORK AND AUTOMATION

The rapid progress made in recent years begs the question as to whether or not new automated equipment should be installed in the office. The way this question is answered will depend upon such factors as the extent of the program the office serves, the amount of clerical work that needs to be done, and the size of the allocated budget.

Automation as used here refers to the processing of data by some mechanical device or system other than typewriters, adding machines, calculators, and photocopiers. Automation can be used in respect to handling such items as accounts payable, cumulative records, health records, inventories, personnel records, schedules, work requests, and transcripts.

Automation can be utilized by an organization either by installing their own machines or by working through some business organization that processes educational data for a fee. Also, the procedure of joining with several other school or college systems for such a service will work very well in some situations. Depending upon the size of the operation, it may be that a job can be done better, the hiring of additional personnel can be eliminated, and the cost will be less without automation.

REFERENCE MATERIALS

An area that high school and college offices should not overlook is the area of reference materials. The elementary, high school, and college offices will find it valuable to develop professional libraries that contain some of the outstanding professional books, periodicals, and standard references for their professional fields. In addition, there should be such references as books and periodicals; bulletins of the state department of education, state department of health, state and national professional organizations; facility references; and catalogues of athletic equipment and supplies.

Although there may be such material in the school library, it may be of value in many locations to have such references in the central office. In this way faculty members utilize them to a greater extent and thus keep up to date with their professional fields.

ADMINISTRATIVE ROUTINE

The administrative routine or manner in which the day-to-day business of the department is carried out by the office represents the basic reason why such a facility exists. Therefore, this matter should receive very careful consideration.

Hours

The office should be open during regular school hours. This usually means from 8 or 9 A.M. to 4 or 5 P.M. During this time there should always be someone present to answer the telephone, greet visitors, and answer students' questions. There may be some exceptions to these hours in a small school, but even in these cases there should be regular office hours that have been publicized as widely as possible.

Teachers should also have regular office hours at which they will be accessible to students, colleagues, and other persons who would like to see them. These office hours should be posted, office personnel informed, and the schedule carefully observed so that requests for information and assistance can be properly handled.

Assignments

All assignments, whether for office personnel or faculty, should be made very clear, be in writing, and be properly publicized. Office personnel may be required to ring electric bells to signal a change in periods, set clocks, take messages, mimeo-

graph daily or weekly bulletins, distribute minor supplies, check the calendar of school events, provide messenger service to teachers and pupils, or assist in the health examination. These details should be clearly understood and carried out at the proper time. Specific responsibilities should be fixed and a schedule of duties prepared so as to prevent any misunderstanding.

Correspondence

Correspondence represents a most effective public relations medium. Letters can be written in a cold, impersonal manner or they can carry warmth and help to interpret what a program expects and is trying to do for a student or other person. Letters should be prepared carefully, using only correct English, and in a neat manner that meets the highest standards of secretarial practice. If a health or physical education teacher has to do his own letters, these same standards should be met. Letters should convey the feeling that the department is anxious to help and to be of assistance wherever possible. Letters should be answered promptly, not placed in a drawer and left for weeks or months. Carbon copies of letters should be made and filed for future reference.

Files and filing

The office should contain steel filing cases for vertical filing. The filing system used will depend upon the number of personnel involved and the person doing the filing, but in any case it should be simple and practical. Files will usually consist of correspondence and informational material. For ease of finding material some form of alphabetical filing should usually be utilized, although numerical filing may at times be practical. The alphabetical files can be done on a name or subject basis, such as "Brown, Charles A.," or "Health Examinations," using a Manila folder for all the material to be filed under the name or subject. Cross references should be included to facilitate finding material. Guide cards can be used to show which divisions of the file pertain to each letter of the alphabet, thus making the search for material much more rapid.

A visible filing system for any records and reports that are used currently and constantly will prove helpful. These are usually prepared on cards, and the visible filing case contains flat drawers that at a moment's notice will show the names or index numbers when pulled outward.

Office files should be kept very accurately. The person doing the filing should be careful to see that the letter or other material gets into the proper folder and that folder into its correct location. Filing should also be kept up to date. A periodic review of the files should be made in order to weed out material that is no longer pertinent to the department. Files that for any reason are removed from the cabinet should be returned. If they are to be kept out for any length of time, an "out" sign should be substituted, showing where they are.

Telephone

The use of the office telephone is a major consideration for good departmental public relations. A few simple rules that should be observed are indicated below.

Promptness. The telephone should be answered as promptly as possible. It should not be allowed to ring for some length of time before the receiver is taken off the hook. Answering promptly reflects efficient office practice and consideration for the person calling.

Professional purposes. The telephone is installed in an office for professional purposes. Secretaries or other office personnel should not be permitted to talk for long periods of time about personal matters that have no relationship to departmental affairs. The telephone should be kept clear for business that is of importance to the achievement of professional objectives.

Courtesy, friendliness, and helpfulness. The person answering the phone should be pleasant in manner and courteous in approach and should desire to be of assistance to whoever is calling. This should be the procedure not only when one is feeling his or her best but at all times. Such a telephone manner represents a professional responsibility that should be carried out with regularity.

Messages. At times faculty or staff members who are being called will not be available. A pencil and telephone pad should be kept at hand for recording calls in such cases, and a definite procedure should be established for relaying these messages to the proper person.

Appointments

Appointments should not be made unless it is believed that they can be kept. Furthermore, all appointments should be kept as nearly at the time scheduled as possible. Many times the person making an appointment has arranged his day with the understanding that he will have his conference at a certain time. If this time is not adhered to it means the schedule has to be altered, and complications frequently arise as a result of such a procedure. The secretary should keep an accurate list of appointments. If no secretary is available, the staff member should keep his own schedule of appointments and check it regularly to see that it is met.

RECORDS AND REPORTS

At times, records and reports are not prepared and maintained accurately because the directions given by the chairman of the department or the teachers are not clear and definite. When complicated reports are to be prepared, oral instructions, by themselves, will usually not be sufficient. Instead, directions should be written, typed, and distributed. The preparation of a sample will also help to ensure better results.

Text continued on p. 600.

B = Boys
G = Girls

	Accident	Adapted program	Application for participation in interscholastic sports	Attendance	Cumulative class record	Equipment	Extracurricular activities	Game reports	Health	Interscholastic sports	Intramurals	Inventory	Medical form for inter-scholastic sports	Medical form for physical education	Parental permission sports	Physical fitness
School 1	B-G			B-G	B-G				B-G	B-G	B-G					B-G
School 2	B-G	B-G			B-G					B-G	B	B-G			B-G	B-G
School 3	B-G	B-G		B-G				B	B-G	B			B		B-G	B-G
School 4	B-G			B-G	B-G	B-G						B-G	B	B-G	B	B-G
School 5					B-G					B			B		B	B-G
School 6	B-G	B-G		B-G				B			B-G				B-G	B-G
School 7	B-G			B-G			B-G			B		B-G				B-G
School 8	B-G		B	B-G	B-G						G	B-G			B-G	B-G
School 9				B-G												
School 10	B-G			B-G					B-G		B-G			B-G	B-G	B-G
School 11	B-G	B-G	B	B-G							B-G	B-G	B-G		B	
School 12				B-G						B	B-G	B-G				B-G
School 13	B-G	B-G		B-G		B-G	B-G			B-G	B-G	B-G			B-G	
School 14	B-G	B-G		B-G		B-G					B-G				B-G	B-G
School 15	B-G		B	B-G				B		B-G						
School 16				B-G	B				B-G						B	
School 17				B		B			B					B		
School 18					B							B-G			B-G	B-G
School 19				B-G					B-G					B-G		B-G
School 20	B-G		B-G	B-G	B-G								B		B-G	B-G
School 21	B-G			B-G		B-G	B-G		B-G	B-G	B-G		B			B-G

Physical education records used in twenty-one schools.

Name

Year

	HT.	WT.	OFF.	HT.	WT.	OFF.	HT.	WT.	OFF.	HT.	WT.	OFF.	HT.	WT.	OFF.	HT.	WT.	OFF.
Hockey																		
Soccer																		
Volleyball																		
Basketball																		
Softball																		
Lacrosse																		
Archery																		
Tennis																		
Badminton																		
Gym club																		
Synchronized swimming																		
Leader's club																		
Junior varsity cheerleader																		
Varsity cheerleader																		
Subtotal																		
Total																		

Comments

(HT.) = Honor team; (WT.) = Winning team; (OFF.) = Officiating.

Girl's physical education extracurricular activity card.

SCHOOL HEALTH EXAMINATION

Please return this report as soon as the examination has been completed. All reports must be in within 30 days after school opens. A physical examination made any time between June 1 and October 1 is acceptable.

Name .... Exam Date ....

Address ....

School..Grade...........Wt............Ht..............

reveals the following defects (leave blank if normal)

Nutrition...

Skin ...   Scalp   Hands   Feet ....

Eyes ....

Ears ....

Nose..

Teeth ....

Tonsils and Adenoids..

Lymphatics ....

Heart ....

Lungs..

Abdomen...

Genito-urinary..

Hernia...

Orthopedic ....

Other...

General Physical and Emotional Status ....

REMARKS: *(Defects and recommendations for care in school to be noted on reverse side.)*

DATES OF IMMUNIZATION: (Not previously recorded):

	Initial	Booster
Smallpox		
Diphtheria		
Pertussis		
Tetanus toxoid		

Polio

Previous illness & operation

X-RAY OF CHEST—Report and date:

....M.D.

(Please print or write legibly)

Phys. Education
yes ☐ no ☐

Address..

Report for school health examination.

NOTICE REGARDING ANNUAL VISION TEST

Pupil's name_____ School_____

Address_____ Nurse _____

To Parent or Guardian:

The results of the annual vision test suggest that your child may have some eye difficulty. We recommend that the child have a complete eye examination in order to determine whether an eye defect exists and, if so, the need for correction or care.

Please ask the examiner to complete this form. We ask that you return the completed form to the school.

* * * * *

To Examiner:

Your diagnosis and recommendations will be appreciated and will assist us in planning this child's school program.

School observations:

Visual acuity   R_____ L_____   Test used _____

Other observations _____

_____

_____

_____   _____

    Supervising Principal   School Nurse or Physician

* * * * *

Examiner's diagnosis and recommendations:

1.   Diagnosis   R_____ L_____

2.   Visual acuity   (a) Without   R _____ (b) With   R _____
                       correction L _____   correction L _____

3.   Are glasses to be worn?   _____Yes   _____ No

4.   If yes, indicate extent of use. _____

5.   Should activities be limited because of eye conditions? _____ Yes _____No

6.   If yes, please specify. _____

7.   Recommendations and remarks. _____

                              _____
                                  Examiner's signature

                              _____
                                         Title

_____   _____
        Date   Address

Health report for vision test.

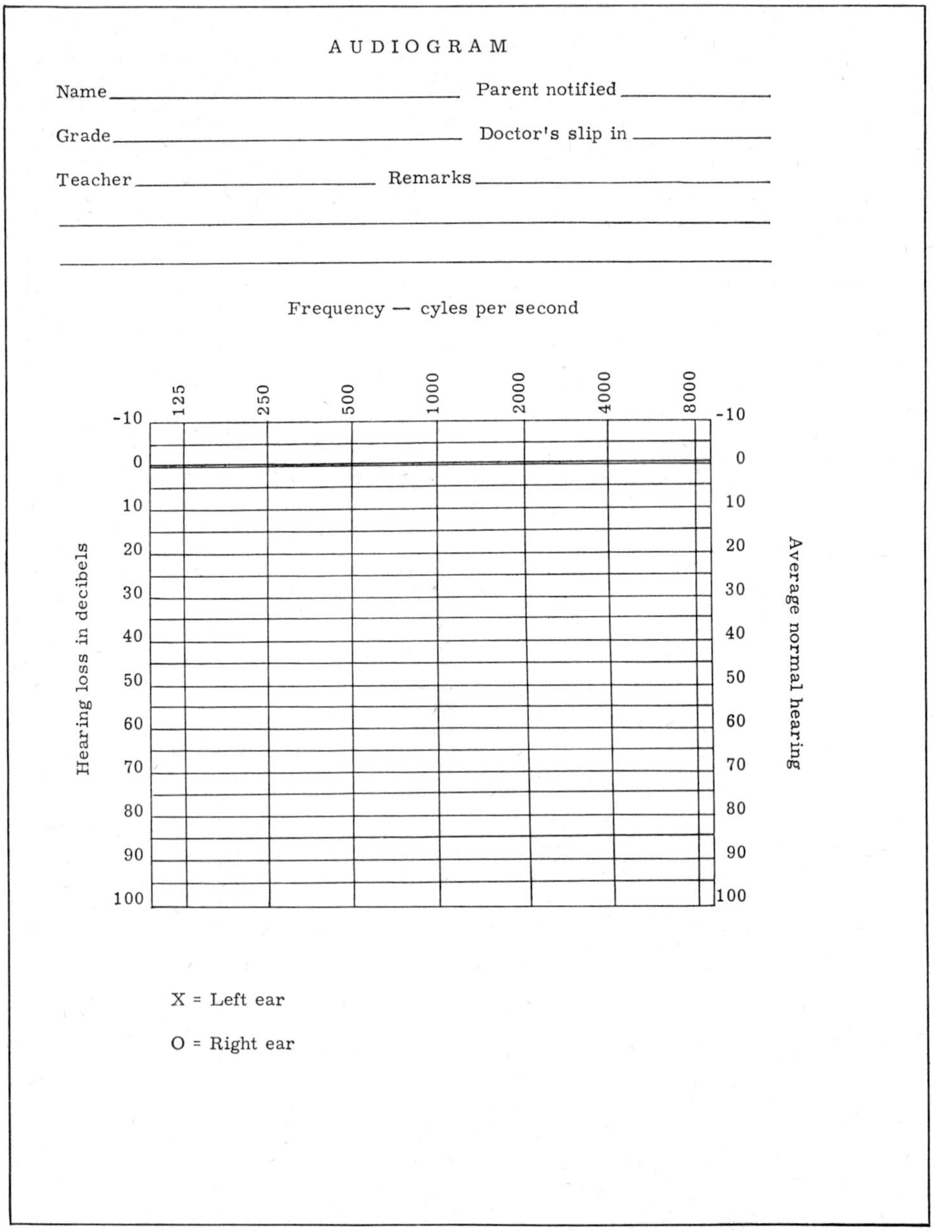

A U D I O G R A M

Name_____   Parent notified _____

Grade_____   Doctor's slip in _____

Teacher_____   Remarks_____

_____

_____

Frequency — cyles per second

Health report form for testing of hearing.

OFFICE OF THE SCHOOL NURSE

Dear Parent:

A recent health appraisal of your child _____

indicates a condition of _____

_____

which we feel warrants more complete diagnostic study and/or treatment

if such is indicated. It is urged that this condition be given immediate

professional attention. If for any reason you are unable to do so, please

advise the school nurse-teacher, who may be able to assist you.

Kindly ask your professional advisor to complete the lower portion

of this notice and return it to me.

_____
School Nurse-Teacher

Telephone No. _____

= =

TO THE EXAMINER

The following information will help us to better understand the health

needs of this child:

Findings: _____

Recommendations given parents: _____ _____

_____

Are any modifications of the school program indicated? If so, what?

_____

Do you wish to see this child again? If so, when? _____

Date _____   _____
                                   Signature of Examiner

                                   Address _____

Health report to parents.

Administrators are often responsible for poorly kept records, inaccurate reports, and late submissions. There should be clear directions, announcements at regular intervals, reminders as to when reports are due, and a prompt checking of reports to see if they are all in and whether there are omissions or other inaccuracies.

A survey was conducted of twenty-one school systems to determine the types of records that were kept in departmental files for health and physical education

SUPPLIES AND EQUIPMENT INVENTORY
(Special Teachers)

Name of teacher _____   School _____

Location of materials*_____   Date _____

Quantity	Description of articles	Condition		
		Good	Fair	Poor

* If the instructor who is preparing this report does not have a homeroom or if equipment used by the instructor is located in cabinets or storage space in more than one room, a notation as to the exact location of articles listed above should be made. If more than one room is used to store supplies, a separate report should be filed to note the contents of each storage location.

(SUBMIT IN DUPLICATE)

Inventory form for supplies and equipment.

personnel. The result of this survey showed that some of the schools were very conscientious in regard to record keeping; others were not. In general, most of the department heads and teachers admitted they should put more time and effort into this phase of health and physical education administration.

In the school systems surveyed, the boys' departments usually kept more records and forms than the girls' departments. See p. 594. This can be explained partially by the fact that athletic programs for boys have many more records associated with it.

The survey showed that in some schools records were kept in the department of health and physical education, while in other schools these same records were kept in another department. For example, in some schools attendance records were kept by the health and physical education department, while in other schools an attendance officer had complete control. In some schools the health and physical education department kept records on health, while in other schools these records were kept by the school nurse. The same was true in regard to budgetary and inventory records.

Pupil's Name .... Gr. ....

Permission is hereby given to .... to
                                                    Pupil's Name
participate in the After-School Play Program for the

.... season. I understand (he) (she) will
          Fall, Winter, Spring

participate in .... on .... of each
                         Activity   *Days*

week from about .... to ....
                              Hour   *Hour*

Date ....
                                                        Parent or Guardian

Enrollment in this program is voluntary. However, once enrolled regular attendance is expected unless prevented for reasons of health or family plans. The pupil is expected to notify the activity supervisor of the reason for each absence.

Details of each season's program are given each pupil to take home in September of each year. Another copy will gladly be sent on request.

5M-7/63-BP

Parental permission form.

Name_____ _____ H. R._____
              Last   First

Lock No._____

Combination_____

Locker No._____

Floor Spot_____

Equipment record.

Some heads of health and physical education departments kept these records, while the business administrator and principals kept them in other schools.

The forms on pp. 595 to 601 show some of the most common types of records kept in the twenty-one school systems surveyed.

Examples of reports and records that are maintained by the health and/or physical education departments include the following:

Health
    Health consultation request
    Medical examination record
    Health history
    Growth records
    Excuse forms
    Exercise card
    Height and weight card
    Body mechanics inspection form
    Films and visual aids list
    Health habits record form
    Accident records

Physical education activity, skill, and squad records and reports
    Basket card
    Physical education record
    Field event report card

Physical education test and achievement forms
    Physical fitness record
    Report to parents
    Résumé of personality traits
    Citizenship guide sheet
    Athletic report

Physical education attendance and excuse records and reports
    Squad card attendance record
    Appointment slip
    Absence report
    Change of program

Physical education equipment forms
    Padlock record
    Equipment record
    Equipment inventory and condition report
    Lost property report

CHECKLIST OF SOME IMPORTANT CONSIDERATIONS FOR OFFICE MANAGEMENT

Space and working conditions   *Yes*   *No*

1. Does the reception room provide ample space for waiting guests? ____ ____
2. Is the clerical space separated from the reception room so that office work is not interrupted by the arrival of guests? ____ ____
3. Are there private offices for the Director of Health and Physical Education and as many of the staff as possible? ____ ____
4. Is there an up-to-date health suite that provides an office and other essential facilities for the school nurse? ____ ____
5. Is there adequate space and equipment for filing? ____ ____
6. Are file drawers arranged so that papers can be inserted and removed easily and with space for future expansion? ____ ____
7. Is the office arranged so that as many workers as possible get the best natural light with glare from sunlight or reflected sunlight avoided? ____ ____
8. Has the office space been painted in accordance with the best in color dynamics? ____ ____
9. Have provisions been made so that unnecessary noise is eliminated, distractions are kept to a minimum, and cleanliness prevails? ____ ____
10. Is there good ventilation, appropriate artificial lighting, and satisfactory heating conditions? ____ ____

CHECKLIST OF SOME IMPORTANT CONSIDERATIONS FOR OFFICE MANAGEMENT–cont'd

Personnel   *Yes*   *No*

11. Is a receptionist available to greet guests and answer queries?
12. Is there a recorded analysis of the duties of each secretarial position?
13. Are channels available for ascertaining causes of dissatisfaction among secretarial help?
14. Do secretaries dress neatly and conservatively?
15. Do secretaries maintain a desk that has an orderly appearance and clear their desks of working papers each day?
16. Do secretaries concern themselves with the efficiency of the office?
17. Are secretaries loyal to the department and staff members?
18. Do staff members have regular office hours?
19. Are appointments kept promptly?

Procedures

20. Is up-to-date reading material furnished for waiting guests?
21. Does the office help continually pay attention to maintaining offices that are neat, with papers, books, and other materials arranged in an orderly manner?
22. Are the secretaries knowledgeable about departmental activities so that they can answer intelligently queries about staff members and activities?
23. Do secretaries wait upon guests promptly and courteously?
24. Are letters typed neatly, well placed on the sheet, properly spaced, free from erasures and smudge and typographical errors?
25. Is correspondence handled promptly?
26. Is the filing system easily learned and is the filing done promptly so that the work does not pile up?
27. Is the office routine efficient of human time and energy with the elimination of duplicate operations or forms?
28. Are the most effective and efficient office methods utilized?
29. Is the clerical output satisfactory, with work starting promptly in the morning and after lunch, breaks taken according to schedule, and work stoppage taking place as scheduled?
30. Has a streamlined procedure been developed so that telephones are answered promptly, guests are courteously treated, and personal argument and gossiping eliminated?
31. Are all essential records properly maintained and kept up to date?
32. Have procedures for typing and duplicating course outlines, committee reports, examinations, bulletins, fliers, letters, announcements, etc., been developed to eliminate uncertainty or confusion on the part of staff members?
33. Are regular office hours for staff posted and known so that office staff can make appointments as needed?
34. Are secretaries acquainted with such details as securing films and other visual aids, obtaining reference material, helping in registration, duplicating material, and obtaining additional forms and records?
35. Is the office covered continuously during working hours?

Questions and exercises

1. Why is good office management essential for good public relations? What are some important reasons why office management is important to a department of physical and/or health education?
2. What three main divisions should office space include? Discuss the physical layout of each of these three divisions.
3. What office personnel should be available in a small high school, in a large high school, and in a college or university?
4. List the equipment and supplies that should be readily available in the average physical education office.
5. What importance can be attributed to a professional list of references in an office? Prepare a list of outstanding references for both the fields of health and physical education.
6. Prepare rules for effective administrative routine in respect to (a) hours, (b) assignments, (c) records and reports, (d) correspondence, (e) files and filing, (f) telephone, and (g) appointments.

Reading assignment in *Administrative Dimensions of Health and Physical Education Programs, Including Athletics:* Selections 16 and 71

Selected references

Courtesy in correspondence, The Royal Bank of Canada Monthly Letter **46:**1, 1965.

Doris, L., and Miller, B.: Complete secretary's handbook, Englewood Cliffs, N. J., 1951, Prentice-Hall, Inc.

Fawcett, W.: Policy and practice in school administration, New York, 1964, The Macmillan Co.

Leffingwell, W. H., and Robinson, E. M.: Textbook of office management, New York, 1950, McGraw-Hill Book Co.

Pittman, J.: Office may become a leader of management, The Office **67:**110, 1968.

Shiff, R. A.: Satellite administrative service centers, Administrative Management **30:**26, 1969.

Siegel, G. B.: Management development and the instability of skills: a strategy, Public Personnel Review **30:**15, 1969.

Measurement programs are gaining increasing prominence in school and college health and physical education programs. In order to show the benefits derived from participation in these programs and in order to conduct them in the most efficient way possible, measurement is an essential consideration.

The term *measurement* is used here to refer to the use of techniques to determine the degree to which a trait, ability, or characteristic exists in an individual.

During the last 35 years many measurement techniques have been developed in the fields of health and physical education. Some of these have been carefully constructed in a scientific manner, but many fall below acceptable standards. The administration should focus its attention on the materials that give valid and reliable results. Furthermore, all interested persons should be encouraged to construct new techniques in areas where shortages exist.

There are measurement techniques other than tests. Some of these are rating scales, checklists, photographic devices, controlled observation, and various measuring instruments.

The Joint Committee on Health Problems in Education of the National Education Association and the American Medical Association† states that the most common instruments or procedures used by health teachers are (1) observations, (2) surveys, (3) questionnaires and checklists, (4) interviews, (5) diaries and other autobiographic records kept by students, (6) health and growth records, (7) other records of health conditions or improvements, (8) samples of students' work, (9) case studies, and (10) health knowledge tests.

PURPOSES OF MEASUREMENT

Many purposes exist to support the utilization of measurement techniques in the administration of school health and physical education programs. A few of these will be discussed.

Measurement helps to determine the progress being made and the degree to which objectives are being met. It aids in discovering the needs of the participants. It identifies strengths and weaknesses of students and teachers, aids in curriculum planning, and shows where emphasis should be placed. It also gives direction and helps to supply information for guidance purposes.

Measurement helps in determining where emphasis should be placed in teaching and the procedures that are effective and ineffective. It also has use in aiding pupils to determine their own progress in respect to health and physical education practices, as a basis for giving grades, and as a means of interpreting programs to administrators and the public in general.

The information provided by measurement techniques can also be utilized in other ways. In the area of measurement, findings can be used for such purposes as grouping individuals according to similar mental, physical, and other traits that will

---

*See also Chapter 11 on Administering School and College Physical Fitness Programs for information on physical fitness tests.

†Joint Committee on Health Problems in Education of National Education Association and American Medical Association: Health education, Washington, D. C., 1961, National Education Association, p. 343.

Table 22-1. Extent of use of pupil evaluation techniques*

Techniques used†	Percent of 38 city school systems	Percent of 44 county school systems
Tests	100.0	100.0
Cumulative records	92.0	77.0
Interviews	89.5	71.0
Case studies	84.2	57.0
Case conferences	81.6	55.0
Group discussion	68.4	68.0
Anecdotal records	63.2	32.0
Observation	60.5	73.0
Files of sample materials	57.9	48.0
Questionnaires	53.3	30.0
Rating scales	44.7	11.0
Checklists	36.8	21.0
Inventories	31.6	18.0
Logs or diaries	13.2	16.0
Sociograms	10.5	2.0

*From Bonney, M. E., and Hampleman, R. S.: Personal-social evaluation techniques, New York, 1962, The Center for Applied Research in Education, Inc. (The Library of Education), pp. 4-5.
†Other techniques mentioned only once by either city, county, or both are the following: followup studies, autobiographies, clinics, case work, stenographic reports, films, recordings, psychiatric consultation, parental interviews, graphs of pupils' progress, interaction content records, and photographs.

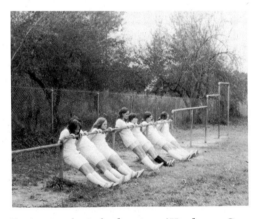

Testing in physical education. (Henderson County Schools, Hendersonville, N. C.)

ensure better instruction. Measurement yields information that can be used as an indication of a person's achievement in various skills and activities. It provides information that can be used to predict future performance and development. It affords data on attitudes that determine whether or not the participant has proper motiva-tion, and it focuses attention on future action that should be taken in the program.

THE COMPUTER AND MEASUREMENT

The computer has many implications for the management of data concerned with pupil achievement in health and physical education programs. It enables the teacher and the administration to reduce the amount of time they devote to the analysis of data. The computer permits the analysis of test scores for thousands of students with comparative ease. It enables the physical educator to identify differentiating characteristics of students, such as scores that are high or low. The computer enables a battery of test items on such characteristics as speed, strength, or power to be analyzed item by item. It is an aid in scheduling in light of the results of measurement, for example, for purposes of grouping students with similar deficiencies into the same class. The computer makes it possible to prepare a profile of each student on the various health and physical education tests that are administered. Test scores of one class of students can be compared with other classes within the same school or with other schools where national norms are available.

These represent only a few examples of how the computer can be of value in the administration of a pupil measurement program. The uses of this device for the imaginative and creative administrator and teacher are limitless. The nation and world are rapidly being run on an electronic basis. Physical education and health education, if they desire to make their measurement programs most effective and meaningful, should examine the possibilities of the computer for their programs.

CRITERIA FOR TEST CONSTRUCTION AND SELECTION

Criteria refer to those particular standards that may be used to evaluate measurement and evaluation materials in the field of education. Such criteria as validity, reliability, objectivity, norms, and administrative economy provide the scientific basis for the selection and construction of tests. Administrators should be particularly concerned that the tests they utilize meet these criteria. If they do, properly interpreted results should aid considerably in developing adequate school health and physical education programs.

A definition of each criterion for test construction and selection and questions that could be asked by the administrator to determine whether or not the tests he desires to use meet the criteria listed are stated here*:

A. Validity

Accuracy in measuring what it claims to measure.

---

*Larson, L. A.: Lecture notes, Course No. 280.62 in Advanced Methods and Materials in Physical Education, Health, and Recreation, New York University, 1946-1947.

1. Does it cover the area for which it is designed?
2. Is it applicable to proper ages and grades?
3. Is the criterion with which material was correlated acceptable?
4. Is the size of the correlation coefficient acceptable?
5. Does the technique give information concerning objectives?
6. Is the sampling adequate, representative, and random?
7. Is evidence cited as to whether it is a classification, achievement, diagnostic, or prognostic technique?
8. Has the technique been tried in the recommended area of application?

B. Reliability

The consistency of measurement and evaluation on the same individual or group under the same conditions and by the same examiner.

1. Is the size of the coefficient correlation acceptable?
2. What are the means of the two tests?
3. What are the conditions under which reliability has been determined?
4. Is the method used for the determination of reliability valid (test-retest, split-halves, parallel forms)?
5. Is the sample adequate, representative, and random?
6. Has the reliability of the technique been determined by using the same group or individuals for which the technique is recommended?

C. Objectivity

The degree to which a technique may be administered to the same individuals or group by a different examiner and obtain the same results.

1. Is there a simple and complete manual of instructions?

2. Is the method used for determination of objectivity valid (test-retest, parallel forms)?
3. Is the sample adequate, representative, and random?
4. Has the objectivity of the technique been determined by using the same group for which the technique is recommended?
5. Are the means cited?
6. What is the difference in the mean scores?
7. Are the conditions under which objectivity has been determined satisfactory?
8. Are the procedures easily understood by the examiner and by the subject?
9. Are alternate forms of tests provided in instances where they are necessary?

D. Norms

Levels of group performance or a statistical average most frequent for a group.

1. What is the basis for construction of the norm (age, grade, ability)?
2. Is the sample adequate, representative, and random?
3. Are norms local or national?
4. Are norms tentative, arbitrary, or experimental?
5. Are all significant extraneous factors eliminated?
6. Is the statistical refinement sufficient?
7. Is the appropriate statistical tool used?

E. Administrative economy

Procedures that deal with the conduct of the program.

1. How much time is required to administer the technique?
2. What is the approximate cost of the equipment used in the administration of the technique?
3. Is the technique easy to administer?

4. How much training is necessary for the examiners?
5. Are the objectives of the test compatible with the objectives of the program?
6. Is the measurement or evaluational technique designed for school or research purposes?
7. How many examiners are needed?
8. Is the technique within the scope of a health or physical educator's training?

FRAMEWORK FOR MEASUREMENT PROCEDURES

To give the reader a clearer knowledge of some of the types of information that can be measured concerning some of the objectives of health and physical education, a partial framework is listed on the following pages. It is presented for the purpose of giving an indication of the vast scope of measurement and how it can influence these specialized programs. Objectives and terms used in framework are defined for purposes of clarification.

Objectives

1. *Organic development objectives* refer to the activity phase of the program that builds physical power in an individual through the development of the various organic systems of the body.
2. *Skill development objective* deals with the phase of the program that develops coordination, rhythm, and poise, through which some particular act may be performed with proficiency.
3. *Mental development objective* deals with the phase of the program that develops a comprehensive knowledge of principles, historical background, rules, techniques, values, and strategies.
4. *Human relations development objective* refers to the phase of the pro-

gram that aids an individual in making personal and group adjustments and in developing desirable standards of conduct essential to good citizenship.

Definitions

1. *Classification information* refers to those elements that can be used as a basis for segregating individuals into homogeneous groups for which they are reasonably well suited mentally, physically, emotionally, and socially.
2. *Achievement information* refers to those elements that can be measured to determine the scope and magnitude of an individual's achievement in organic development, skills, knowledge, and adaptability.
3. *Diagnostic information* refers to those elements that can be used to determine the causal factors of development and performance.
4. *Prognostic information* refers to those elements that can be used as valid forecasters of development and performance.
5. *Basic element* is an aspect of organic, neuromuscular, or mental growth that is a foundation for, and makes possible the development of, a skill.
6. *Fundamental skill* refers to a basic skill that is common to, and essential for participation in, most forms of activity.
7. *Activity skill* refers to a skill that is pertinent to successful participation in a particular activity.

Types of information concerning the objectives

1. *Organic development objective*
   a. Classification information
      (1) Age, weight, height
      (2) Strength
      (3) Posture
      (4) Sensory capacity
      (5) Physical fitness
      (6) Anthropometric measurements
      (7) Mental capacity
      (8) Power
      (9) Energy
      (10) Cardiac efficiency
   b. Achievement information
      (1) Strength
      (2) Endurance
      (3) Speed
      (4) Sensory capacity
      (5) Physical fitness
      (6) Power
      (7) Energy
      (8) Posture
      (9) Cardiac efficiency
      (10) Nutrition
   c. Diagnostic information
      (1) Age, weight, height
      (2) Strength
      (3) Endurance
      (4) Nutrition
      (5) Speed
      (6) Sensory capacity
      (7) Physical fitness
      (8) Power
      (9) Energy
      (10) Cardiac efficiency
      (11) Posture
   d. Prognostic information
      (1) Age, weight, height
      (2) Posture
      (3) Speed
      (4) Endurance
      (5) Sensory capacity
      (6) Physical fitness
      (7) Power
      (8) Energy
      (9) Cardiac efficiency
2. *Skill development objective*
   a. Classification information
      (1) Basic elements (concerned mainly with physical activity— would need development for other types)
         (a) Age, weight, height
         (b) Endurance
         (c) Strength
         (d) Native motor ability

YORKTOWN HEIGHTS ELEMENTARY SCHOOLS

PHYSICAL EDUCATION Progress Record	Grade Weight Height	3				4				5				6			
		Dec. 196....	Grade Average	June 196....	Grade Average	Dec. 196....	Grade Average	June 196....	Grade Average	Dec. 196....	Grade Average	June 196....	Grade Average	Dec. 196....	Grade Average	June 196....	Grade Average
Name																	
CHIN-UPS (Arm strength)																	
JUMPING ROPE - number of jumps completed in 30 seconds (Endurance, leg strength, coordination)																	
STANDING BROAD JUMP (Body movement forward) (feet)																	
JUMPING FOR HEIGHT (Jump - Reach - Body movement upward) (inches)																	
CLIMBING 20-FOOT ROPE (General strength & coordination) (feet)																	
TRAVEL HORIZONTAL LADDER (Arm strength & coordination) (feet)																	
SIT-UPS* (Abdominal strength)																	
50-YARD DASH (Speed) (seconds)																	
SOFTBALL THROW 30 FEET, 10 THROWS (Accuracy)																	
* Maximum sit-ups: 3rd - 20 4th - 30 5th - 50 6th - 50																	

FOUR YEAR FITNESS REPORT CARD

Fitness report card reflects growth and progress. Parents in Yorktown Heights, N. Y., know just how their children did in every phase of the semiannual physical fitness test because they receive fitness report cards twice each year and can check progress and growth. (From Klappholz, L., editor: Successful practices in teaching physical fitness, New London, Conn., 1964, Croft Educational Services. Reprinted by permission.)

    (e) Motor educability
    (f) Reaction time
    (g) Motor interest
    (h) Sensory capacity
 (2) Fundamental skills (mainly concerned with physical activity—other aspects would need to be developed)

    (a) Running
    (b) Throwing
    (c) Kicking
    (d) Jumping
    (e) Dodging
    (f) Leaping
    (g) Vaulting
    (h) Climbing

(i) Skipping
(j) Accuracy
(k) Objective body control
(l) Agility
(m) Timing
(n) Balance
(o) Spring
(p) Hand-eye, foot-eye,
arm-eye coordinations
(3) Activity skills (would need to be broken down into the various components affecting the development of each skill)

b. Achievement information
(1) Basic elements (similar to basic elements under classification information)
(2) Fundamental skills (similar to fundamental skills under classification information)
(3) Activity skills (would need to be broken down into the various components affecting the development of each skill)

c. Diagnostic information
(1) Basic elements
(a) Nutrition
(b) Health habits such as sleep, rest, and mental state
(c) Cardiac efficiency
(d) Sensory capacity
(e) Motor interest
(f) Reaction time
(g) Motor educability
(h) Native motor ability
(i) Strength
(j) Endurance
(k) Age, weight, height
(2) Fundamental skills (similar to fundamental skills under classification information)
(3) Activity skills (would need to be broken down into the various components affecting the development of each skill)

d. Prognostic information
(1) Basic elements (similar to basic

elements under diagnostic information)
(2) Fundamental skills (similar to fundamental skills under classification information)
(3) Activity skills (would need to be broken down into the various components affecting the development of each skill)

3. *Mental development objective*
a. Classification information
(1) Mental capacity
(2) Health education, physical education, and recreation background
(3) Academic background
(4) Moral background
(5) Home environment
b. Achievement information—such knowledge, attitudes, and practices as:
(1) Rules of games
(2) First-aid procedures
(3) General health, health habits, proper living, health knowledge
(a) Personal
(b) Community
(c) Mental
(d) Social
(e) Emotional
(4) Rules of safety
(5) Proper forms in games, athletic events, swimming, dancing, and other physical activities
(6) Etiquette in certain game situations
(7) Team play
(8) Strategy in games and events
(9) Regulations governing meets, tournaments, and other athletic events
(10) Duties of officials
(11) Physical activities
(12) Values of health and physical education
(13) Techniques
(14) Historical background of games and activities

(15) Principles of hygiene and sanitation
(16) Effect of exercise on body
(17) Best kind of exercise to take under certain circumstances

c. Diagnostic information
(1) Mental capacity
(2) Health and physical education background
(3) Academic background
(4) Interest
(5) Home environment
(6) Physical fitness
(7) Achievement records
(8) Health records

d. Prognostic information
(1) Mental capacity
(2) Interest
(3) Physical fitness
(4) Achievement records
(5) Health records

4. *Human relations development objective*

a. Classification information
(1) Character
(2) Personality
(3) Mental health
(4) Social attitudes
(5) Conduct
(6) Habits
(7) Citizenship
(8) Emotions
(9) Drives
(10) Appreciations
(11) Interests
(12) Capacity for leadership
(13) Ability to transfer training
(14) Group living
(15) Sportsmanship
(16) Service to community

b. Achievement information
(1) Character and personality
(a) Honesty
(b) Loyalty
(c) Fair play
(d) Good sportsmanship
(e) Courage
(f) Unselfishness
(2) Leadership

(a) Initiative
(b) Cooperation
(c) Quickness of decision
(d) Fairness and judgment
(e) Vision and imagination
(f) Executive ability
(g) Ability to get along with others
(h) Personal magnetism

(3) Transfer of training
(a) From game situations to other situations in life
(b) Motor transfer—capacity to solve motor situations and to make a new coordinated movement accurately

(4) Habits and practices
(a) Health (eating, sleeping, bathing, and so on)
(b) Exercise and recreation

(5) Attitudes and appreciations
(a) Value of health
(b) Value of physical recreation
(c) Good sportsmanship
(d) Team play
(e) Value of acquiring certain skills
(f) Appreciation of recreation and exercise
(g) Appreciation of health and practicing health habits
(h) Attitude toward cheating
(i) Attitude toward winning
(j) Attitude toward intraschool versus interschool competition
(k) Appreciation of playing with the "dub"
(l) Appreciation of training for competition
(m) Appreciation of ways of spending leisure time
(n) Appreciation of awards and rewards

(6) Social attitudes
(a) Toward individuals of dif-

ferent race, color, and creed
  (b) Toward good citizenship
  (7) Emotions
  (8) Service to community
c. Diagnostic information
  (1) Health and physical education background
  (2) Mental capacity
  (3) Character
  (4) Family background
  (5) Companions
  (6) Personality
  (7) Emotional control
  (8) Drives
  (9) Interests
  (10) Group living
  (11) Sportsmanship
  (12) Physical fitness
d. Prognostic information
  (1) Sportsmanship
  (2) Character
  (3) Personality
  (4) Mental capacity
  (5) Group living
  (6) Leadership
  (7) Emotional control
  (8) Habits
  (9) Attitudes and appreciations
  (10) Physical fitness
  (11) Interests
  (12) Personal ambitions
  (13) Home environment
  (14) Parental influence

TECHNIQUES AND INSTRUMENTS FOR OBTAINING DESIRED INFORMATION ABOUT STUDENTS

There are many techniques and instruments that can be utilized to obtain the various types of classification, achievement, diagnostic, and prognostic information about students. A few examples are listed for each category.

Classification information

An example of an instrument that would yield classification information is McCloy's Classification Index I.* This classification index takes into consideration such items as age, height, weight, and athletic skill, with a simple formula developed for the calculation of the index.

Another example of an instrument that could prove helpful for classification purposes is the Wetzel Grid.† This is valuable in either school health or physical education programs since it takes into consideration such elements as physique, developmental level, and nutritional progress with respect to weight, age, and height.

Achievement information

An example of an instrument that reflects achievement information would be the Indiana Physical Fitness Text.‡ This instrument involves such test items as straddle chins, squat-thrusts, push-ups, and vertical jumps. Norms have been developed for boys and girls.

There are many achievement tests available that can be utilized by school and college programs of health and physical education. Some excellent tests are listed in a later section of this chapter.

Diagnostic information

Examples of diagnostic techniques for a school or college health program would be the health examination, audiometer, and vision tests. These techniques or instruments yield information on an individual's health, including heart, lungs, teeth, hearing, vision, and posture.

An example of a diagnostic instrument

---

*McCloy, C. H., and Young, N. D.: Tests and measurements in health and physical education, ed. 3, New York, 1954, Appleton-Century-Crofts, pp. 59-60.

†Wetzel, N. C.: Grid for evaluating physical fitness, Cleveland, 1948, National Education Association Service, Inc.

‡State of Indiana Department of Public Instruction: High school physical education course of study, Bulletin 222, Indianapolis, 1958, The Department.

in physical education would be the Dyer Backboard Test* for tennis. This test evaluates general tennis ability. It does not analyze the various strokes and elements of the game. It merely consists of volleying a tennis ball as rapidly as possible against a backboard.

Prognostic information

An example of a prognostic instrument would be a sociometric test, which reflects a person's ability to get along with others. Another instrument would be a test of mental capacity to forecast academic achievement. Also, it could be a health record to forecast certain aspects of mental health essential to success in various endeavors. It could be a test of general motor ability to forecast achievement in specific skills. Several types of measurement instruments yield information that would forecast future performance in many of life's activities.

TECHNIQUES AND INSTRUMENTS FOR OBTAINING INFORMATION ABOUT OBJECTIVES

In addition to gaining classification, achievement, diagnostic, and prognostic information about students, it also is necessary to identify particular instruments, materials, resources, and methods for evaluating pupil status in respect to organic, neuromuscular, mental, and social development.

Organic development objective

A medical examination is a valuable technique for obtaining information about the organic development of the pupil. Such an examination should be given at least once a year by a competent physician.

Physical fitness tests will be helpful in determining student status in regard to this objective. Several excellent tests are listed in Chapter 11.

Other tests that should be reviewed as possible instruments for determining the organic development status of pupils are as follows*:

Circulatory-respiratory tests
  Cureton All-Out Treadmill Test
  Henry Tests of Vasomotor Weakness
  MacCurdy-Larson Organic Efficiency Test
  Schneider Cardiovascular Test
  Turner Test of Circulatory Reaction to Prolonged Standing
  Tuttle Pulse-Ratio Test

Anthopometric, posture, and body mechanics measurements
  Cureton Technique for Scaling Postural Photographs and Silhouettes
  Cureton Tissue Symmetry Test
  Cureton-Grover Fat Test
  Cureton-Gunby Conformateur Test of Antero-Posterior Posture
  Cureton-Holmes Tests for Functional Fitness of the Feet
  Cureton-Nordstrom Skeletal Build Index
  Cureton-Wickens Center of Gravity Tests

Muscular strength, power, and endurance tests
  Anderson Strength Index for High School Girls
  Carpenter Strength Test for Women
  Cureton Muscular Endurance Tests
  Larson Dynamic Strength Test for Men
  MacCurdy Test of Physical Capacity
  McCloy Athletic Strength Index
  Rogers Physical Capacity Test and Physical Fitness Index
  Wendler Strength Index

---

*Dyer, J. T.: The backboard test of tennis ability, Supplement to the Research Quarterly 6:63, 1935; Revision of backboard test of tennis ability, Research Quarterly 9:25, 1938.

*These tests may be found in copies of Research Quarterly, American Association of Health, Physical Education, and Recreation, or in one of the measurement and evaluation texts listed in the selected references at the end of this chapter.

Flexibility tests

Cureton Flexibility Tests

Leighton Flexometer Tests

Neuromuscular development objective

Physical skills represent a major part of the physical education program; therefore, appropriate valid tests of physical skills should be utilized. Such qualities as *motor educability, motor capacity, physical capacity, motor ability, and motor efficiency* are terms frequently utilized in connection with neuromuscular development.

Tests have been developed for skills in sports such as archery, badminton, soccer, basketball, bowling, football, golf, handball, field hockey, and ice hockey. Descriptions of these tests are given in some of the source books listed at the end of this chapter. These suggested tests should be studied carefully to determine their suitability or adaptability to a particular school situation. Some of the instruments that should be explored in measuring this objective in students are as follows:

Motor fitness tests

Bookwalter Motor Fitness Tests

Cureton-Illinois Motor Fitness Tests

O'Connor-Cureton Motor Fitness Tests for High School Girls

General motor skills tests

Brace Test of Motor Ability

Carpenter Test of Motor Educability for Primary Grade Children

Cozens Test of General Athletic Ability

Humiston Test of Motor Ability for Women

Iowa Revision of the Brace Motor Ability Test

Johnson Test of Motor Educability

Larson Test of Motor Ability for Men

Metheny Revision of the Johnson Test

Powell-Howe Motor Ability Tests for High School Girls

Scott Test of Motor Ability for Women

Sports skills tests

Borleske Touch Football Test for Men

Cureton Swimming Endurance Tests

Cureton Swimming Tests

Dyer Backboard Test of Tennis Ability

Johnson Basketball Test for Men

Lehsten Basketball Test for Men

Rodgers-Heath Soccer Skills Tests for Elementary Schools

Russell-Lange Volleyball Test for Girls

Schmithals-French Field Hockey Tests for Women

Young-Moser Basketball Test for Women

One of the most significant new developments in the area of skill measurement is being encouraged under the sponsorship of the American Association for Health, Physical Education, and Recreation. During the past few years their Research Council has been working to devise tests and norms for effective evaluation of boys and girls, grades five through twelve, in physical education programs across the United States. This total project includes skill tests for such activities as:

Archery	Football	Softball
Badminton	Golf	Swimming
Baseball	Gymnastics	Tennis
Basketball	Lacrosse	Track and field
Field hockey	Soccer	Volleyball

Administrators should obtain the sports skills test manuals that have been developed. They will be most helpful not only for testing purposes but for instructional suggestions as well. Sample class composite record forms, data, and profile forms are also available from the Association.

Mental development objective

In the field of health education there are several tests for measuring health knowledge and attitudes. Solleder* has compiled a list of several of these instruments

---

*Solleder, M. K.: Evaluation instruments in health education, Washington, D. C., 1965, American Association for Health, Physical Education, and Recreation.

for each educational level. Such tests could be used to evaluate the effectiveness of teaching procedures, weaknesses in the instructional program, and health knowledge of students and for the purpose of grouping students in health classes. They could also be used to determine the impact of health instruction on health knowledge and the attitudes and practices of students, as well as to grade students.

In order to illustrate the types of tests available in health education, one test is listed for each educational level as taken from Solleder's compilation of health evaluating instruments:

Elementary school—Dzenowagis, J. G.: Self-Quiz of Safety Knowledge. This test has been developed to measure safety preparedness of pupils at the fifth- and sixth-grade levels. Available from the National Safety Council, School and College Department, 425 N. Michigan Ave., Chicago, Ill.

Junior high school—Kilander, H. F.: Nutrition Information Test. This test is designed for students in junior high school through college. Norms are available from Dr. H. F. Kilander, Wagner College, Staten Island, N. Y.

Senior high school—Thompson, C. W.: Thompson Smoking and Tobacco Knowledge Test. This test includes the most important physiologic, psychologic, and socioeconomic facts relating to smoking and tobacco. For more information on this test see Thompson, C. W.: Thompson Smoking and Tobacco Knowledge Test, Research Quarterly **35**:60, 1964.

Junior college—Junior College Health Knowledge Test. This multiple-choice test covers eleven areas of health instruction. For more information write to Supervisor of Health Education, P. O. Box 3307, Terminal Annex, Los Angeles, Calif. 90054.

College or university—Dearborn, T. H.: College Health Knowledge Test. For more information write to Stanford University Press, Stanford, Calif.

In the field of physical education, several standardized tests are available for written tests in various sports. Also, some tests may be found in rule books and source books. Some knowledge and understanding tests in physical education that should be explored are the French Tests for Professional Courses in Knowledge and Sports, Hewitt Comprehensive Tennis Knowledge

COMPARISON OF ESSAY AND OBJECTIVE TESTS

Characteristic	Essay test	Objective test
Preparation of test item	Items are relatively easy to construct	Items are relatively difficult to construct
Sampling of the subject matter	Sampling is often limited	Sampling is usually extensive
Measurement of knowledges and understandings	Items can measure both; measurement of understanding is recommended	Items can measure both; measurement of knowledges is emphasized
Preparation by pupil	Emphasis is primarily on larger units of material	Emphasis is primarily on factual details
Nature of response by pupil	Pupil organizes original response	Except for supply test items, pupil selects response
Guessing of correct response by pupil	Successful guessing is minor problem	Successful guessing is major problem
Scoring of pupil responses	Scoring is difficult, time-consuming, and somewhat unreliable	Scoring is simple, rapid, and highly reliable

From Ahmann, J. S.: Testing student achievements and aptitudes, New York, 1962, The Center for Applied Research in Education, Inc. (The Library of Education), p. 35.

Tests, Scott Badminton Knowledge Test, Scott Swimming Knowledge Test, and Scott Tennis Knowledge Test.

Teachers may devise their own tests appropriate to the subject and age level being taught. When teachers develop their own tests, however, they should keep in mind the following principles of test construction:

1. The items selected should stress the most important aspects of the material.
2. The length of the test should be determined in relation to the time available for testing.
3. The test should be appropriately worded and geared for the age level to be tested.
4. Questions or test items should be worded so as to avoid ambiguity.
5. Statements should be simple and direct, not tricky or involved.

Social development objective

There have been several tests developed in the school and college health program to indicate pupil attitudes and behavior. Solleder[*] has listed several of these in her publication. A sampling of these behavior and attitude instruments are as follows:

Elementary school—Yellen, S.: Health Behavior Inventory, 1963. Designed for grades three to six and covers such items as health habits, nutrition, safety, rest, and disease prevention. For more information on this test write to California Test Bureau, Monterey, Calif.

Junior high school—Colebank, A. D.: Health Behavior Inventory, 1963. Designed for grades seven to nine and covers various health information items through a 100-item test. For more information write to California Test Bureau, Monterey, Calif.

Senior high school—Johns, E. B., and Juhnke, W. L.: Health Practice Inventory, 1952. Covers thirteen health areas. Manual of directions and norms also available for senior high students. For more information write to Stanford University Press, Stanford, Calif.

College or university—Leonard, M. L., and

Horton, C. W.: An Inventory of Certain Practices in Health, 1949. Instrument can be used to study health behavior of college students. For more information write to California State Department of Education, Sacramento, Calif.

General tests of social adjustment have also been developed, such as the Bell Adjustment Inventory, Science Research Associates Inventory, Minnesota Multiphasic Personality Inventory, and Bernreuter Personality Inventory. The guidance department in almost any school or college would be a good source of information for many tests of social adjustment.

Attitudes may be measured in different ways. Three techniques utilized in this area are teacher evaluation (observation of students with an anecdotal record being kept by the teacher), opinion polls, and rating scales. The physical education teacher should ask for the assistance of other teachers, particularly of the guidance personnel, in this type of testing.

Sociometrics is being used extensively for measurement of social relationships as determined by use of a sociogram. The sociogram points out the natural leaders in the groups and the outsiders trying to become members. When used more than once with the same group, a comparison of the results indicates social growth or change. A sociogram may be taken, for example, by asking all members of a team to list two people whom they would like to have as their friends, with their choices limited to a given group or team. Results may be pictured with arrows pointing to the names listed.

MINIMUM AND DESIRABLE STANDARDS

Larson and Yocom[*] have developed a list of minimum and desirable standards

---

[*]Solleder, M. K., op. cit.

[*]Larson, L. A., and Yocom, R. D.: Measurement and evaluation in physical, health, and recreation education, St. Louis, 1951, The C. V. Mosby Co., p. 450.

RÉSUMÉ OF PERSONALITY TRAITS

Date_____

| Student | Home Room | Teacher | Subject |

Please check directly above the word or group of words which you think best describes the pupil. Give specific examples, if possible, in parentheses on same line with check or below under COMMENTS if you prefer.

1. INDUSTRY_____|_____|_____|_____|_____
   Needs | Needs | Prepares | Completes | Seeks
   constant | occasional | assigned | supplementary | additional
   prodding | prodding | work | work | tasks

2. STUDY HABITS_____|_____|_____|_____
   Poor | Fair | Good | Excellent

3. RESPONSIBILITY_____|_____|_____|_____
   Unreliable | Somewhat | Usually | Thoroughly | Assumes
   | dependable | dependable | dependable | responsi-
   | | | | bility

4. COOPERATION_____|_____|_____|_____
   Poor | Fair | Good | Excellent

5. HONESTY_____|_____|_____
   Questionable at times | Generally reliable | Completely reliable

6. MATURITY_____|_____|_____
   Immature | Of average maturity | Exceptionally mature

7. EMOTIONAL STABILITY_____|_____|_____
   Usually well balanced | Well balanced | Exceptionally stable

8. MANNERS_____|_____|_____
   Discourteous and | Usually courteous | Always courteous
   inconsiderate | and considerate

9. INFLUENCE_____|_____|_____|_____
   Occasionally | Passive | Average | Generally | Strong
   detrimental | | | beneficial

10. FURTHER COMMENTS: Outstanding personality traits, chief interests, social adjustments, unusual achievements, etc.

Résumé of personality traits. (From Bucher, C. A., Koenig, C. R., and Barnhard, M.: Methods and materials in secondary school physical education, ed. 3, St. Louis, 1970, The C. V. Mosby Co.)

Table 22-2. Minimum and desirable standards for a measurement program in health and physical education

Measurement of program outcomes (product)	Minimum standards	Desirable standards
Organic	Medical examination or a cardio-vascular test Physical (motor) fitness test	Medical examination (including a cardiovascular test) Muscular strength Body build Growth, nutrition, development Posture and body mechanics
Skills	General motor ability	Tests for each sport
Knowledge	Teacher-made tests	Standardized tests and teacher-made tests
Adjustment	Controlled observation	Standardized tests

for a measurement program in health, physical education, and recreation based on the premise that these specialized fields, as pertains to measurement, contribute to the attainment of objectives of organic development, skill or motor development, knowledge or mental development, and adjustment or human relations development. These standards are reproduced in Table 22-2.

Phillips* listed what she considered to be a *minimal program of measurement.* She pointed out that these are stated in general terms and that to prescribe standards for any particular situation, it would be necessary to have information on the quality and/or quantity of such factors as personnel, facilities, equipment, program teacher-pupil ratio. She listed the following six points:

1. A *health examination,* conducted by a medical doctor. The absolute minimum would be for the examination to be given to all incoming freshmen (or sophomores in the 3-year high school). It would be greatly improved if the physical education teacher could administer a posture screening test at the same time.

2. *Tests of neuromuscular skills.* These tests should be given during the final periods of instruction for each motor activity learned. This

provides the teacher and pupil with objective evidence of the pupil's status in the skill and may be used additionally for classification purposes for further instruction and/or for the developing of intramural teams in those cases where the activity is of the intramural type.

3. *Knowledge tests.* These tests should be given at least once a semester and should sample the information and knowledge learned during that time.

4. *Attitude tests.* While no specific recommendation will be made for giving attitude tests in this minimum program, it will be very strongly suggested that the teacher should be constantly alert in observing the behavior of his students. One of the most important of our physical education objectives is the development of good attitudes. The thoughtful teacher will understand that a real effort must be made if this objective is to be realized. Hence, the teacher must carry on a constant program of evaluation in his daily associations with his students and use his observations as a basis for discussion with the individual students.

5. An annual *motor fitness or physical fitness test.* This would provide the teacher and pupil with a yearly check on the progress of the pupil in this vital area of his development.

6. *Self-evaluation.* One of the most important recommendations for this program is one that may not have too much supporting evidence in the formal literature on physical education measurement and evaluation. This is to the effect that the teacher should be carrying on a constant program of self-evaluation, relative to his own professional, personal, and social growth and development, as well as to the quality and effective-

*Letter dated Nov. 15, 1955, from Marjorie Phillips, Indiana University.

ness of the program he is providing for his students.

If the program of self-evaluation is ineffective, then it would be reasonable to expect that the program of pupil evaluation will be equally ineffective.

KEEPING RECORDS AND USING TEST RESULTS

There are many clerical duties associated with the measurement program. For most effective use records should be kept up-to-date and new test results constantly analyzed in terms of student progress and program planning. In some school districts teacher aides and community volunteers have been used to do the clerical work. Also, in today's automation era some schools and colleges have found it advantageous to use IBM cards to record test results. It may also be helpful to maintain a record file of measurement instruments used, adding comments concerning possible success or problems involved in their administration. This would prevent repetition of testing with unsuitable instruments.

The purpose of testing is to help the student and improve the educational program. As pointed out earlier in this chapter, tests can yield classification, achievement, diagnostic, and prognostic information. Therefore, after the testing has been accomplished, the results should be used appropriately.

NEED FOR A STANDARDIZATION OF MEASUREMENT MATERIALS

There are at least three reasons why the need is great for a standardization of measurement materials for the fields of health and physical education.

In the first place, many of the techniques being used today have been developed by individuals who have failed to use or interpret correctly scientific methods of construction. As a result, there are materials being used in our schools and colleges that have either failed to be scientifically evaluated or else have fallen below acceptable standards. In light of these conditions, it is necessary to ensure that only materials that meet acceptable criteria will be used. Standardization would make such a practice possible.

In the second place, it is impossible to make comparisons between individuals of different localities because of the different

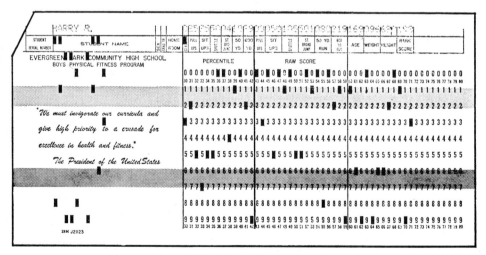

IBM card for recording test results. (From Bucher, C. A., Koenig, C. R., and Barnhard, M.: Methods and materials for secondary school physical education, ed. 3, St. Louis, 1970, The C. V. Mosby Co.)

techniques being used in each section. When a student transfers from one geographic locality to another, the instructor is at a loss to analyze his status, because of the lack of standards for all sections of the country. As a result, the instructor must start from the beginning in determining an individual's physical condition, traits, or characteristics. Standardization would make it possible for records to be interpreted intelligently, regardless of who administers the technique or the locality in which it is administered.

In the third place, it is difficult to measure progress on a national basis without the use of standards. It is imperative that measurement materials be standardized so that the professions can know whether they are meeting the objectives that have been set, can evaluate the various types of programs and instruction, and can know what they are achieving through these programs. Standardization would make it possible to better determine individual and program weaknesses, quality of instruction, and progress achieved. Furthermore, standardization would serve as a means of motivation and comparison.

GRADING

The giving of grades in school programs of health and physical education represents

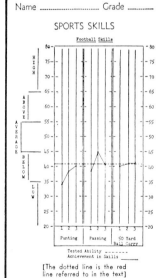

Barrington, Ill., Junior High School Physical Education Progress Report

Name .... Grade ....

SPORTS SKILLS

The chart below indicates the achievement level of the student in performing stunts on gymnastic apparatus. Those in the elementary classification have yet to accomplish all of the fundamental strength building stunts. The intermediate or advanced student is engaged in more difficult phases of the gymnastic activities.

Gymnastic Apparatus

Achievement Level Reached	
Elementary	
Intermediate	✓
Advanced	

Personal Qualities

Cleanliness	
Appearance	
Uniform	
Cooperation	
Courtesy (Manners)	
Promptness	X
Responsibility	
Self-control	X
Sportsmanship	
Team Work	
Aggressiveness	
Courage	
Honor	

A check (X) following any of the qualities shows a need for improvement.
No check indicates performance that is satisfactory or better.

Comments:

The graph above indicates the scores of the student's tested performance and achievement in sports skills compared with his tested ability score. The student's performances should be near or above the horizontal line (dotted) which represents his ability level. It is hoped that his performances on each test indicate some learning and achievement. The vertical lines in each skill column represent each time the student was tested in that skill.

[The dotted line is the red line referred to in the text]

Dear Parent:

This period has been used for the learning and practicing of the basic skills of football and gymnasium apparatus. The boys were tested on their ability to perform the various football skills, individual instruction was given, and vigorous team games giving practice in the skills were played. Making use of its seasonal popularity, football was presented as a means for assisting your boy's physical, mental, and social development and to improve his skill so he may play the game of football with satisfaction and skill if he chooses to select it as a school activity.

Apparatus work on the side horse, parallel bars, traveling rings, trampoline, horizontal bar, flying rings, balance beam, and climbing rope was presented to develop arm and shoulder strength, body control, and courage. It is felt that your boy has made gains in these areas no matter what achievement level he has reached.

Weight training with barbells was also offered to supplement the apparatus exercises.

Experiences in social dancing were presented to give the students the skills necessary for them to enjoy participating at school parties and during the lunch time recreation period.

H. C. Price
Instructor

Signature of parent or guardian

Physical education progress report, Barrington, Ill., Junior High School. (From Bucher, C. A., Koenig, C. R., and Barnhard, M.: Methods and materials for secondary school physical education, ed. 3, St. Louis, 1970, The C. V. Mosby Co.)

an administrative necessity. The purposes for grading include the following:

1. It serves as a means of indicating student achievement in the areas for which the course or experience is offered.
2. It serves as a means of informing such persons as parents, employers, colleges and universities, honorary societies, and other groups of the quality of a pupil's work.

3. It serves as a motivational device for some students.
4. It serves as a guide to program planning and for the grouping of students (grades identify areas of strength and weakness in the curriculum and in the students) and as a basis for counseling students (abrupt changes in a student's grades might be indicative of problems).

Since grading is an established custom

PHYSICAL EDUCATION REPORT CARD
NASHVILLE CITY SCHOOLS

Pupil_____School_____

Homeroom_____Classroom _____Year 19_____ 19_____

GRADE LEVEL	FALL					SPRING					YEAR'S AVERAGE
	1	2	3	Ex	Av	4	5	6	Ex	Av	

Items checked (✔) below need improvement

	1	2	3	4	5	6
Develops co-ordination						
Shows knowledge of rules						
Develops physically						
Strength						
Endurance						
Weight						
Participates						
Dress						
Playing						
Shower						
Attendance (Days absent from class)						
Conduct						

CODE
(Teacher may add plus or minus if she wishes)

A=90 - 100—Consistently does excellent work   C=75 - 81—Does fair work
B =82 - 89—Does good work   D=70 - 74—Low, but passing
    F =Below 70—Failing

Comments enclosed   Date_____ Date_____ Date_____
    Date_____ Date_____ Date_____

Teacher_____

Physical education report card, Nashville city schools. (From Bucher, C. A., Koenig, C. R., and Barnhard, M.: Methods and materials for secondary school physical education, ed. 3, St. Louis, 1970, The C. V. Mosby Co.)

in the educational system of this country, physical education must conform and grant grades or utilize some other method of denoting the progress that has been achieved.

Grades have been issued in physical education in several ways, ranging from granting letter or numeral grades to ranking in a class. These grades have also been based on many factors, many of which have questionable value. Some present practices base grades on such factors as attendance, punctuality, effort, costume, achievement, general attitude, initiative, hygiene, skill, knowledge of rules, cooperation, posture, strength, and endurance. Nationally, there seems to be no set formula or procedure. Each individual instructor establishes the basis on which grades should be granted.

The following recommendations represent some of the more advanced thinking among educators in general. At the elementary level especially, the feeling is increasing that it is not wise to issue a single

ATTITUDES AND PRACTICES	Items checked (✔) below need improvement					
	1	2	3	4	5	6
SOCIAL						
Uses self-control						
Is courteous in speech and action						
Co-operates						
Cares for property (incl. textbooks)						
Is considerate toward others						
Respects and obeys school rules						
WORK						
Makes good use of abilities						
Follows directions promptly						
Completes each task						
Works independently						
Uses initiative						
HEALTH						
Maintains personal cleanliness						
Maintains correct posture						
Obeys safety precautions						

PARENT'S SIGNATURE

1. _____

2. _____

3. _____

4. _____

5. _____

6. _____

For legend see opposite page.

grade or numerical rating. It is felt that a descriptive paragraph telling in more detail what progress is being made by the pupil is much better. Discussing such items as a student's strengths and weaknesses and where he needs to improve is much more meaningful and purposeful. This type of report and talks with parents will better achieve the purpose of showing to what degree educational objectives are being attained and what needs to be accomplished in the future. This method also has implications for grading above the elementary level.

When grades are given, they should be based on the achievement of objectives— the degree to which the student has achieved the desired outcomes. These objectives should be clear in the instructor's and students' minds at the outset of the course so that the desired direction will be known. The individuals getting the best grades would be those students most nearly achieving the objectives that have been listed as desirable goals for the course. In physical education the physical, motor, mental, and human relations objectives would all be kept in mind.

A further recommendation is that, as far as possible, the degree to which desired objectives are achieved should be determined objectively rather than subjectively. This means that wherever possible scientific evaluation and measurement techniques should be utilized. Since there is a dearth of such techniques, some subjective judgments will have to be made.

Grades should be understood by the student. He or she should know how they are arrived at and how the factors that go into the grades are weighed. The grades should also be easily understood by parents, particularly as to how they relate to the objectives of the course the student is taking. As far as possible, the grades should be expressed in the same manner as grades in other subject matter areas throughout the school. This not only facilitates record keeping and transfer of credits but also places health and physical education on the same level as other subjects.

The State Department of Public Instruction at Bismarck, North Dakota, has established some standards for grading in that state. Some excerpts* from their grading policy read as follows:

The hit or miss method of purely subjective grading in physical education so widely used cannot be too strongly condemned. The grade in physical education should be an accurate reflection of how well the pupil has achieved the objectives. It is suggested that the following points be considered in grading:

(a) The system for reporting grades should conform to the system generally used by the school as a whole.

(b) Basis for the grade:
50%, Achievement of physical skill and activity.
30%, Specific health and social qualities.
20%, Knowledge of rules and techniques.

An 'A' student is *superior* in that he:

(a) Is keenly enthusiastic. Persists industriously at his tasks.

(b) Acts intelligently on his own initiative.

(c) Shows positive leadership.

(d) Carries out responsibilities faithfully and honestly.

(e) Displays superior general ability and form.

(f) Is well liked by most of his fellow students, tactful to those in authority and to those he leads.

(g) Is a gracious winner and a good leader and encourages the same in others.

A 'B' student is *excellent* in that he:

(a) Is usually enthusiastic and generally industrious.

(b) Cooperates well with leaders.

(c) Follows directions intelligently without much help.

(d) Generally carries out his share of group activity.

(e) Has good general ability and form.

(f) Has few enemies and gets along well with others.

(g) Seldom displays poor sportsmanship.

---

*Department of Public Instruction: Health education in secondary schools, Bismarck, N. D., 1950, State Department of Public Instruction, pp. 48-49.

A 'C' student is *average* in that he:
  (a) Is passive as a rule. Willing to do as told.
  (b) Is not outstanding in understanding. A little slow at times.
  (c) Usually cooperates. Never assumes leadership.
  (d) Will work with assistance.
  (e) Has some friends and some enemies but none outstanding.
  (f) Has fair ability. Learns slowly at times.
  (g) Displays poor sportsmanship occasionally.

A 'D' student is *below average* in that he:
  (a) Is disinterested and reticent. Tends to avoid work.
  (b) Does not understand directions. Makes frequent errors.
  (c) Must be led and watched.
  (d) Will avoid responsibility frequently.
  (e) Has poor ability and little form. A slow learner.
  (f) Tends to be reclusive or unsociable.

  (g) Is poor in skill. Either has no skill or won't use it.

A student will probably not be completely described by any one of the descriptive groups listed, but as a rule traits above and below the group most descriptive of the individual will level each other into the middle group.

The thinking in regard to grading in physical education is well summarized by the American Association for Health, Physical Education, and Recreation*:

1. Specific goals and objectives should be established with students.

*American Association for Health, Physical Education, and Recreation: Administrative problems in health education, physical education, and recreation, Washington, D. C., 1953, The Association, p. 74.

PASSING OR FAILING IN PHYSICAL EDUCATION*

In response to numerous inquiries from school officials, the following is intended to clarify the statement that boards of education may not refuse graduation or promotion because of failure in physical education.

Physical education is required for all pupils by Education Law and Regulations of the Commissioner of Education. It is expected that each pupil will participate in such classes and that he will exert sufficient effort to enable him to achieve his optimal progress toward all program objectives. If a pupil refuses to attend physical education classes and otherwise does not fulfill course requirements approved by the board of education, and prompt and appropriate notification is given to all concerned, a failing mark may be given and graduation withheld until such time as the deficiency has been removed.

On the other hand, a pupil who fulfills all the requirements and has exhibited acceptable evidence of satisfactory progress in terms of his abilities but who has been unable to meet minimal standards of physical performance may not be given a failing mark in physical education.

Pupils who act in ways deemed undesirable as good school citizens while participating in physical education classes, such as disobeying the teacher, refusing to exert reasonable effort or deliberately violating stated policies and procedures, should be treated as disciplinary cases.

Physical education is an integral part of the school curriculum. It is recognized that achievement of the program's major goals including physical fitness, skills, knowledge, social qualities and attitudes will help provide valuable assets for each pupil. Therefore, every effort should be made to insure that physical education is a meaningful and profitable experience for each boy and girl, particularly for those who possess lower levels of physical ability. One of the most valuable outcomes of a physical education program is the inculcation of a strong appreciation of, desire for and interest in participation in physical activities which will endure throughout life. Would failing in physical education help to reach this goal?

Reviewed and Approved by Division of Law,
State Education Department,
January, 1969

*From New York State Education Department: Curriculum guide: physical education in the secondary school, 1964, p. 21.

Student ....

....

Grade   19............. - 19......

RICHWOODS COMMUNITY HIGH SCHOOL

Progress Report in Physical Education

....	....
Teacher	Counselor

1st pd.	2nd pd.	3rd pd.	Sem. exam	Sem. avg.	4th pd.	5th pd.	6th pd.	Sem. exam	Sem. avg.	Units crdt.

EXPLANATION OF MARKING SYSTEM

Achievement—Grading for actual work done by the student

A—94-100—Excellent   D—70-77—Below Average
B—86- 93—Above Avg.   F—Below 70—Failure
C—78- 85—Average   E—Conditional
                            Inc.—Incomplete

ACTIVITIES INCLUDED IN GRADING PERIODS

ACTIVITIES	PERIOD					
	1	2	3	4	5	6
Flicker Ball						
Flag Football						
Soccer						
*Field Hockey						
*Speed Ball						
*Campcraft						
Basketball (beginning) (advanced)						
Volleyball (beginning) (advanced)						
Tumbling (beginning) (advanced)						
Apparatus (beginning) (advanced)						
Wrestling (beginning) (advanced)						
Handball						
Badminton						
Recreational Games						
*Fundamental Rhythms—Modern Dance						
Track and Field						
Softball						
Archery						
Golf						
Co. P.E. Social Dance						
Co. P.E. Square Dance						
Co. P.E. Volleyball & Rec. Games						
Driver Training (Classroom)						
Health Education (Classroom)						
*Indicates Girls' Activity Only						

GRADING PROCEDURE

The six week grade is evaluated in the following areas:
1. Performance of Skills
2. Knowledge of Skills and Physical Fitness
3. Social Attitudes including cooperation, sportsmanship, and leadership
4. Hygiene conditions (uniforms, showers), and attendance.

PHYSICAL FITNESS TESTS
(Based on National Norms)

	Trial 1 (Fall)		Trial 2 (Spring)	
	Score	% ile	Score	% ile
Pull-Ups (Boys) (shoulder strength)	....	....	....	....
Modified Pull-Ups (Girls) (shoulder strength)	....	....	....	....
Sit-Ups (abdominal strength)	....	....	....	....
Shuttle Run (agility)	....	....	....	....
Standing Broad Jump (leg power)	....	....	....	....
50-Yard Dash (speed)	....	....	....	....
Softball Throw (arm power)	....	....	....	....
600-Yard Run-Walk (endurance)	....	....	....	....

The National Norms and Scores are based on Age, Weight, and Height.

PARENT'S SIGNATURE

Your signature means only that you have seen this report.

1st Period...

2nd Period...

3rd Period...

4th Period...

5th Period...

Each absence, however short, interferes with the student's progress.

Progress report in physical education, Richwoods Community High School, Peoria Heights, Ill. (From Bucher, C. A., Koenig, C. R., and Barnhard, M.: Methods and materials for secondary school physical education, ed. 3, St. Louis, 1970, The C. V. Mosby Co.)

2. Marks should relate to the attainment of these goals and objectives.
3. Students should be informed of how marks will be determined.
4. Marks shall be based upon several factors rather than a single item alone.
5. Evaluation techniques should be valid, reliable, objective, and standardized whenever possible.
6. The place of improvement shall be determined in advance.
7. Personalities shall be removed as a factor in the final mark.
8. The mark should not only inform but it should also suggest ways of improvement.

Table 22-3 outlines a proposed plan by Dr. Lynn McCraw for grading as a means

Table 22-3. Proposed plan for grading*

Components	Weightings	Instruments
Attitude in terms of Attendance Punctuality Suiting out Participation	5% to 25%	Attendance and other records Teacher observation
Skills in terms of Form in execution of skill Standard of performance Application in game situation	20% to 35%	Objective tests Teacher observation Student evaluation
Physical fitness with emphasis on Muscular strength and endurance Cardiovascular-respiratory endurance Agility Flexibility	20% to 35%	Objective tests Teacher observation
Knowledge and appreciation of Skills Strategy Rules History and terms	5% to 25%	Written tests Teacher observation
Behavior in terms of Social conduct Health and safety practices	5% to 25%	Teacher observation Student evaluation

*From McCraw, L. W.: Principles and practices for assigning grades in physical education, Journal of Health, Physical Education, and Recreation **35**:2, 1964.

of assessing the various objectives in an objective manner.

Questions and exercises

1. Define the term *measurement*. Why is it important to the successful administration of any program of health, physical education, or recreation?
2. List as many measurement techniques as possible that are utilized in the schools. Take three of these and describe their use in detail.
3. What is the relationship of measurement to objectives?
4. Why is it important to have classification, achievement, diagnostic, and prognostic information about each individual participating in the program of health, physical education, and/or recreation?
5. What are some general guides in respect to the measurement program that should be known by every administrator and teacher?
6. List and describe the various criteria essential to the construction and selection of scientific tests.
7. How would the standardization of measurement materials contribute to better programs of health, physical education, and recreation?
8. What are the minimum and desirable standards for a measurement program?
9. Develop what you consider to be a satisfactory and practical measurement program for a health, physical education, and/or recreation program.

Reading assignment in *Administrative Dimensions of Health and Physical Education Programs, Including Athletics:* Chapter 17, Selections 91 to 93.

Selected references

Ahmann, J. S.: Testing student achievements and aptitudes, New York, 1952, The Center for Applied Research in Education, Inc. (The Library of Education).

American Association for Health, Physical Education, and Recreation: Research methods applied to health, physical education, and recreation, Washington, D. C., 1949, The Association.

American Association of Health, Physical Education, and Recreation: Sports skills test manuals (archery, basketball, football, softball), 1966, 1967, The Association.

American Association for Health, Physical Education, and Recreation: Grading in physical education, Journal of Health, Physical Education, and Recreation 38:34, 1967.

Bonney, M. E., and Hampleman, R. S.: Personal-social evaluation techniques, New York, 1962, The Center for Applied Research in Education, Inc. (The Library of Education).

Boyd, C. A., and Waglow, I. F.: The individual achievement profile, The Physical Educator 21:3, 1964.

Clarke, H. H.: Application of measurement to health and physical education, ed. 4, Englewood Cliffs, N. J., 1967, Prentice-Hall, Inc.

Fabricius, H., and others: Grading in physical education, Journal of Health, Physical Education, and Recreation 38:5, 1967.

Herman, W. L.: Teaching attitude as related to academic grades and athletic ability of prospective physical education teachers, The Journal of Educational Research 61:40, 1967.

Jensen, C.: Evaluate your testing program, The Physical Educator 21:149, 1964.

Jorndt, L. C.: Point systems—motivational devices, The Physical Educator 23:1, 1966.

Larson, L. A., and Yocom, R. D.: Measurement and evaluation in physical, health, and recreation education, St. Louis, 1951, The C. V. Mosby Co.

Latchaw, M., and Brown, C.: The evaluation process in health education, physical education, and recreation, Englewood Cliffs, N. J., 1962, Prentice-Hall, Inc.

Lawrence, T.: Appraisal of emotional health at the secondary school level, The Research Quarterly 37:2, 1966.

Liba, M. R., and Loy, J. W.: Some comments on grading, The Physical Educator 22:4, 1965.

Link, F. R.: To grade or not to grade, The PTA Magazine 62:10, 1967.

Mathews, D. K.: Measurement in physical education, ed. 2, Philadelphia, 1963, W. B. Saunders Co.

Meyers, C. R., and Blesh, T. E.: Measurement in physical education, New York, 1962, The Ronald Press Co.

National Education Association: Reports to parents, National Education Association Research Bulletin 45:2, 1967.

National Research Council, American Association for Health, Physical Education, and Recreation: Measurement and evaluation materials in health, physical education, and recreation, Washington, D. C., 1950, The Association.

Oxendine, J. B.: Social development—the forgotten objective? Journal of Health, Physical Education, and Recreation 37:5, 1966.

Piscopo, J.: Quality instruction: first priority, The Physical Educator 21:4, 1964.

Smithells, P. A., and Cameron, P. E.: Principles of evaluation in physical education, New York, 1962, Harper & Row, Publishers.

Solleder, M. K.: Evaluation instruments in health education, Washington, D. C., 1965, American Association for Health, Physical Education, and Recreation.

Trump, C.: Meaningful grading, Scholastic Coach 35:44, 1966.

Evaluation as used in this chapter refers to the process of administration. The purpose of evaluation is to improve programs of health and physical education for the students. This includes attention to such items as determining the strengths and weaknesses of the leadership, program, facilities, and activities. A framework of evaluation procedures is discussed below to give the reader a clearer understanding of the types of information that may be evaluated.

FRAMEWORK FOR EVALUATION PROCEDURES

There are many items that can be evaluated in terms of the process of administration. These include an evaluation of various aspects of each category: in administration, this might include policies, finance, publicity, community relationship, and records; in leadership, performance, results, training, and qualifications; in facilities, the various factors that pertain to effective construction, use, and maintenance; in equipment, supply, use, cost, number, and maintenance; in activities, time, facilities, participation, and conduct; and in participation, utilization of facilities, and amount of time permitted.

MEANS FOR EVALUATION

Various means of evaluating educational programs have been devised. These range from very elaborate and detailed checklists, rating scales, and score cards to a list of questions that the administration should ask to determine the relative merit of certain administrative practices and programs.

For example, score cards such as the LaPorte Score Cards have been developed to rate health and physical education programs; Score Card 1 relates to the evaluation of health and physical education programs in the elementary school, and Score Card 2 is used for junior and senior high schools and 4-year high schools. These score cards cover such items as program of activities, class program, and intramural and interschool athletics. Each area can be rated according to a possible score that would represent an excellent program. The score cards have been successfully applied in several thousands of schools. Norms have been developed for purposes of comparison. Also some states, such as Ohio and Indiana, have developed program score cards that are pertinent to their respective states.

Many aspects of evaluation are discussed in this text in chapters that relate to such specific items as facilities, equipment and supplies, class program, health services, and a healthful environment. Therefore, this chapter is designed to cover the broad field of evaluation and to pay particular attention to teacher evaluation, which is of considerable concern to administration today. Recent advances in education have necessitated development of sound methods of rating teachers and their abilities.

TEACHER EVALUATION

In recent years, administrators, parents, teachers, and community have been concerned with developing ways and means of establishing methods to measure teacher effectiveness for the purpose of making sound decisions for retention, salary adjustments, and promotion, as well as to help teachers to improve.

The administration has an important role to play in the evaluation of teachers. Leadership needs to be provided in this area to establish a planned program of evaluation. Teachers need to be helped to improve their own effectiveness. Records should be kept to determine progress.

Some guidelines for the evaluation of teachers are as follows:

1. *Appraisal should involve the teachers themselves.* Evaluation is a cooperative venture and teachers should be involved in the development of the criteria for evaluation and need to understand the process.

2. *Evaluation should be centered on performance.* The job that is to be accomplished should be the point of focus with other extraneous factors omitted.

3. *Evaluation should be concerned with helping the teacher to grow on the job.* The purpose of evaluation is to help the teacher evaluate himself and maintain his strengths and reduce his weaknesses.

4. *Evaluation should look to the future.* It should be concerned with developing a better health program, a better physical education program, and a better school system.

5. *Evaluation of teachers should be well organized and administered,* with the step-by-step approach clearly outlined.

Fawcett* suggests the following outline, which includes some of the broad areas in which a teacher might be evaluated, as a means of initiating an evaluation program.

Interpersonal relations
 Teacher-teacher
 Teacher-students
 Teacher-parents
 Teacher-community
 Teacher-administrators

---

*Fawcett, C. W.: School personnel administration, New York, 1964. The Macmillan Co., pp. 58-59.

Classroom management
 Setting of classroom goals and individual learning goals for each student.
 Assignment and acceptance of individual responsibility by each student in the class.
 Confirmation of desired behavior of students and redirection of undesirable behavior.
 Exercise of authority to secure necessary decisions in the classroom.
 Research behavior of the teacher to keep goals and activities of the classroom consistent with the culture.
 Record-keeping behavior of the teacher essential to the conduct of the classroom.
 Coordination of the instruction in the classroom not only with other instructional activities of the school but with out-of-school learning experiences of the students.
 Inclusion of each student in the learning activities of the class.
 Communication in the classroom not only to make the teacher understand, but to make it possible for each person to share in classroom activities.
 Judgment in the allocation of time and resources to different activities in the classroom.

Teacher-learning
 1. Analysis of students:
  Skills
  Attitudes
  Knowledge
 2. Presentation of subject matter through:
  Lectures
  Group discussions
  Student research
  Programmed learning
 3. Utilization of instructional material and resources:
  Libraries
  Books
  Machines
  Television
  Radio
  Films
  Supplementary materials, organizations, and people of the community
 4. Creation of an efficient learning environment through organization of the physical surroundings in the classroom

Some methods of evaluating teachers are:

1. *Observation of teachers in the classroom or in the gymnasium.* The National Education Association Research Division, in studying this method, reported that the

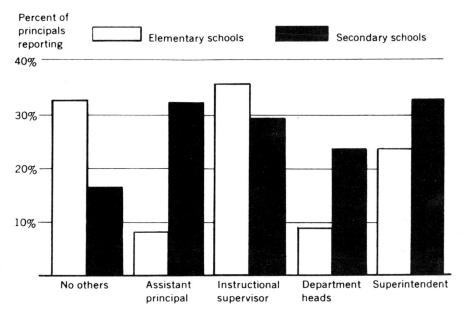

Who shares responsibility for evaluating probationary teachers with the school principal (limited to systems with written evaluations)? (From NEA Research Bulletin **42**:85, 1964.)

median length of time for the most recent observation was 22 minutes, about 25% of the teachers were notified 1 day in advance that the observation would take place, and about 50% of the teachers reported that a conference followed up the observation with the teacher's performance being discussed and evaluated. Nearly one-half of the teachers reported that the observation was helpful to them.

2. *Student progress.* With this method standardized tests are used to determine what progress the student has made as a result of exposure to the teacher.

3. *Ratings.* Ratings vary and may consist of an overall estimate of a teacher's effectiveness or consist of separate evaluations of specific teacher behaviors and traits. Self-ratings may also be used. Ratings may be conducted by the teacher's peers, by students, or by administrative personnel and may include judgments based on observation of student progress. In order to be effective, rating scales must be based on such criteria as objectivity, reliability, sensitivity, validity, and utility.

At college and university levels the evaluation of teacher performance is sometimes more difficult than at precollege levels because of the unwillingness of the faculty to permit members of the administration, or other persons, to observe them. Various methods have been devised in institutions of higher learning to rate faculty members, including statements from department heads, ratings by colleagues, ratings by students, and ratings by deans and other administrative personnel.

A question that frequently arises in the development of any system of teacher evaluation is: what constitutes effectiveness as it relates to a teacher in a particular school or college situation? Several studies have been conducted with some interesting findings. For example, there is only a slight correlation between intelligence and the rated success of an instructor. Therefore, the degree of intelligence a teacher has, within reasonable limits, seems to have little value as a criterion. The relation of knowledge of subject matter to effectiveness appears to relate most in particular

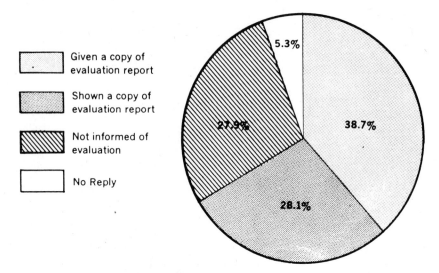

How teachers are informed of their evaluations. (From NEA Research Bulletin **42**:86, 1964.)

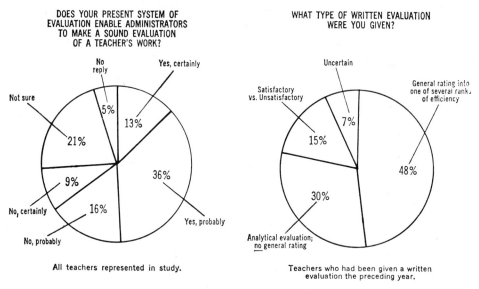

What teachers say about evaluation of teachers. (From NEA Research Bulletin **54**:38, 1965.)

teaching situations. A teacher's demonstration of good scholarship while in college appears to have little positive relationship to good teaching. There is some evidence to show that teachers who have demonstrated high levels of professional knowledge on National Teachers Examinations are more effective teachers. However, the evidence here is rather sparse. The relationship of experience to effectiveness also seems to have questionable value. Experience during the first 5 years of teaching seems to enhance teacher effectiveness but then levels off. There is little, if any, relationship between effectiveness and cultural background, socioeconomic status, sex, and marital status. Finally there is little evidence to show that any specified aptitude for teaching exists. The studies indicate that more research needs to be done in

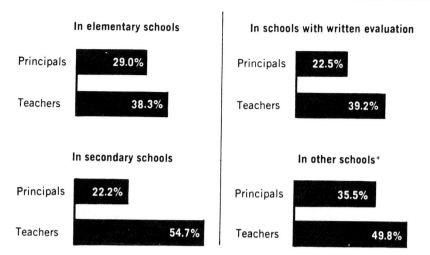

In elementary schools

Principals 29.0%

Teachers 38.3%

In schools with written evaluation

Principals 22.5%

Teachers 39.2%

In secondary schools

Principals 22.2%

Teachers 54.7%

In other schools[a]

Principals 35.5%

Teachers 49.8%

[a] Where there was no written evaluation in the school systems, or teachers did not receive a written evaluation in 1961-62, or were employed in a different school system in 1961-62, or who did not know whether there was written evaluation.

Principals and teachers express doubt or a negative opinion on the system of teacher evaluation. (From NEA Research Bulletin **42**:111, 1964.)

order to establish what constitutes teacher effectiveness on the job.

EVALUATING SCHOOL AND COLLEGE HEALTH PROGRAM ADMINISTRATION

Evaluation of the school or college health program represents a major undertaking. Checklists and other forms have been developed to rate the health instruction, health services, and healthful school or college environment aspects of the total program. Such instruments that have been developed to evaluate various aspects of school and college health programs are as follows:

1. Criteria for evaluating the elementary health program, Sacramento, Calif., 1962, California State Department of Education.
2. Evaluation criteria, health education, Washington, D. C., NSSSD, American Council on Education.
3. Illinois Curriculum Program: Health education program, inventory B; What should we do to strengthen our schools' health education program? Inventory C, Springfield, 1952, Department of Public Instruction.
4. LaPorte, W. A.: Health and physical education scorecard no. 1 and no. 2, College

Book Store, 3413 S. Hoover Blvd., Los Angeles, Calif.
5. Los Angeles City Schools: Health tests (for various grade levels), Los Angeles, 1962, Division of Educational Services, Los Angeles City Schools, School Publication 673.
6. Michigan School Health Association: Appraisal form for studying school health programs, 1962, The Association
7. Oregon State College: A school health program evaluation scale, Corvalis, 1955, Oregon State College.
8. Texas Education Agency: A checklist appraising the school health program, Bulletin 519, Austin, 1955, State Education Department.

To give the reader a clearer understanding of what a checklist for health education is like, a very abbreviated one developed in the state of Colorado is included (p. 635).

Other means of evaluating school and college health programs that have been utilized in addition to checklists and score cards in various parts of the nation are *questionnaires* that have been developed and sent to parents, students, and other individuals; *surveys* of interested groups of people; *expert evaluations* by authorities, such as sanitarians or curriculum special-

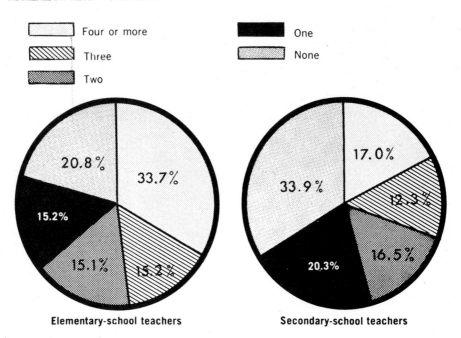

Number of times teachers were observed teaching in their classroom for 5 minutes or more, as reported by teachers from beginning of 1962-1963 term to February 1, 1963. (From NEA Research Bulletin **43**:14, 1965.)

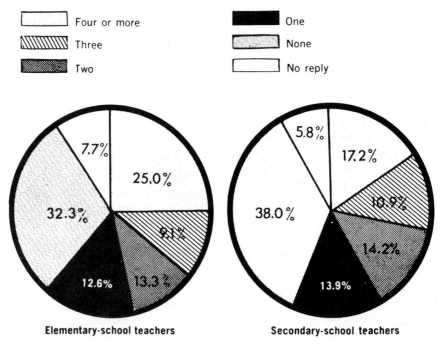

Number of individual conferences of 10 minutes or more that teachers had with principals or other school system official, as reported by teachers from beginning of 1962-1963 term to February 1, 1963. (From NEA Research Bulletin **43**:17, 1965.)

CHECKLIST FOR HEALTH EDUCATION*   *Yes   No*

1. *Sanitary, safe, and wholesome environment*
   a. Are the state-approved medical certificates required for all personnel?   —— ——
   b. Is there a written plan for first-aid care of illness and accidents?   —— ——
   c. Do the buildings and grounds meet state or local sanitary standards?   —— ——
   d. Are cases of communicable disease detected and excluded promptly according to state policy?   —— ——
   e. Are the state policies for busses being followed?   —— ——
   f. Are the state policies for lunchrooms being followed?   —— ——
2. *Graded health and safety education*
   a. Is there a written plan of health instruction throughout all the grades?   —— ——
   b. Is physical education a regular part of the program for all pupils?   —— ——
   c. Are pupils prepared to understand the health services offered in the school and community?   —— ——
   d. Are first-aid courses offered in the high school?   —— ——
3. *Detection of health problems that may diminish effectiveness of the educational program*
   a. Is vision of all pupils periodically checked?   —— ——
   b. Is hearing of all pupils regularly checked?   —— ——
   c. Are you using the new state bulletin on testing vision and hearing?   —— ——
   d. Is attention paid to periodic growth measurements?   —— ——
   e. Are children screened regularly for dental health?   —— ——
   f. Are medical evaluations of all pupils made periodically?   —— ——
   g. Are cumulative health records maintained on all pupils?   —— ——
4. *Guidance on these health problems of individual pupils, including counsel with parents and others*
   a. Is professional follow-up given to known health problems?   —— ——
   b. Are the community health facilities known and used?   —— ——
   c. Are these community facilities adequate for pupil needs?   —— ——
5. *Special facilities for physically, mentally, and emotionally exceptional children who are educable*   —— ——
   a. Are these pupils accurately classified for their learning potential?
   b. Are special programs available for all exceptional children?   —— ——

*From the Colorado Education Association's Journal, October, 1956.

---

ists; *analysis of health records; tests and inventories;* and *interviews and conferences.*

Evaluation is a continuous process to determine if the program is accomplishing the purposes for which it exists.

Johns* points out an evaluation experience with selected schools and colleges in the Los Angeles area where there was a concerted effort to determine the answers to such questions as: How good is the school health program? How well is it being carried out? How well does it compare to what should be done? Evaluations were carried out through self-appraisal as well as by outside consultants and resource persons. Three approaches to evaluation were utilized: (1) appraisals of the health education program, (2) appraisals of behavior changes in pupils as a result of exposure to the program, and (3) appraisals of the process of evaluation. Such procedures were followed as formulating, classifying, defining, and suggesting situations in which the achievement of objectives could be evaluated, tryout of different evaluation methods, developing and evaluating appraisal methods, and interpreting

*Johns, E.: An example of a modern evaluation plan, Journal of School Health 32:5, 1962.

results in light of a more effective health program. A handicapping condition in the study was the lack of available valid appraisal instruments for the total health program. The findings of this study were used to justify the significance of health education in the curriculum. Such an experiment has implications, it seems, for other schools and colleges throughout the United States.

Following is a list of pertinent questions compiled by Smolensky and Bonvechio to evaluate the total school health program:

School health and safety education

1. Which curriculum areas should be emphasized at the various grade levels?
2. What are the most significant present, future, and contemplated health and safety needs of the school-age population?
3. Where and how does health and safety instruction best fit into the crowded school curriculum?
4. What should be the scope and sequence of the health and safety units in the curriculum?
5. What experiences are most conducive to developing health-educated pupils and communities?
6. How can health instruction be best integrated through experiences in the school environment?
7. How can health services be made educational in nature and scope?
8. What instructional techniques and materials are needed?
9. How can in-service staff education be practically accomplished?

School health services

1. How can health appraisal of pupil and school personnel best be accomplished?
2. What is the most effective way to counsel pupils, parents, teachers, and others in interpreting the findings of health appraisal?
3. What can be done to encourage the correction of remediable health defects in children?
4. What is the most effective way to identify, health educate, and generally educate handicapped children?
5. How can the school best control and prevent the spread of disease?
6. What kinds of services, policies, and procedures best meet the needs for emergency services for school children?

7. How can school health service be made educational in nature?
8. What are the responsibilities of the home, school, family physicians, and public health organization for health services?
9. What is the most effective way to ensure communication and coordination between all persons and groups interested in improving child health?
10. Are the duties of the school health team well defined?

Healthful school living (environment)

1. Are all educational programs of the school contributing to the health and safety of the pupils and school employees?
2. Do school administrative policies and procedures contribute to the physical and emotional health of pupils, teachers, and school employees?
3. Is the school's physical and emotional environment conducive to effective learning?
4. Is the school lunch program contributing to nutritional education and good nutrition?
5. How can school sanitation be best maintained, improved, and promoted?
6. Are regular and continuous sanitary inspections made by qualified personnel?

Administration

1. Does the school administrator help to formulate, clarify, and evaluate the goals of the school health program?
2. Does the school administrator coordinate the efforts of all school personnel who work in the school health program?
3. Does he (school administrator) assign the most qualified personnel to the various tasks in the school health program?
4. Does the school make the best possible use of local health resources?
5. Does he (school administrator) adapt the school health program to local needs and interests?
6. Does he (school administrator) motivate others in the school health program through leadership?
7. Does the school have an effective school health council?
8. Does the school district have an effective school health committee?*

---

*Smolensky, J., and Bonvechio, L. R.: Principles of school health, Boston, 1966, D. C. Heath & Co., pp. 101-102 As adapted from Davis, R L: Quality in school health administration, National Elementary Principal 39:8, 1960.

EVALUATING SCHOOL AND COLLEGE PHYSICAL EDUCATION PROGRAM ADMINISTRATION

Evaluation of student achievement in physical education represents only part of the evaluation responsibility. Evaluation of program administration is also important. Such phases of the program as classes, intramurals, interscholastics, intercollegiates, and adapted physical education activities should be evaluated in terms of activities, leadership, equipment, facilities, participation, records, research, and budgetary allotment.

The following are sample questions such as might be formulated for use in evaluation of program administration. They might either be answered with ratings of poor, fair, good, or excellent or be scored on a numerical basis of 1 to 10.

Class program

1. Does the teaching program devote equitable time to team sports, individual sports, rhythms and dance, and gymnastic activities?
2. Are the equipment and facilities adequate to allow maximum student participation?

3. Are reasonable budgetary allotments made for the class teaching program?
4. Are accurate evaluation procedures carried out and worth-while records kept?
5. Are minimal participation requirements met by all students?
6. Are students meeting proper physical education requirements in regard to dressing and showering?
7. Are proper safety measures taken in all activities?
8. Are opportunities for developing student leadership being afforded in the class program?

Adapted program

1. Do adequate screening procedures determine all possible participants in this program?
2. Are adequate facilities, equipment, time, and space made available to the program?
3. Are proper supervision and instruction afforded each individual participant?
4. Is medical approval obtained for each individual's regimen of activity?
5. Do participants engage in some of the regular class work, as well as remedial classes, when advisable?
6. Are careful records and progress notes kept on each student?
7. Is the financial allotment to the program adequate?
8. Does student achievement indicate the value of the program?

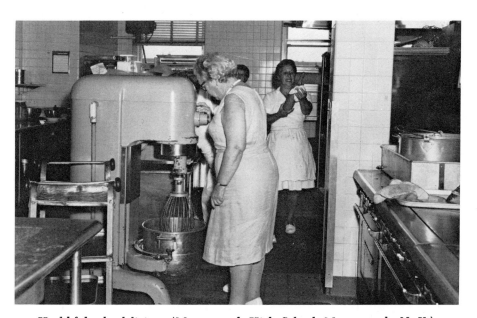

Healthful school living. (Mamaroneck High School, Mamaroneck, N. Y.)

Intramural and extramural programs

1. Are intramural and extramural sports offered to all students in as many activities as possible?
2. Has participation in these programs increased during the past year?
3. Is maximum coaching supervision available to players?
4. Is adequate financial assistance given to this phase of the program?
5. Are accurate records maintained concerning the participants, their honors, awards, and electives?
6. Does the reward or points system emphasize the joys of participation rather than stress the value of the reward?
7. Is equipment well cared for and properly stored to gain the most use from it?
8. Are competitive experiences wholesome and worth while for all participants?

Interscholastic program

1. Is financial support for this program provided by the physical education budget?
2. Is there equitable financial support for all sports in the interscholastic or intercollegiate program?
3. Are interscholastic and intercollegiate sports available to all students, boys and girls alike?
4. Are adequate health standards being met in respect to amount of practices, number of games, fitness of participants, and type of competition?
5. Is competition provided by schools and colleges of a similar size?
6. Is the program justifiable as an important educational tool?
7. Are academic standards for participants maintained?
8. Are good public relations with the community furthered through this program?

Administration

1. Is the teaching staff well qualified and capable of carrying out the program?
2. Is the program run efficiently with little loss of teaching time or space, and is maximum use made of facilities?
3. Are professional standards maintained as to class size and teacher assignment?
4. Is the departmental organization on a democratic basis, with all members sharing in the decisions?
5. Do members of the staff have a professional outlook, attend professional meetings, and keep up with the latest developments in the field?

6. In what areas have scientific tests and research been made for contribution to the profession?*

These sample questions represent only a few that can be used in the evaluation process. The key to successful evaluation of this type lies in the followup steps taken for improvement.

CHECKLIST AND RATING SCALE FOR THE EVALUATION OF THE PHYSICAL EDUCATION PROGRAM

An analysis of evaluation standards required by several state departments of education and those recommended by leading authorities in the field resulted in the formulation of the accompanying checklist and rating scale for evaluating various components of the physical education program. Space prevents a complete and extensive instrument; however, many of the most desirable professional standards are listed. Some of the evaluative criteria may not be directly applicable to a particular program. It is therefore recommended that the criteria be adapted where needed so as to better meet specific local needs.

In regard to scoring, it is recommended that each specific area of the rating form be scored so that a better picture can be gained of a department's strengths and weaknesses in respect to each aspect of the program. The first major section of the checklist and rating scale, "General administrative considerations" requires the checking of appropriate statements where applicable to a particular program of physical education. Each of the statements will be checked if the program meets the professional standards listed. If a statement cannot be checked, consideration should be given to upgrading this aspect of the

---

*Bucher, C. A., Koenig, C., and Barnhard, M.: Methods and materials for secondary school physical education, ed. 2, St. Louis, 1970, The C. V. Mosby Co.

STATE *of* NEBRASKA
DEPARTMENT OF HEALTH
DIVISION, HEALTH EDUCATION
STATE CAPITOL, LINCOLN

....
School's Name

....
Address

....
Signature of Representative

A GUIDE FOR EVALUATING PHYSICAL EDUCATION PROGRAMS

(Adapted from the evaluating criteria of the American Association for Health, Physical Education, and Recreation)

It should be understood that these are minimum standards. It is hoped that many schools will surpass the minimum and will continue to improve each semester.

To qualify for the citation, elementary schools should comply with **FIVE** of the first six standards; secondary schools should comply with **NINE** for the banner. The committee welcomes comments accompanying this application explaining your school's program on the back of this page.

YES   NO

1. Teacher-pupil ratio in a physical education class should not exceed 40 pupils.   ....

   a. Average size physical education class:

   Elementary (K-6)............................ High School (7-12)............................

2. There is balance in the physical education program with emphasis given to individual body building activities as well as to team sports and it is under a professionally qualified physical educator who follows an approved guide.   ....

   a. Person who is general supervisor of physical education classes or teachers:

   Elementary... Secondary...

   b. Basic guide followed:...

   c. Check areas of activity in your program:

Elementary	Secondary	Secondary
☐ 1. Low organized games & relays	☐ 1. Touch or flag football	☐ 11. Calisthenics
☐ 2. Track and field	☐ 2. Track and field	☐ 12. Soccer or speed ball
☐ 3. Self-testing	☐ 3. Testing	☐ 13. Field hockey
☐ 4. Rhythm	☐ 4. Rhythm	☐ 14. Bowling
☐ 5. Basketball	☐ 5. Basketball	☐ 15. Deck tennis
☐ 6. Flag or touch football	☐ 6. Softball	☐ 16. Handball
☐ 7. Softball	☐ 7. Tumbling & Apparatus gymnastics	☐ 17. Fencing
☐ 8. Tumbling	☐ 8. Wrestling	☐ 18. Tennis
☐ 9. Wrestling	☐ 9. Swimming	☐ 19. Shuffleboard
☐ 10. Calisthenics	☐ 10. Golf or tennis	☐ 20. Table tennis

3. Co-educational activities are included in the instructional program and are co-operatively planned and conducted by the men and women instructors.   ....

   a. List some co-educational activities carried out:

4. Modified or adapted activities are provided for students with special needs as based on information from medical data.   ....

   a. Briefly describe some plan you use for taking care of students with special needs:

5. A fitness test is given at least annually (twice per year is desired) and covers such components of fitness as muscular strength, endurance, speed, and agility.   ....

   a. Name of test used............................. b. Dates administered.............................

6. Efforts are made to publicize the physical education activities through demonstrations and public appearances and through local publications or news media.   ....

   a. List several specific instances:

7. Appropriate credit is given for class instruction in physical education and is required for graduation from junior and senior high school.   ....

   a. Amount credit given............................ b. Amount credit accepted for graduation............................

8. Activities such as band, marching, cheerleaders, driver education, and interscholastic athletics are not substituted for physical education.   ....

9. Physical education class participation is required for a minimum of 8 semesters in grades 7-12 and two days each week.   ....

   a. How many semesters of physical education are required 7-12?................................

   b. How many days per week required for each child?................................

10. An intramural program is open to boys and girls and provides competitive participation opportunities.   ....

    a. List two or three activities in which intramural competition is provided:

11. Appropriate uniforms and showering are required of all participants in secondary schools.   ....

These awards are made available by the Woodmen of the World Life Insurance Society, Omaha, Nebraska

A guide for evaluating physical education programs. (Nebraska Department of Health, Division of Health Education, Lincoln, Neb.)

program. The checklist and rating scale that follow, starting with the section on "Considerations in administering physical education programs," provide for a graded scoring system so that the highest rating in each instance would be 5. If rating is less than 5, the school or college system in question may wish to consider upgrading this particular administrative phase of the total physical education program.

CHECKLIST AND RATING SCALE FOR THE EVALUATION OF THE PHYSICAL EDUCATION PROGRAM

General administrative considerations

Philosophy—Physical education and the total school or college program:

——1. Physical education is a part of the total educational program.

——2. Objectives of physical education are a part of and contribute to the achievement of general education objectives.

——3. Physical education is viewed as education of and through the physical.

——4. The students represent the primary point of focus in the physical education program.

——5. Physical education is different from, but allied to, the areas of health, recreation safety, and outdoor education.

——6. The physical education program respects the worth and dignity of each individual.

Objectives—The physical education program strives to meet the following five general objectives:

——1. Physical

——2. Social

——3. Emotional

——4. Intellectual

——5. Personal

Curriculum

——1. The program has a complete, effective, and up-to-date curriculum guide.

——2. The curriculum guide and its related aspects are periodically evaluated and improvements are made on the basis of that evaluation.

——3. The curriculum calls for instruction in all areas as listed under facilities (see Facilities).

General administrative responsibilities

——1. Regular departmental meetings are held and all staff members attend.

——2. Uniform written policies and procedures are in effect for the entire department and are made available to appropriate school personnel.

——3. Other areas of the curriculum, such as driver education, interschool or intercollegiate athletics, band, etc., are not substituted for physical education.

——4. All physical education instructors are involved in program planning and evaluation in a meaningful way.

——5. Organizational structure permits the most efficient scheduling of instructional staff members.

——6. Assignments for class and extraclass activities result in an equitable and reasonable teaching load for all teachers.

——7. The development of a sound accident policy has been carried out, including safety procedures, first aid, hospitalization, reporting, etc.

——8. There is a qualified and designated person to inspect, maintain, and repair equipment.

——9. Individual conferences are held with all students.

——10. Economic, cultural, and social background are considered when screening students.

CHECKLIST AND RATING SCALE FOR THE EVALUATION OF THE PHYSICAL EDUCATION PROGRAM—cont'd

General administrative considerations–cont'd

——11. Lesson plans of a modified or complete nature are required where necessary for those on the instructional staff.

——12. A professional library is available and is continually being updated, including references and resource material.

——13. Periodic reports on the status of equipment and facilities are required.

——14. All committees are required to turn in written reports periodically.

——15. Complete records exist on grades, tests, and performances of each student.

——16. Test results and other evaluative materials are used to improve the program.

Considerations in the administration of physical education programs

Excuses from physical education classes

5 = In writing, by physician only.

3 = In writing, by parents or by decision of school personnel.

1 = By verbal request of student.

Recording attendance

5 = Well-designed and accurate means of determining absences, latenesses, excuses, etc.

3 = Accurate, but time consuming.

1 = Poorly done and lacks authoritativeness.

Provisions for excused students from regular class period

5 = Remedial or adaptive classes as recommended by physician.

3 = Aided and assisted by instructor within limits of physical disability.

1 = Excused from physical education to attend study hall, etc.

Required program

5 = Physical education is required at all grade levels for all pupils and includes adaptive classes.

4 = Physical education is required at all grade levels only for those who can qualify for the regular program.

3 = Physical education is required for all those who do not participate in extramural activities.

2 = Physical education is required only for those who are very low in physical fitness.

1 = Physical education is purely elective in nature.

Required classes per week

5 = Five times per week, not including out-of-class activities, for precollege level and two times per week for college level.

4 = Five times per week supplemented with intramurals or extramurals. (Two times per week supplemented with intramurals or extramurals at college level.)

3 = Four times per week in any combination. (One time per week in any combination at college level.)

2 = Three times per week in any combination. (One time per week in any combination at college level.)

1 = Less than three times per week in any combination. (Less than one time per week in any combination at college level.)

Length of each class

5 = 60 minutes or more.

4 = 50 to 59 minutes.

3 = 40 to 49 minutes.

2 = 30 to 39 minutes.

1 = Less than 30 minutes.

Continued.

CHECKLIST AND RATING SCALE FOR THE EVALUATION OF THE PHYSICAL EDUCATION PROGRAM—cont'd

Considerations in the administration of physical education programs—cont'd

Time provided for showers and dressing
5 = 10 to 12 minutes, including shower.
3 = 13 to 15 minutes, 7 to 9 minutes.
1 = Less than 7 minutes or more than 15 minutes.

Class grouping
5 = By needs and abilities of students.
4 = By physical maturity.
3 = By grades.
2 = By interests (students elect activities).
1 = Haphazardly (for example, whatever period is left after scheduling academic program).

Determining class size
5 = Consideration of personnel, facilities, and activity.
4 = Consideration of two of the above (for example, facilities and activity).
3 = Consideration of one of the above (for example, facility available).
2 = By dividing number of students by number of classes.
1 = Controlled by academic program.

Pupil-teacher ratio in each class
5 = 30 pupils or less.
4 = 31 to 35 pupils.
3 = 36 to 40 pupils.
2 = 41 to 50 pupils.
1 = 51 pupils or more.

Total program financed
5 = Completely through regular school or college budget.
4 = Taxes plus pooling receipts of *all* school or college activities.
3 = Taxes plus gate receipts.
2 = Taxes plus contributions from organizations or individuals and/or gate receipts.
1 = Other.

Extramural program
5 = Administered and controlled by regular school or college authorities.
3 = Administered and controlled by schools and colleges with nonschool or noncollege personnel assisting.
1 = Outside personnel contracted to conduct program.

Public relations
5 = Department makes every effort to keep community informed of the total physical education program.
3 = Full coverage is given to intramural and extramural activities.
2 = Only interscholastic activity news releases are given out for public consumption.
1 = No effort is made by the department to make the community aware of its program.

Athletic standards
5 = Every effort is made to follow league and state eligibility requirements, including setting up individual school standards—also, provide medical examinations, insurance, and supervision when needed.
4 = State and league eligibility requirements conscientiously adhered to, as well as providing medical examinations, insurance, and supervision.
3 = Follow state and league eligibility requirements with modified medical coverage.
2 = State and league eligibility requirements known, occasionally bypassed for the benefit of the student.
1 = Complete disregard of rules and regulations.

CHECKLIST AND RATING SCALE FOR THE EVALUATION OF THE PHYSICAL EDUCATION PROGRAM—cont'd

Considerations in the administration of physical education programs–cont'd

Supervision of intramural and extramural activities

5 = Instructional personnel knowledgeable about given activity plus a background in physical education, including athletic training and first aid.

4 = Instructional personnel knowledgeable about given activity with a background in general education and special training in athletic injuries and first aid.

3 = Instructional personnel knowledgeable about activity and is a classroom teacher without additional preparation.

2 = Instructional personnel knowledgeable about activity but in no other way associated with the school program.

1 = Volunteer from the faculty to coach and/or supervise.

Adjusting teaching schedules to enable effective planning, organizing, and supervising of intramural and extramural programs

5 = Personnel are given released time to adequately prepare for intramural and extramural programs.

3 = Some free time is usually provided to enable some preparation during the school day.

1 = No free time is given personnel during the regular school day to prepare for intramural and extramural activities.

Coeducational instruction and supervision

5 = Both men and women physical educators pool their time and talents to offer a coeducational program.

3 = A limited program for coeducational activities may be offered upon occasion.

1 = No effort is made to offer a coeducational program.

Providing proper equipment

5 = Effort is made to buy the best equipment suitable to the program, and equipment that is wearing out is quickly replaced or rebuilt, taking into consideration high standards and quality.

3 = Usually first quality equipment is purchased. Occasionally, that of a secondary quality is bought so as to stay within the means of the budget.

1 = All efforts are made to buy the best "deal" regardless of quality and long wear but more suited to immediate needs.

The physical education program is supervised by a specially trained professional

5 = The program has a director whose education exceeds the Master's degree, whose major area of study is physical education, and who has a minimum of 5 years' experience.

3 = The director has a major degree in physical education but lacks experience academically (beyond a Bachelor's degree) and professionally (at least 5 years in the field).

1 = There is no director or single person responsible for coordinating the total physical educational program.

Components of the physical education program

Program designed to:

5 = Provide experiences that are related to the normal growth and development of the students, including needs, interests, and abilities.

4 = Offer a variety of activities both of an individual and a dual sport nature so as to appeal to the individual student.

3 = Provide a curriculum of activities that vary but are dependent upon interests and abilities of instructors.

2 = Give the athlete a chance to improve his interscholastic or intercollegiate ability with a general program for the regular student body.

1 = Offer as much physical activity as possible but with a lack of direction.

Continued.

CHECKLIST AND RATING SCALE FOR THE EVALUATION OF THE PHYSICAL EDUCATION PROGRAM—cont'd

Components of the physical education program–cont'd

Specific activities are offered to:

5 = Improve the physical fitness and recreational potential of every individual in the program.

3 = Meet the minimum physical fitness levels *or* to teach recreational games.

1 = Entertain and to gain the approval of the students participating to make physical education more popular.

Activities include:

5 = A variety of activities including *all* of the following: individual and dual sports, rhythms and dances, gymnastics, stunts and self-testing activities, team games, and aquatics.

3 = Basically, a program emphasizing team sports with a few individual activities and dual sports to supplement the program.

1 = Several activities of each nature but lacking any set design.

Aquatics

5 = A full program of aquatics from beginning swimming to life saving as part of the required program.

4 = Part of the required program for beginners and intermediates regardless of grade level.

3 = A required part of the program but only for certain grade levels.

1 = No program offered or available.

Intramural program

5 = Full year-round program.

3 = Part time year-round program.

1 = No program offered.

Interscholastic and intercollegiate activities

5 = Activities are offered which meet the needs of the individual students who have achieved the necessary competencies.

3 = An emphasis on team sports with a few major individual and dual sports offered.

2 = Basically a team sports program.

1 = No interscholastic or intercollegiate program.

A special program of a recreational nature including:

5 = Camping skills, nature hikes, fishing, hunting, etc.—all of which are required.

3 = Several or all of the above but on an elective basis.

1 = No such program available.

A special program of combative activities offered

5 = Judo, wrestling, etc., are part of the required program.

3 = Only a very few combative activities are part of the required program.

2 = Combative activities are not part of the required program but may be elected.

1 = No combative activities offered.

All aspects of the program of physical education should be concerned with the following (all items should be checked if high professional standards prevail):

———1. Designing a program that helps to meet the school's or college's educational objectives.

———2. Achieving specific objectives relative to physical education.

———3. Biologic and sociologic factors when planning the program for the individual.

———4. Physical fitness tests, health appraisal, and health records when classifying for physical education.

———5. The use of visual aids, including slides, films, posters, demonstrations by leaders in the field, etc.

———6. Requiring proper physical education uniforms.

CHECKLIST AND RATING SCALE FOR THE EVALUATION OF THE PHYSICAL EDUCATION PROGRAM—cont'd

Components of the physical education program–cont'd

——7. Providing logical progression and continuity.

——8. Opportunities for student leadership.

——9. Instruction on rules of safety.

——10. A series of warmup drills *directly* related to the activities to be taught.

——11. Providing a series of lectures and discussions to enable the student to understand the human organism, the physiology of exercise, body mechanics, and other related areas.

——12. Showers *required* of all students who are physically able.

——13. Not substituting recess and lunch time for the required physical education program.

——14. Scheduling boys' and girls' classes to achieve maximum efficiency of all facilities.

——15. Offering intramurals for the faculty as well as the students.

——16. An intelligent and *minimal* award system for intramurals and interscholastic athletics.

——17. Sports conducted with concern for sportsmanship, fair play, individual values, etc.

Staff

Members of the instructional staff, having the same status and tenure as other teachers, include the following:

5 = All instructors of physical education classes, intramurals, and interscholastic athletics.

3 = All instructors of the regular class program and intramurals.

1 = Only those involved with the regular class program.

Background preparation includes courses in general liberal education, biologic sciences, social sciences, physical sciences, psychology, and professional courses

5 = Required of all those in the instructional classes, including intramurals and interscholastic athletics.

3 = Required only from those in the regular class program and intramurals.

1 = Required only from those in the regular class program.

All members of the staff (all items should be checked if high professional standards prevail)

——1. Are active participants in educational and professional organizations.

——2. Are working toward improving the professional status (refresher courses, etc.).

——3. Are active participants in inservice training programs.

——4. Are active members of departmental committees, such as committee on evaluation.

——5. Help to plan programs with other content areas of the school when appropriate, such as health, recreation, science, guidance, etc.

——6. Are involved in planning, budgeting and ordering of equipment and supplies.

——7. Maintain a high degree of total fitness for the obvious values inherent in total fitness so as to provide the image to their students of which they profess.

——8. Receive at least one free planning period per day.

——9. Have a teaching load maximum of 5 or 6 clock hours per day (college 15 hours per week).

——10. Have a teaching load with a maximum of 250 pupils per day.

——11. Have a minimum of 20 semester hours in the field of physical education.

Supervision in the locker room

5 = By professionally trained instructor.

3 = By experienced adult.

1 = By student leaders.

Continued.

CHECKLIST AND RATING SCALE FOR THE EVALUATION OF THE PHYSICAL EDUCATION PROGRAM—cont'd

Facilities and equipment (check when applicable—items that can be checked will help to determine if high professional standards prevail)

General facilities meet the following standards:

———1. Facilities are designed for and used by the community as well as the school or college.

———2. Facilities are free from obstruction, free from safety hazards, and meet high standards of health and safety.

———3. Facilities have the necessary safe entrances and exits.

———4. There are a sufficient number and variety of teaching facilities (indoor and outdoor) to permit the realization of all the objectives of the program.

———5. New facilities are planned cooperatively by the physical education department, the school administration, the community, and the architect.

———6. Permanent fixtures (backstops, stall bars, etc.) are placed to afford maximum use and safety.

Indoor facilities include:

———1. Well-designed gymnasia that meet official regulations for specific areas and proper floor markings (for example, basketball court, volleyball area, etc.).

———2. Sound, safe, and practical flooring (no splinters, etc.).

———3. Adequate seating capacity for spectators.

———4. Well-placed drinking fountains and cuspidors.

———5. Adequate and regulation lighting.

———6. Adequate heating and temperature control.

———7. Adequate acoustical features.

———8. A public address system.

———9. Launderette for towel service and the cleaning of certain athletic wear.

———10. Adequate storage space on same level as gymnasia.

———11. An equipment room with:

    ———a. Proper ventilation, temperature, and humidity control.

    ———b. Enough area for storage and efficient dispensing of equipment and supplies.

    ———c. An area for repairing, rebuilding, and checking of equipment and supplies.

    ———d. Room or area for drying athletic gear.

———12. Main gymnasium measuring a minimum of 50 by 80 feet of open space.

———13. Secondary gymnasia for weight-lifting, dancing, etc., measuring at least 15 by 25 feet.

———14. Minimum clearance of 22 feet for ceilings in all gymnasia.

———15. Fixtures recessed and/or protected (such as water fountains, scoreboards, clocks).

———16. Adequate ventilation in all gymnasia.

———17. Areas for:

    ———a. Badminton.

    ———b. Basketball.

    ———c. Dancing.

    ———d. Gymnastics.

    ———e. Ping pong.

    ———f. Swimming pool.

    ———g. Table games (cards, checkers).

    ———h. Volleyball.

    ———i. Weight-lifting.

    ———j. Wrestling.

Major equipment for indoor activities include:

———1. Necessary nets and standards.

———2. High bar.

———3. Low bar.

———4. Balance beam.

———5. Parallel bars.

———6. Side horse.

———7. Long horse.

———8. Trampoline.

———9. Mats.

———10. Vaulting box.

———11. Still rings.

———12. Flying rings.

CHECKLIST AND RATING SCALE FOR THE EVALUATION OF THE PHYSICAL EDUCATION PROGRAM—cont'd

Facilities and equipment–cont'd

——13. Spring boards.
——14. Climbing ropes.
——15. Chalk boards.
——16. Bulletin boards (strategically placed).
——17. Official electric scoring device.
——18. Peg boards.
——19. Stall bars.
——20. Backboards and rims for basketball.
——21. Record library.
——22. Phonograph.
——23. Film library.

Training room includes:
——1. Equipment necessary for the prevention and cure of injuries (whirlpool, diathermy, etc.).
——2. Supplies necessary for sound and safe operation, such as first aid equipment and supplies.

Faculty offices
——1. Separate for men and women.
——2. Includes private locker room facilities.
——3. Appropriately equipped with chairs, desks, shelves, etc.
——4. Window view into locker room and gymnasium or pool.

Locker, shower, and drying rooms include:
——1. Moisture- and shock-proof electric fixtures.
——2. Separate locker rooms for boys and girls.
——3. Individual storage lockers.
——4. One large dressing locker for each student during peak load.
——5. Proper ventilation.
——6. Proper heating.
——7. Proper lighting.
——8. Locker room adjacent to lavatory.
——9. Minimum of 12 square feet per pupil during peak load.
——10. One shower head for every four pupils during peak load.
——11. Gang showers for boys.
——12. Gang showers for girls.
——13. Cubicle stall showers for girls.
——14. One hair dryer to every four girls during peak load.
——15. Urinals, sinks, and toilets in boys' locker room.
——16. Sinks and toilets in girls' locker room.
——17. Drying room between shower and lockers.
——18. Water temperature automatically controlled.
——19. Floor, ceiling, walls, and other permanent fixtures constructed of a type of material that withstands extreme moisture conditions and is sanitary, safe, and easy to maintain.
——20. Proper facilities for visiting teams.
——21. Soap dispensers provided.
——22. Towel service provided.
——23. Proper size permanent benches, mirrors, and open aisle space.

Outdoor facilities include:
——1. Proper equipment intelligently and safely installed (goal posts, back stops, nets, etc.).
——2. Adequate storage space for outdoor facilities.
——3. Being immediately adjacent to school building with safe access to locker rooms.
——4. Grass area on fields.

Continued.

CHECKLIST AND RATING SCALE FOR THE EVALUATION OF THE PHYSICAL EDUCATION PROGRAM—cont'd

Facilities and equipment–cont'd

———5. Safe fencing around all areas.
———6. A minimum of 2½ acres for every 250 pupils.
———7. Areas for the following activities:

———a. Archery.
———b. Badminton.
———c. Basketball.
———d. Baseball.
———e. Croquet.
———f. Cross country.
———g. Cycling.
———h. Field hockey.
———i. Football.
———j. Golf.
———k. Handball.
———l. Horseshoes.

———m. Ice skating.
———n. Lacrosse.
———o. Marching.
———p. Open fields for relays, games, etc.
———q. Shuffleboard.
———r. Skiing.
———s. Soccer.
———t. Softball.
———u. Tennis.
———v. Track and field.
———w. Tetherball.
———x. Volleyball.

———8. Provision for all-year-round activities.
——— 9. Proper surfacing, grading, and drainage.

Measurement and evaluative techniques

The following should be incorporated into a measurement and evaluation of the program, its staff, its students, etc.

Measurement of student status and progress

———1. Standardized tests (knowledge and skill).
———2. Locally designed tests (knowledge and skill).
———3. Medical examination.
———4. Orthopedic screening test.
———5. Motor ability tests.
———6. Observation.
———7. Records on social, mental, and emotional development.
———8. Grading:

———a. Grading is consistent with other subjects in the school program, including credit toward graduation.
———b. Grades are based upon individual ability relative to skills, fitness, knowledge, and health attitudes.
———c. Grading is added by established criteria for measuring student progress.
———d. The final grade indicates the extent to which each pupil has achieved the objectives of the course.

Staff evaluation

———1. Controlled student analysis.
———2. Self-evaluation.
———3. Departmental review.
———4. Academic preparation.
———5. Professional experience.
———6. Inservice participation.
———7. Critical contributions to the school, college, and profession.

Questions and exercises

1. Survey five teachers to determine what they think constitutes the most objective method of evaluation of their performance on the job.
2. Should teachers of health education and of physical education be evaluated in the same way? Why? Why not?
3. What contributions can evaluation make to helping the teacher grow professionally?
4. You are responsible for evaluating a school health program and/or a school physical education program. Select the instrument for evaluation, conduct the evaluation, and report to the class on your findings.
5. What areas of school health and physical education programs, according to your observation and evaluation, need the most professional upgrading?

Reading assignment on *Administrative Dimensions of Health and Physical Education Programs, Including Athletics:* Chapter 18, Selections 94 to 97.

Selected references

Billet, R. E.: Evaluation: the golden fleece, New York State Education **55**:42, 1968.

Brian, G.: Evaluating teacher effectiveness, National Education Association Journal **54**:2, 1965.

Bucher, C. A., Koenig, C., and Barnhard, M.: Methods and materials for secondary school physical education, ed. 3, St. Louis, 1970, The C. V. Mosby Co.

Caldwell, S. F.: Evaluation in the elementary physical education program, The Physical Educator · **22**:153, 1965.

California State Department of Education: Criteria for evaluating the elementary health program, Sacramento, 1962, The Department.

Fawcett, G. W.: School personnel administration, New York, 1964, The Macmillan Co.

Goldman, S.: The school principal, New York, 1966, The Center for Applied Research in Education, Inc. (The Library of Education).

Howsam, R. B.: Facts and folklore of teacher evaluation, The Education Digest **29**:7, 1964.

Johns, E.: An example of a modern evaluation plan, Journal of School Health **32**:5, 1962.

La Porte, W. A.: Health and physical education scorecard no. 1 and no. 2, College Book Store, 3413 S. Hoover Blvd., Los Angeles, Calif. 90056.

Malone, W. C.: A checklist for evaluating coaches, Coach & Athlete **29**:3, 1966.

Michigan School Health Association: Appraisal form for studying school health programs, 1962, The Association.

National Education Association: Methods of evaluating teachers, National Education Association Research Bulletin **43**:1, 1965.

National Education Association: What teachers and administrators think about evaluation, National Education Association Research Bulletin **42**:4, 1964.

Roundy, E. S.: Are our physical education programs meeting todays needs? Journal of Secondary Education **41**:221, 1966.

Simpson, R. H., and Seidman, J. M.: Student evaluation of teaching and learning, Washington, 1962, American Association of Colleges for Teacher Education.

Vander Werf, L. S.: How to evaluate teachers and teaching, New York, 1960, Holt, Rinehart & Winston, Inc.

five

ADMINISTRATION OF RECREATION, CLUB, OUTDOOR EDUCATION, AND CAMPING PROGRAMS

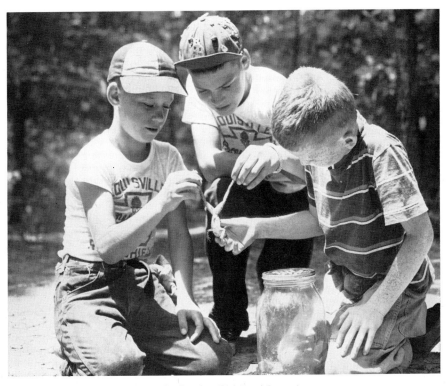

Louisville, Ky., City Division of Recreation.

CHAPTER 24 COMMUNITY AND SCHOOL RECREATION, CLUB, AND ACTIVITY PROGRAMS

Recreation may be defined as that field of endeavor concerned with those socially acceptable and worthwhile activities in which a person voluntarily participates during leisure hours and through which he may better develop physically, mentally, emotionally, and socially.

The key concepts of any form of recreation that is advocated here are five in number. First, the activity must be conducted in hours other than work. It is a *leisure-time activity.* The activity must not be associated with productive labor that is aimed at profit or that is a regular part of one's daily routine as a means of making a living. Second, recreation is an *enjoyable activity.* It is something from which one gains satisfaction, serenity, and happiness. Third, recreation is *constructive* in nature —it is *wholesome.* A person could go out and become inebriated every night and say it is recreation. However, this is not the kind of recreation that is recommended. Recreation should do something to contribute to the individual's physical, mental, emotional, or social welfare. Fourth, recreation is *nonsurvival in nature.* Therefore, such things as sleep cannot be labeled as forms of recreation in the sense that it is discussed in this chapter. Finally, recreation is *voluntary.* The person engages in the activity because he has chosen to participate. There has been no compulsion. He has made the choice freely. These five criteria or concepts must be satisfied if it is the type of recreation that this text is advocating for the benefit of people everywhere.

TYPES OF RECREATION

Some of the better-known kinds of recreation are community, industrial, hospital, school, family, and commercial. The kinds of recreation that will be considered primarily in this chapter are those concerned with community and school recreation.

Community recreation

Community recreation is that in which villages, towns, and cities sponsor a recreation program for their inhabitants. It is controlled, financed, and administered by the community.

Industrial recreation

Industrial recreation is the type wherein an industrial concern, such as Eastman Kodak, Lockheed Aircraft, or other business establishment, sponsors a recreation program for its own employees.

Hospital recreation

Hospital recreation refers to a program that is set up in a veterans, municipal, or other hospital for the benefit of the patients. It includes recreation for the ill and disabled. The therapeutic values of recreation are increasingly being recognized.

School recreation

School recreation refers to the program provided by a board of education for the students that attend a particular school system. Boards of education also provide recreation programs for the adult population of a community.

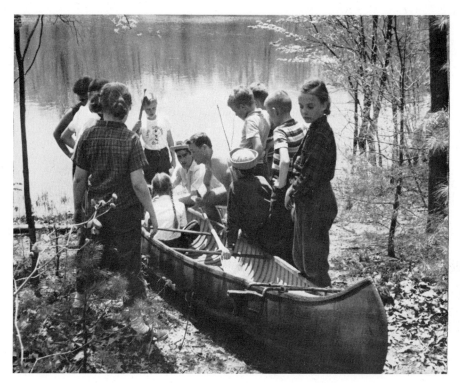

The human relations objective represents a major contribution of recreation to enriched living. "Canoemanship"—one of the activities of recreation course. (University of Connecticut, Storrs, Conn.)

Family recreation

Family recreation means the activities that are engaged in by a family unit during their leisure hours and that have resulted from their own initiative.

Commercial recreation

Commercial recreation is that form of recreation such as is found at amusement parks and that is conducted for profit.

GOALS OF RECREATION

Community recreation is a field of endeavor that deserves increasing recognition for the work that it is doing in enriching individual lives. The goals reflect this contribution. Many goals have been listed for the field of recreation. Some of those that have received attention are the following: physical, mental, emotional, and social health; happiness; satisfaction; balanced growth; creativeness; competition; learning; citizenship; socialization; and the development of one's talents.

Following are six goals for American recreation that have been stated by The Commission on Goals for American Recreation.* They represent one of the best professional statements on recreational goals.

1. *Personal fulfillment.* The democratic ideal is based on the concept that the individual is the most important consideration in our society. To achieve his most important place in our culture, each person needs to fulfill the basic need for adequacy or self-fulfillment. Each person

---

*The Commission on Goals for American Recreation: Goals for American recreation, Washington, D. C., 1964, American Association for Health, Physical Education, and Recreation.

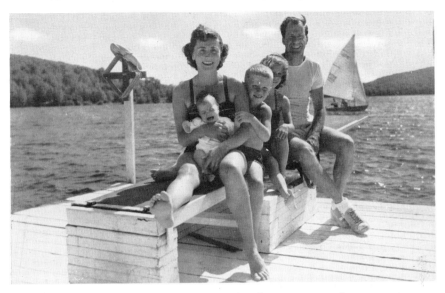

There is insufficient stress on family recreation today.

wants to belong and to feel important. Each person should strive to become all that he is capable of becoming. Therefore, recreation should help each person to achieve full integration of his total personality; contribute to his mental, physical, social, and emotional development; and help to fill in the gaps that work and on-the-job activity do not provide. The many activities offered through a well-organized recreation program can contribute to the self-fulfillment of each person who participates.

2. *Democratic human relations.* The democratic society functions best through associated effort directed and channeled toward the accomplishments of those goals that are in the best interests of the majority. The recreation profession recognizes that its goals exist on the level of the individual as well as on the level of the democratic society of which it is a part. Recreation, therefore, constantly keeps in mind such important tenets as (a) each individual has worth and each personality must be respected, (b) the citizen in a democracy cooperates for the common good, (c) the citizen abides by the laws—rules that have been established to guard

each individual's rights, and (d) the citizen living in a democracy guides his behavior by acceptable moral and ethical values.

3. *Leisure skills and interests.* Recreation is concerned with meeting the interests of those people who voluntarily participate in its programs, developing skills that will provide the incentive, motivation, and medium for spending free time in a constructive and worthwhile manner. As such, recreation must be concerned with a breadth and variety of interests, ranging from physical activities, social activities, and artistic activities to community service programs and learning activities.

4. *Health and fitness.* Recreation is cognizant of the nature of many individuals who live a sedentary existence with the implications this has for poor health and fitness. It also recognizes the importance of a vigorous and active life and seeks to meet the challenge of a society in which mental illness, stress, and inactivity prevail in many quarters.

5. *Creative expression and esthetic appreciation.* There is increased realization today of the need for each individual to give vent to his own personal expression, to creativity, and to the appreciation of the

most beautiful and cultured activities in the various cultures of the world. Recreation seeks to contribute to each individual's desire for creative expression and esthetic appreciation by providing the environment, leadership, materials, and motivation for such experiences, recognizing that creativity can flourish only in a climate that has been properly prepared for its development and growth.

6. *Environment for living in a leisure society.* Recreation recognizes that the environment plays an important role in the determination of the quality and extent of the recreative experience. Therefore, recreation is particularly interested in preserving our natural resources; in the construction of parks, playgrounds, hobby centers, and other recreation centers; in seeing that recreation programs are taken into consideration in city planning; and in awakening the populace to the need for an appreciation of esthetic and cultural values.

I have formulated four objectives for the recreation profession:

1. *The health development objective.* The health development objective is important in the field of recreation. Health to

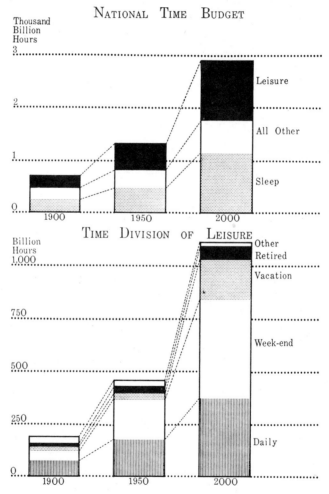

National time budget and time division of leisure—1900, 1950, and 2000. (From The American Academy of Political and Social Science: Leisure in America: blessing or curse? Philadelphia, 1964, The Academy.)

a great degree is related to activity during leisure hours as well as during hours of work. The manner in which a person spends his free time determines in great measure whether his physical, mental, emotional, and spiritual health is of high quality. Through recreation, adaptive physical activity is available that is conducive to organic, mental, emotional, and spiritual health. A range of activities exists that offers opportunities for every individual to promote his organic health. Activities are available in which the individual may relax, escape from the tensions of work, forget about problems, and thereby improve mental health. Activities are planned and conducted that provide individual enjoyment and pleasure and in this way contrib-

ute to emotional health. Activities requiring the participation of many individuals are included and are conducive to better social relations and higher standards of moral and spiritual values, thus promoting spiritual health. Public recreation programs are designed to provide activities that counteract the deteriorating effects of strenuous or routine work or study and thus complement the overall routine that an individual follows. They overcome many of the shortages that exist when the man leaves the office, the child leaves school, or the housewife completes her work. In this way they contribute to the integration and development of the whole individual.

2. *The human relations objective.* The human relations objective represents a ma-

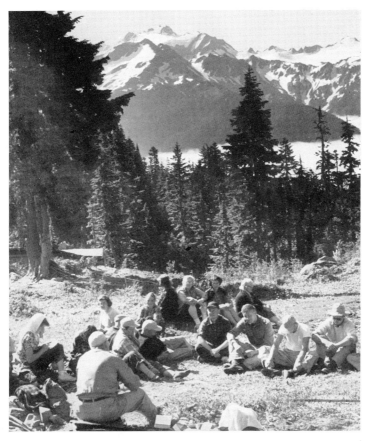

Campcraft class. Mt. Olympus, their ultimate goal, is in the background. (Olympic College, Bremerton, Wash.)

jor contribution of recreation to enriched living. Recreational programs develop many individual qualities that make for better adjustment. Such attributes as courage, justice, patience, tolerance, fairness, and honesty are only a few that are possible of development while individuals are playing and recreating together in the many activities that comprise the total recreation program. Attitudes that promote good human relations are also developed. Wholesome attitudes of social cooperation, loyalty to the group, recognition of the rights of others, and the idea that one receives from a group in direct proportion to what one gives it are a few that make for better relations and enable worthy goals and projects to be accomplished. The growth of family recreation is a trend that also helps to make for a more unified home life. This is very important, since the family group represents the foundation on which good human relations are built. Furthermore, to develop good social traits it is necessary to bring people together in a situation in which there is a feeling of belonging and in which each individual is recognized. There are innumerable opportunities for such interaction in the many recreational programs that exist throughout the country.

3. *The civic development objective.* The civic development objective is a noteworthy goal for recreation. Recreation contributes in many ways to the development of any community. It contributes to community solidarity by uniting people in common projects regardless of race, creed, economic status, or other discriminatory factors. It helps to build the morale of the members of the community. It is a contributing factor in alleviating crime in that it provides settings and activities in which youth and other individuals may engage in constructive, worthwhile activities, rather than in destructive antisocial activities. It helps make the community a safer place in which to live through providing adequate playgrounds and other recreational centers that keep children and youth off the streets. It helps make the community more prosperous by contributing to the health of the individual, by cutting down on the dollar appropriation for crime, and by increasing the total work output of an individual. It helps the growth and development of the individual so that he becomes a more valuable citizen in the community and has more to contribute in its behalf.

4. *The self-development objective.* The self-development objective refers to the potentialities that participation in a program of recreational activities has for developing the individual to his fullest capacity. Recreation does this through a variety of means. It contributes to the balanced growth of an individual. It allows for growth in ways other than in mere production of material things for utilitarian purposes. In other words, it satisfies the human desire for such things as creative music, art, literature, and drama. It allows an individual to create things not for their material value but for the joy, satisfaction, and happiness that go with creating something through one's own efforts. It allows for the development of latent and dormant skills and abilities of the individual until they are aroused by leisure hours with proper settings and leadership. These skills help to make a better-integrated individual.

Recreation provides an avenue for the individual to experience joy and happiness through some activity in which he has the desire to engage. In this chaotic world where there are so many sorrows, heartbreaks, and frowns, it is essential for people to revitalize themselves through the medium of activities. These provide smiles and hearty laughs and release from the tension associated with day-to-day routine. They afford a place for many individuals to excel. Such an urge is many times not satisfied in one's regular job or profession. An opportunity is provided in recreation to satisfy this desire. It offers an educational experience. The participant learns new skills, new knowledges, new techniques, and develops new abilities. He is filing away new and different experiences that will be helpful in facing the situations he will encounter from day to day.

GUIDING PRINCIPLES FOR PLANNING RECREATION PROGRAMS

Recreation programs should not be developed on a "hit-or-miss" basis. Instead, outstanding leaders in recreation have studied very thoroughly and carefully the types of programs that best serve the needs of people and have developed principles that can be used as guides for leaders who are engaged in program planning.

Brightbill* set forth his program principles, which, in adapted form, are as follows:

1. Individual interests, characteristics, needs, and capabilities should be taken into consideration in the planning of recreation programs.

2. The recreational interests and skills of individuals may be determined to some degree as a result of the cultural, economic, religious, and social phenomena that characterize them.

3. Recreation should be planned cooperatively, with the recreator taking into consideration interested individuals, departments, agencies, and organizations.

4. Program planning requires consideration of national standards modified to local conditions.

5. Program planning should take into consideration individual differences in skills and the progressive planning of skill experiences.

6. Creativity and self-expression are considerations in program planning.

7. Opportunities should be made available for individuals to be of service to others so that the personal satisfaction that comes from such service can be realized by such persons.

8. Recreation programs should provide for a wide spectrum of activities.

9. Leadership, financial means, and facilities are essential considerations in program planning.

10. Physical and human resources of the community should be mobilized for the recreation program.

11. The recreation program should seek to provide equality of opportunity for participation for all persons in the community.

12. Flexibility should be possible within a recreation program to provide for such exigencies as changed interests on the part of human beings and other conditions that affect program planning.

13. The health and safety of participants should always be a consideration in planning recreation programs.

14. The recreation program should seek to help each person exemplify acceptable standards of human behavior.

15. The participant in the recreation program should never be exploited for such means as raising money, personal glory, or other similar motives.

16. Recreation should be the object of continual evaluation to determine the measure to which the worthwhile goals are being achieved in light of the investment being made.

Brightbill's goals reflect recreation programs in general, with particular consideration for community recreation. The following principles developed for school recreation by a national conference of experts in this area* are much the same as those established by Brightbill:

1. The recreation program should be characterized by many different activities that are related to the needs and interests of the people they serve.

---

*Langton, C. V., Duncan, R. O., and Brightbill, C. K.: Principles of health physical education, and recreation, New York, 1962, The Ronald Press Co., pp. 251-261.

*National Conference on School Recreation: School recreation, Washington, D. C., 1960, American Association for Health, Physical Education, and Recreation.

2. The welfare of the individual and group should be continually kept in mind when planning the recreation program.

3. The program should be planned so that each individual can realize some of the goals that have been established for recreation.

4. Opportunities should be provided for individuals to participate in the planning of the program. Also, the program should be adapted to local conditions.

5. The recreation program should take into consideration community mores and folkways.

RECREATION ACTIVITIES

The range of recreation activities is infinite in scope. Any activity that meets the criteria listed earlier in the chapter can be a recreational activity. This means that drama, music, art, crafts, games, sports, camping, literature, fairs, nature study, dance, and community work are possible avenues for millions of people to obtain the benefits that recreation can offer.

A list of a few of the possible activities for recreation purposes follows:

Dramatics	*Music*
Clubs	Barber shop quartets
Festivals	Choral groups
Plays	Community sings
	Instrumental
Arts and crafts	Orchestral
Ceramics	
Graphic arts	*Dancing*
Leathercraft	Folk
Metalcraft	Modern
Photography	Social
Plastics	Square
Sewing	
Stenciling and block	*Sports and games*
printing	Archery
	Badminton
Outdoor activities	Bowling
Campfires	Fencing
Camping	Golf
Canoeing	Hopscotch
Conservation	
Fishing	*Miscellaneous*
Orienteering	Cards
Outdoor cooking	Flowers
Woodcraft	Forums
	Hobby clubs

RECREATION AGENCIES

There are three major types of recreation agencies in the United States: (1) public recreation agencies, (2) private or voluntary agencies, and (3) commercial agencies. Some examples of each type are listed:

1. Public recreation agencies
   a. Municipal public agencies—the park department, recreation department, youth commission, education department, and other city or community departments that operate recreation programs
   b. State public agencies—state park departments, state conservation departments, and state education departments
   c. Federal public agencies—national parks, Forestry Service, Children's Bureau, Fish and Wild Life Service, and Tennessee Valley Authority
2. Private or voluntary agencies
   a. Youth-serving organizations—Boys' Clubs of America, Young Men's Christian Associations, Young Women's Christian Associations, Campfire Girls, Boy Scouts, and church centers
   b. Organizations serving an entire population—museums, libraries, athletic clubs, outdoor clubs, and granges
   c. Private voluntary agencies organized around special interests of certain groups—music specialties, photographic specialties, and sports specialties
3. Commercial agencies (operated for profit)—theaters, bowling alleys, art galleries, night clubs, and concert halls

National Recreation and Park Association

A major development in the field of recreation was the unification of five of the national organizations serving laymen and professional recreation. The American Institute of Park Executives, the American Recreation Society, the American Zoological Association, the National Council of State Parks, and the National Recreation Association were merged into a unified national organization known as the *National Recreation and Park Association.* Lawrence S. Rockefeller was elected as the first president of this association. The merger was designed to bring together a single organization supported by private citizens and professional groups and dedicated to helping all Americans to devote their free time to constructive and satisfying activities.

WAYS IN WHICH RECREATION PROGRAMS ARE ADMINISTERED

Recreation programs are not all administered in the same manner in this country. Government agencies, schools, business, and voluntary agencies play a role in many communities. Jenny* has listed five major types of administration of recreation programs in the United States that apply to community recreation.

The recreation board

A recreation board can be set up in any community where enabling legislation exists and permits such action. The board usually consists of five to nine members. The group is frequently composed of representatives of the city government, the school district, the recreation or park department, and the community at large. Terms of office usually run for varying periods of time depending upon the community, and the members usually serve without compensation. Members of the board are either elected or appointed to their positions.

The school board

In many communities the board of education, under a broad interpretation of its powers or under the provisions of state ex-

*Jenny, J. J.: Introduction to recreation education, Philadelphia, 1955, W. B. Saunders Co., pp. 31-35.

tension education laws or enabling acts, conducts recreation programs. In some communities this responsibility is interpreted as providing a program only for its children and youth, whereas other programs are provided for persons of all ages.

The park board

In such cities as Detroit and Seattle, the department of parks administers the recreation program. Since the community parks are used so extensively for recreation purposes, and to avoid duplication of facilities, budgeting, and planning, some citizens feel that the park board is the logical form of administration for community recreation programs. Those opposed to this arrangement, however, point out that recreation does not get priority under such an administrative setup.

The recreation board and the school board

In some communities the recreation board and school board cooperatively work together in administering the recreation program. The school board, for example, may provide the facilities and sometimes the funds, while the recreation board provides the personnel, equipment, and supplies. Regardless of how the responsibilities are shared, a close working relationship is developed between the two groups in providing a recreation program for the inhabitants of the particular geographic locality they serve.

The recreation association, nonprofit agency, and corporation

In villages and other communities where the park, recreation, or school board has not assumed the administration of the recreation program, sometimes recreation associations, clubs, and other organizations provide a program. The Boys' Clubs of America, Young Men's Christian Associations, and Recreation Promotion and Service Corporations are examples of this type of administrative organization. These or-

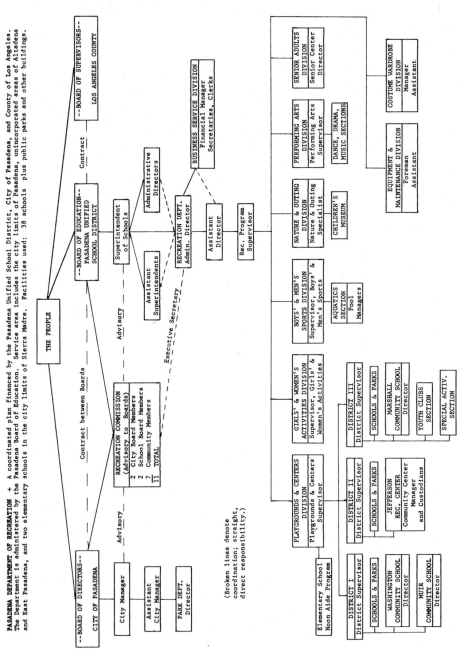

New organization chart of the Pasadena Department of Recreation, Pasadena, Calif.

ganizations have made outstanding contributions in many communities.

THE SCHOOL AND RECREATION

The recommendations of the Second National Conference on School Recreation* included setting forth a series of principles and statements regarding school-centered recreation and municipal-school recreation. These principles and statements are presented in adapted form:

Role of school

1. Schools should accept, as a major responsibility, education for leisure.

2. Schools and colleges should provide their students with opportunities for participation in wholesome, creative activities.

3. The facilities and resources of a school should be made available for recreation purposes when needed.

4. Where community recreation programs are missing or inadequate, the school should take the initiative and provide recreation programs for young and old alike.

5. The school should cooperate with community organizations and agencies interested in or sponsoring recreation programs.

6. The school should appoint a person to act as a community school director; he would be responsible for the recreation-education program in the school.

7. Recreation and education are not identical, but each has its own uniqueness and distinctive features.

8. The community-school director should provide inservice recreation education for his staff.

9. The federal level of government has a responsibility to stimulate recreation programs.

10. Recreation depends upon public understanding and support for its existence.

11. Recreation should be concerned with exploiting the interests of people.

12. The recreation program should consist of many varied activities.

13. Recreation should be concerned with contributing to the mental health of the individual.

Municipal-school recreation

1. The school should accept the responsibility to educate for the worthy use of leisure, contribute to recreation in the instructional program, mobilize community resources, and cooperatively plan facilities for recreation. The college and university should promote research in recreation and provide professional preparation programs in this specialized area.

2. There should be joint planning of municipal school recreation based on stated principles and brought about by state departments of education and local boards of education.

3. School facilities should be available for recreational use.

Some recreation leaders have raised the question as to whether or not recreation should be school centered. Hjelte and Shivers* list some arguments pro and con in respect to this issue.

School-centered recreation

The reasons that Hjelte and Shivers list *for* a school-centered program are as follows: The school possesses the facilities essential to a good recreation program, and duplicating these facilities results in waste and inefficiency. Schools are located within a community in much the same way as recreational centers are located—to meet the needs of the people within a particular geographic area. The school comes in con-

---

*Report of the Second National Conference on School Recreation: Twentieth century recreation, re-engagement of school and community, Nov. 7-9, 1962, Washington, D. C., 1963, American Association for Health, Physical Education, and Recreation.

*Hjelte, G., and Shivers, J. S.: Public administration of parks and recreational services, New York, 1963, The Macmillan Co.

tact with all the children and, therefore, the consumer of recreation can best be helped through this agency. The objectives of schools and the objectives of recreation are similar. The schools are a source of leadership for recreation programs.

Hjelte and Shivers' arguments *against* a school-centered recreation program are as follows: Education should restrict itself to intellectual training and not be concerned with experiences that are only indirectly related to intellectual training. Public schools have too many responsibilities without adding any more. Teachers are poorly paid and facilities are inadequate in many localities, and so a heavier burden should not be placed upon these resources. Recreation is hampered by the formality of the school environment and becomes regimented. Consequently, recreation is able to realize its potentialities to a greater extent through the establishment of a special agency. School facilities, equipment, and supplies are damaged through a recreation program and alterations are necessary, which raises the question as to whether other facilities might not be provided more economically. Finally, in attempting to join the forces of education and recreation, difficulties are encountered in securing financial aid for both. Greater public support can be gained if recreation is not grafted onto the educational program.

Regardless of the arguments for or against school-centered recreation, the schools should play a vital part in the field of recreation. At the present time they are contributing staff and facilities. The program of studies in the schools, however, has a long way to go before it realizes its potentialities for developing resources for leisure.

TEN GUIDELINES FOR THE ADMINISTRATION OF SCHOOL RECREATION*

1. The acceptance and commitment of the administration regarding the role of recreation in education.
2. The establishment of a representative ad hoc committee by the Board of Education to survey recreational needs and interests in the school district. Appropriate funds should be provided for the routine services for such a committee, including secretarial and consultant services.
3. The appointment of a qualified professional staff member, preferably the school district director of health, physical education, and recreation, to serve as coordinator of the study and liaison to the ad hoc committee.
4. The conduct of the study by the committee to determine the status of organized recreation in the school district. This should include: a review of the understanding and philosophy of people in the school district regarding recreation; existing recreational services available.
5. Arranging for technical, professional, consultant services in recreation through recognized agencies for the purpose of appraising the findings of the survey in terms of quality recreation for the school district.
6. Develop, in cooperation with the professional consultant, a proposed plan of recreation for the school district. Such a plan should include a statement of philosophy, principles, policies, procedures, and a financial plan.
7. A review of the ad hoc committee plan by the Board of Education and administration.
8. The acceptance or modification of the plan by the Board of Education.
9. The ratification of the plan and the adjustment of general school district administrative policies to appropriately provide for recreation.
10. The administrative implementation of recreation as officially adopted by the Board of Education, with emphasis on clear communication.

*New York State Department of Education, Albany, N. Y.

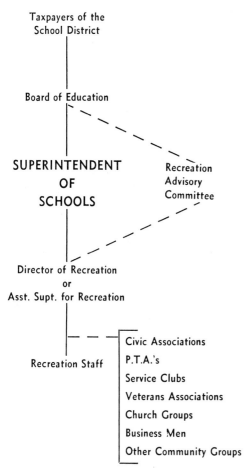

Taxpayers of the
School District

Board of Education

SUPERINTENDENT
OF
SCHOOLS

Recreation
Advisory
Committee

Director of Recreation
or
Asst. Supt. for Recreation

Recreation Staff

Civic Associations
P.T.A.'s
Service Clubs
Veterans Associations
Church Groups
Business Men
Other Community Groups

Recommended organization chart for school-operated recreation programs. (From School recreation, Report of the National Conference on School Recreation, copyrighted 1960.)

Contributions the regular school program can make

All subjects in the educational program have a contribution to make in developing resources for leisure. The school, with wide and varied educational offerings in such fields as science, art, music, physical education, and industrial arts, has infinite opportunities to develop many resources for leisure. During this age of mass production, application of atomic energy to industry, and increasing amounts of leisure, the schools are being challenged to accept this responsibility.

Schools should help young people to adjust to the way of life that they will encounter after leaving school, aid them in solving the problems they will meet, and help them to become responsible citizens. Education most certainly must concern itself with leisure-time education. Leisure hours represent a challenge facing the nation's schools.

Contributions the out-of-class program can make

The school's job does not end when the 3 o'clock bell rings. Its influence extends into the child's life throughout the school day and is also reflected in those activities in which he engages after regular school hours. How the child spends his free time after school and on Saturdays, Sundays, and holidays will influence his health and also his success in life. During his school years he may want to find out more about photography, choral singing, dramatics, or sports. The extracurricular program provides the opportunity to pursue these interests further. Probably one of the greatest values that out-of-school activities have for children is realized in later years. The interests they develop will carry over to adult life and supply them with many happy and profitable hours.

The school can help to enrich leisure

One of the best statements of how the school can help to enrich leisure of students was stated in an editorial by Joy Elmer Morgan, which is as true today as when it was written. He points out that the school can help to enrich leisure:

1. By introducing young people to a wide range of life interests.
2. By teaching the use of books and libraries and developing wholesome reading appetites closely related to each of the great objectives of education and life.
3. By developing appreciation of fine music and skill in singing, playing, and dancing.

4. By having children participate in games and sports which may be easily continued in after years.
5. By providing experience in pleasant social life through school activities.
6. By cultivating in children a love of the out-of-doors—appreciation of flowers, animals, landscape, sky, and stars.
7. By giving children an opportunity to develop hobbies in various creative fields—gardening, mechanics, applied arts, fine arts, architecture, city planning.
8. By making the school and its playfields the center and servant of a wholesome and satisfying neighborhood life.
9. By calling attention to various recreational agencies and the values which they serve—theaters, concerts, libraries, radio, periodicals and newspapers, museums, parks, playgrounds, travel.*

THE RECREATION LEADER

The recreation leader should have most of the qualifications of the health education and physical education specialists and in addition some that are pertinent especially to his field of work.

Qualifications

Various personal attributes are important for the recreation leader who is working with people so much of the time. These include such characteristics as integrity, friendly personality, enthusiasm, initative, organizing ability, and others that will aid in the achievement of recreation objectives.

Recreation leaders should possess a broad cultural background, with an understanding of the needs and problems facing society. This implies a fundamental knowledge of history, sociology, and anthropology. In addition, they should have the skills and competencies necessary for coping with such needs and problems. This would include the communicative arts, knowledge of psychology, and other allied areas.

It is especially important that the recreation leader understand and appreciate human beings. He or she must have respect for the human personality; a broad social viewpoint; the desire to inculcate a high standard of moral and spiritual values; a recognition of the needs, interests, and desires of individuals; an appreciation of the part that recreation can play in meeting these needs and interests; and a desire to serve humanity.

There is special need for an understanding and appreciation of community structure and the place of recreation at the "grass roots" level of this structure. The ability to utilize scientific survey techniques and other methods of social research is also an essential qualification.

There should be ability in the performance of skills in many of the areas with which recreation is concerned. These skills should not be limited to games and sports but in addition should branch out into such areas as arts and crafts, dramatics, camping and outdoor education, music, social recreation, and other important aspects of the total offering.

The philosophy of recreation, with the importance of constructive leisure-time activities to human beings, should be understood. In addition, there is the necessity for the special knowledge, attitudes, and skills concerned with methods and materials, safety, first aid, principles of group work, health, juvenile delinquency, and crime prevention.

Recreation positions and areas of recreation service

The following represent various types of recreation positions for which the aspiring student can prepare and the areas of recreation service:

Recreation positions
    Superintendent of recreation
    Assistant superintendent
    Recreation director
    Consultant
    Field representative
    Executive director

---

*Morgan, J. E.: Editorial, Journal of the National Education Association **19**:1, 1930.

Hospital recreation supervisor
Campus recreation coordinator
Extension specialist
Service club director
Girls' worker—boys' worker
District recreation supervisor
Recreation leader
Supervisor of special activities
Recreation therapist
Recreation educator

Areas of recreation service
Community recreation departments
Park departments
Schools
Service clubs for the armed forces
Churches and religious organizations
Hospitals
Institutions—public and private
Voluntary youth-serving agencies
Rural
Colleges and universities
Industry
State and federal agencies

SCHOOL CLUB AND ACTIVITY PROGRAMS

There are many out-of-class experiences that have educational value for students. Agricultural, cheerleading, music, camping, and journalism clubs and student government represent only a few of these experiences. In some cases these activities are run by the students themselves, whereas in other cases the faculty plays a significant role. The purpose of these programs, however, should be focused on helping the student to obtain a fuller and more total educational experience. Some of the objectives of such clubs are social, service, cultural, recreational, and exploratory in nature. They can provide students with opportunities for self-expression, leadership, constructive use of leisure time, creativity, responsibility, and practice skills.

The school club and activity programs should be planned as unified and integrated programs that dovetail with the curriculum. They should be organized and controlled in a manner that best serves the student's interests, develop special aptitudes and abilities, afford constructive use of leisure time, promote social assets, and provide intellectual and career information. The administration must also recognize that school activities cannot run themselves. They need continuous stimulation and guidance as well as financial support to be successful. The administration should be involved in the process by which the aims of a group are determined, its plans carried out, and the results evaluated to determine if the goals are being met. Problems can develop if the budget is not planned carefully, if qualified personnel are not available to give guidance to the activity, and if inadequate organization and control exist.

School club and activity programs can be a very important part of a well-balanced school program. They can provide opportunities for students to further their education in ways that the formal classroom situation does not permit. If properly administered, they can contribute to cutting down on dropouts, delinquency, and nonconstructive use of leisure hours.

The accompanying checklist highlights some of the important considerations for school club and activity programs.

CHECKLIST FOR SCHOOL CLUB AND ACTIVITY PROGRAMS

	Yes	No
1. Are club activity programs a normal outgrowth of the regular school program?	___	___
2. Are there clearly stated objectives for the club or activity program?	___	___
3. Does the club program supplement the formal curriculum by increasing knowledge and skills?	___	___

Continued.

CHECKLIST FOR SCHOOL CLUB AND ACTIVITY PROGRAMS—cont'd

	Yes	No
4. Are clubs organized in terms of educational value rather than administrative convenience?	—	—
5. Does the administration set adequate policies to guide the program?	—	—
6. Have the aims and objectives of the club or activity program been determined?	—	—
7. Can any student join a club?	—	—
8. Is a student limited to the number of clubs he may join?	—	—
9. Does each club have a simple constitution and bylaws that can guide students in the conduct of the organization?	—	—
10. Do the clubs prepare the student for democratic living?	—	—
11. Do the activities help to develop school spirit?	—	—
12. Does the school schedule club activities so that they do not conflict with regularly scheduled school activities?	—	—
13. Does the school administrator ensure the program of adequate space and funds to carry on a worthwhile program?	—	—
14. Can a student discover and develop special aptitudes and abilities through the club and activity program?	—	—
15. Does the club and activity program offer opportunities for vocational exploration?	—	—
16. Is the individual student able to develop socially acceptable attitudes and ideals through the club program?	—	—
17. Does the club experience provide situations that will contribute to the formation of improved behavior patterns in the student?	—	—
18. Do all club members actively participate in program planning?	—	—
19. Are the projects and activities of the club initiated primarily by the students?	—	—
20. Do the activities performed pertain to the club purposes?	—	—
21. Are students allowed to select clubs and activities according to interests?	—	—
22. Are students issued a calendar of events?	—	—
23. Does the school library make available books and periodicals needed by club and activity groups?	—	—
24. Does the club faculty adviser enlist the confidence of boys and girls?	—	—
25. Is the club faculty adviser willing to give time and thought to making the club or activity program a success?	—	—
26. Is the club faculty adviser able to find his chief satisfaction in pupil growth and not in appreciation of his efforts?	—	—
27. Does the administration of the school evaluate the club periodically?	—	—
28. Does the club allow time for the evaluation of activities?	—	—

Questions and exercises

1. Survey a community recreation program. In the light of this survey list the contributions the program makes to the community, its organization aspects, relation to schools, activities included in its program, and degree to which it is achieving professional objectives.

2. What are the objectives of recreation? Develop a group of guiding principles for the achievement of each of these objectives.

3. To what degree is recreation understood by the American public in general?

4. Discuss what you consider to be the outstanding accomplishments of the recreation profession during the last 50 years.

5. How can the recreation profession turn its shortcomings into accomplishments during the next 50 years?
6. Develop a plan whereby physical education, health education, and recreation can work together most productively in the community.
7. To what extent is your school achieving recreational objectives through its educational offering?
8. Read and critically review one article in *Recreation* magazine.
9. How can television be utilized most advantageously by the recreation profession?
10. Describe what you consider will be a community recreation program in the year 2000.

Reading assignment on *Administrative Dimensions of Health and Physical Education Programs, Including Athletics:* Chapter 19, Selections 98 to 100.

Selected references

American Association for Health, Physical Education, and Recreation: Leisure and the schools, Washington, D. C., 1961.

American Association for Health, Physical Education, and Recreation: Your community-school-community fitness inventory, Washington, D. C., 1959, The Association.

Bentz, C.: Operating a school swimming pool for the benefit of the total community, School Activities **39:**12, 1968.

Brimm, R. P.: The junior high school, New York, 1963, The Center for Applied Research in Education, Inc. (The Library of Education).

Bryant, A.: Activities program beginnings in a new junior college, School Activities **38:**5, 1966.

Bucher, C. A., editor: Methods and materials in physical education and recreation, St. Louis, 1954, The C. V. Mosby Co.

Bullock, N.: Aviation clubs in secondary schools, School Activities **39:**5, 1968.

Bunte, G. V.: Skin diving club, Student Life **27:**20, 1960.

California Association for Health, Physical Education, and Recreation and California State Department of Education: The roles of public education in education, Burlingame, 1960, The Association.

Carlson, R., Deppe, T. R., and Maclean, J. R.: Recreation in American life, Belmont, Calif., 1963, Wadsworth Publishing Co., Inc.

Danford, H. G.: Creative leadership in recreation, Boston, 1964, Allyn & Bacon, Inc.

Douglas, H. R.: Trends and issues in secondary education, New York, 1962, The Center for Applied Research in Education, Inc. (The Library of Education).

Frederick, R. W.: Student activities in American education, New York, 1965, The Center for Applied Research in Education, Inc. (The Library of Education).

Heller, M. P.: School activities need an open door policy, Clearing House **40:**42, 1965.

Hjelte, G., and Shivers, J. S.: Public administration of park and recreational services, New York, 1963, The Macmillan Co.

Kraus, R.: Recreation and leisure in modern society, New York, 1971, Appleton-Century-Crofts.

Kraus, R.: Recreation today—program planning and leadership, New York, 1966, Appleton-Century-Crofts.

Kraus, R. G.: Recreation for rich and poor: a contrast, Teachers College Record **67:**568, 1966.

McKenzie, R. F.: Those extra curricular activities, Texas Outlook **52:**35, 1968.

Meyer, H. D., and Brightbill, C. K.: Community recreation—a guide to its organization, ed. 3, Englewood Cliffs, N. J., 1964, Prentice-Hall, Inc.

Nash, J. B.: Philosophy of recreation and leisure, St. Louis, 1953, The C. V. Mosby Co.

National Conference on School Recreation: School recreation, Washington, D. C., 1960, American Association for Health, Physical Education, and Recreation.

Nelson, R. L.: School recreation, The Physical Educator **20:**111, 1963.

Report of the Second National Conference on School Recreation: Twentieth century recreation, re-engagement of school and community, Washington, D. C., 1963, American Association for Health, Physical Education, and Recreation.

Rodney, L. S.: Administration of public recreation, New York, 1964, The Ronald Press Co.

Shivers, J. S.: Leadership in recreational service, New York, 1963, The Macmillan Co.

The Commission on Goals for American Recreation: Goals for American recreation, Washington, D. C., 1964, American Association for Health, Physical Education, and Recreation.

The International City Managers' Association: Municipal recreation administration, ed. 4, Chicago, 1960, The International City Managers' Association.

Willgoose, C. E.: Recreation—obligation of the schools, Instructor **75:**39, 1966.

Yukic, T. S.: Fundamentals of recreation, New York, 1963, Harper & Row, Publishers.

The pupils of Bowling Green Elementary School in Sacramento, California, experience outdoor learning on their own school grounds where they have a nature center and arboretum. Students at Alberton in western Montana, under a Title III project, developed a 7-day camp for sixth and seventh graders where conservation was stressed by studying such things as timber management, forest fire control, air and water pollution, and the management of animals, plant, and soil. Boys and girls in the public schools of Le Mars, Iowa, go to Camp Quest and participate in an academic curriculum based on the discovery method of learning to stimulate interest in the life and earth sciences. More than 50,000 children have benefited from studying nature's resources at Camp Tyler, Texas, which is operated as part of the school system.

The president* of the Minnesota Outdoor Education Association discussed in the *Journal of the National Education Association* how a kindergarten teacher takes her class outside to study the clouds in the sky, a third-grade class utilizes a compass to measure distances and determine directions preliminary to beginning a map for social studies, a sixth-grade class goes to a park and discovers fossils, and an eighth-grade class finds a spider web and relates it to what they were doing on conservation. Outdoor education is not just nature study but instead represents a vital part of the educational program at all education levels and in all subjects including art, social studies, mathematics, physical education, and industrial arts.

The out-of-doors is nature's laboratory. It is a setting that offers excellent opportunities to learn many knowledges and skills and to develop wholesome attitudes. Experiments and research have shown that boys and girls who use nature's classroom will learn more readily those things that directly relate to the out-of-doors and be more interested in doing so.

Outdoor education and school camping are not synonymous. Outdoor education includes school camping. The camp provides a laboratory by which many facets of the out-of-doors can be studied at first hand. And the camp experience helps to develop qualities important to preparing young people for the lives they will live.

One hundred leaders in education, conservation, and recreation participated in a National Conference on Outdoor Education. This conference reaffirmed the importance of outdoor education and came to the following conclusions*:

1. There is an urgent need during the times in which we live for education in the out-of-doors.
2. There is a need to stress outdoor education in schools and colleges as well as in conservation, recreation, and other agency programs.
3. Those agencies and organizations involved in outdoor education should

---

*Brinley, A.: Classrooms as big as all outdoors, NEA Journal 53:45, 1964.

*Professional Report from the National Conference on Outdoor Education, Journal of Health, Physical Education, and Recreation 33:29, 1962.

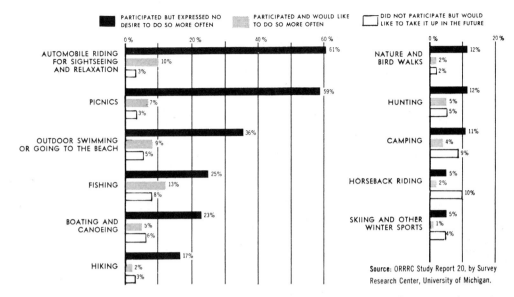

Source: ORRRC Study Report 20, by Survey Research Center, University of Michigan.

Expression of preference of participants and nonparticipants in outdoor activities. (From *Action for Outdoor Recreation for America: A digest of the report of the Outdoor Recreation Resources Review Commission*, with suggestions for citizen action, 1964.)

work cooperatively together to provide as many young people and adults as possible with experiences in this area.

4. The American Association for Health, Physical Education, and Recreation should make provision for outstanding leadership in this field of endeavor.

BEGINNINGS

In May, 1948, representatives of such well-known organizations and agencies as the American Association for Health, Physical Education, and Recreation; United States Office of Education; National Secondary School Principals Association; American Association of School Administrators; and the American Council on Education made recommendations that camping and outdoor education should be a part of every child's educational experience, that cooperative arrangements should be worked out with conservation departments and other agencies directly related to natural resources, and that experimental

camping programs, as a phase of the educational program, should be established in Michigan and any other states that were interested in trying out this educational trend. Since 1948, camping and outdoor education have grown tremendously in this country.

Outdoor education and camping are rapidly being recognized as having an educational value that should be experienced by every boy and girl. Although there are comparatively few camps throughout the United States that are associated with school systems, the trend is more and more in the direction of required camping and outdoor education as part of the educational offering.

Many teacher education institutions preparing teachers of science, elementary education, health education, recreation, and physical education recognize the value of camping and its importance in education. Prospective teachers in some training programs are required to spend one or more sessions at a camp. The experience orients the student in camp living and in the organization and administration of a camp and emphasizes the value of outdoor education. It is also felt by some professional preparing institutions that the student should have a broad understanding of camping in education. This should include a study of the role of camping and outdoor education in the total educational process, the aims and objectives of camping and outdoor education, procedures essential in the conduct of a camp, qualifications and duties of the camp counselor in his relation to the director and to the campers, safety precautions and procedures, the program of activities for all types of weather conditions, and facilities.

SETTINGS FOR OUTDOOR EDUCATION

A publication of the American Association for Health, Physical Education, and Recreation lists some of the significant settings for outdoor education activities*:

1. *School sites and adjacent areas.* The trees, shrubs, streams, ponds, and outdoors in general offer many opportunities to develop outdoor laboratories that can be utilized for experiences related to such areas as science, social studies, arts and crafts, and physical education.

2. *Parks, forests, and farms.* Most communities have parks, farms, or other available outdoor areas nearby that can be utilized for outdoor education.

3. *School farms.* School farms are being developed in some communities and are providing agricultural experiences and a variety of learning situations that revolve around rural living. Such farms offer opportunities for studying birds, animals, conservation, gardening, milk production, home management, care of farm machinery, and community life.

4. *School forests.* School forests or nearby municipal, county, state, or national forests provide excellent outdoor education settings. School experiences relating to art, music, conservation, forestry, zoology, shop, archery, shelter construction, fire protection, camp crafts, and hiking can be provided.

5. *School and community gardens.* The opportunity to till the soil, see plants grow, and other similar activities can be provided for in school and community gardens.

6. *Museums and zoos.* An opportunity to study animals, collections of historic materials, works of art, and other important aspects of our culture is provided by museums and zoos.

7. *School camps.* The utilization of camps, either as a day camp or for an extended period of time, offers opportunities for group living, work experience, development of outdoor skills, and many other experiences important to the well-rounded education of every boy and girl.

VALUES OF OUTDOOR EDUCATION AND SCHOOL CAMPING

The values of outdoor education and school camping are very much in evidence as a result of the many experiments that have been conducted throughout the United States. For purposes of discussion, it might be said that the values of such experiences are threefold: (1) they meet the social needs of the child, (2) they meet the intellectual needs of the child, and (3) they meet the health needs of the child.

A camping experience is an essential part of every child's school experience because it helps to develop the child socially. In a camp setting children learn to live democratically. They mix with children of other creeds or national origin, color, economic status, and ability. They aid in planning the program that will be followed during their camp stay; they assume part

---

*American Association for Health, Physical Education, and Recreation: Leisure and the schools, Washington, D. C., 1961, The Association, p. 108.

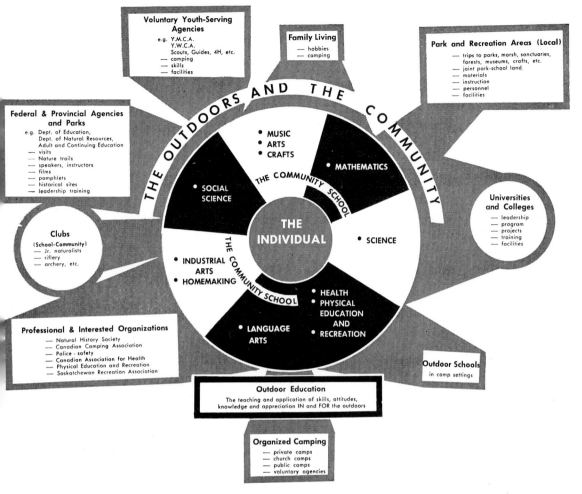

Voluntary Youth-Serving Agencies
e.g. Y.M.C.A.
      Y.W.C.A.
      Scouts, Guides, 4H, etc.
— camping
— skills
— facilities

Family Living
— hobbies
— camping

Park and Recreation Areas (Local)
— trips to parks, marsh, sanctuaries, forests, museums, crafts, etc.
— joint park-school land
— materials
— instruction
— personnel
— facilities

Federal & Provincial Agencies and Parks
e.g. Dept. of Education,
     Dept. of Natural Resources,
     Adult and Continuing Education
— visits
— Nature trails
— speakers, instructors
— films
— pamphlets
— historical sites
— leadership training

THE OUTDOORS AND THE COMMUNITY

• MUSIC
• ARTS
• CRAFTS

• MATHEMATICS

THE COMMUNITY SCHOOL

• SOCIAL SCIENCE

THE INDIVIDUAL

• SCIENCE

THE COMMUNITY SCHOOL

• INDUSTRIAL ARTS
• HOMEMAKING

• HEALTH
• PHYSICAL EDUCATION AND
• RECREATION

• LANGUAGE ARTS

Universities and Colleges
— leadership
— program
— projects
— training
— facilities

Clubs
(School-Community)
— Jr. naturalists
— riflery
— archery, etc.

Professional & Interested Organizations
— Natural History Society
— Canadian Camping Association
— Police - safety
— Canadian Association for Health
— Physical Education and Recreation
— Saskatchewan Recreation Association

Outdoor Schools
in camp settings

Outdoor Education
The teaching and application of skills, attitudes, knowledge and appreciation IN and FOR the outdoors

Organized Camping
— private camps
— church camps
— public camps
— voluntary agencies

The world of outdoor education. (From MacKenzie, J.: Saskatchewan Community 14:4, 1963-1964.)

of the responsibility for the upkeep of the camp, such as making their own beds, helping in the kitchen, sweeping their cabins, and fixing the tennis courts; and they experience cooperative living. The children get away from home and from their parents. They lose their feeling of dependency upon others and learn to do things for themselves. The child learns to rely on his own resources. The camp also provides an enjoyable experience for the child. A child is naturally active and seeks adventure. This experience provides the opportunity to release some of this spirit of adventure and to satisfy the "wanderlust" urge.

A camping experience is an essential part of every child's school experience because it helps to develop the child intellectually. While living in a camp, the child learns about soil, forests, water, and animal and bird life. He learns about the value of the nation's natural resources and how they should be conserved. He learns of ecology, the science concerned with the interrelationship between living organisms and their environment and between organisms themselves. He learns by doing rather than through the medium of textbooks. Instead of looking at the picture of a bird in a book, he actually sees the bird chirping on the branch of a tree. Instead of reading about soil erosion in a textbook, he sees how it actually occurs. Instead of being told about the four basic groups of food, he has the opportunity to live on a diet that meets the right standards. Instead of reading about the value of demo-

cratic living, he actually experiences it. The child experiences many new things that he cannot possibly do at home or within the four walls of a school building. Camping is also of special value to children who do not learn easily from books. In many cases the knowledge accumulated through actual experience is much more enlightening and beneficial.

Camping is an essential part of every

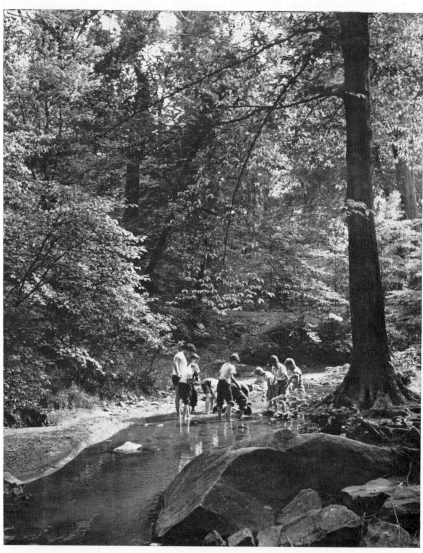

Camping and outdoor education are rapidly being recognized as having an educational value that should be experienced by every boy and girl.

child's school experience because it helps to meet the health needs of the child. Camps are located away from the turmoil, confusion, noise, and rush of urban life. Children experience having their meals at a regular time, obtaining sufficient sleep, and participating in wholesome activity in the out-of-doors. They wear clothing that does not restrict movement, that shields from the sun, and that they are not afraid to get dirty. The food is good. They are doing things that are natural for them to do. It is an outlet for their dynamic personalities. It is much more healthful, both physically and mentally, than living in a "push-button" existence with its lack of recreation, relaxation, and opportunity for enjoyable experiences. It is like living in another world, and children come away refreshed from such an experience.

THE SCHOOL CAMP PROGRAM

The program in most camps consists of such sports activities as swimming, boating, fishing, horseback riding, tennis, badminton, hiking, horseshoes, basketball, and softball; such social activities as campfires, frankfurter and marshmallow roasts, dancing mixers, and cookouts; and opportunities to develop skills and an appreciation in arts and crafts, photography, Indian lore, drama, music, and nature study.

The educational aspects can include a variety of experiences. Some of these are campfires, outdoor cooking, woodcraft, camp sites, canoeing, conservation, astronomy, birds, animals, indoor and outdoor gardening, fishing, hiking, hunting, and orienteering.

A publication of the American Association for Health, Physical Education, and Recreation* points out some experiences

*Joint Committee: Administrative problems in health education, physical education, and recreation, Washington, D. C., 1953, American Association for Health, Physical Education, and Recreation, p. 47.

that might take place and yield educational results:

While the camp program is well integrated with the aims and purposes of general education, there are many implications for essential learnings usually associated with health, physical education, and recreation. A student at a school camp, as a member of a program group made up of boys and girls, might have some of the following experiences: (a) a trip with a cookout; (b) a work project such as planting trees, building shelter for game, repairing boats, and others; (c) responsibility for the common living activities for the day, such as preparation of food, cleaning of the camp, cutting wood for the fire, and the like; (d) participation in activities of interest, such as crafts, dramatics, and music; (e) helping to plan the evening activities for the camp; (f) helping evaluate the day's program; (g) meeting with the camp council; (h) participating in a special campfire program; and (i) countless other kinds of experiences appropriate to the age of the group and the location of the camp.

Julian W. Smith, one of the nation's leaders in the fields of camping and outdoor education, has listed a sample elementary school program (Table 25-1).

SCHOOL CAMPS IN OPERATION

These are some outstanding examples of school systems that are using camping as an effective and worthwhile educational experience.

The sixth-grade children in the city of San Diego and San Diego County, California, have the opportunity to experience one week of camp life at Camp Cuyamaca. This is a former Civilian Conservation Corps Camp and is located in the nearby mountains. Year-round camping is included as part of the education of the boys and girls going to these schools. The staff is made up largely of school personnel, and the financial outlay is assured by the city council and county board of supervisors. From sixty to seventy children at a time experience all sorts of camp activities including arts and crafts, nature study, hikes, and care of living quarters. Teachers accompany the children on camp-

Table 25-1. A sample elementary school camp program*

Day	Teamsters	Cruisers	Lumberjacks
Monday	Planning Hike around lake Cookout Paul Bunyan stories	Planning Hike to abandoned farm Crafts	Planning Camp cruise Tapping trees Square dance
Tuesday	Blacksmiths shop Scavenger hunt Sock hop	Logging Make ice cream Cookout	Treasure hunt Plant trees Fishing
Wednesday	Boiling sap Crafts Square dance	Hike around the lake Fishing Square dance	Fire building Compass hike Crafts
Thursday	Breakfast cookout Compass hike Council fire	Compass hike Plan for council fire Council fire	Cookout Boating Council fire
Friday	Evaluation Clean up and pack Go home	Evaluation Clean up and pack Go home	Evaluation Clean up and pack Go home

*From Smith, J. W.: Outdoor education, Washington, D. C., 1956, American Association for Health, Physical Education, and Recreation, p. 26.

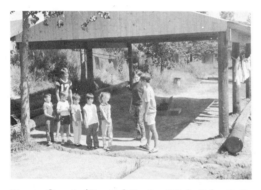

Camp Quest. (Central Junior High School, Le Mars Community School District, Le Mars, Iowa.)

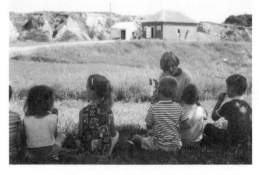

Camp Quest. (Central Junior High School, Le Mars Community School District, Le Mars, Iowa.)

ing trips. One main emphasis in the camp is to have children experience living together with other children in a democratic, healthful, and stimulating environment.

Another notable school camping experience takes place in the public school system of Battle Creek, Michigan, at Saint Mary's Lake Camp. As provided in the arrangements established in this educational setup, children have the opportunity of 2 weeks' camping experience, which may occur at any time during the year. The camp staff is made up of faculty members of the Battle Creek schools. A novel feature of this camp is the banking experience that each child has. All boys and girls deposit their money in the camp bank, and a banking system is established analogous to that used by commercial banks. The campers also run their own post office. The only cost to each child for this valuable experience is the price of the food.

Long Beach, California, also offers a valuable camping experience to the children and faculties of its schools. Their camp, Camp Hi-Hill, is located about 50

Table 25-2. School camping is an extension of the classroom*

Basic scientific understandings and appreciations

How soil is formed
How plants grow
The rain-water cycle
How forest animals live
Dependence of man upon plants and animals
Causes of soil erosion and prevention
Operation of a weather station
Use of map and compass
Significance of fire damage
Study of stars
Meaning of contour, grade, and slope

Study of seasonal changes

Bird, animal, and insect life
Uses of flood control dams
How snow is used for protection and water supply
　for vegetation
Migration, fire hazards
Barometric pressure
Weather observations
How animals use the food they stored
Watersheds

Worthy skills in recreation

Hiking to discover, study, explore, and collect
　native craft materials
Outdoor cooking techniques
Outdoor survival skills
Outdoor sports such as: skiing, boating, canoeing,
　fly-chasing, bait-casting, swimming, skating, and
　mountain climbing
Crafts
Nature workshop
Square dancing
Building outdoor shelters
Appreciating wholesome outdoor recreation

Spiritual values

Experiencing the beauty of nature
Appreciation of living things developed from per-
　sonal contact
Better appreciation of the personal worth of others,
　from living together
Development of finer group unity
Appreciation of the beauty and worth of the out-
　of-doors

Wholesome work experiences

Conservation projects
Planting and terracing to arrest erosion
Repairing trails
Building small check dams
Planting and maintaining a forest nursery
Setting tables
Washing dishes
Cleaning cabins
Caring for animals and pets
Learning safe use and care of simple hand tools

Democratic social living

Cooperative planning by groups
Evaluation by students
Discussing camp safety standards
Living in cabin groups
Participating in campfire activities
Solving problems arising from living together
Understanding duties of the forest ranger
Acting as host, hostess, and hopper at dining table
Improving relationships of pupils and teacher
Enriching and fostering democratic living

Healthful living

Maintaining personal health, cleanliness
Maintaining regular hours of sleeping
Keeping cabin neat and clean
Participating in wholesome exercise
Developing better table manners and eating habits
Planning menus
Practicing first aid

*Adapted from State Board of Education, Concord, N. H.: School camping and outdoor education; and from Division of Instruction, Long Beach, Calif., Public Schools: Guide for the Camp Hi-Hill Program, Long Beach, Calif., June, 1952.

miles from Long Beach in the San Gabriel Mountains. This camp is primarily for sixth graders and faculty members, and the emphasis is on giving these children an opportunity to cope with various problems that arise when a group of individuals start living together in a democratic manner. This camp is also conducted on a year-round basis with winter activities playing just as important a role as summer activities. Table 25-2 shows how the camp experience at Long Beach is an extension of classroom learning activities.

Some states have passed legislation making tax money available to the schools for the support of camping provided for the public school children. This trend in state-level provision for camping in the public schools means that more and more opportunities are going to be made available for children to have this worthwhile experience. For example, in the state of Michigan a bill was passed providing that boards of education, with the exception of those in primary school districts, could operate camps independently or jointly with other boards of education or governing bodies for purposes of recreation and instruction. Provision was made for the charging of fees, if necessary, to cover expenses incurred in maintaining the camp. However, these camps are to be run on a nonprofit basis. Provisions were also made for boards of education to employ personnel to operate these camps, to maintain essential facilities,

and to locate camps on property other than that owned by the board of education, provided that the consent of the owner of said property had been secured. Finally, a provision was made stipulating that the cost of operating a school camp should not be included in the determination of per capita costs of the regular school program.

In the state of New York legislation has provided that boards of education may operate camps on land secured by the school district for camp purposes. The legislature of the state of New York passed the Desmond School Camp Bill, which made it possible for school districts to appropriate funds for instructional programs deemed advisable for school children. Camping is one experience that is being recognized more and more as being an essential for all children of school age.

When historians look back at the twen-

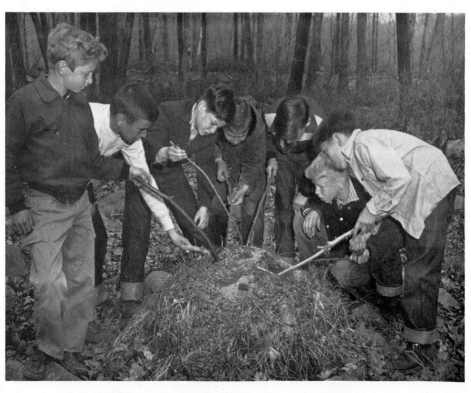

Education in the out-of-doors that is meaningful.

tienth century there is a good possibility they will credit the school camping movement as the greatest educational innovation of the era and acclaim Michigan as one of the pioneer states in proving that nature's classroom helps to prepare the child much more effectively for living in today's world. The history of school camping in this state goes back some 25 years. In the early 1930's Tappan Junior High School in Ann Arbor utilized a camp setting for its junior high school students, and the Cadillac board of education developed a summer camp for its elementary school children. A little later, schools in Battle Creek, Decatur, and Otsego utilized camps in their educational programs. In 1945 the state government passed legislation making it possible for school districts to acquire and operate camps as part of their educational program. In 1946 their Departments of Public Instruction and Conservation, together with the W. K. Kellogg Foundation, joined forces to develop the program further. The late Lee M. Thurston, State Superintendent of Public Instruction, and P. J. Hoffmaster, State Director of Conservation, set as the goal for the state of Michigan: "A week of school camping for every boy and girl in the state."

The rapid development of camping in Michigan has resulted to a great degree because of the educationally significant way in which the program is operated. The groups going to camp usually include fifth- or sixth-graders on the elementary level, or home rooms and special subject matter areas on the secondary level. The camps are run by the teachers and students. Preplanning takes place in the classroom where such essentials as clothing needed, projects to be developed, and job assignments are arranged. The usual procedure is to have two teachers for the average classroom-size group, plus extra help for food preparation and camp maintenance. The parents assume the cost of food, with special provisions being made

for those children whose families are unable to pay the expenses. Any child who wants to go to camp is given the opportunity. Schools assume the instructional cost. The school district or government agency bears the cost of the camp and its facilities.*

Over 100 educational systems include camping in their school programs at the present time in the state of Michigan. This state is pioneering in an educational movement that has many potentialities for furthering the social, mental, physical, and emotional growth of children. The fact that fewer than 10% of the children of camp age in America ever get any type of camp experience presents a challenge for other states to follow Michigan's lead.

The years ahead will undoubtedly find camping becoming more and more a part of the school program. Administrators, teachers, and educators in general should examine the potentialities that camping and outdoor education have for their own school systems.

---

*Smith, J. W.: The Michigan story of camping and outdoor education, The Journal of Educational Sociology 23:508, 1950.

Questions and exercises

1. Prepare a speech to be given to a parent-teacher's association on the importance of camping in education. Point up the values of camping to the children in the community.
2. What is the responsibility of professional preparing institutions in the field of camping and outdoor education?
3. Make a study of the program of camping and outdoor education in the state of Michigan and give a report to the class.
4. Cite specific examples to show how camping and outdoor education can develop a child socially and intellectually.
5. Prepare a report for a board of education to justify taking all the sixth-grade children of a school to camp on school time.
6. What should constitute some of the experiences provided in a camp setting?
7. Make a study of school camping in the fifty states and report to class on the progress that has been made during the last 5 years.

8. How can school camping contribute to the wise use of natural resources?
9. What is meant by enabling legislation? What type of enabling legislation is needed in your state to promote school camping? List a series of logical steps that should be followed to achieve such legislation.
10. Write an essay of 250 words on the subject: School camping is an extension of the classroom.

   Reading assignment in *Administrative Dimensions of Health and Physical Education Programs, Including Athletics:* Chapters 19 and 20, Selections 100 to 103.

Selected references

American Association for Health, Physical Education, and Recreation: Leisure and the schools, Washington, D. C., 1961, The Association.

Brinley, A.: Classrooms as big as all outdoors, NEA Journal 53:45, 1964.

For these children: everything that camp should give, Michigan Education Journal (editorial), 43:26, 1965.

Freeberg, W. H.: Programs in outdoor education, Minneapolis, 1963, Burgess Publishing Co.

Fewer, R. D.: Administrative responsibilities for outdoor education, Illinois Journal of Education 55:7, 1964.

Gabrielson, M. A., and Holtzer, C.: Camping and outdoor education, New York, 1965, The Center for Applied Research in Education, Inc. (The Library of Education).

Hammerman, D. R., and Hammerman, W. M.: Teaching in the outdoors, Minneapolis, 1964, Burgess Publishing Co.

Hammerman, D. R.: Research implications for outdoor education, Journal of Health, Physical Education, and Recreation 35:89, 1964.

Illinois State Superintendent of Public Instruction: Know about outdoor education. Illinois Journal of Education, December, 1964. (Available from Superintendent, Room 302, State Office Building, Springfield.)

Isenberg, R. M.: Education comes alive outdoors, NEA Journal 54:24, 1967.

Report of the Committee on Camping in Education: The place of camping in education, Journal of the American Association for Health, Physical Education, and Recreation 21:15, 1950.

Shanklin, J. F.: Outdoor recreation land, Journal of Health, Physical Education, and Recreation 36:19, 1965.

Shivers, J. S.: Camping — administration counseling, programming, New York, 1971, Appleton-Century-Crofts.

Smith, J. W.: Outdoor education for American youth, Washington, D. C., 1957, American Association for Health, Physical Education, and Recreation.

Appendices

A SOURCES OF EQUIPMENT AND SUPPLIES FOR ATHLETIC, PHYSICAL EDUCATION, RECREATION, OUTDOOR EDUCATION, AND SCHOOL HEALTH PROGRAMS*

AAHPER's seventh annual directory of equipment and supplies is in two parts. The first lists companies and suppliers under sixteen categories. Many of the companies distribute goods in more than one category and are so listed. Only the company name appears under the category heading. Addresses are shown in the second part of the directory, which is an alphabetical listing of suppliers.

Each entry contains the full company name and address, plus a brief description of its services as prepared by the company. The companies listed in this directory have been accepted for advertising in the Journal and for exhibiting at AAHPER national conventions. All have met certain standards of advertising and exhibiting. Those listed in boldface type have advertised and exhibited with AAHPER over a long-term period.

ATHLETIC AND SPORTS EQUIPMENT

AA-Belco All-Automotive Phys-Ed &
   Athletic Laundry Equip. Co.
ADIRONDACK INDUSTRIES, INC.
AMERICAN ATHLETIC EQUIPMENT CO.
American Gym Corporation
ATLAS ATHLETIC EQUIPMENT
   COMPANY
R. E. Austin & Son
BALL-BOY CO.
Benson Optical Company
Bike Athletic Prod. Div., Kendall Co.
Bolco Athletic Co.

*From Journal of Health, Physical Education, and Recreation 40:61-68, 1969.

Brunswick Corp./Bowling Division
Buc-Ol Mfg. Co.
The J. E. Burke Company
CASTELLO FENCING EQUIP. CO. INC.
Chicago Roller Skate Co.
CONVERSE RUBBER COMPANY
COSOM CORPORATION
CRAN BARRY INC.
DAYTON RACQUET CO. INC.
Dekan Timing Devices
DeVac, Inc., Sportation Division
Andy Douglass, Inc.
DUDLEY SPORTS CO. INC.
Exercycle Corporation
Flex-I-Flag Company
The Harry Gill Company
J. E. Gregory Co.
Gulbenkian Swim Inc.
GYM MASTER CO.
Hadar Athletic Mfg. Co.
Hanhart Stop Watch Factory, Ltd.
HARGAL ALL-SPORTS CARRYALL
Harvard Table Tennis Corporation
HILLERICH & BARDSBY CO.
Jayfro Corp.
Adolph Kiefer & Co.—Div. of McNeil Corp.
Kwik-Kold, Inc.
LIND CLIMBER COMPANY
McGregor Company, Consumer Division,
   Brunswick Corp.
MARCY GYMNASIUM EQUIPMENT CO.
Mason City Tent & Awning Co.
McArthur Towels Inc.
Medart Division, Jackes-Evans Mfg. Co.
Mid-Valley Sports Center
3M Company, Recreation & Athletic Products
Mitchell Division/Royal Industries
Monsanto Company—AstroTurf®
   Recreational Surfaces
National Sports Division—Medalist Industries
NISSEN CORPORATION
OCEAN POOL SUPPLY CO. INC.

Oregon Worsted Co.
Pennsylvania Athletic Products
**PHYSICAL EDUCATION SUPPLY
  ASSOCIATES, INC.**
PORT-A-PIT INC.
Premier Products
J. A. PRESTON CORPORATION
Program Aids Inc.
Protection Equipment Sales Division—
  Vogt Mfg. Corp.
Quinton Instruments
Randolph Mfg. Co., Inc.
Rawlings Sporting Goods Company
Saunders Archery Company
Scott & Company-GM Baseball
SEAMLESS
Sells Aerial Tennis Co.
SERON MFG. CO.
Shield Mfg., Inc.
Sorensen-Christian Industries, Inc.
A. G. Spalding & Bros., Inc.
STERLING RECREATION PRODUCTS
Strand Case Co. (Div. of SNR Golf, Inc.)
Top Star Inc.
Universal Athletic Sales Co.
UNIVERSAL BLEACHER CO.
Videonetics, Div. Newell Industries
W. J. VOIT RUBBER CORP.
WILSON SPORTING GOODS CO.
Wittek Golf Range Supply Co., Inc.
Wolverine Sports Supply

ATHLETIC AND SPORTS CLOTHING

M—Men's
W—Women's
B—Both

ALDRICH & ALDRICH INC.—B
Algy Dance Costumes—W
Bike Athletic Prod. Div., Kendall Co.—M
TOM BRODERICK COMPANY, INC.— B
CAPEZIO DANCEWEAR—B
CASTELLO FENCING EQUIP. CO. INC.
CHAMPION PRODUCTS INC.—B
CONVERSE RUBBER COMPANY—B
CRAN BARRY INC.—W
Dolfin Sportswear Company—B
Gulbenkian Swim Inc.—B
GYM MASTER CO.—B
Hanes Sports Division—Hanes Corp.—M
The Hanold Company and its Sylvia
  Putzinger Div.—B
Jean Lee Originals—W
Adolph Kiefer & Co.—Div. of McNeil
  Corp.—B
Loshin's Costume Center, Inc.—W
McArthur Towels Inc.—B

E. R. MOORE CO.— W
National Sports Division—Medalist Industries
New Balance Athletic Shoe Co.—B
NISSEN CORPORATION
OCEAN POOL SUPPLY CO. INC.
**PHYSICAL EDUCATION SUPPLY
  ASSOCIATES, INC.**
Randolph Mfg. Co., Inc.
Rawlings Sporting Goods Company—M
Wheelan and Wheelan, Inc.—W
White Stag-Speedo—B
WILSON SPORTING GOODS CO.
Wilton Mfg. Co. Inc.—B

RESEARCH EQUIPMENT

Warren E. Collins, Inc.
Dekan Timing Devices
E & M Instrument Co., Inc.
Exercycle Corporation
Lafayette Instrument Co.
NISSEN CORPORATION
J. A. PRESTON CORPORATION
Quinton Instruments
Reedco, Inc.
Technology/Versatronics, Inc.

SCOREBOARDS AND TIMERS

R. E. Austin & Son
CRAN BARRY INC.
Dekan Timing Devices
Gulbenkian Swim Inc.
Hanhart Stop Watch Factory, Ltd.
Adolph Kiefer & Co., Div. of McNeil Corp.
NISSEN CORPORATION
Program Aids Inc.
Sorensen-Christian Industries, Inc.
Wolverine Sports Supply

AUDIOVISUAL MATERIALS

ALLYN AND BACON, INC.
American Cancer Society, Inc.
THE ATHLETIC INSTITUTE
R. E. Austin & Son
BALL-BOY CO.
Bowmar Records, Inc.
Stanley Bowmar Co., Inc.
George F. Cram Company, Inc.
Denoyer-Geppert Company
Walt Disney Educational Materials Company
Ealing Corporation
EDUCATIONAL ACTIVITIES, INC.
**EDUCATIONAL RECORDINGS OF
  AMERICA, INC.**
Educators Progress Service, Inc.
Film Distributors International

G. N. Productions
Harcourt, Brace & World, Inc.
HARPER & ROW, PUBLISHERS
D. C. Heath and Company/A Div. of
  Raytheon Education Co.
HOCTOR EDUCATIONAL RECORDS
HOLT, RINEHART AND WINSTON
KIMBO EDUCATIONAL RECORDS
Lafayette Instrument Co.
Marjorie S. Larsen
J. B. Lippincott Company
Loshin's Costume Center, Inc.
Medical Plastics Laboratory, Inc.
FREDA MILLER RECORDS FOR DANCE
3M Company, Visual Products Division
National Dairy Council
The National Foundation—March of Dimes
National Golf Foundation
NISSEN CORPORATION
Physical Education Aids
**PHYSICAL EDUCATION SUPPLY
  ASSOCIATES, INC.**
Popular Science and Audio Visuals, Inc.
Program Aids Inc.
Rhythms Productions Records
School Aid Co., Inc.
Society For Visual Education, Inc.
Syracuse University Film Marketing Division
TAMPAX INCORPORATED
United States Air Force
Videonetics, Div. Newell Industries

FACILITIES

THE ATHLETIC INSTITUTE (planning)
California Products Corporation (surfacing)
DeBourgh Mfg. Co. (lockers)
J. E. Gregory Co.
Adolph Kiefer & Co., Div. of McNeil Corp.
Medart Division Jackes-Evans Mfg. Co.
  (lockers, bleachers)
3M Company—Recreation and Athletic
  Products (Surfacing)
Monsanto Company—AstroTurf® (surfacing)
NISSEN CORPORATION (bleachers)
STERLING RECREATION PRODUCTS
Superior Wire & Iron Products, Inc. (lockers)
Universal Athletic Sales Co.
Universal Bleacher Co.
  (bleachers, port-a-pool)

EDUCATIONAL MATERIALS

AAHPER-USLTA Joint Committee on Tennis
ALLYN AND BACON, INC.
American Cancer Society, Inc.
American Institute of Baking
American Junior Bowling Congress

THE ATHLETIC INSTITUTE
**ATLAS ATHLETIC EQUIPMENT
  COMPANY**
BALL-BOY CO.
Stanley Bowmar Co., Inc.
WM. C. BROWN COMPANY PUBLISHERS
BURGESS PUBLISHING CO.
George F. Cram Company, Inc.
Denoyer-Geppert Company
Walt Disney Educational Materials Company
Ealing Corporation
**EDUCATIONAL RECORDINGS OF
  AMERICA, INC.**
Educators Progress Service, Inc.
Encyclopaedia Britannica, Inc.
Film Distributors International
Harcourt, Brace & World, Inc.
HARPER & ROW, PUBLISHERS
D. C. Heath and Company/A Div. of
  Raytheon Education Co.
HOCTOR EDUCATIONAL RECORDS
HOLT, RINEHART AND WINSTON
Instructional Materials Laboratories, Inc.
KIMBERLY-CLARK CORPORATION
KIMBO EDUCATIONAL RECORDS
LEA & FEBIGER
Licensed Beverage Industries, Inc.
J. B. Lippincott Company
McGraw-Hill Book Co., Webster Division
Medical Plastics Laboratory, Inc.
**CHARLES E. MERRILL PUBLISHING
  COMPANY**
FREDA MILLER RECORDS FOR DANCE
3M Company, Visual Products Division
National Dairy Council
The National Foundation—March of Dimes
National Golf Foundation
National Rifle Association of America
Personal Products Company
The Physical Education Association of
  Great Britain and Northern Ireland
Program Aids Inc.
Reedco, Inc.
Rhythms Productions Records
W. B. SAUNDERS COMPANY
Scott Paper Company
Signal Press
Society For Visual Education, Inc.
Standard Brands Incorporated
Stepping Tones Records
Syracuse University Film Marketing Division
TAMPAX INCORPORATED
Videonetics, Div. Newell Industries

EMBLEMS, AWARDS, TROPHIES

CHAMPION PRODUCTS INC.

CRAN BARRY INC.
Gulbenkian Swim Inc.
**PHYSICAL EDUCATION SUPPLY
ASSOCIATES, INC.**
Program Aids Inc.
Wolverine Sports Supply

PUBLISHERS

Academic Press, Inc.
ALLYN AND BACON, INC.
The W. H. Anderson Company
THE ATHLETIC INSTITUTE
WM. C. BROWN COMPANY PUBLISHERS
BURGESS PUBLISHING CO.
Denoyer-Geppert Company
Ealing Corporation
Educators Progress Service, Inc.
Encyclopaedia Britannica, Inc.
Goodyear Publishing Company, Inc.
Harcourt, Brace & World, Inc.
HARPER & ROW, PUBLISHERS
D. C. Heath and Company
HOCTOR EDUCATIONAL RECORDS
KIMBO EDUCATIONAL RECORDS
LEA & FEBIGER
LIND CLIMBER COMPANY
J. B. Lippincott Company
LYONS & CARNAHAN
THE MACMILLAN COMPANY
McGRAW-HILL BOOK COMPANY
McGraw-Hill Book Co., Webster Division
**CHARLES E. MERRILL PUBLISHING
COMPANY**
FREDA MILLER RECORDS FOR DANCE
THE C. V. MOSBY COMPANY
The National Foundation—March of Dimes
National Sporting Goods Association
O'Brien & O'Brien
The Physical Education Association of
Great Britain and Northern Ireland
Physical Education Aids
**PHYSICAL EDUCATION SUPPLY
ASSOCIATES, INC.**
Program Aids Inc.
Rhythms Productions Records
The Ronald Press Company
W. B. SAUNDERS COMPANY
School Aid Co., Inc.
Charles C Thomas, Publisher
**WADSWORTH PUBLISHING COMPANY,
INC.**

TRAINING ROOM EQUIPMENT AND SUPPLIES

AA-Belco All-Automatic Phys-Ed &
Athletic Laundry Equipment Co.

American Gym Corporation
Bike Athletic Prod Div., Kendall Co.
CRAN BARRY INC.
Exercycle Corporation
Kwik-Kold, Inc.
MARCY GYMNASIUM EQUIPMENT CO.
Master Lock Company
Medical Plastic Laboratory, Inc.
Mitchell Division/Royal Industries
Premier Products
J. A. PRESTON CORPORATION
Program Aids Inc.
Sani-Mist Inc.
SCHOOL HEALTH SUPPLY CO.
SERON MFG. CO.
STERLING RECREATION PRODUCTS
Top Star Inc.
Wolverine Sports Supply

RECREATION AND OUTDOOR EDUCATION EQUIPMENT AND FACILITIES

R. E. Austin & Son
BALL-BOY CO.
Brunswick Corp./Bowling Division
Buc-Ol Mfg. Co.
The J. E. Burke Company
COSOM CORPORATION
Daisy/Heddon, Division Victor
Comptometer Corp.
DeVac, Inc., Sportation Division
Flex-I-Flag Company
J. E. Gregory Co.
Gulbenkian Swim Inc.
Hadar Athletic Mfg. Co.
THE DELMER F. HARRIS CO.
Jayfro Corp.
Adolph Kiefer & Co., Div. of McNeil Corp.
MARCY GYMNASIUM EQUIPMENT CO.
Mason City Tent & Awning Co.
Master Lock Company
Medart Division, Jackes-Evans Mfg. Co.
Mid-Valley Sports Center
3M Company—Recreation and Athletic
Products
Mitchell Division/Royal Industries
Monsanto Company—AstroTurf®
Recreational Surfaces
National Sports Division—Medalist Industries
NISSEN CORPORATION
Pennsylvania Athletic Products
Playground Corporation of America
PORT-A-PIT INC.
Premier Products
J. A. PRESTON CORPORATION
Program Aids Inc.

Saunders Archery Company
SEAMLESS
Shield Mfg., Inc.
Sorensen-Christian Industries, Inc.
STERLING RECREATION PRODUCTS
Superior Wire & Iron Products, Inc.
T. F. Twardzik & Co., Inc.
Universal Athletic Sales Co.
UNIVERSAL BLEACHER CO.
Videonetics, Div. Newell Industries
Wittek Golf Range Supply Co., Inc.
Wolverine Sports Supply

GAMES

COSOM CORPORATION
DAYTON RACQUET CO., INC.
Hanhart Stop Watch Factory Ltd.
Harvard Table Tennis Corporation
Marjorie S. Larsen
Mason City Tent & Awning Co.
PORT-A PIT INC.
J. A. PRESTON CORPORATION
Sells Aerial Tennis Co.
STERLING RECREATION PRODUCTS
R. E. Titus Gym Scooter Co.
T. F. Twardzik & Co., Inc.
Wolverine Sports Supply

CAREER INFORMATION

American Cancer Society, Inc.
Educators Progress Service, Inc.
O'Brien & O'Brien
The Physical Education Association of
    Great Britain and Northern Ireland
United States Air Force
U.S. Army Recruiting Command
U.S. Marine Corps
U.S. Navy
YWCA of the USA

FACILITIES AND EQUIPMENT MAINTENANCE

AA-Belco All-Automatic Phys-Ed &
    Athletic Laundry Equip. Co.
Hillyard Chemical Company
Master Lock Company
McArthur Towels, Inc.
Medart Division Jackes-Evans Mfg. Co.
PELLERIN MILNOR CORPORATION
Sani-Mist Inc.
STERLING RECREATION PRODUCTS

DANCE SUPPLIES

ALDRICH & ALDRICH INC.
Algy Dance Costumes

BALL-BOY CO.
Bowmar Records, Inc.
TOM BRODERICK COMPANY, INC.
CAPEZIO DANCEWEAR
CRAN BARRY INC.
EDUCATIONAL RECORDINGS OF
    AMERICA INC.
J. E. Gregory Co.
HOCTOR EDUCATIONAL RECORDS
KIMBO EDUCATIONAL RECORDS
Kling's Theatrical Shoe Co.
Leo's Advanced Theatrical Co.
Loshin's Costume Center, Inc.
FREDA MILLER RECORDS FOR DANCE
PHYSICAL EDUCATION SUPPLY
    ASSOCIATES, INC.
Rhythms Productions Records
SELVA
Stepping Tones Records
Wheelan and Wheelan, Inc.
Wolff-Fording & Co., Inc.

MISCELLANEOUS

American Junior Bowling Congress
    (bowling programs)
Benson Optical Company
    (athletic eyewear)
COCA-COLA USA (concessions)
CRAN BARRY INC.
    (cheerleading fashions & supplies)
DeBourgh Mfg. Co. (lockers)
Jean Lee Originals
    (cheerleader & majorette fashions)
Mason Candies, Inc. (fund raising)
Master Lock Company (locks)
Monsanto Company—AstroTurf®
    Recreational Surfaces (synthetic turf)
National Sporting Goods Association
    (national trade association for the
    sporting goods industry)
PELLERIN MILNOR CORPORATION
    (laundry machinery)
Reedco, Inc. (tests and measurements)
Superior Wire & Iron Products, Inc.
    (athletic lockers & benches)

A

AA-Belco All-Automatic Phys-Ed &
    Athletic Equipment Co.
P. O. Box 652
Charlotte, North Carolina 28201
Specialized all-automatic physical education and
athletic laundry equipment for doing all gym
uniforms, towels, and game and practice uniforms.

AAHPER-USLTA Joint Committee on Tennis

Norris Gymnasium
University of Minnesota
Minneapolis, Minnesota 55455
Educational materials and teaching aids pertaining
to tennis instruction.

Academic Press, Inc.
111 Fifth Avenue
New York, New York 10003
Texts and reference works in physical education
and health.

ADIRONDACK INDUSTRIES, INC.
McKinley Avenue
Dolgeville, New York 13329
Manufacturer of "Big Stick Bats."

ALDRICH & ALDRICH INC.
1859 Milwaukee Avenue
Chicago, Illinois 60647
Apparel for physical education, pool, and dance.

Algy Dance Costumes
148 West 24 Street
New York, New York 10011
Sequined uniforms for majorettes, cheerleaders,
and twirlers.

ALLYN & BACON, INC.
470 Atlantic Avenue
Boston, Massachusetts 02210
Publishers of preschool through high school and
college textbooks.

AMERICAN ATHLETIC EQUIPMENT CO.
Box 111
Jefferson, Iowa 50129
The manufacturer of gymnasium and gymnastic
equipment.

American Cancer Society, Inc.
219 East 42nd Street
New York, New York 10017
Health-educational teaching aids, films, film cartridges, filmstrips and printed materials.

American Gym Corporation
North Greengate Road
Greensburg, Pennsylvania 15601
American Gym Corp. manufacturers of the Super
Gym Weight Training Machine 8, 9, 10, 11, 13,
14, and 15 Stations.

American Institute of Baking
400 East Ontario Street
Chicago, Illinois 60611
Graded educational literature for teaching nutrition in the health education curriculum.

American Junior Bowling Congress
1572 East Capitol Drive
Milwaukee, Wisconsin 53211
Bowling program for boys and girls.

The W. H. Anderson Company
646 Main Street
Cincinnati, Ohio 46201

THE ATHLETIC INSTITUTE
805 Merchandise Mart
Chicago, Illinois 60654
Audiovisual and published instructional aids on
athletics, physical education, and recreation.

**ATLAS ATHLETIC EQUIPMENT
COMPANY**
2339 Hampton Avenue
St. Louis, Missouri 63139
Gymnasium apparatus and gymnasium mats.

R. E. Austin & Son
705 Bedford Avenue
Bellmore, New York 11710
Quality field and gym athletic equipment.

B

BALL-BOY CO.
27 Milburn Street
Bronxville, New York 10708
New designs—equipment and teaching aids for
sports, athletics, dance.

Benson Optical Company
1812 Park Avenue
Minneapolis, Minnesota 55440
All-American athletic eyewear, all-nylon frame and
safety lenses—comfortable, lightweight, safe.

Bike Athletic Prod. Div., Kendall Co.
309 W. Jackson Boulevard
Chicago, Illinois 60606
Athletic supporters, supports, mouthguards, trainer's tape, trainer's supplies, first aid supplies, and
socks for the prevention and care of injuries.

Bolco Athletic Company
1751 N. Eastern Avenue
Los Angeles, California 90032
Baseball bases, home plates, pitchers plates, base
anchors, helmets.

Bowmar Records, Inc.
622 Rodier Drive
Glendale, California 91201
Music for physical fitness and records of singing,
games, and folk dances.

Stanley Bowmar Co., Inc.
4 Broadway
Valhalla, New York 10595
We sell multi-media materials, including records,
tapes, filmstrips, and transparencies, for all grade
levels.

TOM BRODERICK COMPANY, INC.
2400 Broadway

Parsons, Kansas 67357
Gymwear, poolwear, dancewear, team uniforms.

WM. C. BROWN COMPANY PUBLISHERS
135 South Locust Street
Dubuque, Iowa 52001
Publisher of college textbooks and supplementary materials.

Brunswick Corporation, Bowling Division
69 West Washington
Chicago, Illinois 60602
The finest and most complete line of bowling supplies and equipment including bowling balls, bags, and shoes.

Buc Ol Manufacturing Co.
1017 South Locust Street
Oxford, Ohio 45056
Mac-Col, the safe, all rubber practice golf ball that eliminates the need for nets indoors and large space outdoors.

BURGESS PUBLISHING CO.
426 South 6th Street
Minneapolis, Minnesota 55415
Educational texts and manuals for elementary, high school, and college use.

The J. E. Burke Company
P. O. Box 549
Fond du Lac, Wisconsin 54935
Playground, sports, and recreation equipment.

C

California Products Corporation
169 Waverly Street
Cambridge, Massachusetts 02139
Plexipave tennis courts and Reslite® running tracks.

CAPEZIO DANCEWEAR
1855 Broadway
New York, New York 10023
Dance, theatre, and recreation footwear; leotards, tights, and accessories.

CASTELLO FENCING EQUIP. CO. INC.
30 East 10th Street
New York, New York 10003
Fencing, judo, karate uniforms and equipment.

CHAMPION PRODUCTS INC.
115 College Avenue
Rochester, New York 14607
Athletic knitwear and campus sportswear.

Chicago Roller Skate Co.
4498 West Lake Street
Chicago, Illinois 60624
Boot and clamp-on roller skates, repairs and accessories suitable for physical education programs.

COCA-COLA USA
P. O. Drawer 1734
Atlanta, Georgia 30301
Manufacturers of a complete line of soft drinks—Coca-Cola, Sprite, TAB, Fresca, and Fanta Flavors.

Warren E. Collins, Inc.
220 Wood Road
Braintree, Massachusetts 02184
Ergometers and treadmills for determining work output in mild, moderate, and excessive exercise.

CONVERSE RUBBER COMPANY
392 Pearl Street
Malden, Massachusetts 02148
Manufacturers of tennis, basketball, football, wrestling, and yachting shoes; football and band parkas, warm-up jackets.

COSOM CORPORATION
6030 Wayzata Boulevard
Minneapolis, Minnesota 55416
Safe-T-Play sporting goods—"The First Step in Sports."

George F. Cram Company, Inc.
301 S. LaSalle Street
Indianapolis, Indiana 46206
Anatomical, health, and personality charts and models.

CRAN BARRY INC.
31 Green Street, Box 354
Marblehead, Massachusetts 01945
Complete suppliers of sports equipment and apparel for women.

D

Daisy/Heddon, Division Victor
    Comptometer Corporation
South Highway 71
Rogers, Arkansas 72756
School training programs.

DAYTON RACQUET CO. INC.
302 South Albright Street
Arcanum, Ohio 45304
Steel racquets—tennis, badminton, paddle tennis, and racquet ball.

DeBourgh Mfg. Co.
9300 James Avenue South
Minneapolis, Minnesota 55431
Fully ventilated athletic and physical education lockers and locker room benches.

Dekan Timing Devices
Box 712
Glen Ellyn, Illinois 60137
Automatic performance analyzer, timing automatically and the 1/100th second range with multiple start and stop methods.

Denoyer-Geppert Company
5235 Ravenswood Avenue
Chicago, Illinois 60640
Designed and producer of unbreakable anatomical
models, skeletons, charts, transparencies, and related visual aids for health sciences.

DeVac, Inc., Sportation Division
10122 Highway 55
Minneapolis, Minnesota 55427
Golf machines for direct teaching of proper swing
via muscle memory, non-shanking golf clubs.

Walt Disney Educational Materials
  Company
800 Sonora Avenue
Glendale, California 91201
Upjohn/Disney Health Series: Four Films. This
is Your Health Films: Eight Films.

Dolfin Sportswear Company
South Sterley and Catherine Streets
Shillington, Pennsylvania 19607
Swim suits used for competition, swimming classes,
and practice in general, all around pool, and beach
use.

Andy Douglass, Inc.
2758 Orchid Street
New Orleans, Louisiana 70119
Completely safe weight-lifting machine that eliminates all problems, including safety, economy,
time, and space.

DUDLEY SPORTS CO., INC.
19 West 34th Street
New York, New York 10001
Softballs, baseballs, baseball and tennis machines.

E F

E & M Instrument Co., Inc.
7651 Airport Boulevard
Houston, Texas 77017
Multi-channel, ink-writing recorders and accessories and biotelemetry systems.

Ealing Corporation
2225 Massachusetts Avenue
Cambridge, Massachusetts 02140
Super 8mm, silent, single-concept film loops and
related projection equipment.

EDUCATIONAL ACTIVITIES, INC.
P. O. Box 392
Freeport, New York 11520
Records, tapes, cassettes, filmstrips, and books.

**EDUCATIONAL RECORDINGS OF
  AMERICA, INC.**
P. O. Box 231
Monroe, Connecticut 06468

Everything in educational records—folk, square,
social dance, physical fitness.

Educators Progress Service, Inc.
214 Center Street
Randolph, Wisconsin 53956
Guides to free materials for schools.

Encyclopaedia Britannica, Inc.
Chicago, Illinois
Encyclopaedia Britannica, Great Books of the
Western World, Britannica Junior, and other re-
lated materials.

Exercycle Corporation
630 Third Avenue
New York, New York, 10017
Distributor of Exercycle,® the world's leading
motorized exerciser, the PEP,™ Personal Exerciser
Planner, Torg™ exercise equipment.

Film Distributors International
2223 South Olive Street
Los Angeles, California 90007
16mm films—"Narcotics: Pit of Despair" and "Drug
Abuse: The Chemical Tomb."

Flex-I-Flag Company
2238 N.E. Buchanan
Minneapolis, Minnesota 55418
Inexpensive field flags to be used as boundary
markers for physical education activities.

G H

G. N. Productions
1019 North Cole Avenue
Los Angeles, California 90038
Educational films and film production services.

The Harry Gill Company
201 Courtesy Road
Urbana, Illinois 61801
Track and field equipment.

Goodyear Publishing Company, Inc.
15115 Sunset Boulevard
Pacific Palisades, California 90272
Goodyear Physical Activities Series edited by J.
Tillman Hall.

J. E. Gregory Co.
922 West First
Spokane, Washington 99204
Physical education equipment and supplies.

Gulbenkian Swim Inc.
87 Greenwich Avenue
Greenwich, Connecticut 06830
Nylon swim wear, nylon physical education suits
for swim classes, kickboards, racing lanes, swim
equipment.

GYM MASTER CO.
3200 South Zuni Street
Englewood, Colorado 80110
Gymnasium, gymnastic apparatus, weight lifting equipment, gymnastic clothing.

Hadar Athletic Mfg. Co.
1108 North 13th Street
Humboldt, Iowa 50548
Physical education, track and field, and football equipment.

Hanes Sports Division, Hanes Corp.
Box 3073
Winston-Salem, North Carolina 27102
Manufacturers of athletic and sports clothing.

Hanhart Stop Watch Factory, Ltd.
3 Chestnut Street
Suffern, New York 10901
Hanhart stop watches for timing all sporting events.

Hanold Company and its
Sylvia Putziger Division
Standish, Maine 04084
Sports clothing and gym wear including the Putziger Blazer.

Harcourt, Brace & World, Inc.
757 Third Avenue
New York, New York, 10017
Textbooks and other instructional materials for grades K-12.

HARGAL ALL-SPORTS CARRYALL
Box 1094
Wilmington, California 90744
The Versatile Cart—the kids cannot tear apart.

HARPER & ROW, PUBLISHERS
49 East 33rd Street
New York, New York 10016
Texts and references—health, physical education, recreation.

THE DELMER F. HARRIS CO.
Box 288
Concordia, Kansas 66901
"Swedish Gym" apparatus and other Playmate playground equipment.

Harvard Table Tennis Corporation
265 Third Street
Cambridge, Massachusetts 02142
Table tennis equipment.

D. C. Heath and Company/A Division of
Raytheon Education Company
125 Spring Street
Lexington, Massachusetts 02118
Heath produces films and filmstrips in science, history, and health education for elementary and secondary schools.

HILLERICH & BRADSBY CO.
P. O. Box 506
Louisville, Kentucky 40201
Louisville Slugger bats, golf clubs, and hockey sticks.

Hillyard Chemical Company
302 North 4th Street
St. Joseph, Missouri 64502
All supplies that will make your floors look beautiful yet practical for sports.

HOCTOR EDUCATIONAL RECORDS
115 Manhattan Avenue
Waldwick, New Jersey 07463
Records and manuals for all phases of dance and physical education—Bogen phonographs also.

HOLT, RINEHART AND WINSTON
383 Madison Avenue
New York, New York 10017
Vince Lombardi's The Science and Art of Football
—a series of 12 teaching-training films.

I J

Instructional Materials Laboratories, Inc.
18 East 41st Street
New York, New York 10017
Industry-sponsored school programs in areas of first aid and driver safety.

Jayfro Corp.
P. O. Box 50
Montville, Connecticut 06353
Manufacturers of a top quality line of athletic, gym, and recreation equipment.

Jean Lee Originals
P. O. Box 207
Goshen, Indiana 46526
United States' largest manufacturer and distributor of cheerleader and majorette fashions.

K

Adolph Kiefer & Co., Div. of McNeil Corp.
2741 Wingate
Akron, Ohio 44314
Swimming pool equipment including racing lanes, swimwear, and deck equipment.

KIMBERLY-CLARK CORPORATION
Life Cycle Center
Neenah, Wisconsin 54956
Family life educational booklets and teaching aids.

KIMBO EDUCATIONAL RECORDS
P. O. Box 55
Deal, New Jersey 07723
Educational albums, filmstrips, teacher's manuals for physical education, dance, gymnastics, rhythms, and sports at all grade levels.

Kling's Theatrical Shoe Co.
218 South Wabash Avenue
Chicago, Illinois 60604
Manufacturers and retailers of dance wear.

Kwik-Kold, Inc.
First Federal Building
Moberly, Missouri 65270
Training room supplies including instant cold
packs, Desenex skin protection.

L

Lafayette Instrument Co.
Box 1279
Lafayette, Indiana 47902
Manufacturers of laboratory testing devices.

Marjorie S. Larsen
1754 Middlefield
Stockton, California 95204
Speed-a-Way guide book. Film, audiovisual charts
and tests.

LEA & FEBIGER
600 Washington Square
Philadelphia, Pennsylvania 19106
Distinctive texts in health, physical education, and
recreation, described in new 1969 catalog.

Leo's Advance Theatrical Co.
125 North Wabash Avenue
Chicago, Illinois 60602
Shoes, body garments, records, makeup, tights,
material, costumes for children and adults in dance
and physical education.

Licensed Beverage Industries, Inc.
155 East 44th Street
New York, New York 10017
Free educational reprints for teacher use dealing
with the area of alcohol education as a field of
instruction in schools and colleges.

LIND CLIMBER COMPANY
807 Reba Place
Evanston, Illinois 60202
Gymnastic equipment for elementary schools and
schools for exceptional children, textbook of apparatus activities.

J. B. Lippincott Company
East Washington Square
Philadelphia, Pennsylvania 19105
Books in medicine, dentistry, pharmacy, nursing,
and allied professions.

Loshin's Costume Center, Inc.
215 East 8th Street
Cincinnati, Ohio 45202
Leotards, trunks, tights, dance and recreation footwear, dance and recreation records and manuals.

Lyons & Carnahan
Educational Division/Meredith Corporation
407 East 25th Street
Chicago, Illinois 60616
Publishers of elementary and secondary education
materials.

M

THE MACMILLAN COMPANY
866 Third Avenue
New York, New York 10022
Book publishers in all areas of health, physical
education, and recreation.

MacGregor Company Consumer Division
Brunswick Corporation
I-75 and Jimson Road
Cincinnati, Ohio 45215
Manufacturers of golf equipment and athletic
goods.

MARCY GYMNASIUM EQUIPMENT CO.
1736 Standard Avenue
Glendale, California 91201
Manufacturers of the circuit-trainer™ and complete gym installations.

Mason Candies, Inc.
P. O. Box 500
Mineola, New York 11501
Fill your treasury with Mason Candies' no-risk, no-
investment protected fund raising plan.

Mason City Tent & Awning Co.
403 South Federal Avenue
Mason City, Iowa 50401
Rip Flag is the quality belt and flag set made to
give maximum help to the physical education instructor or coach.

Master Lock Company
2600 North 32nd Street
Milwaukee, Wisconsin 53245
Padlocks and built-in locks for lockers.

McArthur Towels Inc.
Box H
Baraboo, Wisconsin 53913
School gym towels, laundry equipment, related
products.

McGRAW-HILL BOOK COMPANY
330 West 42nd Street
New York, New York 10036
Publishers of outstanding education textbooks.

McGraw-Hill Book Co., Webster Division
Manchester Road
Manchester, Missouri 63011
Physical Education for Life, a physical training
text with film loops on various sports.

Medart Division, Jackes-Evans Mfg. Co.
11737 Administration Drive
St. Louis, Missouri 63141
Telescopic gymseats, basketball backstops, lockers, locks.

Medical Plastics Laboratory, Inc.
P. O. Box 38
Gatesville, Texas 76528
Authentic plastic anatomical reproductions.

CHARLES E. MERRILL PUBLISHING COMPANY
1300 Alum Creek Drive
Columbus, Ohio 43216
Elementary physical education materials and textbooks for prospective elementary and secondary health educators.

Mid-Valley Sports Center
5350 North Blackstone
Fresno, California 93726
The E. Mason "Shorty" Tennis racket—a tennis racket five inches shorter than the regular racket.

FREDA MILLER RECORDS FOR DANCE
Dept. E, Box 383
Northport, New York 11768
Modern dance and rhythms from basic movements to advanced for dance, physical education, and the elementary classroom teacher.

3M Company, Recreation & Athletic Products
3M Center, Adv. Display, 220-6E
St. Paul, Minnesota, 55101
"Tartan" brand surfacing for recreation and athletic playing surfaces.

3M Company, Visual Products Division
3M Center
St. Paul, Minnesota 55101
Complete line of equipment and accessories for overhead projection.

Mitchell Division/Royal Industries
1500 East Chestnut Street
Santa Ana, California 92701
Protective playground cushion and matting products.

Monsanto Company
    Astro Turf® Recreational Surfaces
800 North Lindbergh Boulevard
St. Louis, Missouri 63166
AstroTurf® athletic fields, playgrounds, field houses, golf tees, and greens.

E. R. MOORE CO.
7230 North Caldwell Avenue
Niles (Chicago), Illinois 60648
Gymwear for girls and young women in physical education classes.

THE C. V. MOSBY COMPANY
11830 Westline Industrial Drive
St. Louis, Missouri 63141
Publishers of outstanding college text and reference books in the field of health and physical education.

N O

National Dairy Council
111 North Canal Street
Chicago, Illinois 60606
Publishers of booklets, posters, films, and filmstrips on nutrition education for use in professional, educational, and consumer groups.

The National Foundation—March of Dimes
800 Second Avenue
New York, New York 10017
Free supplementary materials on genetics, birth defects, and prenatal care.

National Golf Foundation
Room 804 Merchandise Mart
Chicago, Illinois 60654
Golf films and publications.

National Rifle Association of America
1600 Rhode Island Avenue, N.W.
Washington, D. C. 20036
National organization promoting marksmanship, firearms safety, hunting safety, and conservation.

National Sporting Goods Association
717 North Michigan Avenue
Chicago, Illinois 60611
National trade association representing sporting goods retailers as well as manufacturers of all types of sporting goods equipment.

National Sports Division Medalist Industries
19 East McWilliams
Fond du Lac, Wisconsin 54935
Complete line of wrestling and gymnasium mats and accessories.

New Balance Athletic Shoe Co.
176 Belmont Street
Watertown, Massachusetts 02172
Athletic-track shoes.

NISSEN CORPORATION
930 27th Avenue S.W.
Cedar Rapids, Iowa 52406
Manufacturing heavy-duty gymnasium equipment for schools and colleges.

O'Brien & O'Brien
Educational Consultants
P. O. Box 271
Buffalo, New York 14221
Guide to Educational Opportunities: Listing of faculty and staff vacancies in universities, colleges, and junior colleges.

OCEAN POOL SUPPLY CO., INC.
17 Stepar Place
Huntington Station, New York 11746
The first and finest in swimwear, equipment, and accessories.

Oregon Worsted Co.
P. O. Box 02098
Portland, Oregon 97202
Manufacture and sale of Flying Fleece balls.

P

PELLERIN MILNOR CORPORATION
P. O. Box 398
Kenner, Louisiana 70062
Manufacturers of heavy duty laundry machinery for school and college use.

Pennsylvania Athletic Products
P. O. Box 951
Akron, Ohio 44309
Athletic products for institutional use.

Personal Products Company
Milltown, New Jersey 08850
Complete program of feminine hygiene instructional materials including motion picture, teacher's guides, and student booklets.

The Physical Education Association of
Great Britain and Northern Ireland
Ling House, 10 Nottingham Place
London, W. 1, England
The professional association of physical educators in Britain and publishers and distributors of a wide variety of books.

Physical Education Aids
P. O. Box 5117
San Mateo, California 94402
Textbooks, wall charts, teaching units for gymnastic and tumbling activities.

**PHYSICAL EDUCATION SUPPLY
ASSOCIATES, INC.**
P. O. Box 292
Trumbull, Connecticut 06611
For the new movement, hoops, balanced jump ropes, magic stretch ropes, wevau balls, wevau ball primer, "Who Can," corrective gymnastics.

Playground Corporation of America
29-16 40th Avenue
Long Island City, New York 11101
Planned physical play environments for children 2-12.

Popular Science Audio Visuals, Inc.
355 Lexington Avenue
New York, New York 10017
Producer-distributor of audiovisual materials.

PORT-A-PIT, INC.
P. O. Box C
Temple City, California 91780
Safety skill development equipment for gymnastics and physical education.

Premier Products
River Vale, New Jersey 07675
Gymnasium, physical education equipment and mats.

J. A. PRESTON CORPORATION
71 Fifth Avenue
New York, New York 10003
Adapted physical education and related research equipment.

Program Aids Inc.
161 MacQuesten Parkway
Mount Vernon, New York 10550
Manufacturers of innovative physical education equipment.

Protection Equipment Sales Division
Vogt Mfg. Corp.
100 Fernwood Avenue
Rochester, New York 14621
Makers of Polvonite wrestling mats and Voplex gym mats.

Q R

Quinton Instruments
3051 44th Avenue West
Seattle, Washington 98199
Treadmills, bicycle ergometers, exercise cardiotachometers, respiratory gas analysis, telemetry equipment.

Randolph Mfg. Co., Inc.
32 South Main Street
Randolph, Massachusetts 02368
Athletic footwear and water sports equipment.

Rawlings Sporting Goods Company
2300 Delmar Boulevard
St. Louis, Missouri 63166
Complete line of athletic goods.

Reedco, Inc.
5 Easterly Avenue
Auburn, New York 13021
Equipment for the testing and teaching of body mechanics and posture.

Rhythms Productions Records
Box 34485
Los Angeles, California 90034
Producers of educational records, audiovisual materials, and folk dance costume picture prints.

The Ronald Press Company
79 Madison Avenue

New York, New York 10016
Books on physical education, sports, gymnastics, and conditioning.

S

Sani-Mist Inc.
3018 Market Street
Philadelphia, Pennsylvania 19104
Foot spray dispenser for the prevention of athletes foot.

Saunders Archery Company
P. O. Box 476
Columbus, Nebraska 68601
Saunders accessories complete your profit picture.

W. B. SAUNDERS COMPANY
West Washington Square
Philadelphia, Pennsylvania 19105
Textbooks, handbooks, and reference books in health and physical education.

School Aid Co., Inc.
911 Colfax Drive
Danville, Illinois 61832
The leader in athletic books.

SCHOOL HEALTH SUPPLY CO.
300 Lombard Road
Addison, Illinois 60101
First aid and athletic training room supplies and equipment.

Scott & Company-GM Baseball
P. O. Box 583
Reseda, California 91335
The GM baseball—finest baseball made.

Scott Paper Company
1133 Avenue of the Americas
New York, New York 10036
World of a Girl—Free educational materials for teaching menstrual hygiene—color, sound film, color illustrated booklets, available in quantity, teaching guides.

SEAMLESS
253 Hallock Avenue
New Haven, Connecticut 06503
Manufacturer of athletic and leisure sports equipment and supplier of tapes and gauzes for trainers.

Sells Aerial Tennis Co.
Box 3042
Kansas City, Kansas 66103
A low-cost indoor, outdoor game, junior high school through adult ages.

SELVA
1607 Broadway
New York, New York 10019
Dance shoes and accessories.

SERON MFG. CO.
15 West Jefferson Street
Joliet, Illinois 60431
Glass-Gard eyeglass holder and other physical education protective products.

The Seven-Up Company
121 South Meramec Avenue
St. Louis, Missouri 63105
7UP, the Uncola and Like, just for girls.

Shield Mfg. Inc.
9 St. Paul Street
Buffalo, New York 14209
Manufacturer of protective mouth guards for all contact sports.

Signal Press
1730 Chicago Avenue
Evanston, Illinois 60201
Materials for teaching the effects of alcohol, narcotics, and tobacco.

Society For Visual Education, Inc.
1345 Diversey Parkway
Chicago, Illinois 60614
Filmstrips, slides, study prints, 8mm loops, and records.

Sorensen-Christian Industries, Inc.
P. O. Box 1
Angier, North Carolina 27501
Metal and electronic products for athletics and recreation.

A. G. Spalding & Bros., Inc.
270 New Jersey Drive
Ft. Washington, Pennsylvania 19034
Manufacturers of quality athletic and field equipment for all major sports.

Standard Brands Incorporated
625 Madison Avenue
New York, New York 10022
Planters Peanuts will offer information and booklets with reference to physical fitness programs for children under 11, and other educational material.

Stepping Tones Records
P. O. Box 64334
Los Angeles, California 90064
Technique for tap, ballet, jazz, training aids—for all grades.

STERLING RECREATION PRODUCTS
7 Oak Place
Montclair, New Jersey 07042
Manufacturers and distributors of full line equipment for all the carry over sports and individual development.

Strand Case Co., Div. of SNR Golf, Inc.
631 East Center Street

Milwaukee, Wisconsin 53212
Team luggage, flag football, athletic, and sports equipment.

Superior Wire & Iron Products, Inc.
16400 South Lathrop Avenue
Harvey, Illinois 60426
Ventilated athletic lockers and locker benches, portable basketball standards.

Syracuse University Film Marketing Division
1455 East Colvin Street
Film Rental Library
Syracuse, New York 13210
Offering seven gymnastics 16mm films for sale—both boys and girls—also super 8 loops.

T

TAMPAX INCORPORATED
161 East 42nd Street
New York, New York, 10017
Free educational materials on menstrual health including student booklets, teaching aids, anatomical charts, and consultant services.

Technology/Versatronics, Inc.
506 South High Street
Yellow Springs, Ohio 45387
Oxygen consumption computer.

Charles C Thomas, Publisher
301-327 East Lawrence Avenue
Springfield, Illinois 62703
Books in the field of health, physical education, and recreation.

R. E. Titus Gym Scooter Co.
1719 Hackney
Winfield, Kansas 67156
Gym scooters and scooter accessories.

Top Star Inc.
P. O. Box 728
Arlington, Texas 76010
Liquid nutrition, ballmate and tiremate sealants, Padphil 4:19 scientific passer development machine.

T. F. Twardzik & Co., Inc.
600 East Center Street
Shenandoah, Pennsylvania 17976
Leases dispensers for table tennis balls and sale of table tennis equipment.

U

United States Air Force
Randolph Air Force Base, Texas 78148
Materials about education and training opportunities in the U.S. Air Force.

UNITED STATES ARMY
RECRUITING COMMAND
Hampton, Virginia 23369
Career and educational opportunities literature.

United States Marine Corps
Commandant of the Marine Corps
(Code DPO)
Headquarters
Washington, D. C. 20380
Career Information.

United States Navy
Bureau of Naval Personnel (Pers-B6e)
Washington, D. C. 20370
Education and occupations available in the U.S. Navy.

Universal Athletic Sales Co.
4707 East Hedges Avenue
Fresno, California 93703
The Universal "Gladiator" gym machine with over 14 exercise positions.

UNIVERSAL BLEACHER CO.
Box 638
Champaign, Illinois 61820
Roll-a-way bleachers, basketball backstops, outdoor bleachers, port-a-pool water safety classrooms.

V W Y

Videonetics, Div. Newell Industries
1216 Kifer Road
Sunnyvale, California 94086
Instant replay stop-action recorder.

W. J. VOIT RUBBER CORP.
Subsidiary of American Machine &
Foundry Company of New York
3801 South Harbor Boulevard
Santa Ana, California 92704
Athletic balls and equipment, exercisers, golf clubs and balls, and scuba diving equipment.

WADSWORTH PUBLISHING COMPANY,
INC.
Belmont, California 94002
Provides textbooks for professionals in recreation and physical education and publishes a series of sports skills instruction books.

Wheelan and Wheelan, Inc.
129 North 12th Street
Philadelphia, Pennsylvania 19107
Manufacturer of girls and women's physical education clothing.

WILSON SPORTING GOODS CO.
2233 West Street
River Grove, Illinois 60171
A complete line of athletic and recreation equipment.

White Stag-Speedo
5203 S.E. Johnson Creek Boulevard
Portland, Oregon 97206
Nylon tank suits for competition and physical education classes, coaches, and lifeguards.

Wilton Mfg. Co., Inc.
Ware, Massachusetts 01082
Athletic clothing and campus wear.

Wittek Golf Range Supply Co., Inc.
3650 Avondale
Chicago, Illinois 60618
World's largest manufacturer and distributor of driving range and miniature equipment.

Wolff-Fording & Co., Inc.

88 Kingston Street
Boston, Massachusetts 02111
Manufacturers of leotards, dance costumes, gym slippers, shoes, and theatrical supplies.

Wolverine Sports Supply
745 State Circle
Ann Arbor, Michigan 48104
Complete line of athletic and playground equipment.

YWCA of the USA
600 Lexington Avenue
New York, New York 10022
Career information for work with private social agency.

B CARE, REPAIR, AND STORAGE OF UNIFORMS AND EQUIPMENT

Following are instructions for the care of uniforms (see also accompanying chart for laundering and cleaning procedures):

1. Clean garments immediately after each wearing. If this is not possible, hang on rust-proof hangers in a well-ventilated room.
2. If garment is saturated with mud and cleaning is to be done immediately, remove excess mud by rinsing under shower.
3. Avoid excessive heat in washing and drying since this will cause shrinkage. Lukewarm water is recommended.
4. Wash white garments separately—do not mix with colored ones.
5. Use a bleaching agent only on white cotton garments.
6. To prevent stains from becoming set, wet-clean or dry-clean garments before they dry.
7. Protect clothing from moisture and dry as soon as possible to prevent mildew.
8. Usually dry-clean brushed or woven wool fabrics.
9. Restore knit goods that may have shrunk to original size by dampening and drying in a stretched condition.
10. When wet garments must be packed, separate jerseys from pants and fold neatly in trunks. Place a layer of plain paper, or a towel, between each jersey. Use same method for pants, but remove knee pads and thigh guards from pants before packing. As soon as possible, unpack and clean or hang to dry.
11. Recommended procedures regarding cleaning of practice equipment is every second or third day under dry conditions. If practice is held during muddy, wet weather, a daily washing should be performed.
12. Send equipment at completion of the season to a reliable cleaner or reconditioner with complete and exact cleaning instructions.
13. Check accessories, such as metal snaps, zippers, slides, and buttons, for rust, breakage, or loss before being stored.
14. Fold repaired garments and pack in storage bins located in cool, dry, well-ventilated area.
15. Store colored textiles in separate containers with napthalene flakes or moth balls.

Following is a chart that indicates the recommended procedures for the care, repair, and storage of various pieces of physical education equipment.

BASEBALL

UNIFORMS		Code
HOF	Wool and Nylon	2
A	Wool and Nylon	2
B	Nylon, Acrilan, Cotton and Orlon	2
F	Cotton, Orlon, Nylon and Rayon	2
H	Nylon, Acrilan, Rayon and Cotton	2
X	Rayon, Cotton, Orlon and Dacron	2
P	Cotton	2
K	Cotton and Nylon Knit	1
JACKETS		
Melton Cloth		5
UNDERSHIRTS		
Wool		2
Cotton		2
Wool and Cotton		2
T-SHIRTS		
Cotton		2

SOFTBALL

SHIRTS	Code
Cotton and Rayon	2
Cotton	2
Fineline Twill	1
PANTS	
Cotton	2

ATHLETIC STOCKINGS

	Code
Worsted	1
Worsted and Cotton	1
Cotton and Rayon	1
Cotton	1
Durene and Nylon	1
Durene and Coylon	1
Durene and Rayon	1
Durene	1
Stretch Nylon	1

WRESTLING

CLOTHING	Code
#24 Stretch Nylon-Spandex	1
#25 Durene Cotton-Nylon-Spandex	1
#28 Stretch Nylon and Cotton Durene	1
#29 Cotton and Nylon	1
#35 Durene Cotton and Nylon	1
#44 Durene Cotton and Nylon	1

TRACK

SHIRTS	Code
Nylon and Durene Cotton	1
Durene Cotton and Rayon	1
PANTS	
Cotton	1
Satin	2
Nyl-Weave	2
MEN'S WARM-UP SHIRTS AND PANTS	
GIRLS' SHIRTS AND PANTS	
Orlon Acrylic	1
Nylon	1
Stretch Nylon and Durene Cotton	1
Durene Cotton and Nylon	1
Durene Cotton and Rayon	1
Cotton and Rayon	1
Nylon and Durene Cotton	1

BASKETBALL

SHIRTS	Code
#19 Stretch Nylon and Durene Cotton	1
#17 Nylon and Durene Cotton	1
#18 Durene Cotton and Nylon	1
#16 Durene Cotton and Rayon	1
#14 Durene Cotton and Rayon	1
#10 Cotton and Rayon	1
PANTS	
Nylon Contact Cloth	1
Nyl-Twill	2
Royal Label Twill	1
Royal Label Satin	2
Nyl-Weave	2
Hi-Glo Acetate Satin	2
WARM-UP JACKETS, SHIRTS AND PANTS	
Brushed Wool	5
Nylon Fleece	1
Orlon Fleece	1
Nyl-Twill	2
Royal Label Twill	1
Nyl-Weave	2
Hi-Glo Acetate Satin	2
Durene Cotton and Nylon	2
Durene Cotton and Rayon	1
Stretch Nylon and Durene Cotton	1

ICE HOCKEY

JERSEYS	
Durene Cotton and Nylon	1
Cotton and Nylon	1
Cotton and Rayon	1
PANT	
Royal Label Twill, Rayon and Cotton	1
Nylon	1
Cotton	1

FOOTBALL

JERSEYS	Code
#12 Nylon and Stretch Nylon	1
#28 Stretch Nylon and Durene	1
#30 Nylon and Durene	1
#33 Stretch Polypropylene and Nylon	1
#35 Durene and Nylon	1
#38 Cotton and Nylon	1
#45 Cotton and Rayon	1
#52 Durene	1

PANTS (half and half)		
(Front)	(Back)	
Nylon Contact Cloth	Stretch Nylon-Spandex	2
Nyl-Knit	Stretch-Nylon-Spandex	2
Nyl-Twill	Stretch Nylon-Spandex	2
Nylon Contact Cloth	Durene Cotton-Nylon-Spandex	2
Nyl-Twill	Durene Cotton-Nylon-Spandex	2
Scrimmage Cloth	Cotton and Nylon	1

KNIT SHELLS	
Stretch Nylon	1
Nyl-Knit	3
Stretch Nylon-Durene	1
Durene and Nylon	1
Cotton and Nylon	1
COACHES PANT	
C. A. Cloth	1
PARKAS AND SIDELINE CAPES	
Vinyl Twill	4

SOCCER

JERSEYS	
Durene Cotton and Nylon	1
Cotton and Nylon	1
PANT	
Cotton	2

LAUNDERING AND CLEANING PROCEDURE

1 Machine wash for 15 minutes with water at 100° Fahrenheit. Use a mild no-bleach detergent. Drip dry at room temperature or use a no-heat dryer.

2 Machine wash for 15 minutes with water at 100° Fahrenheit. Use a mild no-bleach detergent. Drip dry at room temperature.

3 Machine wash for 15 minutes with water at 120° Fahrenheit. Use a mild no-bleach detergent. Drip dry at room temperature.

4 Hand wash using a soft-bristled brush and mild detergent with water at tap-water temperature. Brush should be applied in the direction of the weave of the material. **Do not use cleaning solutions.**

5 Dry clean and steam press.

Chart of laundering and cleaning procedures. (From Rawlings Athletic Equipment Digest, ed. 4, St. Louis, 1966, Rawlings Sporting Goods Co.)

Equipment	Care	Repair	Storage
Archery			
Arrows	1. Carry arrows by pile end so that feathers will not be damaged. 2. Use steel wool for cleaning wooden arrows and then apply a coat of wax. 3. Rub metal piles with oil to prevent rusting. 4. On a wet day collect arrows on ground first and wipe with a tassel. 5. Smooth out arrow feathers that are out of shape. 6. Remove arrows by grasping them in close to target face and pulling straight out while your other hand holds target face against bale.	1. Repair minor splits and cracks by putting cement on both broken edges and then bind tightly with strong thread. 2. Arrows that are broken at pile end can be cut off and new piles applied. 3. Straighten arrow by carefully taking shaft and bending it in opposite direction. 4. Remove a broken pyroxylin nock by using a lighted match; then sand wood to a smooth finish and apply a new nock with a very thin coat of quick-drying cellulose cement. Nock should be perpendicular to cock feather. 5. Cement a loose feather in place and tie with thread until cement is dry. Correctly align feather when tied. 6. Return arrows to manufacturer for refletching, recresting, repolishing, and straightening.	1. Store arrows in racks rather than in boxes. 2. Protect feathers from from moths with a good moth preventive.
Bows Wood	1. Rub Simoniz or Johnson's Wax on bows at end of season to protect finish. 2. Oil leather grip periodically.	1. Send bows to manufacturer for any major repairs.	1. Unbrace bows, hang vertically on wooden pegs, and store in a cool, humid place.
Metal	1. Oil steel occasionally to prevent rusting.		

Special thanks are given to Miss Sharon Irwin of Frostburg State College, Frostburg, Maryland, for her help in the gathering and organizing of this material.

Equipment	Care	Repair	Storage
Archery—cont'd			
Bowstrings	1. Beeswax bowstrings at least once weekly.	1. Replaced badly frayed strings. If only one or two strands are broken, cut them off and wax string. 2. Mark nocking points and replace worn servings. Use carpet thread or dental floss for this.	
Fingertabs and armguards	1. Clean with saddle soap. 2. Oil leather occasionally to keep it from drying out and cracking.	1. Repair broken stitches immediately.	1. Store in cool, humid place.
Targets	1. Cover targets with a waterproof covering if left outside overnight. 2. Reinforce target faces with cardboard or heavy paper backings. 3. Varnish target stand occasionally to protect it from moisture.	No specific recommendations.	1. Keep targets flat and stack or lay singly on a platform several inches from floor. 2. Spread powdered sulfur among the butts to keep animals away.
Athletic shoes			
Canvas shoes	1. Wash with lukewarm water and mild detergent. 2. Keep soles of basketball shoes free of dust and dirt so that maximum gripping action can be maintained.	No specific recommendations.	No specific recommendations.
Leather shoes	1. Allow damp or wet shoes to dry at room temperature after being cleaned of dirt and mud. 2. Place a dry rag in toe of each shoe to aid drying process. 3. Apply leather conditioner, neat's-foot or viscol oil, to shoe— uppers and leather outsoles. 4. Polish shoes regularly.	1. Repair rips and tears immediately to prevent further deterioration. 2. Replace worn-out cleats and spikes to prevent injury and to provide longer wear.	1. Insert shoe trees in shoes to maintain proper form.

Continued.

Equipment	Care	Repair	Storage
Badminton			
Net	1. Check nets regularly for holes, tears, and other damage.	1. Repair immediately with string or very strong thread.	1. Fold nets before they are stored. 2. Lay them flat on a smooth surface protected from dirt and rodents.
Rackets			
Metal	1. Occasionally wipe and strip with oil and then wipe off frame to prevent rusting. Copperplated strings will not rust.	1. Rackets that break may be welded, but are not too satisfactory.	
Wood	1. Apply a thin coat of gut preserver to strings to improve durability. 2. Apply a good brand of wax to wood frame occasionally and polish.	1. Have frame restrung with gut at sports dealers. 2. Broken frame may sometimes be repaired with fiber glass, depending on extent of breakage.	1. Keep in press and in a waterproof case.
Shuttlecock	1. Straighten out feathers of shuttle frequently. 2. Kept shuttles humidified, so that they do not become brittle.	1. Replace a broken feather with a good one by inserting it through stitching and cementing it carefully with a minimum amount of cement so as not to destroy balance.	1. Store shuttlecock in an upright position with base down so that there is no pressure on feathers.
Baseball			
Balls	1. Do not use leather-covered balls on damp ground for longest use. 2. Keep rubber-covered balls inside when not in use since heat and direct sunlight for long periods of time will reduce their durability. 3. Wipe rubber-covered balls with a damp rag.	1. Resew broken threads.	1. Store in dry area and out of direct light. 2. Do not store balls under other objects.

Equipment	Care	Repair	Storage

Baseball—cont'd

Equipment	Care	Repair	Storage
Bases	1. Remove canvas-covered bases after every game to prevent water damage. 2. Brush and reshape bases. 3. Wipe rubber bases with a damp rag.	1. Repair rips in bases as soon as possible.	1. Store bases flat.
Bats	1. Treat bats with linseed oil prior to storage.	1. Repair grips or replace with leather or cork.	1. Store in dry room at normal temperature.
Gloves	1. Dry gloves if they are wet. 2. When leather becomes rough or cracks, treat it with neat's-foot oil. 3. Do not wear a glove made for left hand on right hand since this will destroy pocket and cause padding to move. 4. Occasionally clean gloves with saddle soap, using a moist cloth to rub soap over glove. Wipe off lather with clean cloth.	1. Repair a rip or tear occurring in seam. Cover large rips with a leather patch.	1. Store gloves in a cool, dry place. 2. Do not store under other equipment.

Basketball

Equipment	Care	Repair	Storage
Leather	1. Inflate only to specified pressure; never over-inflate. 2. Moisten inflating needle and insert with rotary motion up to shoulder of needle. 3. Use saddle soap to clean balls.	1. Send a damaged ball to manufacturer.	1. Store balls partially inflated, but with enough air to hold their shape. 2. Store in a cool, dry place.
Rubber	1. Inflate same as leather balls. 2. Wipe ball with damp rag to remove dirt. 3. If ball has mud, oil, or grease on it, use soap and warm water.	1. Return to manufacturer a basketball that is badly punctured. 2. A latex repair might prove sufficient for a small puncture.	1. Reduce pressure to prevent constant strain. 2. Store in a cool, dry place. 3. Do not expose to direct sunlight for a period of time.

Continued.

Equipment	Care	Repair	Storage
Bowling			
Ball	1. Clean ball often with soap and water 2. Use a special bowling ball liquid cleaner if ball has accumulated wax from alley.	No specific recommendations.	1. Keep ball in a bowling bag.
Pins	1. Remove pins that are cracked or broken. 2. Clean both plastic and wood pins as often as necessary.	No specific recommendations.	1. Store in a dry place.
Shoes	1. Wear bowling shoes only while bowling. 2. Give same care as street shoes.	No specific recommendations.	No specific recommendations.
Fencing			
Jackets	1. Wash and fluff jackets regularly.	1. Repair tears or rips immediately.	1. Store in area with maximum ventilation.
Masks	1. Remove lipstick before putting a mask on. 2. Check mask for gaps or rust spots. 3. Wash padding and bibs frequently. 4. Masks that are tinned or chrome plated do not require any treatment other than wiping with soap and water. 5. Clean leather trimming with saddle soap. 6. Wipe leatherette trimming off with warm water and soap. 7. Clean canvas trimming with soap and water.	1. Repaint masks if paint is wearing off.	1. Store masks so that no outside pressure will be exerted on them. 2. Allow for maximum ventilation.
Weapons	1. Secure pommels to prevent guards and blades from rubbing. 2. Put a slight set on blade before using it so that it will always bend in same direction.	1. Remove small nicks in blade with fine emery cloth. 2. Replace broken blades by unscrewing pommel and slipping old blade out.	1. Store foils in a hanging position so that blades are not damaged.

Equipment	Care	Repair	Storage

Fencing—cont'd

Weapons—cont'd

	Care	Repair	Storage
	3. To bend or straighten blade, rub it between shoe sole and floor. Friction heats blade and makes it more pliable. Hands should not be used. 4. Wipe off blade periodically during very humid weather or in damp climates. 5. Oil blade occasionally to prevent it from rusting.	3. A new blade might require filing before fitting properly.	

Field hockey

Equipment	Care	Repair	Storage
Balls	1. Reenamel leather-covered balls when protective covering is worn. 2. If match is played on a wet surface use a number of balls.	1. Before paint is applied, scrape off all old paint. Use denatured alcohol or a paint thinner and medium-coarse steel wool for this purpose. 2. A board in which nails have been driven will serve as a ball rack for wet balls. 3. If a leather-covered ball has ripped at seams, it might be repaired at a shoe repair shop.	1. Store away from dampness.
Goalie pads and shin guards	1. Allow wet guards to dry at normal room temperature before putting them away. 2. Remove dirt and mud with a stiff brush. 3. Oil leather straps occasionally to prevent drying out and cracking.	1. Leather straps, elastic understraps, and buckles that have come loose can be repaired at a shoe repair shop.	1. Attach matching guards by buckling and store in pairs on a flat surface. 2. Store goalie pads in a dry, well-ventilated area.
Stick	1. Keep head of stick clean. Scrape off mud or dirt with a knife or steel wool; then wipe blade with a slightly dampened cloth.	1. Sandpaper and wax a stick that has frayed at edges. 2. If stick splinters, shave down, working toward open end of splinter.	1. Store sticks away from dampness and heat. 2. Store sticks flat without pressure of other sticks on them.

Continued.

Equipment	Care	Repair	Storage
Field hockey—cont'd			
Stick—cont'd	2. Wipe off blades of new sticks with linseed oil to preserve wood. 3. Repeat this procedure occasionally during season. 4. At end of season remove excess dirt with steel wool, rub blade with beeswax, and paint it with shellac or varnish. 5. Avoid sitting or leaning on stick when testing its resiliency. 6. Wipe stick immediately after use in rain or on wet ground.	Then sand and protect with a piece of adhesive tape. Use only one layer of tape since heavy taping will cause an unbalance of stick. 3. Replace if rubber grip rots and dries.	
Football			
Ball	Same as for basketball	Same as for basketball.	Same as for basketball.
Football pads	1. Allow thorough drying after each use. 2. Wash pads that have fiber parts sewn on by hand with a soft bristle brush with soap and water, then rinse entire pad in clear water. Dry fabric at normal temperature in well-ventilated room. 3. Brush-coat fiber parts with clear lacquer. 4. Clean Armorlite parts with soap or detergent and water, rinsing thoroughly. 5. Remove pads from pockets before washing girdle pads. 6. Clean pads with no exposed fiber parts by wrapping any exposed metal with cloth or tape (to prevent damage to washer); then wash in automatic washer with detergent.	1. Send to a qualified renovator for major repairs.	1. Store in a dry, well-ventilated room. 2. Do not stack pads on each other since this will distort their form. 3. Do not hang by elastic straps since this will weaken strap. 4. Store hip pads by hanging from buckle.

Equipment	Care	Repair	Storage

Football—cont'd

Football pads—
cont'd

Dry under room temperature in well-ventilated room.

Helmet

1. Several times during season clean padding in each helmet with saddle soap.
2. Work up a heavy lather on brush or cloth; then scrub leather surface to loosen dirt. Wipe off surface with clean cloth; then apply light coating of castor oil to leather lining to keep it from becoming harsh.
3. Make sure chin strap is always in position shaped to chin contour when not in use.

1. When refinishing a helmet, use steel wool or fine sand paper to thoroughly remove surface dirt or loose paint.
2. Replace worn straps and snaps.
3. Use a thin coat of clear lacquer on outside of helmet to restore glossy appearance.

1. Store helmets in a cool, dry area.
2. Store on helmet hangers, on helmet racks, or in their original boxes.

Golf

Bag

1. Clean with detergent and water.

1. Replace broken straps or mend them with leather and rivets.

1. Store at normal room temperature.

Balls

1. Wash balls frequently.
2. Paint practice balls.

Clubs
Irons

1. If grips of any clubs have become loose, or if a change in thickness is desired, remove string at top and bottom of leather and then unwind.
2. Little care is required to maintain irons other than drying and oiling occasionally to prevent rusting.
3. File club nicks smooth when they appear on surface.
4. Clean iron heads occasionally with fine grade steel wool and detergent.

1. Replace damaged or worn grips at pro shop.
2. If head of wooden-shafted iron becomes loose, taken it to a club maker.

1. Store at normal room temperature.

Continued.

Equipment	Care	Repair	Storage
Golf—cont'd Irons—cont'd	5. When playing, clean grooves in head with tee after each use. 6. Clean shaft with a moistened cloth and detergent. Dry immediately.		
Woods	1. If club has been used in rain or wet grass, wipe with an oily rag. 2. Occasionally wash with mild soap and water and clean grooves on faces with a soft brush or a wooden tee. 3. Wax (paste wax) wooden clubheads to prevent warping and cracking. 4. Apply a light oil to steel shaft. 5. Head covers protect head from scarring. 6. Check sole plates frequently to see that they remain tight. 7. Use a file to smooth out nicks to prevent damage to balls 8. Rub leather grips lightly with neat's-foot oil several times a year.		1. When storing, put a few drops of linseed oil on a cloth and wipe club thoroughly. 2. Use another cloth with a mixture of a few drops of oil and shellac and give wooden heads of clubs a vigorous rubbing. This will coat surface and help repel moisture. 3. Store at normal room temperature.
Gymnastic equipment Balance beam	1. Sand wood balance beam. 2. When original lacquer sealer is worn, apply another coat 3. Be careful not to build up a high gloss heavy finish since this will make it slippery.	No specific recommendations.	No specific recommendations.

Equipment	Care	Repair	Storage
Gymnastic equipment—cont'd			
Horizontal bar	1. Sand steel horizontal cross bars with emery cloth to keep them bright and to keep rust and chalk from accumulating. 2. Check mechanical connections regularly.	1. Refinish metal bases of all these pieces with spray enamels.	No specific recommendations.
Horse	1. Pommels need no finish and excess chalk can be sanded off. 2. A periodic application of saddle soap to clean horse body is recommended to keep leather soft.	1. When leather becomes badly worn, have it replaced by manufacturer.	No specific recommendations.
Mats	1. Wash vinyl-covered mats with ordinary soap and water. 2. Clean canvas mats every week with a vacuum cleaner. 3. Repair small rips and tears immediately. 4. Send badly worn mats back to factory where they will be recovered using old filler.	1. In repairing rubber mats, roughen rubber surface and cut a patch with the sides rounded. Roughen one surface of patch with sandpaper and apply coat of cement with a brush to both mat surface and rough side of patch. Allow about 5 to 10 minutes for cement to dry and then apply second and third coats, allowing each time to dry thoroughly. Roll cemented side of patch onto prepared cemented place on mat. Also cement a patch on opposite side of mat cover, using same technique. Allow 40 hours for the cement to cure fully at room temperature.	1. Hang mats on mat hangers when not in use or stacked upon each other. 2. Keep them in a rolled position.
Parallel bars	1. Leave rails unfinished and smooth. Use 6/0 or 8/0 sandpaper to maintain texture and remove excess chalk.	No specific recommendations.	No specific recommendations.

Continued.

Equipment	Care	Repair	Storage
Gymnastic equipment—cont'd			
Parallel bars —cont'd	2. Do not use waxes and preservatives on wood. 3. Clean paint finish on most apparatus with a mild solvent. 4. To keep adjustment staffs moving freely, use a spray can of silicone product sparingly.		
Rings	1. Wipe leather covering with a moist cloth and allow time to dry. 2. Check all mechanical connections regularly.	No specific recommendations.	No specific recommendations.
Ropes	1. Check constantly for frayed areas. Also, check connections for support. 2. Replace worn ropes.	No specific recommendations.	No specific recommendations.
Trampoline	1. Wash trampoline beds with cold water and mild soap and put back on trampoline under spring tension while they are still wet. Never use warm water or harsh detergent on nylon trampoline beds.	No specific recommendations.	1. Fold and store out of way.
Lacrosse			
Balls	1. Rinse balls in a warm, soapy solution and dry.	No specific recommendations.	1. Store in an area with low humidity and normal room temperature.
Gloves	1. When gloves become wet, allow drying to take place at normal room temperature. Mineral or vegetable oil will remove harshness caused by drying. 2. Clean with saddle soap only. Apply saddle soap with a moist cloth by rubbing cloth over soap to work up a cream on cloth. Rub soiled leather with cloth until a lather	1. Repair broken stitches.	1. Store at normal room temperature.

Equipment	Care	Repair	Storage
Lacrosse—cont'd Gloves—cont'd	has been worked up and dirt is loosened. Wipe off dirty lather with a clean cloth and rub leather briskly with a clean cloth.		
Goalie pads	Refer to instructions for field hockey goalie pads.	Refer to instructions for field hockey goalie pads.	Refer to instructions for field hockey goalie pads.
Helmet	Refer to instructions for football helmet.	Refer to instructions for football helmet.	Refer to instructions for football helmet.
Nets	1. Moisture-proof leather portions of net with coat of Lexol. 2. Tarred nets are best for damp areas.	No specific recommendations.	No specific recommendations.
Stick	1. Loosen lead string after play. 2. Wipe crosse with a dry rag after playing. 3. Oil wood with linseed oil after rain and about once a month. This should be just enough to moisten the rub. 4. Use petroleum jelly or leather conditioner on thongs and gut. 5. Occasionally apply varnish or furniture wax to protect wood from moisture. 6. Place tongue depressors vertically in gut wall when it becomes wet after play in inclement weather.	1. Sandpaper any wood surface that has splintered. Tape small breaks with a very light tape, used sparingly so as not to disturb balance of crosse. 2. Mend broken gut by making a split in broken end as well as in one end of piece being used for repair; then thread one end through other. 3. Tape angles that have split. This may not prove satisfactory if crosse is put to hard use.	1. When crosses are stored at end of season, insert small sticks in guard, parallel to short strings. A thin coat of shellac applied to guard will stiffen it and hold it in place. After shellac dries, remove sticks. 2. In order to avoid pressure on bridge or guard, hang crosses on a peg or nail, with weight of crosse resting against peg. Crosses can also be placed on a shelf in horizontal position, wood down, with space between crosses. 3. Store crosses in a place protected from rodents at normal room temperature.
Skiing Boots	1. Remove excess snow or surface moisture at end of the day with a soft cloth. If moisture has seeped inside of boot, a temporary stuffing of	No specific recommendations.	1. Insert ski boot trees to maintain proper form.

Continued.

Equipment	Care	Repair	Storage
Skiing—cont'd Boots—cont'd	newspaper will help to absorb it quickly. 2. Never dry boots next to direct heat. 3. When boots are dry, check their surface for cuts and scrapes, massage immediately, preferably with the fingers with wax. Polish all over as often as necessary to maintain protective finish of leather.		
Poles	1. Check cane poles for splits and loose laminations.	1. Use only water-resistant glue in regluing.	1. Cover metal with a thin coat of oil before storing. 2. Oil all leather parts carefully.
Skis	1. Thoroughly scrape skis with sandpaper, a knife, or steel wool and wax base with a liquid wax containing pine tar. Following this they should be surfaced waxed. 2. Use "wax wax" for powdered snow and "tar wax" for wet snow. Use paraffin as a final application. 3. Wax can be applied in several ways—by hand, with an iron, with a cork, or in liquid form with a brush. Brush method is most durable. Apply the wax in lengthwise strokes from tail to tip. 4. Two or three coats of ski lacquer are recommended for skis that do not have plastic bottoms. 5. Wax tops of skis with a good floor wax to prevent snow collecting on them.	No specific recommendations.	1. Place skis back to back and fastened together with ski ties near tips and near tails. A 2 × 4 inch block of wood sandwiched between them at level of binding will preserve their camber and their shape.

Equipment	Care	Repair	Storage
Skiing—cont'd Skis—cont'd	6. Never bring skis directly from a warm place into contact with snow since running surface will freeze.		
Soccer Ball	Refer to basketball.	Refer to basketball.	Refer to basketball.
Net	Refer to lacrosse.	Refer to lacrosse.	Refer to lacrosse.
Softball	Refer to baseball.	Refer to baseball.	Refer to baseball.
Squash Ball	No specific recommendations.	No specific recommendations.	1. Store balls in a cool, dry place.
Racket	Refer to instructions for badminton rackets. 1. After play wash squash racket in a mild soap and water solution to remove dirt and perspiration.	Refer to instructions for badminton rackets.	Refer to instructions for badminton rackets.
Tennis Ball	1. Brush off dirt and dust before putting away. 2. Allow sufficient time for drying if balls are wet before putting away. 3. Replace balls that become damp during play.	No specific recommendations.	1. Store balls in can with a cap on it. 2. Store at normal room temperature.
Net	1. Take twine nets indoors when weather is damp or wet. 2. Slacken rope cables at end of day. 3. During dry seasons and at end of a season, wash nets with a hose to remove dust and dirt. 4. Dip cord nets into commercial creosote once during season and before storing. 5. Wipe steel cable occasionally with an oily rag, and remove rust with emery cloth dipped in kerosene.	1. Repair holes or tears using a fisherman's knot.	1. Be sure that nets are thoroughly dry before storing them at end of season. 2. Store nets in a cool, dry place away from rodents.

Continued.

Equipment	Care	Repair	Storage
Tennis—cont'd			
Net—cont'd			
	6. Occasionally wipe metal nets with an oily rag.		
Racket			
Metal	Same as for badminton.	No specific recommendations.	No specific recommendations.
Wood	Same as for badminton.	Same as for badminton.	Same as for badminton.
Track and field			
Discus	1. Clean and polish metal rim of discus. 2. Varnish wood portion to prevent water absorption.	No specific recommendations.	No specific recommendations.
Javelin	1. Check binding and steel points for looseness. A loose wrapping will interfere with throwing, and a loose point may cause the javelin to snap.		1. Store javelins in a dry place and hang them from a nail or hook.
Shot	1. Clean shot with kerosene and emery cloth.		1. Oil and store in a dry place.
Vault pole	1. Replace worn or torn tape. Do not add more tape than is needed for a satisfactory grip since tape adds weight. 2. Catch poles after jump to avoid splintering (bamboo) or denting (aluminum).		1. Store poles in a rack in a horizontal position.
Volleyball			
Ball	Same as for basketball.	Same as for basketball.	Same as for basketball.
Net	Same as for badminton.	Same as for badminton.	Same as for badminton.

C SCHOOL LAWS AND REGULATIONS ON THE TEACHING OF HEALTH, SAFETY, DRIVER, OUTDOOR, AND PHYSICAL EDUCATION

State	Total	Specific law (M)	Course of study (MC)	Permissive (P and PI)	Total	Auth. state board	Auth. state dept.	Law	Reg.	Grade or level	Law	Reg.	Grade or level
		Laws			Regulations			Health education (separate subject) Authorization			Health and physical education (combined subject) Authorization		
_1_	_2_	_3_	_4_	_5_	_6_	_7_	_8_	_9_	_10_	_11_	_12_	_13_	_14_
Total laws and regulations: States and D. C.	216	138	23	55	81	49	32	11	22	—	20	17	—
Outlying areas	1	1	0	0	7	3	4	1	3	—	0	1	—
Aggregate U. S.	217	139	23	55	88	52	36	12	25	—	20	18	—
Alabama	2	2	0	0	2	2	0	—	(SB[1])	1-9	—	—	—
Alaska	2	2	0	0	1	1	0	([2])	—	—	—	—	—
Arizona	2	1	0	1	1	0	1	—	—	—	—	(SD[3])	E
Arkansas	4	4	0	0	1	1	0	—	—	—	(M[3])	—	E-S
California	10	7	1	2	1	1	0	(MC[4])	—	E	—	—	—
Colorado	2	1	0	1	0	0	0	—	—	—	—	—	—
Connecticut	5	4	1	0	0	0	0	—	—	—	(MC[5])	—	E-S
Delaware	4	2	1	1	2	0	2	—	SB	E-S	—	—	—

*From State school laws and regulations for health, safety, driver, outdoor, and physical education, Washington D. C., 1964, D
†E, Elementary; M, mandatory, required by specific law; MC, required by law through specific mention among subjects to be incl
secondary; SB, state board of education; SD, state department of education; 0, zero in colums 2 through 8; and —, zero in col

Physical education (separate subject)			Safety education (separate subject)			Driver education			Outdoor education			Special health and/or safety topics			
Authorization			Authorization			Authorization			Authorization				Authorization		
Law	Reg.	Grade or level	Law	Reg.	Grade or level	Law	Reg.	Grade or level	Law	Reg.	Grade or level	Topic	Law	Reg.	Grade or level
15	16	17	18	19	20	21	22	23	24	25	26	27	28	29	30
17	28	—	8	5	—	33	7	—	6	0	—	—	121	2	
0	3	—	0	0	—	0	0	—	0	0	—	—	0	0	
17	31	—	8	5	—	33	7	—	6	0	—	—	121	2	
M	SB	E-S	—	[1]	—	—	—	—	—	—	—	Fire drills	M	—	E-S
—	SB	S	—	—	—	—	—	—	—	—	—	Alcohol and narcotics	(M[2])	—	E-S
												Fire drills	M	—	E-S
—	—	—	—	[3]	—	—	—	—	—	—	—	Alcohol and narcotics	M	—	E-S
												Use of firearms and safe hunting	P	—	E-S
—	SB	S	[3]	—	—	—	—	—	—	—	—	Alcohol and narcotics	M	—	3-8
												Fire drills	M	—	E-S
												Fire prevention	M	—	E
M[4])	—	E-S	(M[4])	—	E-S	(M[4])	—	S	(P[4])	—	E-S	Alcohol and narcotics including manners and morals	M	—	E-S
	SB	S	—	—	—	—	—	—	—	—	—	Fire drills	M	—	E-S
												School safety patrol	P	—	E-S
												Fire prevention	M	—	E-S
—	—	—	—	—	—	P	—	S	—	—	—	First-aid instruction	M	—	S
												Physiology and hygiene, including alcohol and narcotics	M	—	E-S
—	—	—	—	—	—	M	—	S	—	—	—	Alcohol and narcotics	M	—	E-S
												Fire drills	M	—	E-S
												Highway safety	M	—	E-S
M	SB	E-S	—	—	—	PI	—	S	—	—	—	Physiology and hygiene, including alcohol, stimulants, and narcotics	MC	—	E-S
												Fire drills	M	—	E-S

rtment of Health, Education, and Welfare.
d in course of study; P, permissive law; PI, permissive by implication—law implies recognition of school's responsibility; S, is 9 through 29.

Continued.

State	All subjects in this table							Health education (separate subject)			Health and physical education (combined subject)		
	Laws				Regulations			Authorization			Authorization		
		Mandatory		Permissive (P and PI)									
	Total	Specific law (M)	Course of study (MC)		Total	Auth. state board	Auth. state dept.	Law	Reg.	Grade or level	Law	Reg.	Grade or level
1	2	3	4	5	6	7	8	9	10	11	12	13	14
Florida	3	1	1	1	3	3	0	—	SB	E-S	—	—	—
Georgia	3	3	0	0	1	1	0	—	SB	S	(M[3])	—	E-S
Hawaii	1	0	0	1	3	0	3	—	(SD[6])	E-S	—	—	—
Idaho	3	2	0	1	2	2	0	—	SB	S	—	—	—
Illinois	7	3	0	4	1	0	1	—	—	—	M	—	E-S
Indiana	7	6	0	1	3	3	0	—	SB	S	—	—	—
Iowa	3	3	0	0	0	0	0	—	—	—	M	—	E-S
Kansas	1	0	1	0	2	0	2	MC	—	E	—	SD	S
Kentucky	2	1	0	1	3	3	0	—	(SB[3])	E	—	(SB[3])	S
Louisiana	2	1	1	0	1	1	0	(MC[9])	—	E	—	—	—

Physical education (separate subject)			Safety education (separate subject)			Driver education			Outdoor education						
Authorization			Authorization			Authorization			Authorization						
Law	Reg.	Grade or level	Law	Reg.	Grade or level	Law	Reg.	Grade or level	Law	Reg.	Grade or level	Topic	Law	Reg.	Grade or level
15	16	17	18	19	20	21	22	23	24	25	26	27	28	29	30
—	SB	E-S	—	SB	E-S	P	—	S	—	—	—	Alcohol and narcotics	MC	—	E-S
												Fire drills	M	—	E-S
—	—	—	([3])	—	—	—	—	—	—	—	—	Alcohol on human health and behavior, social and economic conditions	M	—	E-S
												Temperance day designated	M	—	E-S
—	SD	E-S	—	([6])	—	PI	—	S	—	—	—	Fire drills	—	SD	E-S
—	SB	S	—	—	—	P	—	S	—	—	—	Physiology and hygiene, including alcohol, stimulants, and narcotics	M	—	E-S
												Alcohol, narcotics, and tobacco	M	—	E-S
—	SD	E-S	P	—	E-S	(P[7])	—	S	P	—	E-S	Physiology and hygiene, including alcohol and narcotics	M	—	E-S
												Highway safety	(M[7])	—	E-S
												School safety patrol	P	—	E-S
M	—	E-S	M	—	8	(P[8])	—	S	—	—	—	Alcoholic drinks, tobacco, sedatives, and narcotics	M	—	4-8
—	SB	S	—	([8])	—	—	SB	S				Fire drills	M	—	E-S
												Moral instruction	M	—	E-S
												Hygiene and sanitary science	M	—	5
—	—	—	—	—	—	—	—	—	—	—	—	Physiology and hygiene, including stimulants, narcotics, and poisonous substances	M	—	E-S
												Fire drills	M	—	E-S
—	—	—	—	—	—	—	—	—	—	—	—	Fire drills	—	SD	E
—	SB	E	—	([3])	—	—	—	—	—	—	—	Alcohol and narcotics	M	—	4-10
												Moral instruction	P	—	E-S
—	SB	E-S	—	—	—	—	—	—	—	—	—	Alcohol and narcotics	(M[9])	—	E-S

Continued.

State	All subjects in this table							Health education (separate subject)			Health and physical education (combined subject)		
		Laws				Regulations		Authorization			Authorization		
		Mandatory											
	Total	Specific law (M)	Course of study (MC)	Permissive (P and PI)	Total	Auth. state board	Auth. state dept.	Law	Reg.	Grade or level	Law	Reg.	Grade or level
1	2	3	4	5	6	7	8	9	10	11	12	13	14
Maine	4	3	0	1	2	2	0	—	SB	E-S	(M³)	—	E-S
Maryland	5	3	1	1	0	0	0	—	—	—	—	—	—
Massachusetts	4	1	1	2	0	0	0	—	—	—	(MC¹¹)	—	E-S
Michigan	4	3	0	1	0	0	0	—	—	—	M	—	E-S
Minnesota	7	4	0	3	2	0	2	—	SD	E-S	M	—	E-S
Mississippi	4	2	1	1	0	0	0	—	—	—	(M¹²)	—	E-S
Missouri	2	2	0	0	1	1	0	—	—	—	—	—	—

Physical education (separate subject)			Safety education (separate subject)			Driver education			Outdoor education			Special health and/or safety topics			
Authorization			Authorization			Authorization			Authorization				Authorization		
Law	Reg.	Grade or level	Law	Reg.	Grade or level	Law	Reg.	Grade or level	Law	Reg.	Grade or level	Topic	Law	Reg.	Grade or level
15	16	17	18	19	20	21	22	23	24	25	26	27	28	29	30
—	SB	1-11	(³)	—	—	P	—	S	—	—	—	Physiology and hygiene, including alcohol, stimulants, and narcotics	M	—	E-S
												Temperance day designated	M	—	E-S
M¹⁰)	—	E-S	—	—	—	P	—	S	—	—	—	Physiology and hygiene, including alcohol and narcotics	M	—	E-S
												Hygiene and sanitation	MC	—	E
												Fire drills	M	—	E-S
—	—	—	(¹¹)	—	—	(P¹¹)	—	S	—	—	—	Fire drills	M	—	E-S
												School safety patrols	P	—	E-S
—	—	—	—	—	—	P	—	S	—	—	—	Physiology and hygiene, including alcohol and narcotics	M	—	E-S
												Fire drills	M	—	E-S
—	SD	E-S	—	—	—	PI	—	S	P	—	E-S	Alcohol on human system and character and upon society	M	—	E-S
												Morals, physiology and hygiene, narcotics, and stimulants	M	—	E-S
												School safety patrol	P	—	E-S
												Fire drills	M	—	E-S
—	—	—	—	—	—	P	—	9-12	—	—	—	Physiology and hygiene, including alcohol and narcotics, home and community sanitation; highway safety	(MC¹²)	—	E-S
												Fire drills	M	—	E-S
M	SB	E-S	—	—	—	—	—	—	—	—	—	Physiology and hygiene, including tobacco, alcohol, narcotics, and stimulants	M	—	E-S

Continued.

State	All subjects in this table							Health education (separate subject)			Health and physical education (combined subject)		
		Laws				Regulations		Authoriza-tion			Authoriza-tion		
			Mandatory										
	Total	Specific law (M)	Course of study (MC)	Permis-sive (P and PI)	Total	Auth. state board	Auth. state dept.	Law	Reg.	Grade or level	Law	Reg.	Grade or level
1	2	3	4	5	6	7	8	9	10	11	12	13	14
Montana	5	4	1	0	1	1	0	—	—	—	(M[13])	SB	E-S
Nebraska	3	2	0	1	0	0	0	(M[9])	—	E-S	—	—	—
Nevada	6	5	0	1	1	2	0	M	SB	E	—	—	—
New Hampshire	5	2	0	3	0	0	0	—	—	—	—	—	—
New Jersey	5	3	0	2	0	0	0	—	—	—	(M[3])	—	E-S
New Mexico	5	4	0	1	4	4	0	—	SB	E	(M[15]) (SB[15])	—	E-S 1-8
New York	7	5	0	2	3	0	3	M	SD	1-8 E-S	—	—	—

Physical education (separate subject) Authorization			Safety education (separate subject) Authorization			Driver education Authorization			Outdoor education Authorization			Special health and/or safety topics	Authorization		
Law	Reg.	Grade or level	Law	Reg.	Grade or level	Law	Reg.	Grade or level	Law	Reg.	Grade or level	Topic	Law	Reg.	Grade or level
5	16	17	18	19	20	21	22	23	24	25	26	27	28	29	30
												Narcotics, drugs, use and abuse	M	—	E-S
—	—	—	—	—	—	—	—	—	—	—	—	Physiology and hygiene, including alcohol, stimulants, and narcotics	MC	—	E-S
												Fire prevention	M	—	E
												Fire drills	M	—	E-S
						PI	—	S				Fire prevention	M	—	E-S
(10)	—	S	—	—	—	P	—	S				Physiology and hygiene, including stimulants and narcotics	M	—	E-S
	SB	E-S										Fire drills	M	—	E-S
												Fish and game laws	M	—	E-S
(14)	—	E-S	—	—	—	PI	—	E-S				Physiology and hygiene, including alcohol and narcotics	M	—	E-S
		E										Use of firearms and safe hunting	P	—	E-S
			(3)	—	—	PI	—	S				Alcohol and narcotics	M	—	E-S
												Fire drills	M	—	E-S
												School safety patrol	P	—	E-S
	SB	E-S	—	—	—	P	—	9-12				Physiology and hygiene, including alcohol and narcotics	M	—	E-S
							SB	S				Fire prevention	M	—	E-S
												Fire drills	M	—	E-S
1	SD	E-S	—	(SD7)	E-S	—	—	—	P	—	E-S	Physiology and hygiene, including alcohol, narcotics, and drugs	(M7)	—	3-9 / 9-12
												Fire prevention	M	—	E-S
												Fire drills	M	—	E-S
												Highway safety, traffic regulations, safety patrols	P	—	E-S
												Use of firearms and safe hunting	MC	—	E-S

Continued.

State	All subjects in this table							Health education (separate subject)			Health and physical education (combined subject)	
	Laws				Regulations			Authorization			Authorization	
		Mandatory										
	Total	Specific law (M)	Course of study (MC)	Permissive (P and PI)	Total	Auth. state board	Auth. state dept.	Law	Reg.	Grade or level	Law	Reg.
1	2	3	4	5	6	7	8	9	10	11	12	13
North Carolina	4	2	1	1	4	0	4	(M[11])	SD	E-S 1-8	—	SD
North Dakota	6	4	1	1	1	0	1	—	—	—	—	—
Ohio	2	0	1	1	4	4	0	—	SB	E	(MC[17])	SB
Oklahoma	3	0	1	2	3	0	2	—	(SD[18])	E	(MC[18])	SD
Oregon	3	2	0	1	1	1	0	—	—	—	—	SB
Pennsylvania	4	2	1	1	3	0	3	—	(SD[19])	E	(MC[19])	SD
Rhode Island	6	5	0	1	0	0	0	M	—	E-S	M	—
South Carolina	8	7	1	0	3	3	0	(M[20])	SB	E-S	—	—
South Dakota	1	0	1	0	5	5	0	—	(SB[21])	7-8	—	SB

Physical education (separate subject)			Safety education (separate subject)			Driver education			Outdoor education			Special health and/or safety topics			
Authorization			Authorization			Authorization			Authorization				Authorization		
w	Reg.	Grade or level	Law	Reg.	Grade or level	Law	Reg.	Grade or level	Law	Reg.	Grade or level	Topic	Law	Reg.	Grade or level
15	16	17	18	19	20	21	22	23	24	25	26	27	28	29	30
11)	SD	E-S 1-8	(11)	—	—	(P11)	SD	S	—	—	—	Alcohol and narcotics	MC	—	E-S
												Fire prevention, fire drills, fire prevention day	M	—	E-S
	—	E-S	—	(16)	—	PI	(SD16)	S	—	—	—	Physiology and hygiene, including alcohol, narcotics, and tuberculosis	MC	—	E-S
												Temperance day designated	M	—	E-S
												Fire drills	M	—	E-S
												Moral instruction	M	—	E-S
	SB	E-S	(17)	(SB17)	E	PI	—	S	—	—	—	—	—	—	—
8)	—	E-S	(18)	—	—	(18)	—	E-S	—	—	—	—	—	—	—
	—	—	—	—	—	P	—	S	—	—	—	Alcohol, narcotics, and moral instruction	M	—	E-S
												Fire dangers and drills	M	—	E-S
	SD	E	(19)	—	—	P	—	E-S	—	—	—	Physiology and hygiene, including alcohol, narcotics, and tuberculosis	M	—	E-S
												Fire drills	M	—	E-S
	—	—	—	—	—	P	—	S	—	—	—	Physiology and hygiene, including alcohol, stimulants, and narcotics	M	—	E-S
												Fire prevention	M	—	E-S
												Fire drills	M	—	E-S
	SB	E-S / E-S	(20) (20)	(20)	E	—	(SB20)	S	—	—	—	Physiology and hygiene, including alcohol, narcotics, and moral instruction	MC	—	E-S
												Alcohol and narcotics	M	—	E-S
												Traffic laws	M	—	E-S
												Fire prevention	M	—	E
												Fire drills	M	—	E-S
	SB	7-8 and 9-12 optional	—	SB	S	—	SB	S	—	—	—	Alcoholic drinks and narcotics, including moral temperance	MC	—	E-S

Continued.

State	All subjects in this table							Health education (separate subject)			Health and physical education (combined subject)	
	Laws				Regulations			Authorization			Authorization	
		Mandatory										
	Total	Specific law (M)	Course of study (MC)	Permissive (P and PI)	Total	Auth. state board	Auth. state dept.	Law	Reg.	Grade or level	Law	Reg.
1	2	3	4	5	6	7	8	9	10	11	12	13
Tennessee	5	4	1	0	2	2	0	—	(SB[22])	E-S	(MC[22])	—
Texas	3	1	1	1	2	2	0	(M[23])	—	E-S	—	(SB[23])
Utah	6	4	0	2	2	2	0	—	SB	S	—	—
Vermont	6	2	2	2	0	0	0	—	—	—	(MC[5])	—
Virginia	7	4	1	2	1	1	0	—	SB	1-7	M	(SB[24])
Washington	5	3	1	1	1	0	1	—	—	—	—	SD

Physical education (separate subject)			Safety education (separate subject)			Driver education			Outdoor education			Special health and/or safety topics			
Authorization			Authorization			Authorization			Authorization				Authorization		
Law	Reg.	Grade or level	Law	Reg.	Grade or level	Law	Reg.	Grade or level	Law	Reg.	Grade or level	Topic	Law	Reg.	Grade or level
15	16	17	18	19	20	21	22	23	24	25	26	27	28	29	30
M	(SB[22])	E-S	M	—	S	—	([22])	—	—	—	—	Temperance day designated	M	—	E-S
												Fire drills	M	—	E-S
M	SB	E-S 7-8	—	([23])	—	(PI[3])	—	E-S 9-12	—	—	—	—	—	—	—
—	SB	S	—	—	—	P	—	9-12	—	—	—	Physiology and hygiene, including stimulants and narcotics	M	—	E-S
												Sanitation and prevention of diseases	M	—	8-12
												Alcohol, narcotics, and tobacco; school safety patrol	M	—	E-S
—	—	—	—	—	—	—	—	—	—	—	—	Physiology and hygiene	MC	—	E
												Physiology and hygiene, including alcohol and narcotics	M	—	E-S
												Alcohol education	M	—	E-S
												Firearms, game laws, and hunting	P	—	E-S
												Fire drills	M	—	E-S
												School safety patrol	P	—	E-S
—	—	—	(M[24])	—	E-S	(P[24])	—	S	P	—	E-S	Physiology and hygiene, including alcohol and narcotics	M	—	E-S
												Physiology and hygiene	MC	—	E
												Fire drills	M	—	E-S
M	—	E-S	—	—	—	—	—	—	—	—	—	Physiology and hygiene, including alcohol, stimulants, and narcotics	MC	—	E-S
												Temperance and citizenship day, including alcohol and narcotics	M	—	E-S
												School safety patrol	P	—	E-S
												Fire drills	M	—	E-S

Continued.

State	Total	Specific law (M)	Course of study (MC)	Permissive (P and PI)	Total	Auth. state board	Auth. state dept.	Law	Reg.	Grade or level	Law	Reg.	Gr o lev
					All subjects in this table			Health education (separate subject)			Health and physical education (combined subject		
		Laws			Regulations			Authorization			Authorization		
		Mandatory											
1	2	3	4	5	6	7	8	9	10	11	12	13	1
West Virginia	3	2	0	1	5	0	5	([25])	SD	E	—	(SD[25])	F
Wisconsin	9	6	0	3	0	0	0	—	—	—	—	—	—
Wyoming	4	3	0	1	1	1	0	PI	—	E-S	—	SB	
District of Columbia	2	1	0	1	2	0	2	—	—	—	—	SD	E
Canal Zone	0	0	0	0	2	0	2	—	SD	E-S	—	—	
Guam	0	0	0	0	0	0	0	—	—	—	—	—	
Puerto Rico	1	1	0	0	2	0	2	(M[27])	SD	E	—	—	
Virgin Islands	0	0	0	0	3	3	0	—	(SB[28])	E	—	SB	

[1]Combined subjects of health, science, and safety.

[2]Law on alcohol and narcotics refers to health education by implication in elementary schools.

[3]Combined subjects of health, physical education, and safety.

[4]Combined subjects of training in healthful living, morals, and manners; outdoor science and conservation education; safety and accident prevention. Driver education required to be offered in secondary schools.

[5]Combined subjects of health and physical education, alcohol and narcotics.

[6]Combined subjects of social studies, science, health, and safety—elementary grades only; health (separate subject) in secondary grades.

[7]Highway safety—on elementary level strong emphasis in traffic safety; on secondary level strong emphasis on driver education.

[8]Combined subjects of health and safety. Driver education—established division of school traffic safety in state department of education to initiate, promote, and supervise the development and expansion of driver education.

[9]Combined subjects of health, alcohol, and narcotics.

[10]Combined subjects of physical education and training.

[11]Law on driver education refers to safety education. Combined subjects of health and physical education, physiology and hygiene, physical education and good behavior, alcohol, stimulants, and narcotics.

[12]Combined subjects of hygiene, health training through physical exercise, games, recreation, and athletics; special health and/or safety topics.

[13]Combined subjects of health, physical education, and recreation.

[14]Combined subjects of military drills and physical exercises. Physical exercises must be included in the program.

[15]Combined subjects of physiology and hygiene, morals, health, and physical exercises. (Regulation—combined subjects with recreation.)

[16]Combined subjects of driver education and safety education.

Physical education (separate subject)			Safety education (separate subject)			Driver education			Outdoor education			Special health and/or safety topics			
Authorization			Authorization			Authorization			Authorization				Authorization		
Law	Reg.	Grade or level	Law	Reg.	Grade or level	Law	Reg.	Grade or level	Law	Reg.	Grade or level	Topic	Law	Reg.	Grade or level
15	16	17	18	19	20	21	22	23	24	25	26	27	28	29	30
—	SD	S	—	(SD[25])	E	P	SD	S	—	—	—	Scientific temperance, including alcohol and narcotics			
												Fire prevention	M	—	E-S
M	—	E-S	(M[26])	—	E-S	PI	—	S	P	—	E-S	Physiology and hygiene, including stimulants and narcotics	M	—	E-S
												Fire drills	M	—	E-S
												Fire prevention	M	—	E-S
												Dairy products—vitamin content	M	—	E-S
												School safety patrol	P	—	E-S
—	—	—	M	—	E-S	—	—	—	—	—	—	Alcohol and narcotics	M	—	E-S
												Fire drills	M	—	E-S
—	SD	S	—	—	—	PI	—	S	—	—	—	Physiology and hygiene, including alcohol and narcotics	M	—	E-S
—	SD	S	—	—	—	—	—	—	—	—	—	—	—	—	—
—	—	—	—	—	—	—	—	—	—	—	—	—	—	—	—
—	SD	E-S	—	—	—	—	—	—	—	—	—	—	—	—	—
—	SB	E	—	([28])	—	—	—	—	—	—	—	—	—	—	—

ombined subjects of health and physical education, alcohol, and narcotics, first aid, safety, and fire prevention.

nbined subjects of first aid, safety, and fire prevention.

ombined subjects of health and safety. Combined subjects of health and physical education, fitness and safety, ohol, narcotics, and driver education (high school only). Combined subjects of military training, athletic training, physical examinations.

ombined subjects of health, physical education, and safety. Health education—combined subject with science or arate subject.

ombined subjects of health and safety. Combined subjects of driver education and safety, cigarettes.

ealth education—may be combined with science or physical education.

n secondary level, health education course includes physical education and driver education. Combined subjects of lth and physical education, hygiene and sanitation, alcohol, narcotics, and cigarettes.

ombined subjects of health, physiology, alcohol and narcotics; health, physical education, and safety; driver education and traffic safety.

ombined subjects of safety, accident prevention, highway and motor vehicle safety (high school only). Driver edu-on as part of health and physical education curriculum.

w on special health topics refers to health education by implication. Combined subjects of health and physical cation, first aid, and safety.

ombined subjects of safety, accident prevention, and highway safety; physiology and hygiene, including stimulants narcotics—½ school term, grades 6, 7, or 8.

ivision of school hygiene "to carry out a complete program of health and physical development of pupils."

nits on health and safety are included in general science and biology courses in grades 7 to 10, and home nomics courses, grades 8 to 12.

D FIELD AND COURT DIAGRAMS

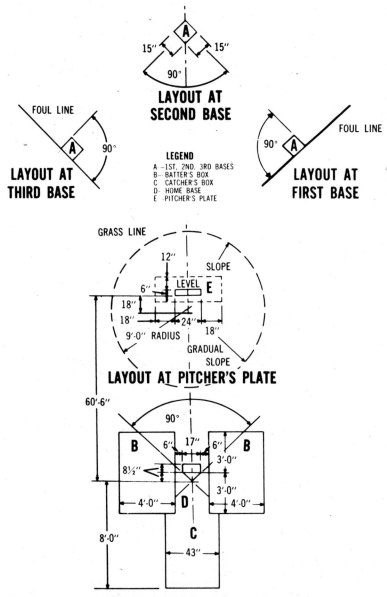

15" 15"
90°

LAYOUT AT SECOND BASE

FOUL LINE

90°

LAYOUT AT THIRD BASE

LEGEND
A —1ST, 2ND, 3RD BASES
B—BATTER'S BOX
C CATCHER'S BOX
D HOME BASE
E —PITCHER'S PLATE

FOUL LINE

90°

LAYOUT AT FIRST BASE

GRASS LINE

12"
SLOPE
6" LEVEL E
18"
18" 24"
9'-0" RADIUS 18"
GRADUAL SLOPE

LAYOUT AT PITCHER'S PLATE

60'-6"

90°

B 6" 17" 6" B
3'-0"
8½"
3'-0"
4'-0" D 4'-0"

8'-0" C

43"

Reprinted courtesy McGregor-Consumer Division, Brunswick Company, Cincinnati, Ohio.

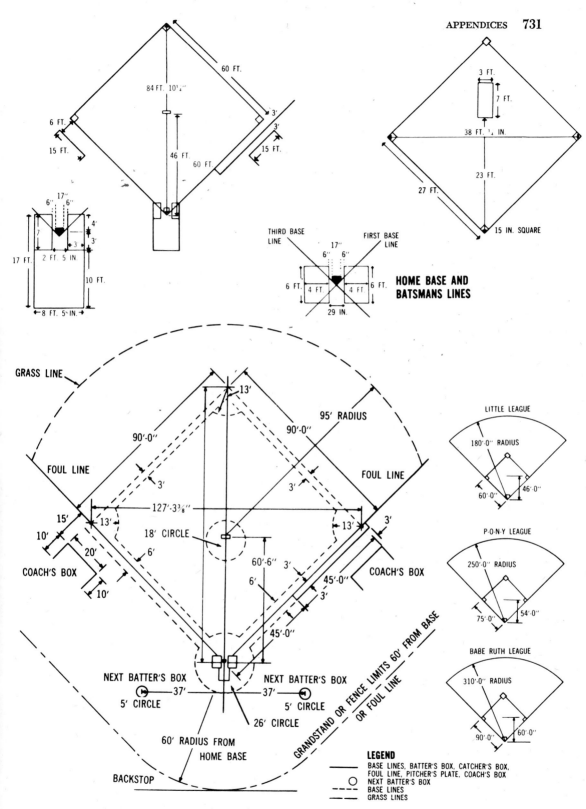

HOME BASE AND BATSMANS LINES

LITTLE LEAGUE
180'-0" RADIUS
60'-0"
46'-0"

P-O-N-Y LEAGUE
250'-0" RADIUS
75'-0"
54'-0"

BABE RUTH LEAGUE
310'-0" RADIUS
90'-0"
60'-0"

LEGEND
BASE LINES, BATTER'S BOX, CATCHER'S BOX, FOUL LINE, PITCHER'S PLATE, COACH'S BOX
O   NEXT BATTER'S BOX
BASE LINES
GRASS LINES

Reprinted courtesy McGregor-Consumer Division, Brunswick Company, Cincinnati, Ohio.

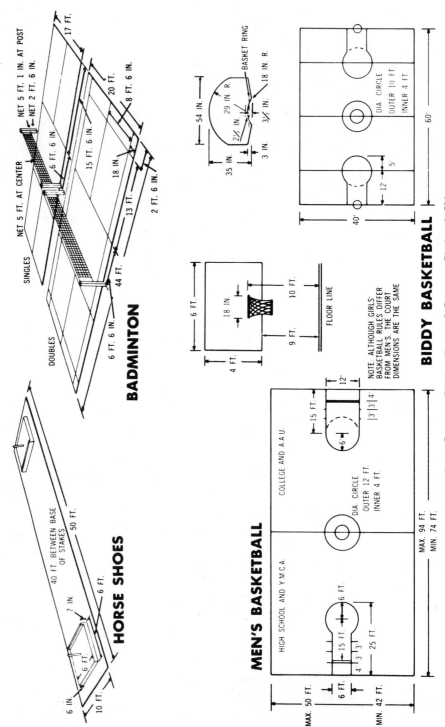

BADMINTON

HORSE SHOES

MEN'S BASKETBALL

BIDDY BASKETBALL

NOTE: ALTHOUGH GIRLS' BASKETBALL RULES DIFFER FROM MEN'S. THE COURT DIMENSIONS ARE THE SAME

Reprinted courtesy McGregor–Consumer Division, Brunswick Company, Cincinnati, Ohio.

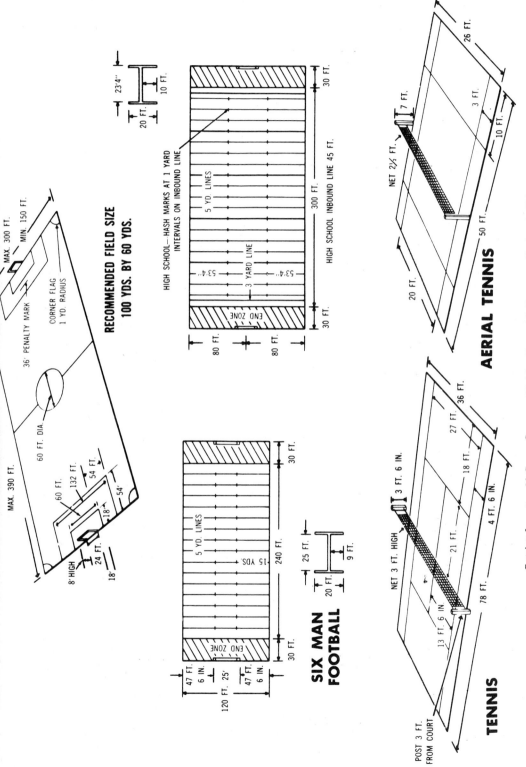

MAX. 300 FT.

MIN. 150 FT.

CORNER FLAG
1 YD. RADIUS

36' PENALTY MARK

60 FT. DIA.

MAX. 390 FT.

60 FT.

132 FT.

54 FT.

54'

18'

8' HIGH

24 FT.

18'

RECOMMENDED FIELD SIZE
100 YDS. BY 60 YDS.

2¾"

10 FT.

20 FT.

30 FT.

HIGH SCHOOL—HASH MARKS AT 1 YARD
INTERVALS ON INBOUND LINE

5 YD. LINES

53'4"

3 YARD LINE

53'4"

300 FT.

HIGH SCHOOL INBOUND LINE 45 FT.

30 FT.

END ZONE

80 FT.

80 FT.

30 FT.

5 YD. LINES

15 YDS.

240 FT.

END ZONE

30 FT.

25 FT.

20 FT.

9 FT.

47 FT.
6 IN.

25'

120 FT.

47 FT.
6 IN.

SIX MAN
FOOTBALL

26 FT.

3 FT.

10 FT.

7 FT.

NET 2½ FT.

50 FT.

20 FT.

AERIAL TENNIS

36 FT.

27 FT.

18 FT.

3 FT. 6 IN.

NET 3 FT. HIGH

21 FT.

4 FT. 6 IN.

13 FT. 6 IN

78 FT.

POST 3 FT.
FROM COURT

TENNIS

Reprinted courtesy McGregor-Consumer Division, Brunswick Company, Cincinnati, Ohio.

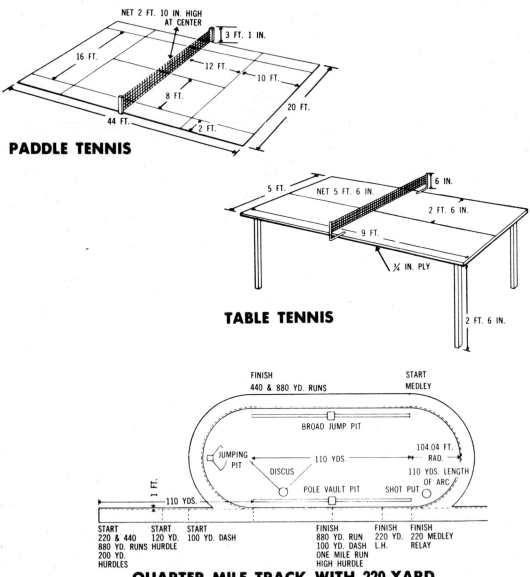

PADDLE TENNIS

NET 2 FT. 10 IN. HIGH AT CENTER

3 FT. 1 IN.

16 FT.

12 FT.

10 FT.

8 FT.

20 FT.

44 FT.

2 FT.

TABLE TENNIS

5 FT.

NET 5 FT. 6 IN.

6 IN.

2 FT. 6 IN.

9 FT.

¾ IN. PLY

2 FT. 6 IN.

QUARTER MILE TRACK WITH 220-YARD STRAIGHTAWAY

FINISH
440 & 880 YD. RUNS

START
MEDLEY

BROAD JUMP PIT

104.04 FT. RAD.

JUMPING PIT

110 YDS.

DISCUS

110 YDS. LENGTH OF ARC

POLE VAULT PIT

SHOT PUT

1 FT.

110 YDS.

START
220 & 440
880 YD. RUNS
200 YD.
HURDLES

START
120 YD.
HURDLE

START
100 YD. DASH

FINISH
880 YD. RUN
100 YD. DASH
ONE MILE RUN
HIGH HURDLE

FINISH
220 YD.
L.H.

FINISH
220 MEDLEY
RELAY

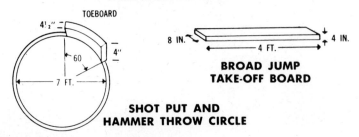

TOEBOARD

4½"

60

4"

7 FT.

8 IN.

4 FT.

4 IN.

BROAD JUMP TAKE-OFF BOARD

SHOT PUT AND HAMMER THROW CIRCLE

Reprinted courtesy McGregor-Consumer Division, Brunswick Company, Cincinnati, Ohio.

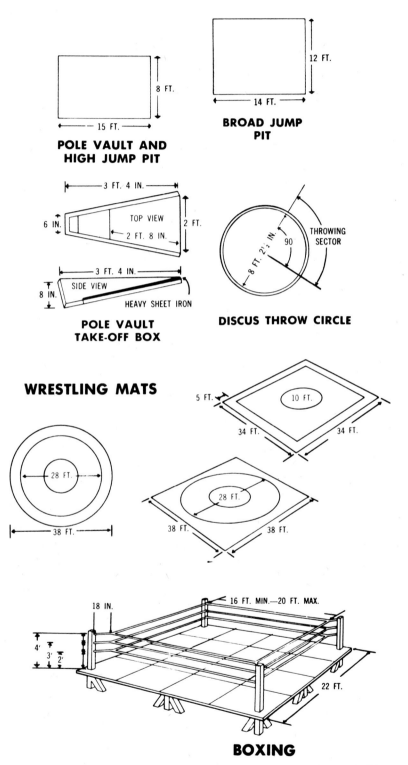

POLE VAULT AND HIGH JUMP PIT

BROAD JUMP PIT

POLE VAULT TAKE-OFF BOX

DISCUS THROW CIRCLE

WRESTLING MATS

BOXING

Reprinted courtesy McGregor-Consumer Division, Brunswick Company, Cincinnati, Ohio.

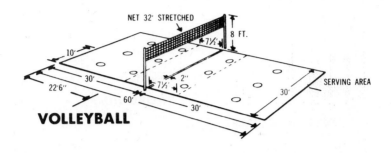

VOLLEYBALL

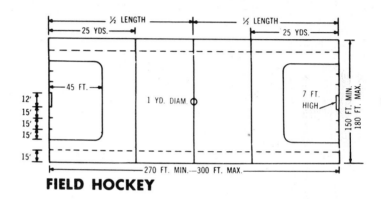

FIELD HOCKEY

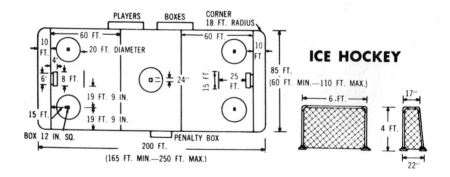

ICE HOCKEY

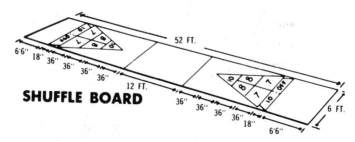

SHUFFLE BOARD

Reprinted courtesy McGregor-Consumer Division, Brunswick Company, Cincinnati, Ohio.

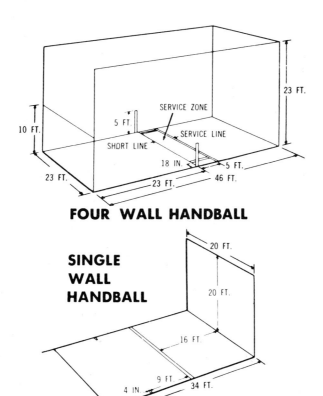

FOUR WALL HANDBALL

SINGLE WALL HANDBALL

Reprinted courtesy McGregor-Consumer Division, Brunswick Company, Cincinnati, Ohio.

Index